Refugee, Migrant and Ethnic Minority Health

Refugee, Migrant and Ethnic Minority Health

Special Issue Editors

Aristomenis Exadaktylos
David Shiva Srivastava
Osnat Keidar
Emmanouil Pikoulis

MDPI • Basel • Beijing • Wuhan • Barcelona • Belgrade

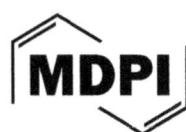

Special Issue Editors
Aristomenis Exadaktylos
Universitat Bern
Switzerland

David Shiva Srivastava
Universitat Bern
Switzerland

Osnat Keidar
Universitat Bern
Switzerland

Emmanouil Pikoulis
University of Athens
Greece

Editorial Office
MDPI
St. Alban-Anlage 66 4052
Basel, Switzerland

This is a reprint of articles from the Special Issue published online in the open access journal *International Journal of Environmental Research and Public Health* (ISSN 1660-4601) from 2018 to 2019 (available at: https://www.mdpi.com/journal/ijerph/special_issues/refugee_migrant_health).

For citation purposes, cite each article independently as indicated on the article page online and as indicated below:

LastName, A.A.; LastName, B.B.; LastName, C.C. Article Title. *Journal Name* **Year**, *Article Number*, Page Range.

ISBN 978-3-03921-644-4 (Pbk)
ISBN 978-3-03921-645-1 (PDF)

Cover image courtesy of Master Course "Global Health—Disaster Medicine" and the National and Kapodistrian University of Athens (NKUA).

© 2019 by the authors. Articles in this book are Open Access and distributed under the Creative Commons Attribution (CC BY) license, which allows users to download, copy and build upon published articles, as long as the author and publisher are properly credited, which ensures maximum dissemination and a wider impact of our publications.
The book as a whole is distributed by MDPI under the terms and conditions of the Creative Commons license CC BY-NC-ND.

Contents

About the Special Issue Editors xi

Osnat Keidar, David S. Srivastava, Emmanouil Pikoulis and Aristomenis K. Exadaktylos
Health of Refugees and Migrants—Where Do We Stand and What Directions Should We Take?
Reprinted from: *Int. J. Environ. Res. Public Health* **2019**, *16*, 1319, doi:10.3390/ijerph16081319 ... 1

Ana Cristina Lindsay, Qun Le and Mary L. Greaney
Infant Feeding Beliefs, Attitudes, Knowledge and Practices of Chinese Immigrant Mothers: An Integrative Review of the Literature
Reprinted from: *Int. J. Environ. Res. Public Health* **2018**, *15*, 21, doi:10.3390/ijerph15010021 9

Jan Ilhan Kizilhan
Trauma and Pain in Family-Orientated Societies
Reprinted from: *Int. J. Environ. Res. Public Health* **2018**, *15*, 44, doi:10.3390/ijerph15010044 24

Zelalem B. Mengesha, Janette Perz, Tinashe Dune and Jane Ussher
Preparedness of Health Care Professionals for Delivering Sexual and Reproductive Health Care to Refugee and Migrant Women: A Mixed Methods Study
Reprinted from: *Int. J. Environ. Res. Public Health* **2018**, *15*, 174, doi:10.3390/ijerph15010174 ... 31

Michèle Twomey, Ana Šijački, Gert Krummrey, Tyson Welzel, Aristomenis K. Exadaktylos and Marko Ercegovac
Strengthening Emergency Care Systems to Mitigate Public Health Challenges Arising from Influxes of Individuals with Different Socio-Cultural Backgrounds to a Level One Emergency Center in South East Europe
Reprinted from: *Int. J. Environ. Res. Public Health* **2018**, *15*, 501, doi:10.3390/ijerph15030501 ... 43

Subin Park, Yeeun Lee and Jin Yong Jun
Trauma and Depression among North Korean Refugees: The Mediating Effect of Negative Cognition
Reprinted from: *Int. J. Environ. Res. Public Health* **2018**, *15*, 591, doi:10.3390/ijerph15040591 ... 49

Ourania S. Kotsiou, David S. Srivastava, Panagiotis Kotsios, Aristomenis K. Exadaktylos and Konstantinos I. Gourgoulianis
The Emergency Medical System in Greece: Opening Aeolus' Bag of Winds
Reprinted from: *Int. J. Environ. Res. Public Health* **2018**, *15*, 745, doi:10.3390/ijerph15040745 ... 59

Kevin Claassen and Pia Jäger
Impact of the Introduction of the Electronic Health Insurance Card on the Use of Medical Services by Asylum Seekers in Germany
Reprinted from: *Int. J. Environ. Res. Public Health* **2018**, *15*, 856, doi:10.3390/ijerph15050856 ... 73

Teresa Dalla Zuanna, Martina Del Manso, Cristina Giambi, Flavia Riccardo, Antonino Bella, Maria Grazia Caporali, Maria Grazia Dente, Silvia Declich and The Italian Survey CARE Working Group
Immunization Offer Targeting Migrants: Policies and Practices in Italy
Reprinted from: *Int. J. Environ. Res. Public Health* **2018**, *15*, 968, doi:10.3390/ijerph15050968 ... 84

Karl Puchner, Evika Karamagioli, Anastasia Pikouli, Costas Tsiamis,
Athanasios Kalogeropoulos, Eleni Kakalou, Elena Pavlidou and Emmanouil Pikoulis
Time to Rethink Refugee and Migrant Health in Europe: Moving from Emergency Response to
Integrated and Individualized Health Care Provision for Migrants and Refugees
Reprinted from: *Int. J. Environ. Res. Public Health* **2018**, *15*, 1100, doi:10.3390/ijerph15061100 . . . **98**

Flavia Riccardo, Jonathan E. Suk, Laura Espinosa, Antonino Bella, Cristina Giambi,
Martina Del Manso, Christian Napoli, Maria Grazia Dente, Gloria Nacca and Silvia Declich
Key Dimensions for the Prevention and Control of Communicable Diseases in Institutional
Settings: A Scoping Review to Guide the Development of a Tool to Strengthen Preparedness
at Migrant Holding Centres in the EU/EEA
Reprinted from: *Int. J. Environ. Res. Public Health* **2018**, *15*, 1120, doi:10.3390/ijerph15061120 . . . **104**

Alexandra Jablonka, Christian Dopfer, Christine Happle, Georgios Sogkas, Diana Ernst,
Faranaz Atschekzei, Stefanie Hirsch, Annabelle Schäll, Adan Jirmo, Philipp Solbach,
Reinhold Ernst Schmidt, Georg M. N. Behrens and Martin Wetzke
Tuberculosis Specific Interferon-Gamma Production in a Current Refugee Cohort in
Western Europe
Reprinted from: *Int. J. Environ. Res. Public Health* **2018**, *15*, 1263, doi:10.3390/ijerph15061263 . . . **120**

Georgios Schoretsanitis, Sarah Eisenhardt, Meret E. Ricklin, David S. Srivastava,
Sebastian Walther and Aristomenis Exadaktylos
Psychiatric Emergencies of Asylum Seekers; Descriptive Analysis and Comparison with
Immigrants of Warranted Residence
Reprinted from: *Int. J. Environ. Res. Public Health* **2018**, *15*, 1300, doi:10.3390/ijerph15071300 . . . **128**

Donna Angelina Rade, Gemma Crawford, Roanna Lobo, Corie Gray and Graham Brown
Sexual Health Help-Seeking Behavior among Migrants from Sub-Saharan Africa and
South East Asia living in High Income Countries: A Systematic Review
Reprinted from: *Int. J. Environ. Res. Public Health* **2018**, *15*, 1311, doi:10.3390/ijerph15071311 . . . **138**

Dominic Kaeser, Rebekka Guerra, Osnat Keidar, Urs Lanz, Michael Moses, Christian Kobel,
Aristomenis K. Exadaktylos and Meret E. Ricklin
Verbal and Non-Verbal Aggression in a Swiss University Emergency Room:
A Descriptive Study
Reprinted from: *Int. J. Environ. Res. Public Health* **2018**, *15*, 1423, doi:10.3390/ijerph15071423 . . . **160**

Georgios Schoretsanitis, Dinesh Bhugra, Sarah Eisenhardt, Meret E. Ricklin,
David S. Srivastava, Aristomenis Exadaktylos and Sebastian Walther
Upon Rejection: Psychiatric Emergencies of Failed Asylum Seekers
Reprinted from: *Int. J. Environ. Res. Public Health* **2018**, *15*, 1498, doi:10.3390/ijerph15071498 . . . **167**

Atefeh Fathi, Usama El-Awad, Tilman Reinelt and Franz Petermann
A Brief Introduction to the Multidimensional Intercultural Training Acculturation Model
(MITA) for Middle Eastern Adolescent Refugees
Reprinted from: *Int. J. Environ. Res. Public Health* **2018**, *15*, 1516, doi:10.3390/ijerph15071516 . . . **176**

Manish Pareek, Teymur Noori, Sally Hargreaves and Maria van den Muijsenbergh
Linkage to Care Is Important and Necessary When Identifying Infections in Migrants
Reprinted from: *Int. J. Environ. Res. Public Health* **2018**, *15*, 1550, doi:10.3390/ijerph15071550 . . . **190**

Olena Ivanova, Masna Rai and Elizabeth Kemigisha
A Systematic Review of Sexual and Reproductive Health Knowledge, Experiences and Access
to Services among Refugee, Migrant and Displaced Girls and Young Women in Africa
Reprinted from: *Int. J. Environ. Res. Public Health* **2018**, *15*, 1583, doi:10.3390/ijerph15081583 . . . **194**

Elena Rodriguez-Alvarez, Nerea Lanborena and Luisa N. Borrell
Obesity Inequalities According to Place of Birth: The Role of Education
Reprinted from: *Int. J. Environ. Res. Public Health* **2018**, *15*, 1620, doi:10.3390/ijerph15081620 . . . **206**

Subin Park, Soo Jung Rim and Jin Yong Jun
Related Factors of Suicidal Ideation among North Korean Refugee Youth in South Korea
Reprinted from: *Int. J. Environ. Res. Public Health* **2018**, *15*, 1694, doi:10.3390/ijerph15081694 . . . **216**

Kevin Pottie, Tamara Lotfi, Lama Kilzar, Pamela Howeiss, Nesrine Rizk, Elie A. Akl, Sonia Dias, Beverly-Ann Biggs, Robin Christensen, Prinon Rahman, Olivia Magwood, Anh Tran, Nick Rowbotham, Anastasia Pharris, Teymur Noori, Manish Pareek and Rachael Morton
The Effectiveness and Cost-Effectiveness of Screening for HIV in Migrants in the EU/EEA: A Systematic Review
Reprinted from: *Int. J. Environ. Res. Public Health* **2018**, *15*, 1700, doi:10.3390/ijerph15081700 . . . **224**

Ourania S. Kotsiou, Panagiotis Kotsios, David S. Srivastava, Vaios Kotsios, Konstantinos I. Gourgoulianis and Aristomenis K. Exadaktylos
Impact of the Refugee Crisis on the Greek Healthcare System: A Long Road to Ithaca
Reprinted from: *Int. J. Environ. Res. Public Health* **2018**, *15*, 1790, doi:10.3390/ijerph15081790 . . . **247**

Jolanta Klukowska-Röetzler, Maria Eracleous, Martin Müller, David S. Srivastava, Gert Krummrey, Osnat Keidar and Aristomenis K. Exadaktylos
Increased Urgent Care Center Visits by Southeast European Migrants: A Retrospective, Controlled Trial from Switzerland
Reprinted from: *Int. J. Environ. Res. Public Health* **2018**, *15*, 1857, doi:10.3390/ijerph15091857 . . . **265**

Daniel T Myran, Rachael Morton, Beverly-Ann Biggs, Irene Veldhuijzen, Francesco Castelli, Anh Tran, Lukas P Staub, Eric Agbata, Prinon Rahman, Manish Pareek, Teymur Noori and Kevin Pottie
The Effectiveness and Cost-Effectiveness of Screening for and Vaccination Against Hepatitis B Virus among Migrants in the EU/EEA: A Systematic Review
Reprinted from: *Int. J. Environ. Res. Public Health* **2018**, *15*, 1898, doi:10.3390/ijerph15091898 . . . **278**

Christian Dopfer, Annabelle Vakilzadeh, Christine Happle, Evelyn Kleinert, Frank Müller, Diana Ernst, Reinhold E. Schmidt, Georg M. N. Behrens, Sonja Merkesdal, Martin Wetzke and Alexandra Jablonka
Pregnancy Related Health Care Needs in Refugees—A Current Three Center Experience in Europe
Reprinted from: *Int. J. Environ. Res. Public Health* **2018**, *15*, 1934, doi:10.3390/ijerph15091934 . . . **297**

Lotte De Schrijver, Tom Vander Beken, Barbara Krahé and Ines Keygnaert
Prevalence of Sexual Violence in Migrants, Applicants for International Protection, and Refugees in Europe: A Critical Interpretive Synthesis of the Evidence
Reprinted from: *Int. J. Environ. Res. Public Health* **2018**, *15*, 1979, doi:10.3390/ijerph15091979 . . . **309**

Christina Greenaway, Iuliia Makarenko, Claire Nour Abou Chakra, Balqis Alabdulkarim, Robin Christensen, Adam Palayew, Anh Tran, Lukas Staub, Manish Pareek, Joerg J. Meerpohl, Teymur Noori, Irene Veldhuijzen, Kevin Pottie, Francesco Castelli and Rachael L. Morton
The Effectiveness and Cost-Effectiveness of Hepatitis C Screening for Migrants in the EU/EEA: A Systematic Review
Reprinted from: *Int. J. Environ. Res. Public Health* **2018**, *15*, 2013, doi:10.3390/ijerph15092013 . . . **326**

Osnat Keidar, Sabrina N. Jegerlehner, Stephan Ziegenhorn, Adam D. Brown, Martin Müller, Aristomenis K. Exadaktylos and David S. Srivastava
Emergency Department Discharge Outcome and Psychiatric Consultation in North African Patients
Reprinted from: *Int. J. Environ. Res. Public Health* **2018**, *15*, 2033, doi:10.3390/ijerph15092033 . . . 350

Charles Hui, Jessica Dunn, Rachael Morton, Lukas P. Staub, Anh Tran, Sally Hargreaves, Christina Greenaway, Beverly Ann Biggs, Robin Christensen and Kevin Pottie
Interventions to Improve Vaccination Uptake and Cost Effectiveness of Vaccination Strategies in Newly Arrived Migrants in the EU/EEA: A Systematic Review
Reprinted from: *Int. J. Environ. Res. Public Health* **2018**, *15*, 2065, doi:10.3390/ijerph15102065 . . . 361

Martin Wetzke, Christine Happle, Annabelle Vakilzadeh, Diana Ernst, Georgios Sogkas, Reinhold E. Schmidt, Georg M. N. Behrens, Christian Dopfer and Alexandra Jablonka
Healthcare Utilization in a Large Cohort of Asylum Seekers Entering Western Europe in 2015
Reprinted from: *Int. J. Environ. Res. Public Health* **2018**, *15*, 2163, doi:10.3390/ijerph15102163 . . . 374

Liliane Costa, Sónia Dias and Maria do Rosário O. Martins
Fruit and Vegetable Consumption among Immigrants in Portugal: A Nationwide Cross-Sectional Study
Reprinted from: *Int. J. Environ. Res. Public Health* **2018**, *15*, 2299, doi:10.3390/ijerph15102299 . . . 383

Agata Vitale and Judy Ryde
Exploring Risk Factors Affecting the Mental Health of Refugee Women Living with HIV
Reprinted from: *Int. J. Environ. Res. Public Health* **2018**, *15*, 2326, doi:10.3390/ijerph15102326 . . . 397

Matt Driedger, Alain Mayhew, Vivian Welch, Eric Agbata, Doug Gruner, Christina Greenaway, Teymur Noori, Monica Sandu, Thierry Sangou, Christine Mathew, Harneel Kaur, Manish Pareek and Kevin Pottie
Accessibility and Acceptability of Infectious Disease Interventions Among Migrants in the EU/EEA: A CERQual Systematic Review
Reprinted from: *Int. J. Environ. Res. Public Health* **2018**, *15*, 2329, doi:10.3390/ijerph15112329 . . . 415

Asha Jama, Mona Ali, Ann Lindstrand, Robb Butler and Asli Kulane
Perspectives on the Measles, Mumps and Rubella Vaccination among Somali Mothers in Stockholm
Reprinted from: *Int. J. Environ. Res. Public Health* **2018**, *15*, 2428, doi:10.3390/ijerph15112428 . . . 437

Eva Morawa and Yesim Erim
Health-Related Lifestyle Behavior and Religiosity among First-Generation Immigrants of Polish Origin in Germany
Reprinted from: *Int. J. Environ. Res. Public Health* **2018**, *15*, 2545, doi:10.3390/ijerph15112545 . . . 446

Eric N. Agbata, Rachael L. Morton, Zeno Bisoffi, Emmanuel Bottieau, Christina Greenaway, Beverley-A. Biggs, Nadia Montero, Anh Tran, Nick Rowbotham, Ingrid Arevalo-Rodriguez, Daniel T. Myran, Teymur Noori, Pablo Alonso-Coello, Kevin Pottie and Ana Requena-Méndez
Effectiveness of Screening and Treatment Approaches for Schistosomiasis and Strongyloidiasis in Newly-Arrived Migrants from Endemic Countries in the EU/EEA: A Systematic Review
Reprinted from: *Int. J. Environ. Res. Public Health* **2019**, *16*, 11, doi:10.3390/ijerph16010011 463

Elizabeth B. Moran, Mark A. Katz, Orel-Ben Ari, Nadav Davidovitch and Oren Zwang
For What Illnesses Do Asylum Seekers and Undocumented Migrant Workers in Israel Seek Healthcare? An Analysis of Medical Visits at a Large Urgent Care Clinic for the Uninsured in Tel Aviv
Reprinted from: *Int. J. Environ. Res. Public Health* **2019**, *16*, 252, doi:10.3390/ijerph16020252 . . . **503**

About the Special Issue Editors

Aristomenis Exadaktylos, professor and chair of Emergency Medicine, director of the Department of Emergency Medicine at Inselspital Bern, University of Bern, Switzerland, has 22 years of experience in emergency medicine. Dr. Exadaktylos leads a team of physicians and researchers to conduct research on medicine for refugees, migrants, and minorities. Dr. Exadaktylos is well known for his work on health systems analysis and health decisions, for developing guidelines, and for exploring the research–policy interface in health systems. Dr. Exadaktylos has co-authored more than 270 scientific papers. Dr. Exadaktylos obtained his MD degree from the Martin Luther University, Germany, and his MSc in Translational Medicine from the University of Edinburgh, UK. Dr. Exadaktylos is a Fellow of the Royal College of Emergency Medicine and the co-president of the Swiss Society of Emergency and Rescue Medicine.

David Shiva Srivastava, MD, MBA is currently the Head of the Fast Track unit and Senior Attending Specialist in the Department of Emergency Medicine at the University Hospital of Bern, Switzerland. He is a board-certified Emergency Physician and holds an MBA in International Healthcare Management. His research focuses on Refugees, Migrants, and Minorities in the Emergency Department and he has led multiple projects in this area. David Srivastava obtained his MD at the Albert-Ludwigs University of Freiburg, Germany and received his MBA from the Frankfurt School for Finance and Management in Frankfurt, Germany.

Osnat Keidar, PhD, MPH, B.Ed holds a Master's degree and a Doctorate from the school of Public Health, the Hebrew University and Hadassah Hospital, Israel. Osnat currently works as a Senior Research Associate in the Department of Emergency Medicine, Inselspital, Bern University Hospital, with a focus on migrant and refugee health. She has about 20 years of experience in field work as well as research, with a focus on the planning, implementation, and evaluation of health-promoting programs in various settings. She teaches in the School of Public Health at the Hebrew University and is affiliated as Associate Fellow to the African Population and Health Research Center in Nairobi.

Emmanouil Pikoulis, MD, PhD, DMCC, FACS, FEBS, is Professor of Surgery and Chairman of the 3rd Department of Surgery (Attiko hospital), School of Medicine, National and Kapodistrian University of Athens, Greece. He also serves as Adjunct Professor of Surgery at USUHS, Bethesda, Maryland, USA. Since 2016, he is Scientific Director of the MSc "Global Health—Disaster Management" at the same University and leads a multidisciplinary team of physicians, other healthcare professionals, and social scientists to develop educational curricula and conduct research on acute and disaster medicine and management as well as international medicine, with a specific focus on refugees health. His areas of expertise include general and acute surgery, themes that he teaches to medical students, residents, and fellows. He has received numerous awards and grants. He is Editorial Board Member of many peer-reviewed journals and has numerous publications in national and international journals. He has presented extensively on topics related to trauma and acute surgery training both nationally and internationally and he is the author and co-author of many relevant books.

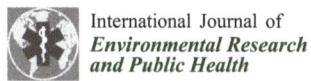

Editorial

Health of Refugees and Migrants—Where Do We Stand and What Directions Should We Take?

Osnat Keidar [1,*], David S. Srivastava [1], Emmanouil Pikoulis [2] and Aristomenis K. Exadaktylos [1]

1 Department and Emergency Medicine, Inselspital, Bern University Hospital, University of Bern, 3010 Bern, Switzerland; DavidShiva.Srivastava@insel.ch (D.S.S.); Aristomenis.Exadaktylos@insel.ch (A.K.E.)
2 3rd Department of Surgery, "Attikon" University General Hospital, National and Kapodistrian, University of Athens (NKUA), 11527 Athens, Greece; mpikoul@med.uoa.gr
* Correspondence: osnat.keidar@insel.ch

Received: 2 April 2019; Accepted: 3 April 2019; Published: 12 April 2019

1. Introduction

International migration, particularly to Europe, has increased in the last few decades, making research on aspects of this phenomenon, including numbers, challenges, and successes, particularly vital. Accordingly, we are pleased to introduce a Special Issue of *International Journal of Environmental Research and Public Health* on the health of refugees, migrants, and ethnic minorities.

Discussions of a topic must begin with foundational definitions:

A "migrant" is any individual who moves across international borders away from his or her country of origin, regardless of legal status or cause [1].

A "refugee" is any person who, resulting from a well-founded fear of persecution for reasons of race, religion, nationality, membership of a particular social group or political opinion, is outside the country of his/her nationality and is either unable or too scared to avail himself/herself of the protection of that country [2].

An "asylum seeker" (AS) is someone who has applied for protection as a refugee and is awaiting the determination of his or her status [3]. The above definitions may vary according to country and local law; however, there remain fundamental distinctions between a migrant and a refugee. In comparison with migrants, refugees have not chosen to leave their country but have fled in response to a crisis. They are more likely to leave family behind, travel without proper documents, have little choice on their country of arrival, and will probably never return home [4]. These unique characteristic impact how migrants and refugees should be considered in terms of both needs and health outcomes.

Sustainable Development Goals (STGs) aim to decrease disparities within populations by 2030. For example, SDG 10 incorporates Target 10.7: "Facilitate orderly, safe, regular and responsible migration and mobility of people, including through the implementation of planned and well-managed migration policies"; this is intended to guide state members in taking measurable steps to attain these goals [5].

Having provided necessary definitions, some relevant data on migrants, refugees, and asylum seekers includes the following: As of 2017, the estimated number of international migrants has reached 258 million, in comparison with 220 million in 2010 and 173 million in 2000 [6]. As of 2017, Europe and Asia together host 62% of total international migrants [6].

At the end of 2016, the total number of refugees and AS in the world was estimated at 25.9 million, which corresponds to 10.1% of all international migrants. Turkey recorded the largest refugee population and hosts approximately 3.1 million refugees and AS, with the most significant increase in the world since 2000 [6].

During 2015 and 2016, more than 2.5 million people applied for asylum in the European Union (EU). To put such numbers in context, more than 2030 people are thought to have lost their lives in the Mediterranean during the first six months of 2017. In 2015 and 2016, more than 2.3 million illegal crossings were detected by Frontex, the EU border surveillance agency. Within Europe, Germany hosts the greatest number of refugees: approximately 1.2 million, including 222,560 in-process AS requests [7].

The Dublin Regulation establishes the responsibility of a member state to examine the asylum application; the Regulation's objective is to ensure rapid access to asylum procedures and to guarantee that the merits of the application are examined by a single, clearly determined member state. Criteria for establishing responsibility run, in hierarchical order, from family considerations, to recent possession of a visa or residence permit in a member state, to whether the applicant has entered the EU regularly or irregularly [8].

These figures may spark humanitarian, security, and ethical concerns and may oblige European countries to support the absorption of these refugees. Making the outmost effort to support their new life is not only a humanitarian issue but also an essential obligation of the European countries for both economic and practical reasons. Most of these refugees will, in some years, become migrants and later residents. An effective supportive process will enable them to become an integral and contributing work force in their host countries. However, if this process fails, these new residents may pose a significant economic and security burden on society, as can already be observed in some countries. Unemployment, health disparities, mental problems, and addictions are only some of the outcomes of the failure to create a supportive and effective process for AS, migrants, and refugees. Recent studies indicate that countries with a higher integration score for migrants present better socio-economic and health outcomes for these communities. Therefore, research on these phenomena is essential, including the presentation of needs and assets of these diverse populations as well as suggestions for possible policies, interventions, and subsequent evaluation of these programs.

This Special Issue highlights this necessary and relevant area of research. The Special Issue is not intended solely for academic purposes. Policy makers may use the suggested policies and interventions to improve existing programs.

2. Review of Articles in the Special Issue

There are 37 articles in the current special issue, including studies on diverse topics relating to the health of refugees, migrants, and ethnic minorities.

Most articles (28 of them) present studies focusing on European host countries, including Germany, Greece, Italy, Switzerland, Spain, Portugal, and Sweden. The focus on Europe is justified if we take into consideration the increase in numbers of refugees and migrants who have come to Europe in recent years. However, there are also articles which present studies from countries in other continents.

Topics discussed in the Issue's articles are summarized in Table 1, and include healthcare (HC) utilization, infectious diseases, mother and child health, mental health, and chronic diseases.

Table 1. Summary of special issue manuscripts, arranged according to principle topics.

Topic	Main Findings	Number of Articles
Infectious diseases	<ul><li>Early detection of infections is important to prevent morbidity and mortality.</li><li>The most important issues include the effectiveness and cost effectiveness of screening for HIV, hepatitis B and C, schistosomiasis and strongyloidiasis [9–13].</li><li>Older people are at greater risk of developing active tuberculosis, so that new and better policies and strategies are needed for the detection and treatment of tuberculosis in older people [14].</li><li>In migrant centers, the staff numbers and their various skills, together with physical infrastructure (including poor hygiene, lack of electricity and heating) are crucial in preventing and mitigating outbreaks [13].</li><li>A review on interventions to increase vaccine intake found that they had little impact on vaccine uptake [15].</li><li>Factors associated with accessibility and acceptability of interventions to prevent infectious disease included knowledge of the disease and the related stigma, as well as migrants' interaction with HC providers [16].</li><li>HC providers must possess culture-sensitive communication skills when planning interventions [16]. They must focus on social mobilization and community outreach when planning vaccination programs and educational campaigns [15].</li></ul>	11 [9–19]

Table 1. Cont.

Topic	Main Findings	Number of Articles
Mental health	• Migrants face traumatic events that impact their mental health, with various risk factors, including association between early trauma and depression symptoms and feelings of personal failure [20]. • In comparison to controls, North Korean refugees with suicide ideation had lower levels of family cohesion, lower self-esteem, lower resilience and higher post-traumatic stress disorder [21]. • AS with rejected applications showed high levels of psychiatric emergencies and higher stress levels [22]. • In women with HIV infection, mental health was impaired by multiple factors, including stigma, racial discrimination and resettlement adversities [23].	6 [20–25]
Healthcare utilization	• Primary care is most often accessed in the first period directly after arrival [26]. • In comparison with the local population, migrants (mainly from North Africa) use ER more often and for less urgent complaints and are more often discharged as outpatients; young males more often consulted psychiatrists [27]. • Migrants are more often involved in hospital-related aggression [28]. • The health insurance card increased the use of outpatient care [29]. • It is important to develop guidelines, policy and resources to support the health system; NGOs' support is essential for successful integration [30].	10 [26–35]
Mother and child health	• An increased need for reproductive health services. Barriers faced by women to access services include language, stigma, direct and indirect cost, lack of cultural competency within health services, distance and difficulty in navigating health services [36,37]. • Healthcare providers emphasize the unique needs of migrant and refugee women in sexual and reproductive health, and the lack of proper training to address them [38]. • Sexual violence is highly frequent in migrants and refugees in Europe [39]. • Displaced or migrant girls and young women in Africa possessed limited knowledge of contraceptive methods, STIs and HIV/AIDS. This poses a risk to gender and sex-based violence and abuse [40]. • Need to train healthcare providers', in order to increase culturally-tailored health services [36,38].	7 [36–42]
Lifestyle and chronic diseases	• Being a migrant woman was a risk factor for obesity, while migrant men of low educational level in the Spanish population were relatively protected [43]. • Older and educated women consumed more vegetables and fruits than men [44]. • Intrinsic religiosity is a protective factor for smoking and alcohol consumption in Polish migrants in Germany [45].	3 [43–45]

2.1. Infectious Diseases

Infectious diseases are a frequent topic in this Special Issue, which features six systematic reviews and one commentary, all written as part of ECDC publications. These reviews discuss the effectiveness and cost effectiveness of screening for HIV, hepatitis B and C, schistosomiasis, and strongyloidiasis. The articles also discuss the effectiveness of interventions (including vaccinations) and their cost effectiveness in migrants in the EU/EEA (Table 1) [9–12,15,16]. These have led to a recent publication of the European Center for Disease Prevention and Control (ECDC) entitled "Public health guidance on screening and vaccination for infectious diseases in newly arrived migrants within the EU/European Economic Area (EEA)" [46].

2.2. Mental Health

Mental health is also an important topic and is a major concern within migrant and refugee populations (Table 1). Prevention and treatment are essential. High rates of mental health issues are likely impacted by the trauma experienced during crises, travel time to the host country and the many different challenges related to migrant experiences, including separation from family, difficulties in proper use of the health services as a result of cultural differences, lack of knowledge of the new health system, and language barriers [20–25].

2.3. Health Care Utilization

This issue also documents how migrants and refugees access health services and some of their health care outcomes [26–35]. Studies in this special issue emphasize the need for well-structured policies and guidelines in the EU to ensure the proper integration of AS and refugees within health systems. Studies indicate that there are differences in health service consumption among migrant communities in comparison with the host population of a country, with more frequent outpatient discharges, walk-in visits, visits for less urgent reasons, and an increased need for access to psychiatric consultation among migrant populations (Table 1).

2.4. Mother and Child Health

Within the refugee and migrant population, children and women are particularly vulnerable. The increase in health service consumption for women poses great challenges and is significantly impacted by differences in culture diversity. This topic requires professional and targeted adaptation of health services if such services are to properly face this challenge and overcome barriers to both appropriate use and better service. Women and girls, as well as health care providers, must be instructed on these issues (Table 1) [36–42].

2.5. Lifestyle and Chronic Diseases

Chronic diseases and lifestyles are briefly presented in this issue in three articles. As seen in Table 1, migrant status does not necessarily pose a risk factor. Other sociodemographic factors, such as gender, age, education, and religious adherence were found to be associated with obesity and overall quality of diet, such as consumption of vegetables and fruit as well as alcohol consumption [43–45].

3. Discussion

The numerous articles in this Special Issue illustrate the increased interest and new data on the unique needs of migrant and refugee populations. Migrant and refugee status poses increased risk and health challenges; host countries are encouraged to integrate policies and interventions to accommodate these gaps.

The Ottawa charter and the social determinants of health are linked to migration. Within the total migrant population, refugees and asylum seekers are at greater risk of poor health outcomes. Most refugees come from low income countries, with a high burden of both disease and civil unrest. They suffer from unfortunate conditions during their transit and, occasionally, following their arrival in the host country. Other challenges include legal status, sometimes lack of culturally competent health and social services, lack of social support and isolation, and difficult working and living conditions [47–49].

Other factors that impact migrant and refugee health include social and cultural barriers to integration, stress, exclusion and discrimination, poor socioeconomic status, loss of supportive networks, and changes in lifestyle and diet. This has encouraged the WHO and other organizations to include migration as a social determinant of health and to promote inter-sectorial HP initiatives to address these determinants [47,50,51].

A holistic approach is required for interventions that aim to improve migrant health. Such an approach must be inclusive and take into consideration the beliefs, values, capacities, needs, and social context of all migrants and refugees. It also must support integration by using participatory approaches [47,52,53] and be adopted by decision makers [54,55]. Areas for interventions should include the five action areas of the Ottawa charter [56]:

- Ensuring that there are policies within all sectors of government which aim to promote the health of refugees and migrants;
- Improvements in social services, and the quality of physical and social environments, prioritizing community-centered approaches that build local capacities;

- Investment in language support and health literacy initiatives to develop personal skills;
- Promotion of approaches to health care that are sensitive to culture and diversity;
- Development of a culturally competent health workforce [47,57].

However, additional research is required, as discussed in both the articles of the Special Issue and elsewhere [55,58]. More studies are needed that use both qualitative and quantitative methods to enhance our understanding of the current situation and the various factors which impact migrant and refugee health. Many studies focus on specific countries or populations, which implies that their conclusions may not be applicable to global migrant communities. As evaluation of HP interventions has been inadequate, both process and impact evaluation should be incorporated in all programs. This is to assess the effectiveness of such initiatives, and to support the improvement and focus for sub-groups from various backgrounds, languages, and cultures.

It is our ethical responsibility, as both providers and policy makers, to integrate these approaches and focuses in our daily work to help to support the health gaps and to promote equity.

4. Conclusions

Migrant and refugee health poses a significant challenge. Further development of guidelines and policies at both local and international levels is needed. Priorities must be set by encouraging and funding in-depth research that aims to evaluate the impact of existing policies and interventions. Such research will help us formulate recommendations for the development of strategies and approaches that improve and strengthen the integration of migrants and refugees into the host countries.

Author Contributions: Conceptualization: O.K, A.K.E. and D.S.S. Writing of original draft: O.K. Review and editing of original draft- O.K., A.K.E., D.S.S. and E.P.

Funding: This research received no external funding.

Conflicts of Interest: The authors declare no conflict of interest.

References

1. International Organization for Mogration (IOM). Who Is a Migrant? Available online: https://www.iom.int/who-is-a-migrant (accessed on 28 January 2019).
2. The UN Refugee Agency (UNHCR). The 1951 Convention Relating to the Status of Refuges L Geneva, Switzerland. Available online: https://www.unhcr.org/1951-refugee-convention.html (accessed on 28 January 2019).
3. United Nations Educational, Scientific and Cultural Organization (UNESCO). Asylum Seeker. Available online: http://www.unesco.org/new/en/social-and-human-sciences/themes/international-migration/glossary/asylum-seeker/ (accessed on 11 March 2019).
4. Ministry of Health. *Refugee Health Care: A handbook for Health Professionals*; Ministry of Health: Wellington, New Zealand, 2012; ISBN 978-0-478-37346. Available online: https://www.health.govt.nz/publication/refugee-health-care-handbook-health-professionals (accessed on 28 January 2019).
5. United Nations. Sustainable Development Goals. Sustainable Development Goals. Available online: https://sustainabledevelopment.un.org/?menu=1300 (accessed on 11 March 2019).
6. International Organization for Migration (IOM). *World Migration Report 2018*; International Organization for Migration: Geneva, Switzerland, 2018. Available online: https://www.iom.int/wmr/world-migration-report-2018 (accessed on 11 March 2019).
7. European Parliament. *EU Migrant Crisis: Facts and Figures*; European Parliament: Strasbourg, France, 2017. Available online: http://www.europarl.europa.eu/news/en/headlines/priorities/refugees/20170629STO78630/eu-migrant-crisis-facts-and-figures (accessed on 11 March 2019).
8. European Commission. *Common European Asylum System*; Migration and Home Affairs: Brussels, Belgium, 2013. Available online: https://ec.europa.eu/home-affairs/what-we-do/policies/asylum/ (accessed on 11 March 2019).
9. Agbata, E.N.; Morton, R.L.; Bisoffi, Z.; Bottieau, E.; Greenaway, C.; Biggs, B.A.; Montero, N.; Tran, A.; Rowbotham, N.; Arevalo-Rodriguez, I.; et al. Effectiveness of Screening and Treatment Approaches for Schistosomiasis and Strongyloidiasis in Newly-Arrived Migrants from Endemic Countries in the EU/EEA: A Systematic Review. *Int. J. Environ. Res. Public Health* **2018**, *16*, 11. [CrossRef] [PubMed]

10. Greenaway, C.; Makarenko, I.; Chakra, C.N.A.; Alabdulkarim, B.; Christensen, R.; Palayew, A.; Tran, A.; Staub, L.; Pareek, M.; Meerpohl, J.; et al. The Effectiveness and Cost-Effectiveness of Hepatitis C Screening for Migrants in the EU/EEA: A Systematic Review. *Int. J. Environ. Res. Public Health* **2018**, *15*, 2013. [CrossRef]
11. Myran, D.T.; Morton, R.; Biggs, B.A.; Veldhuijzen, I.; Castelli, F.; Tran, A.; Staub, L.; Agbata, E.; Rahman, P.; Pareek, M.; et al. The Effectiveness and Cost-Effectiveness of Screening for and Vaccination against Hepatitis B Virus among Migrants in the EU/EEA: A Systematic Review. *Int. J. Environ. Res. Public Health* **2018**, *15*, 1898. [CrossRef] [PubMed]
12. Pottie, K.; Lotfi, T.; Kilzar, L.; Howeiss, P.; Rizk, N.; Akl, E.; Dias, S.; Biggs, B.A.; Christensen, R.; Rahman, P.; et al. The Effectiveness and Cost-Effectiveness of Screening for HIV in Migrants in the EU/EEA: A Systematic Review. *Int. J. Environ. Res. Public Health* **2018**, *15*, 1700. [CrossRef] [PubMed]
13. Riccardo, F.; Suk, J.E.; Espinosa, L.; Bella, A.; Giambi, C.; Del Manso, M.; Napoli, C.; Dente, M.; Nacca, G.; Declich, S. Key Dimensions for the Prevention and Control of Communicable Diseases in Institutional Settings: A Scoping Review to Guide the Development of a Tool to Strengthen Preparedness at Migrant Holding Centres in the EU/EEA. *Int. J. Environ. Res. Public Health* **2018**, *15*, 1120. [CrossRef] [PubMed]
14. Jablonka, A.; Dopfer, C.; Happle, C.; Sogkas, G.; Ernst, D.; Atschekzei, F.; Hirsch, S.; Schäll, A.; Jirmo, A.; Solbach, P.; et al. Tuberculosis Specific Interferon-Gamma Production in a Current Refugee Cohort in Western Europe. *Int. J. Environ. Res. Public Health* **2018**, *15*, 1263. [CrossRef]
15. Hui, C.; Dunn, J.; Morton, R.; Staub, L.P.; Tran, A.; Hargreaves, S.; Greenaway, C.; Biggs, B.; Christensen, R.; Pottie, K. Interventions to Improve Vaccination Uptake and Cost Effectiveness of Vaccination Strategies in Newly Arrived Migrants in the EU/EEA: A Systematic Review. *Int. J. Environ. Res. Public Health* **2018**, *15*, 2065. [CrossRef]
16. Driedger, M.; Mayhew, A.; Welch, V.; Agbata, E.; Gruner, D.; Greenaway, C.; Noori, T.; Sandu, M.; Sangou, T.; Mathew, C.; et al. Accessibility and Acceptability of Infectious Disease Interventions Among Migrants in the EU/EEA: A CERQual Systematic Review. *Int. J. Environ. Res. Public Health* **2018**, *15*, 2329. [CrossRef]
17. Jama, A.; Ali, M.; Lindstrand, A.; Butler, R.; Kulane, A. Perspectives on the Measles, Mumps and Rubella Vaccination among Somali Mothers in Stockholm. *Int. J. Environ. Res. Public Health* **2018**, *15*, 2428. [CrossRef]
18. Pareek, M.; Noori, T.; Hargreaves, S.; van den Muijsenbergh, M. Linkage to Care Is Important and Necessary When Identifying Infections in Migrants. *Int. J. Environ. Res. Public Health* **2018**, *15*, 1550. [CrossRef] [PubMed]
19. Dalla, Z.T.; Del Manso, M.; Giambi, C.; Riccardo, F.; Bella, A.; Caporali, M.G.; Dente, M.; Declich, S.; Italian Survey CARE Working Group. Immunization Offer Targeting Migrants: Policies and Practices in Italy. *Int. J. Environ. Res. Public Health* **2018**, *15*, 968.
20. Park, S.; Lee, Y.; Jun, J.Y. Trauma and Depression among North Korean Refugees: The Mediating Effect of Negative Cognition. *Int. J. Environ. Res. Public Health* **2018**, *15*, 591. [CrossRef]
21. Park, S.; Rim, S.J.; Jun, J.Y. Related Factors of Suicidal Ideation among North Korean Refugee Youth in South Korea. *Int. J. Environ. Res. Public Health* **2018**, *15*, 1694. [CrossRef] [PubMed]
22. Schoretsanitis, G.; Bhugra, D.; Eisenhardt, S.; Ricklin, M.E.; Srivastava, D.S.; Exadaktylos, A.; Walther, S. Upon Rejection: Psychiatric Emergencies of Failed Asylum Seekers. *Int. J. Environ. Res. Public Health* **2018**, *15*, 1498. [CrossRef]
23. Vitale, A.; Ryde, J. Exploring Risk Factors Affecting the Mental Health of Refugee Women Living with HIV. *Int. J. Environ. Res. Public Health* **2018**, *15*, 2326. [CrossRef]
24. Kizilhan, J.I. Trauma and Pain in Family-Orientated Societies. *Int. J. Environ. Res. Public Health* **2017**, *15*, 44. [CrossRef]
25. Schoretsanitis, G.; Eisenhardt, S.; Ricklin, M.E.; Srivastava, D.S.; Walther, S.; Exadaktylos, A. Psychiatric Emergencies of Asylum Seekers; Descriptive Analysis and Comparison with Immigrants of Warranted Residence. *Int. J. Environ. Res. Public Health* **2018**, *15*, 1300. [CrossRef] [PubMed]
26. Wetzke, M.; Happle, C.; Vakilzadeh, A.; Ernst, D.; Sogkas, G.; Schmidt, R.E.; Behrens, G.; Dopfer, C.; Jablonka, A. Healthcare Utilization in a Large Cohort of Asylum Seekers Entering Western Europe in 2015. *Int. J. Environ. Res. Public Health* **2018**, *15*, 2163. [CrossRef] [PubMed]
27. Keidar, O.; Jegerlehner, S.N.; Ziegenhorn, S.; Brown, A.D.; Muller, M.; Exadaktylos, A.K.; Srivastava, D. Emergency Department Discharge Outcome and Psychiatric Consultation in North African Patients. *Int. J. Environ. Res. Public Health* **2018**, *15*, 2033. [CrossRef] [PubMed]

28. Kaeser, D.; Guerra, R.; Keidar, O.; Lanz, U.; Moses, M.; Kobel, C.; Exadaktylos, A.; Ricklin, M. Verbal and Non-Verbal Aggression in a Swiss University Emergency Room: A Descriptive Study. *Int. J. Environ. Res. Public Health* **2018**, *15*, 1423. [CrossRef]
29. Claassen, K.; Jager, P. Impact of the Introduction of the Electronic Health Insurance Card on the Use of Medical Services by Asylum Seekers in Germany. *Int. J. Environ. Res. Public Health* **2018**, *15*, 856. [CrossRef]
30. Kotsiou, O.S.; Kotsios, P.; Srivastava, D.S.; Kotsios, V.; Gourgoulianis, K.I.; Exadaktylos, A.K. Impact of the Refugee Crisis on the Greek Healthcare System: A Long Road to Ithaca. *Int. J. Environ. Res. Public Health* **2018**, *15*, 1790. [CrossRef]
31. Klukowska-Roetzler, J.; Eracleous, M.; Muller, M.; Srivastava, D.S.; Krummrey, G.; Keidar, O.; Exadaktylos, A. Increased Urgent Care Center Visits by Southeast European Migrants: A Retrospective, Controlled Trial from Switzerland. *Int. J. Environ. Res. Public Health* **2018**, *15*, 1857. [CrossRef]
32. Puchner, K.; Karamagioli, E.; Pikouli, A.; Tsiamis, C.; Kalogeropoulos, A.; Kakalou, E.; Pavlidou, E.; Pikoulis, E. Time to Rethink Refugee and Migrant Health in Europe: Moving from Emergency Response to Integrated and Individualized Health Care Provision for Migrants and Refugees. *Int. J. Environ. Res. Public Health* **2018**, *15*, 1100. [CrossRef]
33. Kotsiou, O.S.; Srivastava, D.S.; Kotsios, P.; Exadaktylos, A.K.; Gourgoulianis, K.I. The Emergency Medical System in Greece: Opening Aeolus' Bag of Winds. *Int. J. Environ. Res. Public Health* **2018**, *15*, 745. [CrossRef]
34. Twomey, M.; Sijacki, A.; Krummrey, G.; Welzel, T.; Exadaktylos, A.K.; Ercegovac, M. Strengthening Emergency Care Systems to Mitigate Public Health Challenges Arising from Influxes of Individuals with Different Socio-Cultural Backgrounds to a Level One Emergency Center in South East Europe. *Int. J. Environ. Res. Public Health* **2018**, *15*, 501. [CrossRef]
35. Moran, E.B.; Katz, M.A.; Ari, O.B.; Davidovitch, N.; Zwang, O. For What Illnesses Do Asylum Seekers and Undocumented Migrant Workers in Israel Seek Healthcare? An Analysis of Medical Visits at a Large Urgent Care Clinic for the Uninsured in Tel Aviv. *Int. J. Environ. Res. Public Health* **2019**, *16*, 252. [CrossRef]
36. Dopfer, C.; Vakilzadeh, A.; Happle, C.; Kleinert, E.; Muller, F.; Ernst, D.; Schmidt, R.; Behrens, G.; Merkesdal, S.; Wetzke, M.; et al. Pregnancy Related Health Care Needs in Refugees—A Current Three Center Experience in Europe. *Int. J. Environ. Res. Public Health* **2018**, *15*, 1934. [CrossRef]
37. Rade, D.A.; Crawford, G.; Lobo, R.; Gray, C.; Brown, G. Sexual Health Help-Seeking Behavior among Migrants from Sub-Saharan Africa and South East Asia living in High Income Countries: A Systematic Review. *Int. J. Environ. Res. Public Health* **2018**, *15*, 1311. [CrossRef]
38. Mengesha, Z.B.; Perz, J.; Dune, T.; Ussher, J. Preparedness of Health Care Professionals for Delivering Sexual and Reproductive Health Care to Refugee and Migrant Women: A Mixed Methods Study. *Int. J. Environ. Res. Public Health* **2018**, *15*, 174. [CrossRef]
39. De Schrijver, L.; Vander Beken, T.; Krahe, B.; Keygnaert, I. Prevalence of Sexual Violence in Migrants, Applicants for International Protection, and Refugees in Europe: A Critical Interpretive Synthesis of the Evidence. *Int. J. Environ. Res. Public Health* **2018**, *15*, 1979. [CrossRef]
40. Ivanova, O.; Rai, M.; Kemigisha, E. A Systematic Review of Sexual and Reproductive Health Knowledge, Experiences and Access to Services among Refugee, Migrant and Displaced Girls and Young Women in Africa. *Int. J. Environ. Res. Public Health* **2018**, *15*, 1583. [CrossRef]
41. Lindsay, A.C.; Le, Q.; Greaney, M.L. Infant Feeding Beliefs, Attitudes, Knowledge and Practices of Chinese Immigrant Mothers: An Integrative Review of the Literature. *Int. J. Environ. Res. Public Health* **2017**, *15*, 21. [CrossRef]
42. Fathi, A.; El-Awad, U.; Reinelt, T.; Petermann, F. A Brief Introduction to the Multidimensional Intercultural Training Acculturation Model (MITA) for Middle Eastern Adolescent Refugees. *Int. J. Environ. Res. Public Health* **2018**, *15*, 1516. [CrossRef]
43. Rodriguez-Alvarez, E.; Lanborena, N.; Borrell, L.N. Obesity Inequalities According to Place of Birth: The Role of Education. *Int. J. Environ. Res. Public Health* **2018**, *15*, 1620. [CrossRef]
44. Costa, L.; Dias, S.; Martins, M. Fruit and Vegetable Consumption among Immigrants in Portugal: A Nationwide Cross-Sectional Study. *Int. J. Environ. Res. Public Health* **2018**, *15*, 2299. [CrossRef]
45. Morawa, E.; Erim, Y. Health-Related Lifestyle Behavior and Religiosity among First-Generation Immigrants of Polish Origin in Germany. *Int. J. Environ. Res. Public Health* **2018**, *15*, 2545. [CrossRef]

46. European Center for Disease Prevention and Control (ECDC). *Public Health Guidance on Screening and Vaccination for Infectious Diseases in Newly Arrived Migrants within the EU/EEA*; European Center for Disease Prevention and Control: Stockholm, Sweden, 2018. Available online: https://ecdc.europa.eu/sites/portal/files/documents/Public%20health%20guidance%20on%20screening%20and%20vaccination%20of%20migrants%20in%20the%20EU%20EEA.pdf (accessed on 11 March 2019).
47. World Health Organization (WHO) Regional Office for Europe. *Health Promotion for Improved Refugee and Migrant Health (Technical Guidance on Refugee and Migrant Health)*; WHO: Copenhagen, Denmark, 2018; ISBN 978 92 890 5380. Available online: http://www.euro.who.int/en/publications/abstracts/health-promotion-for-improved-refugee-and-migrant-health-2018 (accessed on 28 January 2019).
48. Helgesson, M.; Johansson, B.; Vingård, E.; Svartengren, M. 1.1-O2The Healthy Migrant Effect among migrants to Sweden. *Eur. J. Public Health* **2018**, *28* (Suppl. 1), cky047-002. [CrossRef]
49. Thomas, S.L.; Thomas, S.D. Displacement and health. *Br. Med Bull.* **2004**, *69*, 115–127. [CrossRef]
50. Castañeda, H.; Holmes, S.M.; Madrigal, D.S.; Young, M.-E.D.; Beyeler, N.; Quesada, J. Immigration as a Social Determinant of Health. *Annu. Rev. Public Health* **2015**, *36*, 375–392. [CrossRef]
51. Fleischman, Y.; Willen, S.S.; Davidovitch, N.; Mor, Z. Migration as a social determinant of health for irregular migrants: Israel as case study. *Soc. Sci. Med.* **2015**, *147*, 89–97. [CrossRef]
52. Razum, O.; Spallek, J. Addressing health-related interventions to immigrants: Migrant-specific or diversity-sensitive? *Int. J. Public Health* **2014**, *59*, 893–895. [CrossRef]
53. Renzaho, A.M.N.; Halliday, J.A.; Mellor, D.; Green, J. The Healthy Migrant Families Initiative: Development of a culturally competent obesity prevention intervention for African migrants. *BMC Public Health* **2015**, *15*, 272. [CrossRef]
54. Zimmerman, C.; Kiss, L.; Hossain, M. Migration and health: A framework for 21st century policy-making. *PLoS Med.* **2011**, *8*, e1001034. [CrossRef]
55. Abubakar, I.; Devakumar, D.; Madise, N.; Sammonds, P.; Groce, N.; Zimmerman, C.; Aldridge, R.W.; Clark, J.; Horton, R. UCL-Lancet Commission on Migration and Health. *Lancet* **2016**, *388*, 1141–1142. [CrossRef]
56. World Health Organization (WHO). The Ottawa Charter for Health Promotion Ottawa. In Proceedings of the First International Conference on Health Promotion, Ottawa, ON, Canada, 11 November 1986. Available online: https://www.who.int/healthpromotion/conferences/previous/ottawa/en/ (accessed on 28 January 2019).
57. McElfish, P.A.; Post, J.; Rowland, B. A Social Ecological and Community-Engaged Perspective for Addressing Health Disparities among Marshallese in Arkansas. *Int. J. Nurs. Clin. Pract.* **2016**, *3*, 2016. [CrossRef]
58. Wickramage, K.; Vearey, J.; Zwi, A.B.; Robinson, C.; Knipper, M. Migration and health: A global public health research priority. *BMC Public Health* **2018**, *18*, 987. [CrossRef]

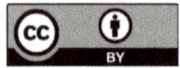

© 2019 by the authors. Licensee MDPI, Basel, Switzerland. This article is an open access article distributed under the terms and conditions of the Creative Commons Attribution (CC BY) license (http://creativecommons.org/licenses/by/4.0/).

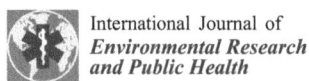

Review

Infant Feeding Beliefs, Attitudes, Knowledge and Practices of Chinese Immigrant Mothers: An Integrative Review of the Literature

Ana Cristina Lindsay [1,2,*], Qun Le [1] and Mary L. Greaney [3]

[1] Department of Exercise and Health Sciences, University of Massachusetts Boston, Boston, MA 02125, USA; Qun.Le001@umb.edu
[2] Department of Nutrition, Harvard T. H. Chan School of Public Health, Boston, MA 02115, USA
[3] Health Studies and Department of Kinesiology, University of Rhode Island, Kingston, RI 02881, USA; mgreaney@uri.edu
* Correspondence: Ana.Lindsay@umb.edu; Tel.: +617-287-7579

Received: 30 November 2017; Accepted: 20 December 2017; Published: 23 December 2017

Abstract: Chinese are a fast-growing immigrant population group in several parts of the world (e.g., Australia, Canada, Europe, Southeast Asia, United States). Research evidence suggests that compared to non-Hispanic whites, individuals of Asian-origin including Chinese are at higher risk of developing cardiovascular disease and type 2 diabetes at a lower body mass index (BMI). These risks may be possibly due to genetic differences in body composition and metabolic responses. Despite the increasing numbers of Chinese children growing up in immigrant families and the increasing prevalence of obesity among Chinese, little research has been focused on children of Chinese immigrant families. This integrative review synthesizes the evidence on infant feeding beliefs, attitudes, knowledge and practices of Chinese immigrant mothers; highlights limitations of available research; and offers suggestions for future research. Using the Preferred Reporting Items for Systematic Review and Meta-Analyses (PRISMA) guidelines, we searched four electronic academic/research databases (CINAHL, Medline, PsycINFO, and PubMed) to identify peer-reviewed, full-text papers published in English between January 2000 and September 2017. Only studies with mothers 18+ years old of normally developing infants were included. Of the 797 citations identified, 15 full-text papers were retrieved and 11 studies (8 cross-sectional studies, 3 qualitative studies) met the inclusion criteria and were included in this review. Reviewed studies revealed high initiation rates of breastfeeding, but sharp declines in breastfeeding rates by six months of age. In addition, reviewed studies revealed that the concomitantly use of breast milk and formula, and the early introduction of solid foods were common. Finally, reviewed studies identified several familial and socio-cultural influences on infant feeding beliefs and practices that may increase risk of overweight and obesity during infancy and early childhood among Chinese children of immigrant families. Nonetheless, as only 11 studies were identified and because the majority of studies (*n* = 8) were conducted in Australia, additional research including longitudinal studies, and studies conducted in countries with large Chinese immigrant population are needed to further identify and understand influences on Chinese immigrant mothers' beliefs, attitudes, and practices related to infant feeding that may increase risk of child overweight and obesity. This information is needed to develop interventions tailored to the beliefs and needs of this fast-growing immigrant group and aimed at promoting healthy infant feeding practices to prevent childhood overweight and obesity.

Keywords: breastfeeding; complementary feeding; Chinese; immigrant mothers; infant; obesity

1. Introduction

Childhood overweight and obesity are significant global public health problems [1,2] and prior research documents increased risk of overweight and obesity among racial/ethnic minority children of immigrant families [3,4]. More specifically, evidence suggests that children from racial/ethnic minority, immigrant families with low incomes are at elevated risk of obesity in the first two years of life [5–11]. Lower socio-economic status, limited education language barriers, cultural beliefs, and inadequate access to health care have been found to be associated with increased risk of overweight and obesity among children of immigrant parents [6–12].

Chinese are a fast-growing immigrant population group in several parts of the world (e.g., Australia, Canada, Europe, Southeast Asia, United States (U.S.)). Research evidence suggests that compared to non-Hispanic whites individuals of Asian-origin including Chinese develop cardiovascular disease and type 2 diabetes at a lower body mass index (BMI). This difference may be due to genetic differences in body composition and metabolic responses [13,14]. Despite the increasing numbers of Chinese children of immigrant families, and the overall increasing prevalence of obesity among Chinese immigrants, until recently children of Chinese immigrants have received little attention in the childhood obesity research literature [15–18].

Infancy is a crucial developmental period that has long-term impact on children's health status [19–21]. Identifying modifiable risk factors amenable to interventions during this early life stage is critical for preventing childhood obesity and its associated co-morbidities [21–23]. Parents, especially mothers, make or directly influence the early feeding decisions and practices that impact their children's healthy eating habits, food preferences, ability to self-regulate food intake, and ultimately risk of overweight and obesity in early childhood and later life [24–30]. Evidence suggests that non-exclusive and limited breastfeeding (less than four months) and the early introduction of foods (e.g., serving juices, adding cereal to the bottle) are associated with rapid growth in the first six months of life and increased risk of obesity in infancy and early childhood, which may carry into later life stages [27,28,31–38]. Nonetheless, the worldwide prevalence of exclusive breastfeeding (EBF) is low and early introduction of complementary feeding is high [22].

Several national and international organizations recommend EBF infants until six months of age, then continuing breastfeeding until at least one year of age with nutritious solid foods being introduced at about six months [24,38]. Parents' decision to breastfeed is one of the first feeding decisions they make and this decision may have a lasting impact on their children's weight and health status [39]. Results of research examining the effects of breastfeeding on risk of child obesity are not consistent, with some research indicating that breastfeeding protects against overweight and obesity during childhood [33,39]. Results of some studies, however, indicate that breastfeeding has minimal [40] or no impact [41] on children's weight status.

Complementary feeding, the process of gradual introduction of foods and beverages to breastfed or formula-fed infants, is an important feeding transition that has been linked to eating habits, food preferences and risk of excessive weight gain and obesity in children [28,30,33,34]. Research evidence suggests that introduction of complementary foods before four months of age (risk may be even stronger among formula-fed infants) is a risk factor for obesity [42,43].

It is important to identify factors associated with infant feeding beliefs, attitudes and practices that may inhibit children developing healthy eating habits and weight so interventions to prevent and reduce child obesity can be developed. Interventions that offer parents guidance on healthy infant feeding practices may be an important strategy to promote children's healthy weight status [23–26]. Given that Chinese are at increased risk of cardiovascular disease and type 2 diabetes at a lower BMI [13–18], and the growing evidence linking early feeding practices to the risk of childhood obesity [44,45], the purpose of this integrative literature review were to: (1) identify and summarize findings from existing studies examining infant feeding beliefs, attitudes, knowledge and practices of Chinese-born immigrant mothers; (2) highlight the limitations of reviewed studies; and (3) generate suggestions for future research.

2. Materials and Methods

The methods employed during this review were informed by those developed by Whittemore and Knafl [46] and allowed for the inclusion of qualitative, quantitative, and mixed methods studies. The review included three key steps: (1) a systematic literature search; (2) data evaluation involving a thematic analysis process—data reduction, data display, drawing and verifying conclusions; and (3) presentation of conclusions. In addition, we used the reporting guidelines of the Preferred Reporting Items for Systematic Reviews and Meta-Analysis (PRISMA) statement [47] to guide the inclusion and exclusion of research papers. The PRISMA statement comprises guidelines that include a four-phase flow diagram to systematically guide the inclusion and exclusion of research papers. In addition, the guidelines provide a 27-item checklist that describes the requirements per review section (e.g., title, abstract, introduction, methods, results, discussions, funding) to ensure that systematic reviews are properly conducted and reported [47].

2.1. Search Strategy

We searched four electronic databases—PubMed, Medline, PsycINFO, and Cumulative Index to Nursing and Allied Health Literature (CINAHL). The search, conducted between December 2016 and September 2017, was limited to full-text, peer-reviewed articles published in English between January 2000 and September 2017. Search terms included: (1) infan* OR newborns OR child*; (2) 'breastfeeding' OR 'breast milk feeding' OR 'breast milk' OR 'human milk' OR 'nursing' OR 'lactation'; (3) 'formula feeding' OR formula; (4) 'complementary feeding' OR 'complementary food' OR 'supplementary food'; (5) weaning; (6) 'infant feeding'; (7) 'feeding practices' OR 'feeding behavior' OR 'feeding strategy'; (8) parent* OR caregiver OR mother; (9) immigrant; and (10) Chinese OR China.

Two authors (ACL, QL) independently examined the titles and abstracts of all identified citations and studies were excluded when both authors determined that the study did not meet the inclusion criteria. Next, these same two authors independently reviewed the full article of studies that were not excluded based on titles or abstracts. Furthermore, to identify additional potentially eligible studies, these two authors searched the reference lists of existing full articles that satisfied the inclusion criteria. The two authors agreed upon a final set of articles and examined the articles to extract the relevant information pertaining to the objectives of this review. The search strategy using the PRISMA flow diagram is illustrated in Figure S1.

2.2. Study Selection

This review was limited to studies that included normally developing children (i.e., not born preterm, not diagnosed with physical or mental complications, etc.) of Chinese immigrants. Qualitative and quantitative studies were eligible for inclusion if they met the following criteria: (1) peer-reviewed, full-text articles published in English between January 2000 and June 2017; (2) sample included Chinese immigrant parents (18+ years old); and (3) in the case of multi-ethnic samples, at least 25% of the total sample was Chinese-born immigrant mothers.

2.3. Data extraction and Data Synthesis

The 11 identified eligible studies were analyzed and synthesized using the Matrix Method [48]. Two authors (ACL, QL) independently read all articles and completed a data extraction form created to gather the following: (1) authors; (2) study setting; (3) study aim(s); (4) study population; (5) study design; (6) measure(s) of infant feeding practices; and (7) study findings. The two sets of completed data extraction forms were compared, and discrepancies were resolved with feedback from a third author. Due to the inclusion of studies using qualitative and quantitative designs conducting a meta-analysis of the data was not appropriate, and results of this review are presented as a narrative summary.

2.4. Quality Assessment of Included Studies

Included studies were evaluated using two quality frameworks. Using the Strengthening in the Reporting of Observational Studies in Epidemiology (STROBE) guidelines [49], two authors assessed observational studies (*n* = 8) for possible bias and methodological areas that may have been inadequately addressed using a quality checklist created for this review. The checklist consisted of nine questions (see Table S1) designed to be answered with either "yes", or "no." Each "yes" response was assigned 1 point, and a score of 0 was given to "no" response). Total scores (range of scores 0–9) were then used to assign a rating of the study as strong (score > 7), moderate (score between 7 and 5), or weak (score < 5). Qualitative studies were assessed using the Critical Appraisal Skills Program (CASP) [50], a nine-question appraisal tool (see Table S2). Two researchers (ACL, QL) independently assessed the studies included in this review using these checklists and discussed and resolved any differences in scoring.

3. Results

3.1. Search

The search strategy generated 797 unique articles (see Figure S1). After exclusion, 11 research articles were deemed eligible and included in this integrative review [51–61].

3.2. Summary of Included Studies

Of the 11 included studies, all focused on breastfeeding and/or formula feeding beliefs, attitudes, knowledge and practices (initiation and duration) [51–61], while five also examined complementary feeding beliefs and practices [54,56,57,60,61]. The 11 studies took place in four countries—eight in Australia, one in Canada, one Ireland, and one in the United States. Of the 11 reviewed studies, eight employed quantitative methods, and all were cross-sectional [51–55,57–59]. Sample sizes ranged from 15 to 506. Three quantitative studies (3/8) [51,52,57] used questionnaires specifically developed for the study, either alone or in combination with medical records [52], while three (3/8) [53–55] used the Perth Infant Feeding Study (PIFS) questionnaire [62], and two (2/8) [58,59] used the Iowa Infant Feeding Attitudes Survey (IIFAS) [63] translated and adapted for Chinese.

Three studies employed qualitative methods [56,60,61], and all three used semi-structured in-depth interviews. Further details of included studies are presented in Table S3, while Table S4 provides the synthesized information on methodology and main findings of included studies.

3.2.1. Initiation and Duration of Breastfeeding

Seven studies, all conducted in Australia, examined initiation and duration of breastfeeding [51–55,58,59]. These studies found high breastfeeding initiation rates (53.2%–94.1%) among Chinese immigrant mothers, but lower rates of breastfeeding duration in comparison to initiation rates. For example, one study conducted in Australia [51] showed that only 34% of mothers were breastfeeding when baby was three months of age. Similarly, two other studies conducted in Australia [54,55,58] showed sharp decline in breastfeeding (any breastfeeding) rates at six months of age—6% [55] and 55.6% [54]. Similarly, another study conducted in Australia showed that only 33.8% of Chinese immigrant mothers reported "fully breastfeeding" at six months of age [58].

Several studies indicated that most mothers do not EBF for the first six months of life, and use formula concomitantly with breast milk [52–55,58,59]. One cross-sectional study [55] conducted in Australia found that 88.5% of women initiated breastfeeding; however, only 55.6% reported breastfeeding six-month postpartum. The majority of studies reported that the mean duration of exclusive breastfeeding was below the recommended about six months, with mean duration ranging from two to five months postpartum. Moreover, one study [54] found that duration of breastfeeding was associated with the age at which the infant was introduced to formula or cow's milk, with a later the introduction being associated with a longer the duration of breastfeeding.

Two cross-sectional studies using data from the same sample [53,54] showed that the most often cited reason for bottle-feeding was a perceived lack of breast milk. Another common reason for stopping breastfeeding reported was mother going back to work [53,54].

3.2.2. Beliefs, Attitudes, and Knowledge about Breastfeeding

All 11 reviewed studies [51–61] examined mothers' beliefs related to infant feeding. These studies found that most believed that "breastfeeding was natural" and "provided the best nutrition for infants' health and growth". Positive beliefs were found to be associated with breastfeeding initiation in some studies [51,54,57].

Moreover, four studies (4/11) found that mothers' decision to breastfeed was partially influenced by her perceptions and personal assessment of infant's health and growth [56,57,60,61]. For example, one qualitative study conducted in Canada [56] revealed that mother's perceptions of their babies weight and size were used to assess whether her baby "was being fed high quality milk" and "enough milk". Similarly, a qualitative study conducted in Australia [61] revealed that mothers' who perceived their infants growth to be unsatisfactory (below 50%) were not confident that their milk supply was sufficient and that their infant was getting enough nutrition from breast milk alone.

In addition, despite studies indicating that women believed that breastfeeding is the best feeding mode, some studies reported that mothers often expressed doubts about being able to produce "enough breast milk" and perceived that breast milk alone would not satiate their baby, especially when infant's growth "tracked down" [56,60,61]. A common belief among mothers was that a "fat baby is a healthy baby" [56,61]. This belief was associated with the decision to formula feed exclusively or in combination (mixed feeding) with breastfeeding [56,60,61].

Nine studies [51–57,60,61] assessed mothers' attitudes towards breastfeeding, and overall these studies revealed that most mothers held favorable attitudes towards breastfeeding, and that most chose to breastfeed due to a sense of fulfillment, joy, love, and attachment to their baby. Nonetheless, several studies also reported common negative attitudes towards breastfeeding including breastfeeding being an embarrassing practice in pubic, adverse to mother's figure, father feels left out, bottle feeding reduces risk of neonatal infection, breastfeeding babies become "too attached" to the mother [51,53–55,57,60,61]. In addition, four studies (4/9) found that mothers who held negative attitudes towards breastfeeding were less likely to breastfeed, and breastfed for shorter duration [54,57,60,61]. Moreover, some studies showed that mothers practiced mixed feeding (breast and formula feeding), and introduced formula in the first three months of infants' life as they thought this would "familiarize their baby with formula" and prevent problems when breastfeeding was reduced or stopped [54,60,61].

Four studies assessed mothers' knowledge of breastfeeding [51,53,55,57]. Overall, these studies revealed that Chinese immigrant mothers were aware of the health benefits of breast milk and advantages of breastfeeding their infants, although several misconceptions about breastfeeding existed [51,53,55,57]. A cross-sectional study conducted in Australia [53] found that more than half of the mothers (68.4%) believed in the importance of breast milk as the first feed for all infants and that infant formula should not be used as an initial food. Furthermore, a couple of studies (2/4) reported that mothers recognized colostrum as being nutritionally important and that the benefits of breast milk last after weaning [53,55]. Another cross-sectional study of Chinese mothers living in Australia found that although mothers were knowledgeable about the health benefits of breastfeeding, they also held several misconceptions such as bottle-feeding causes less neonatal infection, breastfed babies become "too attached" to the mother, and breastfeeding affects the healing of the episiotomy wound [51]. Similarly, a cross-sectional study conducted in Ireland [57] revealed that most Chinese immigrant mothers (approximately 82%) believed that breast milk is the ideal food for infants, over 70% were conscious of the unique health benefits of breast milk and more than 60% recognized that breastfeeding offered some disease protective effects. Nevertheless, some studies found that mothers held several misconceptions mothers held such as the benefits of breast milk last only until the baby is weaned, mothers should not breastfeed if have a cold, and infant formula should be fed to all newborns [51,56,57,61].

3.2.3. Complementary Feeding (Introduction of Solids)

Five of the 11 included studies reported information on complementary feeding practices (i.e., introduction of solid foods) [54,56,57,60,61]. Finding of these studies conducted in three countries—Australia [54,61], Canada [56], Ireland [57], and the US [60] found that mothers introduced solid foods earlier than recommended. In addition, a cross-sectional study conducted in Australia [54] showed that Chinese immigrant mothers introduced solid foods earlier than Australian-born mothers. Two qualitative studies [60,61] showed that many of the infants' solid foods introduced were traditional Chinese foods and that most were introduced before six months, most often at around three months of age. Mothers who introduced traditional Chinese solid foods to infants early did this as they perceived that that the benefits of this included strengthening bone development, children learning how to swallow foods other than milk, prolonged satiety, steady or accelerated growth, and improved digestive system based on the appearance of infants' feces [60,61].

3.2.4. Influence of Socio-Demographics, Economic and Cultural Factors on Infant Feeding

Nine of the 11 included studies examined the influence of socio-demographics, economic and acculturation factors on infant feeding beliefs and practices [51–57,60,61]. Two (2/9) cross-sectional studies conducted in Australia [53,54] found that higher family income was associated with mothers' less preference for breastfeeding. Furthermore, two studies conducted in Australia [53,54] determined that mother's level of education was positively associated with the initiation and increased duration of breastfeeding. Several studies documented that mothers from lower socio-economic and educational backgrounds more often reported misconceptions about breastfeeding and formula feeding than women with greater education and higher income [51,53,54,57]. Moreover, better employment opportunity for mothers in the country of immigration was found to be associated with shorter breastfeeding duration [54,57].

Cultural influences on infant feeding beliefs and practices were reported in several studies [51,56,57,60,61]. Four studies found that Chinese immigrant mothers' breastfeeding practices (initiation and duration) are tied to traditional cultural health beliefs such as the *yin-yang* theory (hot-cold theory) and *zuo yuezi* ("doing the month" or "sitting in for the first month") [56,57,60,61]. In addition to the belief about the consumption of "hot" or "warm" (e.g., protein rich) and "cold" (e.g., fruits and vegetables) foods during *zuo yuezi*, some studies also showed that mothers' consumed specific protein-rich foods (e.g., fish, chicken, pork, duck, rabbit) to address breastfeeding issues such as low milk supply [56,57,60,61]. Moreover, one qualitative study [56] conducted in Canada found that mothers' perception about breast milk was determined by their beliefs of physical health and restoring balance of the body.

Mothers' level of acculturation to Western culture was found in both quantitative [52,54,57] and qualitative studies [56,60] to influence infant feeding practices. For example, some studies (5/11) found that mothers who had lived in the country of immigration longer were more likely to adopt infant feeding practices of that country, which in turn resulted in more positive infant feeding practices, including immediate initiation and longer duration of breastfeeding [52,54,60], and delayed introduction of solids foods [54,57].

3.2.5. Family Support and Influence of Husbands and Grandparents on Infant Feeding Method

All 11 studies reported on the influence of family support on mothers' infant feeding beliefs and practices, with studies documenting the critical influence of husbands and grandparents on mothers' infant feeding beliefs and practices [51–61]. Three quantitative studies found that husband's preference for breastfeeding was associated with breastfeeding initiation [53–55]. In addition, three other studies, two qualitative [60,61] and one quantitative [57] reported that grandparents in China often visit the mother's new country and stay for several months to take care of the mother and the newborn. Two qualitative studies [60,61] showed that grandparents had a major influence on infant feeding decisions and practices, reporting that mothers often negotiated infant feeding choices, seeking agreement and support from extended family to align recommendations received from health professionals and extended family, in particular grandparents [60,61].

3.2.6. Support from Healthcare Professionals

Four studies conducted in Australia reported on the influence of healthcare professionals on mothers' infant feeding practices [53–55,61]. Three studies [53–55] using survey data from the same sample reported that Chinese women delivering in Australia received more breastfeeding support and assistance from health professionals and that these mothers were more likely to have breastfeed immediately after birth compared with women delivering in China. In addition, doctors' support of breastfeeding had a positive influence on the initiation and duration of breastfeeding [53–55]. A qualitative study [61] revealed that mothers valued and respected the advice of health professionals such as doctors, nurses and midwives and relied on their advice to better understand the best infant feeding practices for healthy growth.

4. Discussion

Childhood obesity is a growing global public health epidemic [1,2]. The incidence of childhood obesity has increased in most high-income countries in the past decades, and more recently, the same trend is being observed in middle- and low-income countries [1,2]. Recent research documents increases in the prevalence of obesity in China [64–66] and among Chinese immigrants living outside China [67–72]. Despite some observed decreases in childhood obesity in high-income countries, racial/ethnic minority immigrant groups in these countries remain at increased risk [1,2,5–12]. Changing social and physical environments coupled with socioeconomic, language and cultural barriers, as well as limited access to, or inadequate utilization of healthcare represent additional risk factors for immigrant populations in a new country [27,73–82].

Maternal infant feeding practices are influential on infant' and child's growth, and could possibly explain obesity rates across generations [30,33,39,83]. A small, but increasing body of research conducted primarily in Western countries, has examined infant feeding practices of ethnic minority immigrant mothers [84–87], but limited attention has been paid to Chinese immigrant mothers, a large and growing group in several countries. Therefore, the purpose of this integrative review was to identify and synthesize information from studies examining infant feeding practices conducted among Chinese immigrant mothers in order to describe and highlight factors influencing infant feeding practices of this immigrant group that may be used to inform the design of interventions.

Overall, findings of studies included in this integrative review showed high initiation rates of breastfeeding, but sharp decline in rates of breastfeeding by six months of age [51–55,58,59]. The limited duration of EBF is concerning, as a longer duration is associated with positive health outcomes for infant and mother [19,27,30,33,34,38,40].

Findings of studies included in this review showed that overall Chinese immigrant mothers hold positive beliefs about breastfeeding [51,53–56,58–61]. Nonetheless, reviewed studies also documented negative beliefs and misconceptions such as bottle feeding causes less neonatal infections, breastfed babies become "too attached" to the mother, etc. [51–53,55,56,58,60] that may influence mothers' decision to supplement infant feeding with formula. Furthermore, several studies found that most Chinese immigrant mothers do not EBF, and that the concomitantly use of formula feeding is common [53,55,58,60,61]. These findings are in agreement with findings from studies conducted in China [88–91]. Interventions designed to promote healthy infant feeding practices among Chinese immigrant mothers and families should take this information into account. Moreover, obesity prevention and control efforts among Chinese children of immigrant families should target early feeding practices including practices during infancy, as these practices may be closely related to the early origins of obesity risk in this population group.

Cultural, socioeconomic, and psychological factors shape mothers' perceptions of and practices related to infant feeding [27,30,33]. Cultural dietary and feeding beliefs are particularly important for immigrant populations, which often hold on to these cultural beliefs across generations to keep a close relationship with their country and cultural origins [88–91]. In agreement with prior research conducted in a range of cultural settings [92,93], findings from studies included in this review documented the influence of culture beliefs on mothers' infant feeding practices [51,53–61]. Evidence shows that many traditional medical practitioners in China encourage exclusive breastfeeding during the practice of *zuo yuezi* for the benefit of both mother and infant [88–91]. These findings suggest the importance of understanding and incorporating cultural beliefs common in the Chinese culture when developing interventions to promote healthy infant feeding practices targeting Chinese immigrant mothers and families. Moreover, findings from a few reviewed studies suggest the influence of acculturation levels on Chinese immigrant mothers' infant feeding beliefs and practices [54,56,58–61], and indicate the importance of taking into account acculturation levels. Interventions developed to promote healthy infant feeding practices targeting Chinese immigrant mothers should be designed taking social and cultural changes faced by families and mothers, as well as acculturation levels within Chinese immigrant families.

Like previous studies with other ethnic groups, findings from studies included in this review indicate that mothers' infant feeding beliefs and practices are influenced by the broader family context [93–96]. Findings from studies reviewed showed that husbands and grandparents are important influences on Chinese immigrant mothers' infant feeding beliefs and practices, which is in agreement with previous research conducted in China suggesting that family roles in Chinese culture influence mother's choice to breastfeed [97–100]. Studies conducted in China indicate that in Chinese culture, the baby's father and paternal grandmother have significant influence on the choice of infant feeding method [88–90,98,99]. In the case of Chinese immigrant mothers, the husband might be particular influential on the decision to breastfeed [91]. These findings are important and suggest that effective interventions targeting Chinese immigrant mothers must address the promotion of healthy infant feeding practices within the context of the family, and take into account the influence of family members, especially husbands and grandparents, who should also be considered targets for health promotion interventions.

Although findings from studies included in this review documented the influence of socio-demographic and economic factors on Chinese immigrant mothers' infant feeding practices [51–56,58–61], the mothers participating in the majority of the studies (8/11) were from relatively affluent backgrounds. Overall, the majority of Chinese immigrant mothers participating in the majority of the reviewed studies conducted in Australia (7/11) [51–55,58,59,61] and Ireland (1/11) [57] were highly educated (50%–80% participants had completed college), and most were relatively affluent (middle income or higher). Mothers' ages ranged from 22 to 59 years old, the majority had resided in the country of immigration for more than five years, and most were housewives. Nonetheless, in agreement with research conducted among other ethnic minority groups [27,33,42,74,79,82,87,98], findings from reviewed studies suggest the importance of taking into account socio-demographic and economic factors when designing interventions for Chinese immigrant children and families.

Mirroring findings from research conducted with other ethnic groups [43,83–87,94], findings from studies included in this review showed that early introduction of solids is a common practice [54,56,57,60,61], and that cultural beliefs might influence this practice [57,60,61]. Furthermore, a few of reviewed studies showed that some mothers were not knowledgeable about the long-term benefits of breastfeeding, which may result in the early introduction of solids [54,56,57]. Conflicting evidence exists for the association between timing of introduction of solid foods and risk of subsequent obesity [34,42,94,101–103]. Some studies suggest that early introduction of solid foods is associated with subsequent obesity in childhood, and that the association vary by whether an infant is breastfed or formula-fed [34,42,101,102]. While some studies have found that breastfeeding and delaying complementary foods yield lower likelihood of obesity and greater probability of healthy weight status [19,34,38,42], other studies have not found a significant association between early introduction of solids and risk of obesity in childhood [43].

Our evaluation of the methodologies of studies included in this integrative review suggests some possible limitations, which warrant caution in the interpretation of study findings. All included quantitative studies (8/8) examining infant feeding practices were cross-sectional. Additional longitudinal studies are needed to better understand infant feeding practices, and the relationship between these practices and risk of overweight and/or obesity in children in Chinese immigrant families. All included quantitative studies employed self-reported or administered questionnaires for the assessment of infant feeding practices, which may result in misclassification. A methodological strength was the use of well-known, validated questionnaires to assess infant feeding knowledge, attitudes and practices including the PIFS [62] and the IIFAS [63] in six of the reviewed studies [53–55,57–59].

Only three qualitative studies were identified and included in this review [56,60,61], and these studies were conducted in three countries including Australia [61], Canada [56], and the U.S. [60]. Given the dearth of information on Chinese immigrant mothers' infant feeding practices, additional qualitative studies are needed to further explore factors identified by available qualitative and quantitative studies conducted among this population group.

Finally, the majority (8/11) studies examining infant feeding practices were conducted among Chinese immigrants in Australia [51–55,58–61], with only three studies conducted in three other countries (i.e., Canada, Ireland, and the U.S.) [56,57,60]. Although several countries with large Chinese immigrant populations (e.g., Australia, Canada, Ireland, and U.S.) were represented in studies included in this review, other countries with large Chinese immigrant populations (e.g., Thailand, Singapore, Malaysia, Indonesia, Europe) were not. It is probable that Chinese immigrants in countries not included in this review are influenced by similar factors that Chinese immigrants in countries represented in this review, even though some social contextual factors may differ. Furthermore, the paucity of studies examining infant feeding practices of immigrant Chinese mothers in countries with large Chinese immigrant populations such as Canada and the U.S. is a concern given the evidence from research linking infant feeding to increased risk of child obesity during early childhood [19,34–40], and evidence that children of racial/ethnic minority families living in high-income countries are at increased risk of obesity [5–12]. Finally, it is possible that we did not identify all relevant articles due to studies being published in other formats, such as country reports, alternative databases, or in other languages not included in this review. The use of systematic criteria (i.e., PRISMA) [47] to identify and select studies and modified quality assessment tools for the critical appraisal of papers are strengths of this study (i.e., STROBE and CASP) [49,50].

In summary, additional studies are needed to further explore and understand multiple influences on Chinese immigrant mothers' infant feeding decisions and practices and to quantify the effects of these practices on child's weight status in infancy and early childhood. Future research should also include both qualitative and quantitative research methods and longitudinal study designs and further explore the role of psychosocial and cultural factors in influencing infant feeding practices of Chinese immigrant parents. In addition, studies employing multiple methods for assessing infant feeding practices including direct observations are needed to further examine infant feeding practices associated with increased risk of overweight and obesity in children of Chinese immigrant families. This information will be important to identify factors among this ethnic group amenable to intervention.

5. Conclusions

Information about factors associated with parental feeding practices is needed to promote healthy infant feeding practices aimed at the prevention of child overweight and obesity [103].

Several modifiable infant feeding beliefs and practices were identified in the present integrative review. Findings from the synthesis of studies included in this integrative review suggest direction for further research, as well as potential targets for interventions aimed at promoting healthy infant feeding practices and preventing and decreasing disparities in early childhood obesity among Chinese children of immigrant families. Given the growing evidence suggesting the link between infant feeding practices and increased risk of overweight and obesity in children, additional research examining these associations in Chinese immigrant children in various geographical location (i.e., Asia, Australia, Europe and North America) is needed due to the paucity of research identified and the increasing prevalence of overweight and obesity rates in Chinese children of immigrant families in several countries across the globe. This information is needed to develop culturally relevant interventions that can change influences in these modifiable risky practices and that are likely to help prevent and reduce risk of child obesity in Chinese children of immigrant families.

Supplementary Materials: The following are available online at www.mdpi.com/1660-4601/15/1/21/s1, Figure S1: PRISMA flow diagram, Table S1: Quality assessment of included quantitative studies using adapted "Strengthening the Reporting of Observational Studies in Epidemiology (STROBE)" statement; Table S2: Quality assessment of included qualitative studies using the Critical Appraisal Skills Program (CASP); Table S3: Description of studies included in systematic review; Table S4: Characteristics of studies examining infant feeding beliefs, attitudes, knowledge and practices of Chinese immigrant mothers included in integrative review.

Acknowledgments: The authors are grateful for library assistance provided by Teresa Maceira, Head Reference Librarian at the University of Massachusetts Boston.

Author Contributions: The following co-authors contributed to the work: Ana Cristina Lindsay in study design, data collection, data analysis, and manuscript preparation and review. Qun Le in data collection, analysis, manuscript preparation and review. Mary L. Greaney in manuscript preparation and review. All authors read and approved the final manuscript.

Conflicts of Interest: The authors declare no conflict of interest.

References

1. De Onis, M.; Blössner, M.; Borghi, E. Global prevalence and trends of overweight and obesity among preschool children. *Am. J. Clin. Nutr.* **2010**, *92*, 1257–1264. [CrossRef] [PubMed]
2. Ng, M.; Fleming, T.; Robinson, M.; Thomson, B.; Graetz, N.; Margono, C.; Gakidou, E. Global, regional, and national prevalence of overweight and obesity in children and adults during 1980–2013: A systematic analysis for the Global Burden of Disease Study 2013. *Lancet* **2014**, *384*, 766–781. [CrossRef]
3. Ogden, C.L.; Carroll, M.D.; Flegal, K.M. Prevalence of obesity in the United States. *JAMA* **2014**, *312*, 189–190. [CrossRef] [PubMed]
4. Strauss, R.S.; Pollack, H.A. Epidemic increase in childhood overweight, 1986–1998. *JAMA* **2001**, *286*, 2845–2848. [CrossRef] [PubMed]
5. Kimbro, R.T.; Brooks-Gunn, J.; McLanahan, S. Racial and ethnic differentials in overweight and obesity among 3-year-old children. *Am. J. Public Health* **2007**, *97*, 298–305. [CrossRef] [PubMed]
6. Sanchez-Vaznaugh, E.V.; Kawachi, I.; Subramanian, S.V.; Sánchez, B.N.; Acevedo-Garcia, D. Differential effect of birthplace and length of residence on body mass index (BMI) by education, gender and race/ethnicity. *Soc. Sci. Med.* **2008**, *67*, 1300–1310. [CrossRef] [PubMed]
7. Ebenegger, V.; Marques-Vidal, P.M.; Nydegger, A.; Laimbacher, J.; Niederer, I.; Bürgi, F.; Puder, J.J. Independent contribution of parental migrant status and educational level. Journal of Human Lactation 33 to adiposity and eating habits in preschool children. *Eur. J. Clin. Nutr.* **2011**, *65*, 210–218. [CrossRef] [PubMed]
8. Singh, G.K.; Siahpush, M.; Hiatt, R.A.; Timsina, L.R. Dramatic increases in obesity and overweight prevalence and body mass index among ethnic-immigrant and social class groups in the United States, 1976–2008. *J. Community Health* **2011**, *36*, 94–110. [CrossRef] [PubMed]
9. Dixon, B.; Peña, M.M.; Taveras, E.M. Lifecourse approach to racial/ethnic disparities in childhood obesity. *Adv. Nutr. Int. Rev. J.* **2012**, *3*, 73–82. [CrossRef] [PubMed]
10. Pan, L.; Grummer-Strawn, L.M.; McGuire, L.C.; Park, S.; Blanck, H.M. Trends in state/territorial obesity prevalence by race/ethnicity among U.S. low-income, preschool aged children. *Pediatr. Obes.* **2016**, *11*, 397–402. [CrossRef] [PubMed]

11. Waters, E.; Ashbolt, R.; Gibbs, L.; Booth, M.; Magarey, A.; Gold, L.; Kai Lo, S.; Gibbons, K.; Green, J.; O'Connor, T.; et al. Double disadvantage: The influence of ethnicity over socioeconomic position on childhood overweight and obesity: Findings from an inner urban population of primary school children. *Int. J. Pediatr. Obes.* **2008**, *3*, 196–204. [CrossRef] [PubMed]
12. Oza-Frank, R.; Cunningham, S.A. The weight of US residence among immigrants: A systematic review. *Obes. Rev.* **2010**, *11*, 271–280. [CrossRef] [PubMed]
13. Razak, F.; Anand, S.S.; Shannon, H.; Vuksan, V.; Davis, B.; Jacobs, R.; Teo, K.K.; McQueen, M.; Yusuf, S. Defining obesity cut points in a multiethnic population. *Circulation* **2007**, *115*, 2111–2118. [CrossRef] [PubMed]
14. World Health Organization. Appropriate body-mass index for Asian populations and its implications for policy and intervention strategies. *Lancet* **2004**, *363*, 157–163.
15. Aris, I.M.; Chen, L.W.; Tint, M.T.; Pang, W.W.; Soh, S.E.; Saw, S.M.; Shek, L.P.; Tan, K.H.; Gluckman, P.D.; Chong, Y.S.; et al. Body mass index trajectories in the first two years and subsequent childhood cardio-metabolic outcomes: A prospective multi-ethnic Asian cohort study. *Sci. Rep.* **2017**, *7*, 8424. [CrossRef] [PubMed]
16. Aris, I.M.; Bernard, J.Y.; Chen, L.W.; Tint, M.T.; Pang, W.W.; Lim, W.Y.; Soh, S.E.; Saw, S.M.; Godfrey, K.M.; Gluckman, P.D.; et al. Infant body mass index peak and early childhood cardio-metabolic risk markers in a multi-ethnic Asian birth cohort. *Int. J. Epidemiol.* **2017**, *46*, 513–525. [CrossRef] [PubMed]
17. Oza-Frank, R.; Ali, M.K.; Vaccarino, V.; Narayan, K.M. Asian Americans: Diabetes prevalence across U.S. and World Health Organization weight classifications. *Diabetes Care* **2009**, *32*, 1644–1646. [CrossRef] [PubMed]
18. Ye, J.; Rust, G.; Baltrus, P.; Daniels, E. Cardiovascular risk factors among Asian Americans: Results from a National Health Survey. *Ann. Epidemiol.* **2009**, *19*, 718–723. [CrossRef] [PubMed]
19. Baker, J.L.; Michaelsen, K.F.; Rasmussen, K.M.; Sorensen, T.I. Maternal prepregnant body mass index, duration of breastfeeding, and timing of complementary food introduction are associated with infant weight gain. *Am. J. Clin. Nutr.* **2004**, *80*, 1579–1588. [PubMed]
20. Institute of Medicine, Food and Nutrition Board. *Examining a Developmental Approach to Childhood Obesity: The Fetal and Early Childhood Years—Workshop Summary*; National Academies Press: Washington, DC, USA, 2015.
21. Fewtrell, M.S.; Haschke, F.; Prescott, S.L. (Eds.) *Preventive Aspects of Early Nutrition*; 85th Nestle Nutrition Institute Workshop Series; Karger AG Basel: London, UK, 2014. [CrossRef]
22. World Health Organization. *Report of the First Meeting of the Ad Hoc Working Group on Science and Evidence for Ending Childhood Obesity*; World Health Organization: Geneva, Switzerland, 2014.
23. Lumeng, J.C.; Taveras, E.M.; Birch, L.; Yanovski, S.Z. Prevention of obesity in infancy and early childhood: A National Institutes of Health workshop. *JAMA Pediatr.* **2015**, *169*, 484–490. [CrossRef] [PubMed]
24. Anzman, S.L.; Rollins, B.Y.; Birch, L.L. Parental influence on children's early eating environments and obesity risk: Implications for prevention. *Int. J. Obes.* **2010**, *34*, 1116–1124. [CrossRef] [PubMed]
25. Lindsay, A.C.; Sussner, K.M.; Kim, J.; Gortmaker, S. The role of parents in preventing childhood obesity. *Future Child.* **2006**, *16*, 169–186. [CrossRef] [PubMed]
26. Sleddens, S.F.; Gerards, S.M.; Thijs, C.; De Vries, N.K.; Kremers, S.P. General parenting, childhood overweight and obesity-inducing behaviors: A review. *Int. J. Pediatr. Obes.* **2011**, *6* (Suppl. 3), e12–e27. [CrossRef] [PubMed]
27. Singh, G.; Kogan, M.; Dee, D.L. Nativity/immigrant status, race/ethnicity, and socioeconomic determinants of breastfeeding initiation and duration in the United States, 2003. *Pediatrics* **2007**, *119* (Suppl. 1), S38–S46. [CrossRef] [PubMed]
28. Birch, L.L. Learning to eat: Behavioral and psychological aspects. *Nestle Nutr. Inst. Workshop Ser.* **2016**, *85*, 125–134. [CrossRef] [PubMed]
29. Ventura, A.K. Associations between Breastfeeding and Maternal Responsiveness: A Systematic Review of the Literature. *Adv. Nutr.* **2017**, *8*, 495–510. [CrossRef] [PubMed]
30. DiSantis, K.I.; Hodges, E.A.; Johnson, S.L.; Fisher, J.O. The role of responsive feeding in overweight during infancy and toddlerhood: A systematic review. *Int. J. Obes. (Lond.)* **2011**, *35*, 480–492. [CrossRef] [PubMed]
31. Ong, K.K.; Loos, R.J. Rapid infancy weight gain and subsequent obesity: Systematic reviews and hopeful suggestions. *Acta Paediatr.* **2006**, *95*, 904–908. [CrossRef] [PubMed]
32. Monteiro, P.O.; Victora, C.G. Rapid growth in infancy and childhood and obesity in later life—A systematic review. *Obes. Rev.* **2005**, *6*, 143–154. [CrossRef] [PubMed]

33. Weng, S.F.; Redsell, S.A.; Swift, J.A.; Yang, M.; Glazebrook, C.P. Systematic review and meta-analyses of risk factors for childhood overweight identifiable during infancy. *Arch. Dis. Child.* **2012**, *97*, 1019–1026. [CrossRef] [PubMed]
34. Pearce, J.; Taylor, M.A.; Langley-Evans, S.C. Timing of the introduction of complementary feeding and risk of childhood obesity: A systematic review. *Int. J. Obes.* **2013**, *37*, 1295–1306. [CrossRef] [PubMed]
35. Thompson, A.L.; Bentley, M.E. The critical period of infant feeding for the development of early disparities in obesity. *Soc. Sci. Med.* **2013**, *97*, 288–296. [CrossRef] [PubMed]
36. Gross, R.S.; Mendelsohn, A.L.; Fierman, A.H.; Hauser, N.R.; Messito, M.J. Maternal infant feeding behaviors and disparities in early child obesity. *Child. Obes.* **2014**, *10*, 145–152. [CrossRef] [PubMed]
37. Koletzko, B.; von Kries, R.; Closa, R.; Escribano, J.; Scaglioni, S.; Giovannini, M.; Beyer, J.; Demmelmair, H.; Anton, B.; Gruszfeld, D.; et al. Can infant feeding choices modulate later obesity risk? *Am. J. Clin. Nutr.* **2009**, *89*, 1502S–1508S. [CrossRef] [PubMed]
38. American Academy of Pediatrics, Committee on Nutrition. Complementary feeding. In *Pediatric Nutrition*, 7th ed.; Kleinman, R.E., Greer, F., Eds.; American Academy of Pediatrics: Elk Grove Village, IL, USA, 2013.
39. Yang, Z.; Huffman, S.L. Nutrition in pregnancy and early childhood and associations with obesity in developing countries. *Matern. Child Nutr.* **2013**, *9*, 105–119. [CrossRef] [PubMed]
40. Hancox, R.J.; Stewart, A.W.; Braithwaite, I.; Beasley, R.; Murphy, R.; Mitchell, E.A. ISAAC Phase Three Study Group. Association between breastfeeding and body mass index at age 6–7 years in an international survey. *Pediatr. Obes.* **2015**, *10*, 283–287. [CrossRef] [PubMed]
41. van der Willik, E.M.; Vrijkotte, T.G.; Altenburg, T.M.; Gademan, M.G.; Kist-van Holthe, J. Exclusively breastfed overweight infants are at the same risk of childhood overweight as formula fed overweight infants. *Arch. Dis. Child.* **2015**, *100*, 932–937. [CrossRef] [PubMed]
42. Wang, J.; Wu, Y.; Xiong, G.; Chao, T.; Jin, Q.; Liu, R.; Hao, L.; Wei, S.; Yang, N.; Yang, X. Introduction of complementary feeding before 4 months of age increases the risk of childhood overweight or obesity: A meta-analysis of prospective cohort studies. *Nutr. Res.* **2016**, *36*, 759–770. [CrossRef] [PubMed]
43. Barrera, C.M.; Perrine, C.G.; Li, R.; Scanlon, K.S. Age at Introduction to Solid Foods and Child Obesity at 6 Years. *Child. Obes.* **2016**, *12*, 188–192. [CrossRef] [PubMed]
44. Tian, H.; Xie, H.; Song, G.; Zhang, H.; Hu, G. Prevalence of overweight and obesity among 2.6 million rural Chinese adults. *Prev. Med.* **2009**, *48*, 59–63. [CrossRef] [PubMed]
45. He, Y.; Pan, A.; Wang, Y.; Yang, Y.; Xu, J.; Zhang, Y.; Liu, D.; Wang, Q.; Shen, H.; Zhang, Y.; et al. Prevalence of overweight and obesity in 15.8 million men aged 15–49 years in rural China from 2010 to 2014. *Sci. Rep.* **2017**, *7*, 5012. [CrossRef] [PubMed]
46. Whittemore, R.; Knafl, K. The integrative review: Updated methodology. *J. Adv. Nurs.* **2005**, *52*, 546–553. [CrossRef] [PubMed]
47. Moher, D.; Liberati, A.; Tetzlaff, J.; Altman, D.; PRISMA Group. Preferred reporting items for systematic reviews and meta-analyses: The PRISMA statement. *PLoS Med.* **2009**, *6*, e1000097. [CrossRef] [PubMed]
48. Garrard, J. *Health Sciences Literature Review Made Easy: The Matrix Method*, 3rd ed.; Aspen Publishers: Gaithersburg, MD, USA, 2010.
49. Von Elm, E.; Altman, D.G.; Egger, M.; Pocock, S.J.; Gøtzsche, P.C.; Vandenbroucke, J.P. Strengthening the reporting of observational studies in epidemiology (STROBE) statement: Guidelines for reporting observational studies. *BMJ* **2007**, *335*, 806–808. [CrossRef] [PubMed]
50. Critical Appraisal Skills Programme (CASP). *Qualitative Research: Appraisal Tool Public Health Resource Unit*; Oxford University Press: Oxford, UK, 2006.
51. Diong, S.; Johnson, M.; Langdon, R. Breastfeeding and Chinese mothers living in Australia. *Breastfeed. Rev.* **2000**, *8*, 17–23. [PubMed]
52. Homer, C.S.; Sheehan, A.; Cooke, M. Initial infant feeding decisions and duration of breastfeeding in women from English, Arabic and Chinese speaking backgrounds in Australia. *Breastfeed. Rev.* **2002**, *10*, 27–32. [PubMed]
53. Li, L.; Zhang, M.; Binns, C.W. Chinese mothers' knowledge and attitudes about breastfeeding in Perth, Western Australia. *Breastfeed. Rev.* **2003**, *11*, 13–19. [PubMed]
54. Li, L.; Zhang, M.; Scott, J.A.; Binns, C.W. Factors associated with the initiation and duration of breastfeeding by Chinese mothers in Perth, Western Australia. *J. Hum. Lact.* **2004**, *20*, 188–195. [CrossRef] [PubMed]

55. Li, L.; Zhang, M.; Scott, J.A.; Binns, C.W. Infant feeding practices in home countries and Australia: Perth Chinese mothers survey. *Nutr. Diet.* **2005**, *62*, 82–88. [CrossRef]
56. Chen, W.L. Understanding the cultural context of Chinese mothers' perceptions of breastfeeding and infant health in Canada. *J. Clin. Nurs.* **2010**, *19*, 1021–1029. [CrossRef] [PubMed]
57. Zhou, Q.; Younger, K.M.; Kearney, J.M. An exploration of the knowledge and attitudes towards breastfeeding among a sample of Chinese mothers in Ireland. *BMC Public Health* **2010**, *10*. [CrossRef] [PubMed]
58. Chen, S.; Binns, C.W.; Zhao, Y.; Maycock, B.; Liu, Y. Breastfeeding by Chinese mothers in Australia and China: The healthy migrant effect. *J. Hum. Lact.* **2013**, *29*, 246–252. [CrossRef] [PubMed]
59. Chen, S.; Binns, C.W.; Liu, Y.; Maycock, B.; Zhao, Y.; Tang, L. Attitudes towards breastfeeding the Iowa Infant Feeding Attitude Scale in Chinese mothers living in China and Australia. *Asia Pac. J. Clin. Nutr.* **2013**, *22*, 266–269. [CrossRef] [PubMed]
60. Lee, A.; Brann, L. Influence of Cultural Beliefs on Infant Feeding, Postpartum and Childcare Practices among Chinese-American Mothers in New York City. *J. Community Health* **2015**, *40*, 476–483. [CrossRef] [PubMed]
61. Kuswara, K.; Laws, R.; Kremer, P.; Hesketh, K.D.; Campbell, K.J. The infant feeding practices of Chinese immigrant mothers in Australia: A qualitative exploration. *Appetite* **2016**, *105*, 375–384. [CrossRef] [PubMed]
62. Scott, J.A.; Aitkin, I.; Binns, C.W.; Aroni, R.A. Factors associated with the duration of breastfeeding amongst women in Perth, Australia. *Acta Paediatr. Scand.* **1999**, *88*, 416–421. [CrossRef]
63. De la Mora, A. The Iowa Infant Feeding Attitude Scale: Analysis of Reliability and Validity. *J. Appl. Soc. Psychol.* **1999**, *29*, 2362–2380. [CrossRef]
64. Wildman, R.P.; Gu, D.; Muntner, P.; Wu, X.; Reynolds, K.; Duan, X.; Chen, C.S.; Huang, G.; Bazzano, L.A.; He, J. Trends in overweight and obesity in Chinese adults: Between 1991 and 1999–2000. *Obesity (Silver Spring)* **2008**, *16*, 1448–1453. [CrossRef] [PubMed]
65. He, Y.; Pan, A.; Yang, Y.; Wang, Y.; Xu, J.; Zhang, Y.; Liu, D.; Wang, Q.; Shen, H.; Zhang, Y.; et al. Prevalence of Underweight, Overweight, and Obesity Among Reproductive-Age Women and Adolescent Girls in Rural China. *Am. J. Public Health* **2016**, *106*, 2103–2110. [CrossRef] [PubMed]
66. Reynolds, K.; Gu, D.; Whelton, P.K.; Wu, X.; Duan, X.; Mo, J.; He, J. Inter ASIA Collaborative Group. Prevalence and risk factors of overweight and obesity in China. *Obesity (Silver Spring)* **2007**, *15*, 10–18. [CrossRef] [PubMed]
67. Bolton, K.A.; Kremer, P.; Hesketh, K.D.; Laws, R.; Campbell, K.J. The Chinese-born immigrant infant feeding and growth hypothesis. *BMC Public Health* **2016**, *16*, 1071. [CrossRef] [PubMed]
68. Chomitz, V.R.; Brown, A.; Lee, V.; Must, A.; Chui, K.K.H. Healthy Living Behaviors among Chinese-American Preschool-Aged Children: Results of a Parent Survey. *J. Immigr. Minor. Health.* **2017**. [CrossRef] [PubMed]
69. Pai, H.L.; Contento, I. Parental perceptions, feeding practices, feeding styles, and level of acculturation of Chinese Americans in relation to their school-age child's weight status. *Appetite* **2014**, *80*, 174–182. [CrossRef] [PubMed]
70. Zhou, N.; Cheah, C.S.; Van Hook, J.; Thompson, D.A.; Jones, S.S. A cultural understanding of Chinese immigrant mothers' feeding practices. A qualitative study. *Appetite* **2015**, 160–167. [CrossRef] [PubMed]
71. Liu, W.H.; Mallan, K.M.; Mihrshahi, S.; Daniels, L.A. Feeding beliefs and practices of Chinese immigrant mothers. Validation of a modified version of the child feeding questionnaire. *Appetite* **2014**, *80*, 55–60. [CrossRef] [PubMed]
72. Chang, L.Y.; Mendelsohn, A.L.; Fierman, A.H.; Au, L.Y.; Messito, M.J. Perception of Child Weight and Feeding Styles in Parents of Chinese-American Preschoolers. *J. Immigr. Minor. Health* **2017**, *19*, 302–308. [CrossRef] [PubMed]
73. Jain, A.; Mitchell, S.; Chirumamilla, R.; Zhang, J.; Horn, I.B.; Lewin, A.; Huang, Z.J. Prevalence of obesity among young Asian-American children. *Child. Obes.* **2012**, *8*, 518–525. [CrossRef] [PubMed]
74. Caprio, S.; Daniels, S.R.; Drewnowski, A.; Kaufman, F.R.; Palinkas, L.A.; Rosenbloom, A.L.; Schwimmer, J.B. Influence of race, ethnicity, and culture on childhood obesity: Implications for prevention and treatment. *Obesity* **2008**, *16*, 2566–2577. [CrossRef] [PubMed]
75. Antecol, H.; Bedard, K. Unhealthy assimilation: Why do immigrants converge to American health status levels? *Demography* **2006**, *43*, 337–360. [CrossRef] [PubMed]
76. Diep, C.S.; Baranowski, T.; Kimbro, R.T. Acculturation and weight change in Asian-American children: Evidence from the ECLS-K: 2011. *Prev. Med.* **2017**, *99*, 286–292. [CrossRef] [PubMed]

77. Yeh, M.C.; Parikh, N.S.; Megliola, A.E.; Kelvin, E.A. Immigration status, visa types, and body weight among new immigrants in the United States. *Am. J. Health Promot.* **2016**. [CrossRef] [PubMed]
78. Baquero, B.; Molina, M.; Elder, J.; Norman, G.; Ayala, G. Neighborhoods, social and cultural correlates of obesity risk among Latinos living on the U.S.-Mexico border in Southern California. *J. Health Care Poor Underserved* **2016**, *27*, 700–721. [CrossRef] [PubMed]
79. Melius, J.; Cannonier, C. Exploring, U.S. Hispanic parents' length of time in the United States: Influences on obesity outcomes among U.S. Hispanic children. *Soc. Work Health Care* **2016**, *55*, 826–842. [CrossRef] [PubMed]
80. Power, T.G.; O'Connor, T.M.; Orlet Fisher, J.; Hughes, S.O. Obesity Risk in Children: The Role of Acculturation in the Feeding Practices and Styles of Low-Income Hispanic Families. *Child. Obes.* **2015**, *11*, 715–721. [CrossRef] [PubMed]
81. Delavari, M.; Sonderlund, A.L.; Swinburn, B.; Mellor, D.; Renzaho, A. Acculturation and obesity among migrant populations in high income countries—A systematic review. *BMC Public Health* **2013**, *13*, 458. [CrossRef] [PubMed]
82. Goodell, L.S.; Wakefield, D.B.; Ferris, A.M. Rapid weight gain during the first year of life predicts obesity in 2–3 year olds from a low income, minority population. *J. Community Health* **2009**, *34*, 370–375. [CrossRef] [PubMed]
83. Wood, C.T.; Skinner, A.C.; Yin, H.S.; Rothman, R.L.; Sanders, L.M.; Delamater, A.M.; Perrin, E.M. Bottle Size and Weight Gain in Formula-Fed Infants. *Pediatrics* **2016**, *138*. [CrossRef] [PubMed]
84. Rios-Ellis, B.; Nguyen-Rodriguez, S.T.; Espinoza, L.; Galvez, G.; Garcia-Vega, M. Engaging Community with Promotores de Salud to Support Infant Nutrition and Breastfeeding among Latinas Residing in Los Angeles County: Salud con Hyland's. *Health Care Women Int.* **2015**, *36*, 711–729. [CrossRef] [PubMed]
85. Bartick, M.C.; Jegier, B.J.; Green, B.D.; Schwarz, E.B.; Reinhold, A.G.; Stuebe, A.M. Disparities in Breastfeeding: Impact on Maternal and Child Health Outcomes and Costs. *J. Pediatr.* **2017**, *181*, 49–55. [CrossRef] [PubMed]
86. Evans, K.; Labbok, M.; Abrahams, S.W. WIC and breastfeeding support services: Does the mix of services offered vary with race and ethnicity? *Breastfeed. Med.* **2011**, *6*, 401–406. [CrossRef] [PubMed]
87. Mihrshahi, S.; Battistutta, D.; Magarey, A.; Daniels, L.A. Determinants of rapid weight gain during infancy: Baseline results from the NOURISH randomised controlled trial. *BMC Pediatr.* **2011**, *11*, 99. [CrossRef] [PubMed]
88. Xu, F.; Binns, C.; Yu, P.; Bai, Y. Determinants of breastfeeding initiation in Xinjiang, PR China, 2003–2004. *Acta Paediatr.* **2007**, *96*, 257–260. [CrossRef] [PubMed]
89. Raven, J.H.; Chen, Q.; Tolhurst, R.J.; Garner, P. Traditional beliefs and practices in the postpartum period in Fujian Province, China: A qualitative study. *BMC Pregnancy Childbirth* **2007**, *7*. [CrossRef] [PubMed]
90. Qui, L.; Zhao, Y.; Binns, C.W.; Lee, A.H.; Xie, X. Initiation of breastfeeding and prevalence of exclusive breastfeeding at hospital discharge in urban, suburban and rural areas of Zhejiang China. *Int. Breastfeed. J.* **2009**, *4*. [CrossRef]
91. Donaldson, H.; Kratzer, J.; Okutoro-Ketter, S.; Tung, P. Breastfeeding among Chinese immigrants in the United States. *J. Midwifery Women Health* **2010**, *55*, 277–281. [CrossRef] [PubMed]
92. Kim, J.H.; Fiese, B.H.; Donovan, S.M. Breastfeeding is natural but not the cultural norm: A mixed-methods study of first-time breastfeeding, African-American mothers participating in WIC. *J. Nutr. Educ. Behav.* **2017**, *49*, S151–S161. [CrossRef]
93. Kong, S.K.; Lee, D.T. Factors influencing decision to breastfeed. *J. Adv. Nurs.* **2004**, *46*, 369–379. [CrossRef] [PubMed]
94. Lindsay, A.C.; Wallington, S.F.; Greaney, M.L.; Hasselman, M.H.; Tavares Machado, M.M.; Mezzavilla, R.S. Brazilian Immigrant Mothers' Beliefs and Practices Related to Infant Feeding: A Qualitative Study. *J. Hum. Lact.* **2017**, *33*, 595–605. [CrossRef] [PubMed]
95. Lindsay, A.C.; Sussner, K.M.; Greaney, M.L.; Peterson, K.E. Latina mothers' beliefs and practices related to weight status, feeding, and the development of child overweight. *Public Health Nurs.* **2011**, *28*, 107–118. [CrossRef] [PubMed]
96. Melgar-Quiñonez, H.R.; Kaiser, L.L. Relationship of child-feeding practices to overweight in low-income Mexican– American preschool-aged children. *J. Am. Diet. Assoc.* **2004**, *104*, 1110–1119. [CrossRef] [PubMed]

97. Xu, F.; Qui, L.; Binns, C.W.; Liu, X. Breastfeeding in China: A review. *Int. Breastfeed. J.* **2009**, *4*. [CrossRef] [PubMed]
98. Zhao, J.; Zhao, Y.; Du, M.; Binns, C.W.; Lee, A.H. Maternal education and breastfeeding practices in China: A systematic review and meta-analysis. *Midwifery* **2017**, *50*, 62–71. [CrossRef] [PubMed]
99. Li, B.; Adab, P.; Cheng, K.K. The role of grandparents in childhood obesity in China—Evidence from a mixed methods study. *Int. J. Behav. Nutr. Phys. Act.* **2015**, *12*. [CrossRef] [PubMed]
100. Dahlen, H.G.; Homer, C.S. Infant feeding in the first 12 weeks following birth: A comparison of patterns seen in Asian and non-Asian women in Australia. *Women Birth.* **2010**, *23*, 22–28. [CrossRef] [PubMed]
101. Zalewski, B.M.; Patro, B.; Veldhorst, M.; Kouwenhoven, S.; Crespo Escobar, P.; Calvo Lerma, J.; Koletzko, B.; van Goudoever, J.B.; Szajewska, H. Nutrition of infants and young children (one to three years) and its effect on later health: A systematic review of current recommendations (EarlyNutrition project). *Crit. Rev. Food Sci. Nutr.* **2017**, *57*, 489–500. [CrossRef] [PubMed]
102. Harrison, M.; Brodribb, W.; Hepworth, J. A qualitative systematic review of maternal infant feeding practices in transitioning from milk feeds to family foods. *Matern. Child Nutr.* **2017**. [CrossRef] [PubMed]
103. Nader, P.R.; Huang, T.T.; Gahagan, S.; Kumanyika, S.; Hammond, R.A.; Christoffel, K.K. Next steps in obesity prevention: Altering early life systems to support healthy parents, infants, and toddlers. *Child. Obes.* **2012**, *8*, 195–204. [CrossRef] [PubMed]

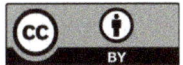

© 2017 by the authors. Licensee MDPI, Basel, Switzerland. This article is an open access article distributed under the terms and conditions of the Creative Commons Attribution (CC BY) license (http://creativecommons.org/licenses/by/4.0/).

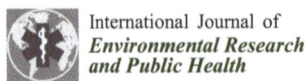

Commentary

Trauma and Pain in Family-Orientated Societies

Jan Ilhan Kizilhan [1,2,3]

1. Mental Health and Addiction, Co-operative State University Baden-Württemberg, Schramberger Str. 26, 78054 Villingen-Schwenningen, Germany; kizilhan@dhbw-vs.de
2. Institute for Psychotherapy and Psychotraumatology, University of Duhok, 42001 Duhok, Irak
3. Department of Transcultural Psychosomatic, MediClin-Klinik am Vogelsang Donaueschingen, 78166 Donaueschingen, Germany

Received: 4 December 2017; Accepted: 26 December 2017; Published: 28 December 2017

Abstract: People from family-oriented societies in particular, in addition to having a post-traumatic stress disorder (PTSD) suffer from chronic pain and physical complaints. Such people have a different understanding of physical illness and pain and, compared to patients from western societies, have different ideas on healing, even when confronted with the therapist. Hitherto, these factors have not been sufficiently taken into account in modern, multi-module therapy approaches. Trauma can be perceived via pain and physical complaints, whereby the pain is not restricted to one part of the body but is seen as covering the body as a whole. Therefore, in the treatment and above all in the patient-therapist relationship, it is necessary to understand what importance is attached to the perceived pain in relation to the trauma. The afflicted body expresses the trauma in the shape of its further-reaching consequences such as the patient's social, collective, economic and cultural sensitivity. Therefore, for the effective treatment of trauma and chronic pain, it is necessary to use a multi-modal, interdisciplinary, and culture-sensitive approach when treating patients from traditional cultural backgrounds.

Keywords: post-traumatic stress disorder (PTSD); pain; pain perception; understanding of illness; culture; family-oriented societies

1. Introduction

As a result of the increasing numbers of people from other cultures who flee and migrate for political, religious or economic reasons or because of war—in recent years, mainly refugees from Asia and Africa—doctors and therapists are reporting that traumatized refugees from family-oriented societies—such as Syria, Iraq, or Afghanistan—in addition to mental complaints caused by traumatization, complain of pain more than patients from the western world [1,2]. They believe that psychotherapy is not very suitable on its own and think that medication or even an operation would be the better course of treatment [3]. In addition to flashbacks, intrusions, fears, etc. total body pain is at the forefront and this indicates a different perception and processing of traumatic experiences [4].

Unlike the western society, which puts impetus on 'individualism', the traditional family oriented society is 'collectivistic' in that it promotes interdependence and co-operation, with the family forming the focal point of this social structure. The traditional family oriented society families like in Syria, Iraq, Afghanistan and some part of south European countries are therefore far more involved in caring of its members, and also suffer greater illness burden than their western counterparts.

In family-oriented societies the mention of psychotherapy can give rise to the feeling that they are in some way 'mad' and that they are ostracized and that medication or 'resting the body' can reduce the pain. A further reason for rejecting psychotherapy is the collective thinking in which the family plays a superordinate role. For this reason, personal feelings and inner mental symptoms are often not expressed; to adapt to the social environment is considered a sign of personal maturity [5].

The human body is 'allowed' one illness however, which is why both physical and mental complaints are expressed via the body. On examination, therefore, it is initially relatively difficult to establish whether the patient is suffering from a physical or a mental illness or both.

The literature describes the treatment and relationship structure of patients with PTSD and a pain disorder from family-oriented societies as difficult [1,4,6] and therefore this article will offer an overview of the understanding of trauma and pain perception and the cultural differences surrounding trauma and pain disorders and will outline some possible new treatment strategies.

2. Culture, Trauma, and Pain

The diagnostics of mental disorders and the consequences of PTSD orient towards the criteria of ICD-10 and DSM-V. This assumes that all people display comparable stress and reactions following a traumatic experience. This is, however, not substantiated by clinical experience and the findings of transcultural psychiatry [7].

The link between PTSD and chronic pain has been proven in numerous studies. In a study with general psychiatric outpatients Villano and colleagues [8] found that 46% of those examined fulfilled the criteria of a PTSD, 40% reported chronic pain, and 24% of the patients were diagnosed with both. The results of an examination of war veterans showed a comorbidity rate for PTSD and chronic pain of 66% [9]. Other studies with war veterans showed that, in parts, well over 80% of those examined fulfilled the criteria for both disorders [10]. The data of a very comprehensive Canadian random test with 36,984 test persons (Canadian Community Health Survey Cycle) show a considerable discrepancy with regard to chronic pain between people with and without a diagnosed PTSD: of the PTSD patients, 46% suffered from chronic back pain (compared to 20.6% of those examined who did not have PTSD), and 33% suffered from migraine (compared to 10%) [11].

According to Otis and colleagues [9] the prevalence of pain among PTSD patients is 34–80% significantly higher than the other way round, where the PTSD prevalence among pain patients is 10–50%. This imbalance can be explained in part by the fact that traumatic experiences are often linked to physical pain and that these represent a kind of post-traumatic disorder [4].

A study by Norman and colleagues [12] with patients at a trauma centre at the University of California showed that pain immediately after the traumatic incident was a risk factor for developing PTSD. According to the authors, the link may be the result of a more negative assessment of the trauma recollection as a result of the pain and increased stress associated with the trauma. In comparison to German women who had been victims of sexualized violence, female victims of sexualized violence from Turkey complained more about physical pain and somatic ailments than the German women and in some cases developed a cleansing compulsion [13].

The literature indicates a high degree of co-occurrence between pain and PTSD, regardless of whether the pain is being assessed in patients with PTSD or PTSD is being assessed in patients with chronic pain. Also, they may interact in such a way as to negatively affect the course and outcome of treatment of either disorder [9]. The high comorbidity between these disorders has been postulated as being due to either shared vulnerability or mutual maintenance [14,15].

Every culture has developed its own management strategies appropriate to their own values and norms to cope with physical ailments in connection with pain. The Irish, for example, shrank rather from any contact with others because they thought it was indelicate to show pain [16]. North Americans went the doctor's as early as possible and described their symptoms without showing any emotion so that the doctor could immediately initiate a rational treatment [16]. Southern Europeans expressed their pain loudly and clearly so that those around them could sympathize. Filipinos acquiesced to their fate in a fatalistic manner [16].

Psychological problems following trauma manifest themselves, amongst other things, in the form of physical disorders appropriate to the person's cultural imprint [17]. Nigerians, when they report fear and depression, talk of "a sensation of heat" in their head, "writhing maggots", as well as a "biting sensation" in their whole body [18]. In psychiatric clinics in China they report "weak nerves" along with fatigue, headache, vertigo, and gastrointestinal disorders [17,19]. Many people from South America and the Mediterranean react to psychological burdens with headaches and muscle pain, heat sensations and pins and needles in the feet, heart problems, and stomach complaints [18]. In some parts of India and the Middle East, rheumatic and rheumatoid pains are described as "wind" pains. Also reported are "wandering" pains which manifest themselves in a different part of the body each day [16].

Patients from family-orientated societies, predominantly from rural Turkey, Iraq, or Syria, report pain disorders significantly more often than western patients and this explains the high number of pain diagnoses [6]. Those affected speak of all complaints as if they were physical, i.e., the sufferers seem to be stuck in an archaic idea of illness. Subjective suffering can be expressed symbolically with fatigue, crying, walking with aids, etc. The patients present themselves as broken and weak people. As a rule, they remain consistent to this regressive and appellative stance so that they remain inactive even in their home environment.

This severe fixation with total-body pains, the cause of which is often difficult to elicit, frequently leads to problems of diagnosis and treatment [16].

3. Diagnostics

Fundamentally, the concepts of PTSD and cognitive behavioral therapy are applicable to all ethnic groups. However, the varying perceptions of health and disease and the cultural, traditional, medical treatment for dealing with traumatic experiences require alternative concepts or additions.

The culture-specific aspects of patients from traditional cultures are their knowledge of the anatomy and physiology of their own body and their concept of pain (seen as magic, a curse, punishment, etc.). The experiencing of pain is not limited to one part of the body but is seen holistically i.e., over the body as a whole. Therefore, even when initially documenting the pain—i.e., localization, quality, time pattern, and cause—the patients give other details than those to be expected from northern European patients [4]. For example, ethnic Turkish patients, in contrast to German ones, see fate or extreme environmental factors as responsible for their illness. In addition to their war traumatization, some refugees are so bitter that they try to escape the injustice they feel as a kind of regression through physical pain [4,20]. The way in which people report their pain or in some cases do not speak about it has an important influence on how the therapist takes down their case history and consequently correctly diagnoses the complaints.

Understanding illness is especially important, both for the diagnosis and for the treatment. The comparative study on ethnic Turkish and German patients in a psychosomatic clinic revealed that significantly fewer ethnic Turkish patients were able to describe their illness [7]. It is necessary to analyze the circumstances of the onset or aggravation of the pain and to consider the individual and collective biography in doing so (e.g., ostracism because of the ethnic and/or religious denomination in their country of birth, migration, culture and generation conflicts, etc.) in order to elucidate the indications for the triggering factors. The aim is to find out what diminishes or intensifies the pain and what restrictions arise as a result [20].

However, this pain patient must feel that his complaints and ailments are being taken seriously; otherwise he will stop the therapy [8]. In general, patients from traditional societies do not present their problems very chronologically so that what they say, viewed initially superficially, does not seem to relate clearly to their complaint.

The aim of psychological pain therapy is to reduce the patient's impairment since this normally leads to a reduction in the subjective pain intensity. Since patients from traditional societies have a pain model reduced to somatic variables and a specific understanding of anatomy, the treatment setting has to be somewhat modified for them. Their causal and control attributions are determined in part, for example, by simple biomedical assumptions originating in the Arabic—Greek medicine of the "Four Humours Theory" and magical connotations [20]. The way in which patients from family-oriented societies present their complaints together with their different ideas of anatomy and its functions with respect to mental illnesses are to be considered when diagnosing. Consequently, a suitable treatment and explanation model must be developed with the patient, which is appropriate to their level of education and cultural perceptions [16].

4. Treatment

On the whole, in the case of a large number of patients from family-oriented societies the activity spectrum appears to be significantly limited. As a result, their life revolves around the pain; it becomes the focus of their thinking and behavior [16,19]. Their assumption that the body has to rest when it experiences pain leads to a passive relieving posture. It therefore presents a great challenge if we wish to increase the room for manoeuvre necessary to counteract the patient's restrictions: behavioral (little movement), emotional (reduction of depression and helplessness) and cognitive (limitation to pain). Breaking down avoidance behavior is therefore a high priority when carrying out the therapy.

Owing to the various ways pain is presented, the passive relieving posture, language problems, and possible ethnic-cultural behavioral differences, it is important to form a relationship based on trust with the patient. With patients from family-oriented societies the physician (the clinical psychologist too, is regarded as a physician/"doctor") is traditionally seen as a father-like family friend [20]. He represents a figure of authority who cultivates an active, knowing, and advisory role with the patient and his family. He must accept this cultural role if he does not wish to considerably unsettle the patient.

Whereas with a German patient the main focus is on mobilising the individual's potential, the patients mentioned above expect more help from the person in authority and this must be offered [21]. This means, however, that the therapist must develop an awareness of his own cultural attachment and should be able, from this position, via his (counter-) transpositions (individual and social prejudices and stereotypes) to "de-actualize" his attitudes and avoid presenting them to the patient before they affect the therapy in a destructive way. Only then will the patient be willing to alter his behavior at a mental and physical level [19].

The traditional exposition therapy is not always effective with victims of political oppression and with people suffering from complex and cumulative traumatization [20,21]. It can even be counter-productive and reduce compliance, increase pain perception and also the drop-out rate. There are reports that not all, but some, patients find it more helpful, as a first step, to concentrate on the pain and its treatment rather than dealing directly with the traumatizing incidents. It is also necessary to discuss whether repression and avoidance, in other words keeping up the pain, would not present a better coping strategy [7]. In some cultures, living with pain and suppressing the trauma is regarded as a successful coping mechanism. This is particularly prevalent in collective societies in which social harmony is the highest priority [22]. Here, in particular, the healing process is determined by the cultural and social context, and care is taken to make sure that the victim does not 'lose face'. This applies especially to politically-motivated violence [23]. A conversation with these patients on the topic of stress is normally avoided.

Case Casuistry

Yasemin is a Yazidi and her family were persecuted and taken hostage by the "Islamic State" (ISIL). She was repeatedly raped and sold before she was able to escape from the hands of her tormentors. She reports how the IS fighters took her prisoner; she talks of violence, rape, escape, and unimaginable suffering. She says she was sold 12 times to IS fighters in Iraq and Syria, and beaten and raped again and again.

Finally, after eight months of captivity, she managed to flee from Syria. She says more than 20 members of her family were murdered by the ISIL. She had to watch her husband being executed. She is nervous, desperate and shows me a bag full of pain killers and sleeping pills because she has pain all over her body and cannot sleep. "If only I didn't have this pain, I would be much better. The doctors say my body is all right. The pains are due to my mental state. I don't understand that.

I am in pain, I can feel it all over my body." As regards the pain, she has the feeling that her body is besmirched. She feels she has to shower several times every day and yet she still has the feeling that her body is unclean.

Just how far psychotherapeutic trauma work is possible seems also to depend on how a society deals with the topic of sexualized violence. In this context, patients often report of a considerable feeling of insecurity, not to say viewing the topic as an absolute taboo. High moral ideas and restrictions, especially in women, lead to considerable worry and fear since they are particularly at risk of being ostracized by the collective. In this respect, feelings of shame play a special part. This is due to the fact that, in a so-called shame culture, the actual event and the violation of a norm are of less importance than the desire to keep one's face. For example, the collective may regard the rape of a young woman as shameful and the victim ostracized. The fact that the perpetrator is also seen as violating a norm is of secondary importance in the collective.

From the psychodynamic perspective, discussing traumatic incidents via *statements of pain* [24] offers people with severe traumatic experiences the possibility of transferring the ostracism, social affront, feelings of guilt and inferiority away from their conscious experience and on to a physical level. In this way they maintain their self-esteem and at the same time hope that the doctor and medicine can help them [7,11].

In addition to feelings of mental and physical tension, the perception of pain is also influenced by increased inactivity and avoidance behavior. As a result, the fear of possible consequences, so-called "catastrophe thinking" and "fear avoidance beliefs" the cycle of pain results in an increase of inactivity, avoidance behavior and depression.

The crucial link between the PTSD and the pain chain is avoidance/inactivity and the associated depression. These factors have a crucial influence on the development and maintenance of both the PTSD and chronic pain [25,26].

Following the diagnostics, a further treatment model is psycho-education as a necessary integral part of the therapy. Psycho-education is designed to reinforce the patient's own self-efficacy beliefs. This can be in the form of media such as self-help brochures and videos in the patient's mother tongue. One essential target of this education is to demonstrate to the patient that physical and mental processes are intertwined. In doing so, the culture-specific aspects and the patient's level of education should be taken into account [27].

5. Conclusions

A culture-sensitive approach to the treatment of traumatized individuals with chronic pain and physical ailments from family-oriented societies is indicated when the patient is severely restricted and needs medical help; when psychological factors influence his perception of pain and this impairment can be verified in the diagnosis; when conventional treatment does not work sufficiently well on the patient due to his different understanding of illness and how to cope with trauma and pain.

An individual and culture-sensitive treatment which takes the relationship structure between the patients and therapist into consideration is especially important, whereby traumatologists and doctors co-operate with other professional groups (sport therapists, physiotherapists, creative therapists, etc.) and look at the patient's state of the art cultural imprint [3,17].

If language, cultural, and migration-specific aspects are included in the consultation, treatment and social support of patients from family-oriented societies with PTSD and chronic pain, it is possible to fundamentally improve their care and integration [28]. Therefore, on the part of both the therapist and the health institutes, specific transcultural knowledge and the consideration of the social and political structures of the health institutes are necessary to be able to treat these patients early enough and adequately and in this way, for instance, to prevent a chronification of the illness [24]. In addition to multicultural teams of therapists, it is above all necessary to make all staff aware of the need to take a transcultural, culturally-sensitive perspective [29,30].

Treating patients with PTSD and chronic pain from family-oriented societies is not about learning a new form of psychotherapy. It is about registering and learning skills of the culture-sensitive use of psychotherapeutic treatment in general and especially in behavioral trauma therapy and chronic pain methods [24]. Individual therapy is also about concentrating on people from different cultures, with a different concept of illness and how to deal with it [1,2,31]. This requires being willing to reflect and possessing a critical attitude to one's own work whilst at the same time remaining impartial and open to the patients' concerns. Transcultural competence is needed and means that it is necessary to reflect on one's own culture in order to understand other cultures [17,31].

When dealing with patients from family-oriented societies with PTSD and chronic pain it is necessary to consider cultural, historical (trauma) and socio-political aspects, the perception of illness and dealing with it and the way in which a relationship can be formed with the patient [21,25]. In addition, alternative therapy approaches are important, involving an interdisciplinary and culturally-sensitive focus in the psychiatrists and psychotherapists, as is close co-operation with other professional groups and the patient's state-of-the-art cultural imprint.

Conflicts of Interest: The authors declare no conflict of interest.

References

1. Hassan, G.; Ventvoegel, P.; Jeffee-Bahloul, H. Mental health and psychosocial wellbeing of Syrians affected by armed conflict. *Epidemiol. Psychiatr. Sci.* **2016**, *25*, 129–141. [CrossRef] [PubMed]
2. Hinton, D.; Kirmayer, L.J. The flexibility hypothesis of healing. *Cult. Med. Psychiatry* **2016**. [CrossRef] [PubMed]
3. Kizilhan, J.I. Zum psychotherapeutischen arbeiten mit migrantinnen und migranten in psychosomatisch-psychiatrischen kliniken. *Psychotherapeutenjournal* **2011**, *10*, 21–27. (In German)
4. Kizilhan, J.I. *Kultursensible Psychotherapie*; VWB-Verlag für Wissenschaft und Bildung: Berlin, Germany, 2012. (In German)
5. Heine, P.; Assion, H.J. Traditionelle Medizin in islamischen Kulturen. In *Migration und Seelische Gesundheit*; Assion, J., Ed.; Springer: Berlin, Germany, 2005; pp. 29–42. (In German)
6. Schiltenwolf, M.; Pogatzki-Zahn, E.M. Schmerzmedizin aus einer interkulturellen und geschlechterspezifischen Perspektive. *Schmerz* **2005**, *29*, 569–575. (In German) [CrossRef] [PubMed]
7. Schouler-Ocak, M. *Trauma and Migration: Cultural Factors in the Diagnosis and Treatment of Traumatised Immigrants*; Springer: Berlin, Germany, 2015.
8. Villano, C.L.; Rosenblum, A.; Magura, S. Prevalence and correlates of posttraumatic stress disorder and chronic severe pain in psychiatric outpatients. *J. Rehabil. Res. Dev.* **2007**, *44*, 167–177. [CrossRef] [PubMed]
9. Otis, J.D.; Keane, T.M.; Kerns, R.D. An examination of the relationship between chronic pain and posttraumatic stress disorder. *J. Rehabil. Res. Dev.* **2003**, *40*, 397–406. [CrossRef] [PubMed]
10. Shipherd, J.C.; Keyes, M.; Jovanovic, T.; Ready, D.J.; Baltzell, D.; Worley, V.; Gordon-Brown, V.; Hayslett, C.; Duncan, E. Veterans seeking treatment for posttraumatic stress disorder: What about comorbid chronic pain? *J. Rehabil. Res. Dev.* **2007**, *44*, 153–165. [CrossRef] [PubMed]
11. Broeckman, B.F.P.; Olff, M.; Boer, F. The genetic background to PTSD—Review. *Neurosci. Biobehav. Rev.* **2007**, *31*, 348–362. [CrossRef] [PubMed]
12. Dunmore, E.; Clark, D.M.; Ehlers, A. A prospective investigation of the role of cognitive factors in persistent posttraumatic stress disorder (PTSD) after physical or sexual assault. *Behav. Res. Ther.* **2001**, *39*, 1063–1084. [CrossRef]
13. Ehlers, A.; Clark, D.M. A cognitive model of persistent posttraumatic stress disorder. *Behav. Res. Ther.* **2000**, *38*, 319–345. [CrossRef]
14. Kizilhan, J.I. Interaktion von trauma und reinigungszwang und religion bei patientinnen mit einer PTSD. Eine vergleichende studie. *Verhaltensmed. Verhaltensther.* **2010**, *31*, 307–322. (In German)
15. Asmundson, G.J.G.; Coons, M.J.; Taylor, S.; Katz, J. PTSD and the experience of pain: Research and clinical implications of shared vulnerability and mutual maintenance models. *Can. J. Psychiatry* **2002**, *47*, 930–937. [CrossRef] [PubMed]

16. Sharp, T.J.; Harvey, A.G. Chronic pain and posttraumatic stress disorder: Mutual maintenance? *Clin. Psychol. Rev.* **2001**, *21*, 857–877. [CrossRef]
17. Kizilhan, J.I. Patient form middle east and the impact of culture on psychological pain-treatment. *Fibrom Open Access* **2017**. Available online: https://www.omicsonline.org/open-access/patient-form-middle-east-and-the-impact-of-culture-on-psychological-paintreatment.pdf (accessed on 27 December 2017).
18. Edigbo, P. A cross sectional study of somatic complaints of Nigerian females using the Enugu Somatization Scale. *Cult. Med. Psychiatry* **1986**, *10*, 167–186.
19. Poundja, J.; Fikretoglu, D.; Brunet, A. The co-occurence of posttraumatic stress disorder symptoms and pain: Is depression a mediator? *J. Trauma. Stress* **2006**, *19*, 747–751. [CrossRef] [PubMed]
20. Gatchel, R.; Peng, Y.; Peters, M.; Fuchs, P.; Turk, D. The biopsychosocial approach to chronic pain: Scientific advances and future direction. *Psychol. Bull.* **2007**, *133*, 581–624. [CrossRef] [PubMed]
21. Kizilhan, J.I. Die deutung des schmerzes in anderen Kulturen. *Schmerz* **2016**, *30*, 346–351. (In German) [CrossRef] [PubMed]
22. Pagotto, L.F.; Mendlowicz, M.V.; Coutinho, E.S.; Figueira, I. The impact of posttraumatic symptoms and comorbid mental disorders on the health-related quality of life in treatment-seeking PTSD patients. *Compr. Psychiatry* **2015**, *58*, 68–73. [CrossRef] [PubMed]
23. Machleidt, W.; Gül, K. Kulturelle und transkulturelle Psychotherapie—Tiefenpsychologische Behandlung. In *Praxis der Interkulturellen Psychiatrie und Psychotherapie*; Machleidt, W., Heinz, A., Eds.; Elsevier: München, Germany, 2010; pp. 401–413. (In German)
24. Norman, S.B.; Stein, M.B.; Dimsdale, J.E.; Hoyt, D.B. Pain in the aftermath of trauma is a risk factor for posttraumatic stress disorder. *Psychol. Med.* **2007**. [CrossRef]
25. Kira, I.A. Etiologyand treatment of post-cumulative traumatic stress disorders in different cultures. *Traumatology* **2010**, *16*, 128–141. [CrossRef]
26. Kizilhan, J.; Utz, K.S.; Bengel, J. Transkulturelle Aspekte bei der Behandlung der Posttraumatischen Belastungsstörung. In *Traum(a) Migration—Aktuelle Konzepte zur Therapie traumatisierter Flüchtlinge und Folteropfer*; Feldmann, R.E., Jr., Siedler, G.H., Eds.; Psychosozial-Verlag: Gießen, Germany, 2013; pp. 261–279. (In German)
27. Miranda, R.; Meyerson, L.A.; Marx, B.P.; Tucker, P.M. Civilian-based posttraumatic stress disorder and physical complaints: Evaluation of depression as a mediator. *J. Trauma. Stress* **2002**, *15*, 297–301. [CrossRef] [PubMed]
28. Kirmayer, L.J.; Young, A. Culture and somatization: Clinical, epidemiological and ethnographic perspectives. *Psychosom. Med.* **1998**, *60*, 420–430. [CrossRef] [PubMed]
29. Buhmann, C.B. Traumatized refugees: Morbidity, treatment and predictors of outcome. *Dan. Med. J.* **2014**, *61*, 48–71.
30. Droidek, B. How do we salve our wounds? Intercultural perspectives an individual and collective strategies of making peace with own past. *Traumatology* **2010**, *16*, 5–16. [CrossRef]
31. Slobodin, O.; De Jong, T.J. Mental health interventions for traumatized asylum seekers and refugees: What do we know about their efficacy? *Int. J. Soc. Psychiatry* **2015**, *61*, 17–26. [CrossRef] [PubMed]

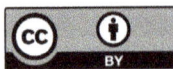

© 2017 by the author. Licensee MDPI, Basel, Switzerland. This article is an open access article distributed under the terms and conditions of the Creative Commons Attribution (CC BY) license (http://creativecommons.org/licenses/by/4.0/).

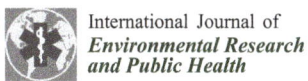

Article

Preparedness of Health Care Professionals for Delivering Sexual and Reproductive Health Care to Refugee and Migrant Women: A Mixed Methods Study

Zelalem B. Mengesha [1,*], Janette Perz [1], Tinashe Dune [1,2] and Jane Ussher [1]

1. Translational Health Research Institute (THRI), School of Medicine, Western Sydney University, Penrith, NSW 2751, Australia; J.perz@westernsydney.edu.au (J.P.); t.dune@westernsydney.edu.au (T.D.); J.ussher@westernsydney.edu.au (J.U.)
2. School of Science and Health, Western Sydney University, Penrith, NSW 2751, Australia
* Correspondence: Z.mengesha@westernsydney.edu.au; Tel.: +61-2-4620-3669

Received: 8 December 2017; Accepted: 16 January 2018; Published: 22 January 2018

Abstract: Past research suggests that factors related to health care professionals' (HCPs) knowledge, training and competency can contribute to the underutilisation of sexual and reproductive health (SRH) care by refugee and migrant women. The aim of this study was to examine the perceived preparedness of HCPs in relation to their knowledge, confidence and training needs when it comes to consulting refugee and migrant women seeking SRH care in Australia. A sequential mixed methods design, comprising an online survey with 79 HCPs (45.6% nurses, 30.3% general practitioners (GPs), 16.5% health promotion officers, and 7.6% allied health professionals) and semi-structured interviews with 21 HCPs, was utilised. HCPs recognised refugee and migrant women's SRH as a complex issue that requires unique skills for the delivery of optimal care. However, they reported a lack of training (59.4% of nurses, 50% of GPs, and 38.6% of health promotion officers) and knowledge (27.8% of nurses, 20.8% of GPs, and 30.8% of health promotion officers) in addressing refugee and migrant women's SRH. The majority of participants (88.9% of nurses, 75% of GPs, and 76% of health promotion officers) demonstrated willingness to engage with further training in refugee and migrant women's SRH. The implications of the findings are argued regarding the need to train HCPs in culturally sensitive care and include the SRH of refugee and migrant women in university and professional development curricula in meeting the needs of this growing and vulnerable group of women.

Keywords: refugee and migrant women; sexual and reproductive health; training; knowledge; confidence; health care professionals

1. Introduction

Health care professional (HCP) interactions with patients from refugee and migrant backgrounds are increasing, due to growing diversity in migration to countries such as Australia [1]. In addition to clinical training and knowledge, caring for refugee and migrant patients requires an understanding of factors in the broader socio-ecological environment that impact the level and type of care to be provided, such as migration circumstances, cultural backgrounds and language needs [2]. Previous research suggests that cross-cultural training increases HCPs' interest in seeing migrant patients [3]. Furthermore, HCPs who received cultural competency training were more likely to use professional interpreters to improve communication and understanding [4,5] and to make changes in their practices to accommodate migrant clients [5]. The HCP's cultural awareness also improves communication, understanding and treatment compliance in consultations with people from refugee and migrant backgrounds [6]. Despite having these benefits, there is a growing concern in migrant resettlement countries that HCP education is not responding to the changing demographics of the population, with many HCPs not satisfied with their knowledge and understanding in providing appropriate health care to patients from refugee and migrant backgrounds [2,7,8].

There are several issues particular to refugee and migrant women that have bearing on their interpersonal interactions with HCPs within a SRH context. For example, some refugee and migrant women have experienced rape and other forms of sexual abuse before and after resettlement in host countries [9,10]. Consequently, they may experience SRH and psycho-social problems [11], such as unsafe abortion, sexually transmitted diseases, including HIV, and trauma [12]. Furthermore, talking about sex and menstruation is taboo among many women from refugee and migrant backgrounds, which may present a challenge for HCPs who are trying to understand the women's needs during consultations [13,14]. Some refugee and migrant women also attend SRH consultations with their husbands which pose challenges for HCPs to provide care as male partners commonly dominate the consultation leaving women unable to disclose their SRH needs in the presence of their partners [15]. This suggests that HCPs require skills in broaching SRH and navigating patient relationships in ways that allow them to satisfy refugee and migrant women's SRH needs. Without this acuity, the level of care that HCPs are able to offer to these women is reduced [16].

A number of studies in Australia have examined the provision of cross-cultural training to HCPs who have day-to-day interactions with people from refugee and migrant backgrounds. For example, Watt and colleagues report that only 23.8% of General Practice (GP) registrars received cross-cultural training, despite more than half of their patients coming from a cultural background different from the provider [17]. In another study, GPs reported acquiring cross-cultural knowledge and competency mainly through exposure to patients, as opposed to formal training [18]. These studies did not examine the type of health care provision, or the range of migrant populations seen by GPs or other health care providers. A comprehensive socio-ecological analysis of HCP's perceptions and experiences regarding their multi-cultural training and competency is lacking.

Research into the provision of SRH care to refugee and migrant women in countries of resettlement is growing [19]. This research has concentrated on understanding the experiences of HCPs regarding language barriers and interpreter use [20], communication [21,22], expectations around language services, cultural competency and type of care [23], structural barriers to providing care [24], and the women's familiarity with services [22]. One of the remaining gaps in knowledge is the perceived preparedness of HCPs in relation to their training, knowledge and confidence when it comes to consulting refugee and migrant women seeking SRH care. The aim of this mixed-methods study was to address this gap, in order to: (1) assess the perceived knowledge and confidence of HCPs in their ability to work with refugee and migrant women seeking SRH care; and (2) examine HCP's training experiences and needs with respect to the provision of SRH care to refugee and migrant women in Australia.

Theoretical Approach

Health care provision requires the involvement and coordination of several micro systems in the broader health system [25]. As such, a systematic approach which considers influences beyond the individual level is relevant to have a broader understanding of factors that impact health care access and utilisation [25]. The socio-ecological model is most central to this process as it recognises multiple domains of influence in an individual's social environment that impact health care access and provision [26,27]. With this in mind, the socio-ecological model was selected as a framework to systematically analyse factors that influence HCP's preparedness for providing SRH care to refugee and migrant women in Australia at four levels: Individual, Interpersonal, Organisational, and Societal levels. The model is also appropriate for mixed methods research. The quantitative component in this study considers the individual level factors while the qualitative data further explores these factors across the four levels of the socio-ecological framework. The important conceptualisation is that, as the four levels of the socio-ecological model are interconnected, so too are quantitative and qualitative data collected to examine the HCP's preparedness to provide SRH care [28].

2. Methods

This sequential mixed methods study involved the collection, analysis and interpretation of quantitative and qualitative data to achieve the research objectives [29]. An online survey was conducted with a diverse group of HCPs to assess their knowledge, confidence, training needs and experience in relation to the provision of SRH care to refugee and migrant women. Semi-structured interviews were then conducted to explain and elaborate upon issues identified within the survey [30]. Ethical approval was obtained from the Human Research Ethics Committee at Western Sydney University (Approval Number H11034) and informed consent was obtained from all individual participants included in the study.

2.1. Participants

Seventy-nine HCPs participated in this research. HCPs were a convenient sample recruited through advertisements in nursing and public health professional association newsletters and email lists, family planning clinics, and snowball sampling. To advertise the study, a leaflet which contained information about the proposed study and the opportunity to participate in a survey and semi-structured interviews was used. Table 1 presents the socio-demographic and work experience profile of the HCPs who responded to the survey. The vast majority were women (96.2%) with a mean age of 47.1 years (+12.12). HCPs included nurses (45.6%), GPs (30.3%), health promotion officers (16.5%) and allied health professionals (7.6%). They had an average work experience of 11.2 years in the health sector ranging between 2 and 41 years. The majority (58.2%) reported seeing 1–5 women daily from refugee and migrant backgrounds in their practices. HCPs reported that SRH services that refugee and migrant women most commonly sought were: contraception (64.56%), gynaecological concerns (60.46%), pregnancy related (41.77%) and infertility (40.51%). These experiences were widely distributed across women from several countries which included Afghanistan (41.33%), Sudan (40%) and Iran (40%).

Table 1. Socio-demographic and work experience characteristics.

	Characteristic	Frequency (n)	Percentage (%)
Gender	Women	76	96.2
	Men	3	3.8
Occupation	Nurse/Midwife	36	45.6
	GP	24	30.3
	Health promotion officer *	13	16.5
	Allied health professionals **	6	7.6
Work experience in years	1–10	33	41.8
	11–20	25	31.6
	21 and above	21	26.6
Refugee and migrant women seen daily	0	27	34.1
	1–5	46	58.2
	>6	6	7.7
SRH services refugee and migrant women commonly accessed	Contraception	51	64.56
	Pregnancy related (Antenatal care, delivery and postnatal care)	33	41.77
	Abortion	29	36.71
	Sexually transmitted infections (Information, screening and treatment)	29	36.71
	Screening (Chlamydia and Cervical cytology)	36	45.57
	Infertility	32	40.51
	Safer sex options	17	21.52
	Sexual pain and discomfort	30	37.97
	Sexual violence and unwanted sex	17	21.52

Table 1. Cont.

Characteristic		Frequency (n)	Percentage (%)
Background of women seen	Afghanistan	31	41.33
	Iran	30	40
	Sudan	30	40
	Iraq	29	38.67
	Myanmar/Burma	19	25.33
	Somalia	18	24
	Bhutan	6	8
	Congo (DRC)	6	8
	Others ***	36	48

* Health promotion officer includes bilingual health educators and health educator managers. ** Allied health professionals include psychologists and sex therapists. *** Others include South East Asia, Zimbabwe, Turkey, Saudi Arabia, and Egypt.

2.2. Procedure

2.2.1. Survey

HCPs completed the survey online which consisted of 24 closed and open-ended items. The survey covered many issues which include: knowledge and confidence to provide SRH care to refugee and migrant women; past training experiences and current needs in relation to refugee and migrant women's SRH; and barriers to the SRH care of these women. In addition, demographic questions (i.e., gender, age, years of experience, first language, country of birth, country where they received their professional training and approximate number of refugee and migrant women seen in their practice) were also included.

2.2.2. Semi-Structured Interviews

After the HCPs completed the online survey they were asked to participate in a follow up interview about their experiences of providing SRH care to refugee and migrant women. Of the 79 survey participants, 32 responded positively to the invitation. Then, 21 were purposefully selected and interviewed. These participants included nurses (8), GP (5), health promotion officers (5), sexual therapists (2) and a midwife. The HCPs interviewed had an average work experience of 21 years across the public (5), private (2), public/private (4) and non-profit/NGO (10) sectors, with work experience ranging from 2 and 41 years. Individual semi-structured interviews were conducted by the first author via telephone and one face-to-face. Topics included the HCP's perceptions of refugee and migrant women as well as their knowledge, competencies, training needs, experiences, and preferences; their use of interpreters; perceived support needs of HCPs and refugee and migrant women to facilitate access to care. The interviews were audio-recorded and lasted an average of 50 min. All the interviews were professionally transcribed with subsequent integrity checking undertaken for accuracy. To enhance clarity and readability of the results, irrelevant sentences and words were deleted and replaced by sentence ellipses (" … "). For longer quotes, pseudonyms, profession and years of work experience are also given.

2.3. Operational Definitions

To better explore the perspectives of HCPs operationalising what is meant by various, and overlapping, terms is helpful. As such, in this paper the following definitions were used.

Preparedness: HCP's perceived ability to provide SRH care to refugee and migrant women where having appropriate knowledge, training and confidence is perceived as being "prepared".

Knowledge: the perceived facts, information, and skills acquired through experience or education that enable HCPs provide SRH care to refugee and migrant women [31].

Confidence: the perceived feeling or belief that one can provide SRH care to women from refugee and migrant backgrounds [32].

2.4. Analysis

Descriptive statistical analyses were employed to evaluate quantitative data such as demographic variables, training history, current needs and experiences and perceived confidence for providing SRH care to refugee and migrant women. Analyses were run using SPSS 24 Statistical Software (IBM Corporation, New York, NY, USA). Chi-square tests were conducted to test for differences between the professional groups in relation to their knowledge, confidence, training needs and experience.

Thematic analysis according to Braun and Clarke [33] was used to analyse semi-structured interviews and open-ended survey responses. This process started with the first author reading and re-reading the interview transcripts resulting in the identification of first order codes such as "HCP's deficiencies", "Strengthening GP service", and "Training needs". The other authors also read the transcriptions and collectively contributed to the development of the coding frame. The entire data set was then coded using NVivo, a qualitative data management and organisation software. Through attentive reading and examination of the coded data, the codes were grouped into preliminary themes. This was followed by the development of conceptual themes such as "Knowledge and confidence to provide SRH care" and "Training needs and experiences in the SRH care of refugee and migrant women" through a process which involved examining patterns, similarities and differences across the codes and preliminary themes by all the authors. Finally, the results of the survey and qualitative analyses were combined through a process of triangulation that enabled the authors to connect and interpret both data sets simultaneously through convergence and corroboration [29]. The socio-ecological model which was introduced after data analysis to make sense of the results in the broader framework helped us to identify factors that impact the HCP's preparedness for providing SRH care to refugee and migrant women across the four levels.

3. Results

The results are presented thematically, addressing the aims of the study: (1) knowledge and confidence: "Providers don't want to deal with it or they can't deal with it"; and (2) training experience and needs: "It's an entirely different topic not covered in the universities". Within each theme, a number of factors were identified at individual, organisational and societal levels of the socio-ecological model. These factors interact across levels to influence HCP's preparedness for providing SRH care to refugee and migrant women. For example, at individual level the data indicated that work experience in SRH care, cross-cultural knowledge, on job training and confidence to initiate and discuss SRH influenced HCP's ability to provide SRH care to refugee and migrant women. At the organisational level, university education/curricula and training availability in refugee and migrant women's SRH care impacted HCP's knowledge and confidence in SRH care provision. Influential societal level factors included SRH taboo, health system priorities of providing resources instead of training in SRH care, and emphasis on aboriginal cultural training. These suggest that HCP preparedness to provide SRH care to refugee and migrant women is influenced by multiple factors across the socio-ecological model, and multiple and multilevel interventions are necessary. Figure 1 shows a summary of factors at each level. In the presentation of the two major themes below, the ways in which the identified factors across the socio-ecological model were constructed to influence HCP's preparedness to provide SRH care to refugee and migrant women are discussed.

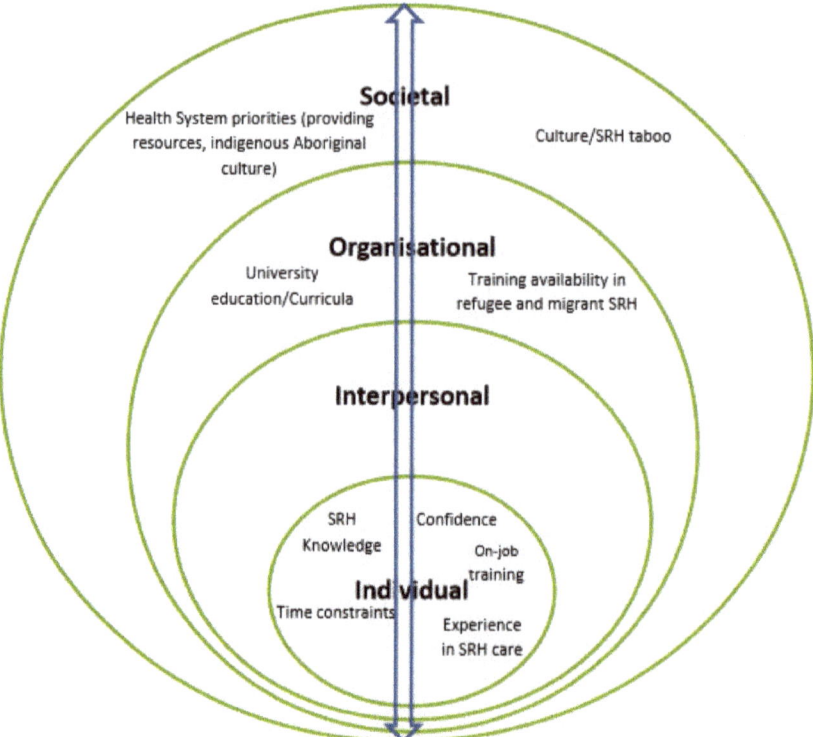

Figure 1. A socio-ecological analysis of factors that influence provider preparedness for delivering SRH care to refugee and migrant women in Australia.

3.1. Knowledge and Confidence: "Providers Don't Want to Deal with It or They Can't Deal with It"

Although no significant differences were observed between professional groups in relation to perceived knowledge and confidence, more than a quarter (26%) of HCPs rated their knowledge of refugee and migrant women's SRH as very low or low, and 16.4% of HCPs rated their confidence to provide SRH care as low or very low (Table 2). A number of areas where HCPs across all occupational groups described their knowledge and confidence to provide SRH care to refugee and migrant women as inadequate were also identified from the semi-structured interviews. For example, many HCPs explained that engaging in SRH conversations was difficult:

> Broaching the subject is the challenge I face because lots of women tell you "oh, I don't want to talk about it." So it's a challenge to be able to break that barrier to let them know that it's important to talk about what's going on because you need to help them in regards to not having any problem now or in the future. (Alice, GP, 35)

This perceived difficulty demonstrates the challenges and cultural barriers on which HCPs need more training to effectively raise discussions about SRH, as Hannah (GP, 31) indicated:

> Hell, the majority of them (HCPs) can't do (talk about) sexual and reproductive health to these women ... You can't sit there and giggle and say, "oh I'm sorry I've got to ask you a personal question." The challenge is getting them (the women) to bring it up as they are not going to say "I have got a discharge."

This may hinder the HCP's ability to understand the women's needs and provide appropriate SRH care. According to some of the HCPs, the difficulty in discussing sexual health was related to their lack of awareness about the women's attitude towards sexual health: "I don't know their attitude towards sexual pleasure or towards sexual practice to talk about it" (Emma, sex therapist, 6). Consequently, some HCPs may just refer refugee and migrant women to specialist services to avoid the difficulty: "Often GPs will just refer (women) to sexual health (clinics) because they don't want to deal with it (difficulty of raising SRH discussions) or they can't deal with it" (Amy, nurse, 17). This implies that HCPs may miss opportunities to gain experience in SRH care provision to refugee and migrant women.

Table 2. HCP's knowledge, confidence, training needs and experience with refugee and migrant women's SRH care.

Variable		Occupation			Test of Group Difference	
		Nurse	GP	HPO	χ^2	p
Knowledge	Very low/low	10 (27.8%)	5 (20.8%)	4 (30.8%)	2.04	0.73
	Moderate	15 (41.7%)	13 (54.2%)	4 (30.8%)		
	High	11 (30.6%)	6 (25.0%)	5 (30.8%)		
Confidence	Very low/low	7 (19.4%)	3 (12.5%)	2 (15.4%)	1.95	0.74
	Moderate	18 (50.0%)	14 (58.3%)	5 (38.5%)		
	High	11 (30.6%)	7 (29.2%)	6 (46.2%)		
Previous training	Yes	11 (30.6%)	12 (50%)	8 (61.5%)	4.58	0.10
	No	25 (69.4%)	12 (50%)	5 (38.5%)		
Need for further training	Yes	32 (88.9%)	18 (75%)	10 (76.9%)	2.04	0.33
	No	4 (11.1%)	6 (25%)	23.1%)		

Not all HCPs described themselves as inadequately prepared to discuss SRH with refugee and migrant women. Few nurses indicated that they were confident talking to refugee and migrant women about SRH, with their confidence stemming from previous training in SRH care provision: "I've done a number of courses as part of my work and I'm very comfortable talking about sexuality" (Alex, nurse, 42). Others reported that their confidence stemmed from their extensive work experience in SRH:

> "I have worked in sexual health for a long time. So to me it's no different to addressing the health of their eyes or their lungs or their feet or anything else. There is no cultural group that I can't discuss these (sexual health) issues with." (Amy, nurse, 17)

This indicates that extended work experience in SRH care improves the HCP's confidence to initiate and discuss SRH topics with women from refugee and migrant backgrounds. A number of HCPs shared strategies they had found effective in helping to overcome the difficulty of initiating SRH discussions with refugee and migrant women. They emphasised the need to prepare the women, by starting the discussion by highlighting the benefits of engaging in an open conversation with HCPs:

> "Generally no one likes talking about that area of their health. So the way I do it is prepare them first, that I would like to ask them these questions, and give them a benefit to answering those questions for themselves. So for example, I ask this for your health. I want to make sure you're all right. There is a positive in it for them." (Amy, nurse, 17)

This result highlights the importance of how HCPs initiate SRH discussions with refugee and migrant women seeking SRH care. It is imperative that HCPs use different approaches to discuss SRH as societal taboos associated with this topic may hinder the women from seeking information and service leading to misconceptions and knowledge gaps.

3.2. Training Experiences and Needs: Moving across Levels of Influence

HCPs in this study recognised refugee and migrant women's SRH as a "more complex" and "entirely different topic". They also reported that SRH care provision to refugee and migrant women requires a "different skill set to give these messages to these ladies". Despite these acknowledgements, the majority of nurses (59.4%), 50% of GPs and 38.6% of health promotion officers had not undertaken any training or professional development that specifically addressed refugee and migrant women's SRH (Table 2). The absence of HCP training in refugee and migrant women's SRH was also identified by many participants across all professional groups in the interviews. HCPs provided many reasons why they had not received training in refugee and migrant women's SRH. Some participants described refugee and migrant women's SRH as "not covered in the universities" and that HCPs are "not taught as much as (they) could be during training". For example, Grace (nurse, 13) explained that "there is more emphasis on providing resources than educating HCPs about refugee and migrant health issues" in the health system. Another nurse stated that "something that's easily accessible and affordable education about these cultural issues is not available for migrant and refugee groups" (Harper, 19). Where cross-cultural training exists in the healthcare system, some HCPs reported that it focused on Indigenous Aboriginal health with little attention to refugee and migrant health:

> "There is now a huge push for us to learn about the Aboriginal culture and it's become mandatory that we do some of the training on that. But there's nothing really to—along similar lines to educate us about these other cultures and about some of the traumas and such that people go through." (Grace, nurse, 13)

Whilst some of the HCPs did not mind having more training on the SRH of refugee and migrant women, others reported a lack of time to undertake additional training:

> "So time constraint is a big issue for health professionals. Because they're always short of time, I think that they don't spend the time or don't put the time aside to do extra training in terms of sexual and reproductive health care, and when training does come up, often they can't go because they're so short of time, or because they just don't want to do it because it's too hard." (Amy, nurse, 17)

Consequently, many HCPs noticed that they were underprepared to provide SRH care to refugee and migrant women: "We're taught some and we're taught not enough in so many areas (of refugee and migrant women's SRH). There are a lot of areas that I feel inadequate in" (Hannah, GP, 31). Finally, several HCPs suggested areas where additional training is needed. For instance, Chloe (nurse, 13) explained that with "cultural awareness training … I like to know what messages I'm conveying subconsciously. I would like to improve that and be able to convey my messages a bit more clearly". Importantly knowing the women's cultural background is reported to be important in delivering SRH messages. Grace (GP, 13) added, "We need more education on the cultures, cultural norms and the cultural expectations of these migrant and refugee women and some understanding of how they would like care to be provided when it's care around sexuality and sexual health". Learning about the role of culture and ethnicity in refugee and migrant women's SRH was viewed by many as facilitating self-reflection and analysis and leading to better patient care:

> "Sometimes you can be having a consultation—it's all going well, and then something just changes. I think I would really like to know why in some of those cases. Some of them you can sit back and think, oh, I shouldn't have said that or I should have said this differently, or I should have backed off and asked that in a different way. I think having increased knowledge helps to do that sort of analysis afterwards." (Chloe, nurse, 13)

HCPs described increased SRH knowledge as an imperative to improved service delivery versus being elective with regards to professional development. Tayla (GP, 22) noted, "All GPs (need) to be adequately trained in sexual and reproductive health, rather than regarding it as an optional extra for those with special interest". Few participants also recommended training to medical support staff such as receptionists to help them understand the contexts of refugee and migrant women and assist the women in booking and re-booking appointments:

> "I guess that's the same for even potentially medical receptionists as well, because if a woman misses her appointments a couple of times, or comes extremely late for an appointment, sometimes that can be quite frustrating for receptionists who have to re-book their appointments, yet they don't actually understand the reasons why that might be occurring." (Kokob, health promotion officer, 8)

Given that 88.9% of nurses, 75% of GPs and 76% of health promotion officers reported need for and demonstrated willingness to engage with further training in this area, the modes of delivering for such training are important. The majority of the HCPs preferred online self-directed learning (66.67%), workshop methodologies (65.22%) and professionally accredited courses (43.48%). These results imply that HCP SRH education programs in the health system need to consider their audience, scope, timing, content, accessibility and recognition relating to modes of training delivery.

4. Discussion

Previous research has recommended the need to prepare the health workforce and the health system to effectively respond to the changing demography in major refugee and migrant resettlement countries such as Australia [34–36]. Whilst there have been efforts in the health system to improve cultural competency for healthier living and environments [37,38], less effort has addressed the preparedness of HCPs in relation to their knowledge, confidence and training to provide SRH care to referee and migrant women.

HCPs in this study reported a lack of knowledge regarding refugee and migrant women's SRH issues that may impact the quality of care they are able to offer these women [16]. Similarly, HCPs in other multicultural societies reported that their undergraduate and postgraduate studies had not prepared them to provide care for women from refugee and migrant backgrounds [39]. The finding that HCPs who received training in refugee and migrant women's SRH were comfortable with their knowledge and confidence suggests that further training would likely result in improved knowledge and competency in this area [2,5]. This implies the need to improve cultural competency training in higher education institutions and training in culture, sexuality and health and core concepts of working with refugee and migrant women as they are pertinent to the care of these women in SRH [40]. The SRH issues of refugee and migrant women should also be incorporated in higher education and other professional development curricula for HCPs.

Another important finding at individual level was the enthusiasm of the majority of HCPs to undertake further training/professional development activities in refugee and migrant women's SRH. This finding highlights the key role that HCPs can take in informing the development of effective and relevant cross cultural training in SRH [5]. The areas identified for additional training included cultural sensitivity and awareness and health issues specific to refugees and migrant women. The training needs expressed by the HCPs can be associated with the perceived challenges of providing SRH care to refugee and migrant women [4]. For instance, majority of the HCPs in this study reported having difficulties in effectively initiating and discussing SRH with refugee and migrant women due to societal taboos associated with this topic. This may mean that the SRH needs of these women are to some extent under addressed [41]. Past research suggests training of HCPs working in cross-cultural care to improve interpersonal communication and understanding with patients from refugee and migrant backgrounds [42].

This study has a number of strengths and limitations. The sequential mixed methods design was strength as it helped us to better explain and elaborate issues raised in relation to the HCP's knowledge, confidence and training to provide SRH care to refugee and migrant women. A limitation was that

HCPs may have provided socially desirable responses as they self-rated their knowledge, training and confidence to provide SRH care to refugee and migrant women. As such, the HCP's knowledge, confidence and training may have been inflated. Due to response bias, HCPs who participated in this study might also be those who were more interested in refugee and migrant women's SRH. Majority of the HCPs were also women which makes it difficult to ascertain if provider gender influences their preparedness. As a result, generalisation of the findings to all HCPs in Australia could not be drawn. Further research on how refugee and migrant health and SRH is being taught in universities and professional development courses; whether it is integrated into the curriculum; and how students feel about their knowledge and skills to provide care to women from refugee and backgrounds is recommended.

5. Conclusions

This study has provided evidence that a significant proportion of HCPs in Australia may not be providing optimal SRH care to refugee and migrant women even though many put efforts to accommodate them. This is mainly attributed to the broader interplay of influencing factors at individual, organisational and system levels suggesting the need for multilevel strategies to improve the provision of SRH care to refugee and migrant women. The policy implications of the findings are argued regarding the need to train HCPs in culturally sensitive care and include the SRH of refugee and migrant women in university and professional development curricula. These interventions are vital to the provision of gender-sensitive and culturally appropriate SRH care to this growing and vulnerable group of Australia's population [11,13,43].

Acknowledgments: The authors would like to acknowledge the Multicultural Centre for Women's Health and Family Planning NSW that provided support in the recruitment of research participants. Our acknowledgement also goes to HCPs who provided their time and voices to this project.

Author Contributions: Zelalem B. Mengesha conceived and designed the study with continuous support from Janette Perz. Zelalem B. Mengesha collected the data. Zelalem B. Mengesha, Janette Perz, Tinashe Dune and Jane Ussher involved in data analysis and interpretation. Zelalem B. Mengesha drafted the manuscript. Janette Perz, Tinashe Dune and Jane Ussher read and revised the manuscript. All authors have read and approved the submission.

Conflicts of Interest: The authors declare no conflict of interest.

References

1. Phillips, C.B.; Travaglia, J. Low levels of uptake of free interpreters by Australian doctors in private practice: Secondary analysis of national data. *Aust. Health Rev.* **2011**, *35*, 475–479. [CrossRef] [PubMed]
2. Alpern, J.D.; Davey, C.S.; Song, J. Perceived barriers to success for resident physicians interested in immigrant and refugee health. *BMC Med. Educ.* **2016**, *16*, 178. [CrossRef] [PubMed]
3. Hudelson, P.; Perron, N.J.; Perneger, T.V. Measuring physicians' and medical students' attitudes toward caring for immigrant patients. *Eval. Health Prof.* **2010**, *33*, 452–472. [CrossRef] [PubMed]
4. Vázquez Navarrete, M.L.; Terraza Núñez, R.; Vargas Lorenzo, I.; Lizana Alcazo, T. Perceived needs of health personnel in the provision of healthcare to the immigrant population. *Gac. Sanit.* **2009**, *23*, 396–402. [CrossRef] [PubMed]
5. Papic, O.; Malak, Z.; Rosenberg, E. Survey of family physicians' perspectives on management of immigrant patients: Attitudes, barriers, strategies, and training needs. *Patient Educ. Couns.* **2012**, *86*, 205–209. [CrossRef] [PubMed]
6. Harmsen, H.; Meeuwesen, L.; van Wieringen, J.; Bernsen, R.; Bruijnzeels, M. When cultures meet in general practice: Intercultural differences between GPs and parents of child patients. *Patient Educ. Couns.* **2003**, *51*, 99–106. [CrossRef]
7. Pieper, H.-O.; MacFarlane, A. I'm worried about what I missed: GP Registrars' Views on Learning Needs to Deliver Effective Healthcare to Ethnically and Culturally Diverse Patient Populations. *Educ. Health* **2011**, *24*, 494.

8. Dias, S.; Gama, A.; Cargaleiro, H.; Martins, M.O. Health workers' attitudes toward immigrant patients: A cross-sectional survey in primary health care services. *Hum. Resour. Health* **2012**, *10*, 14. [CrossRef] [PubMed]
9. Freedman, J. Sexual and gender-based violence against refugee women: A hidden aspect of the refugee "crisis". *Reprod. Health Matters* **2016**, *24*, 18–26. [CrossRef] [PubMed]
10. Keygnaert, I.; Vettenburg, N.; Temmerman, M. Hidden violence is silent rape: Sexual and gender-based violence in refugees, asylum seekers and undocumented migrants in Belgium and The Netherlands. *Cult. Health Sex.* **2012**, *14*, 505–520. [CrossRef] [PubMed]
11. The United Nations Children's Fund. *Sexual and Gender-Based Violence against Refugees, Returnees and Internally Displaced Persons-Guidelines for Prevention and Response*; United Nations High Commissioner for Refugees: Geneva, Switzerland, 2003.
12. Austin, J.; Guy, S.; Lee-Jones, L.; McGinn, T.; Schlecht, J. Reproductive health: A right for refugees and internally displaced persons. *Reprod. Health Matters* **2008**, *16*, 10–21. [CrossRef]
13. Ussher, J.M.; Perz, J.; Metusela, C.; Hawkey, A.J.; Morrow, M.; Narchal, R.; Estoesta, J. Negotiating Discourses of Shame, Secrecy, and Silence: Migrant and Refugee Women's Experiences of Sexual Embodiment. *Arch. Sex. Behav.* **2017**, *46*, 1901–1921. [CrossRef] [PubMed]
14. Metusela, C.; Ussher, J.; Perz, J.; Hawkey, A.; Morrow, M.; Narchal, R.; Estoesta, J.; Monteiro, M. In My Culture, We Don't Know Anything about That: Sexual and Reproductive Health of Migrant and Refugee Women. *Int. J. Behav. Med.* **2017**, *24*, 836–845. [CrossRef] [PubMed]
15. Mengesha, Z.; Perz, J.; Dune, T.; Ussher, J. Refugee and migrant women's engagement with sexual and reproductive health care in Australia: A socio-ecological analysis of health care professional perspectives. *PLoS ONE* **2017**, *12*, e0181421. [CrossRef] [PubMed]
16. Utting, S.; Calcutt, C.; Marsh, K.; Doherty, P. *Women and Sexual and Reproductive Health*; Australian Women's Health Network: Drysdale, Australia, 2012.
17. Watt, K.; Abbott, P.; Reath, J. Cross-cultural training of general practitioner registrars: How does it happen? *Aust. J. Prim. Health* **2016**, *22*, 349–353. [CrossRef] [PubMed]
18. Watt, K.; Abbott, P.; Reath, J. Cultural competency training of GP Registrars-exploring the views of GP Supervisors. *Int. J. Equity Health* **2015**, *14*, 89. [CrossRef] [PubMed]
19. Suphanchaimat, R.; Kantamaturapoj, K.; Putthasri, W.; Prakongsai, P. Challenges in the provision of healthcare services for migrants: A systematic review through providers' lens. *BMC Health Serv. Res.* **2015**, *15*, 390. [CrossRef] [PubMed]
20. Newbold, K.B.; Willinsky, J. Providing family planning and reproductive healthcare to Canadian immigrants: Perceptions of healthcare providers. *Cult. Health Sex.* **2009**, *11*, 369–382. [CrossRef] [PubMed]
21. Degni, F.; Suominen, S.; Essen, B.; El Ansari, W.; Vehvilainen-Julkunen, K. Communication and cultural issues in providing reproductive health care to immigrant women: Health care providers' experiences in meeting the needs of (corrected) Somali women living in Finland. *J. Immigr. Minor. Health* **2012**, *14*, 330–343. [CrossRef] [PubMed]
22. Lyons, S.M.; O'Keeffe, F.M.; Clarke, A.T.; Staines, A. Cultural diversity in the Dublin maternity services: The experiences of maternity service providers when caring for ethnic minority women. *Ethn. Health* **2008**, *13*, 261–276. [CrossRef] [PubMed]
23. Ng, C.; Newbold, K.B. Health care providers' perspectives on the provision of prenatal care to immigrants. *Cult. Health Sex.* **2011**, *13*, 561–574. [CrossRef] [PubMed]
24. Tobin, C.L.; Murphy-Lawless, J. Irish midwives' experiences of providing maternity care to non-Irish women seeking asylum. *Int. J. Women's Health* **2014**, *6*, 159–169. [CrossRef] [PubMed]
25. Pruitt, S.D.; Epping-Jordan, J.E. Preparing the 21st century global healthcare workforce. *BMJ* **2005**, *330*, 637–639. [CrossRef] [PubMed]
26. McLeroy, K.R.; Bibeau, D.; Steckler, A.; Glanz, K. An ecological perspective on health promotion programs. *Health Educ. Q.* **1988**, *15*, 351–377. [CrossRef] [PubMed]
27. Bronfenbrenner, U. The ecology of human development: Experiments by nature and design. *Am. Psychol.* **1979**, *32*, 513–531. [CrossRef]
28. Onwuegbuzie, A.J.; Collins, K.M.; Frels, R.K. Foreword: Using Bronfenbrenner's ecological systems theory to frame quantitative, qualitative, and mixed research. *Int. J. Mult. Res. Approaches* **2013**, *7*, 2–8. [CrossRef]
29. Creswell, J.W.; Klassen, A.C.; Plano Clark, V.L.; Smith, K.C. *Best Practices for Mixed Methods Research in the Health Sciences*; National Institutes of Health: Bethesda, MD, USA, 2011; pp. 2094–2103.

30. Ivankova, N.V.; Creswell, J.W.; Stick, S.L. Using mixed-methods sequential explanatory design: From theory to practice. *Field Methods* **2006**, *18*, 3–20. [CrossRef]
31. Hilpinen, R. Knowing that one knows and the classical definition of knowledge. *Synthese* **1970**, *21*, 109–132. [CrossRef]
32. Confidence in Psychology Today. 2017. Available online: https://www.psychologytoday.com/basics/confidence (accessed on 17 August 2017).
33. Braun, V.; Clarke, V. Using thematic analysis in psychology. *Qual. Res. Psychol.* **2006**, *3*, 77–101. [CrossRef]
34. Mengesha, Z.; Perz, J.; Dune, T.; Ussher, J. Challenges in the provision of sexual and reproductive health care to refugee and migrant women: A Q methodological study of health professional perspectives. *J. Immigr. Minor. Health* **2017**. [CrossRef] [PubMed]
35. National Health and Medical Research Council. *Increasing Cultural Competency for Healthier Living & Environments: Discussion Paper*; National Health and Medical Research Council: Canberra, Australia, 2005.
36. Whelan, A.M. Consultation with non-English speaking communities: Rapid bilingual appraisal. *Aust. Health Rev.* **2004**, *28*, 311–316. [CrossRef] [PubMed]
37. National Health and Medical Research Council. *Cultural Competency in Health: A Guide for Policy, Partnerships and Participation*; National Health and Medical Research Council: Canberra, Australia, 2006.
38. Royal Australian College of General Practitioners. *Royal Australian College of General Practitioners Curriculum for Australian General Practice*; Multicultural Health: Melbourne, Australia, 2011.
39. Kurth, E.; Jaeger, F.N.; Zemp, E.; Tschudin, S.; Bischoff, A. Reproductive health care for asylum-seeking women—A challenge for health professionals. *BMC Public Health* **2010**, *10*, 659. [CrossRef] [PubMed]
40. Mengesha, Z.; Dune, T.; Perz, J. Culturally and linguistically diverse women's views and experiences of accessing sexual and reproductive health care in Australia: A systematic review. *Sex. Health* **2016**, *13*, 299–310. [CrossRef] [PubMed]
41. Ussher, J.M.; Perz, J.; Gilbert, E.; Wong, W.K.; Mason, C.; Hobbs, K.; Kirsten, L. Talking about sex after cancer: A discourse analytic study of health care professional accounts of sexual communication with patients. *Psychol. Health* **2013**, *28*, 1370–1390. [CrossRef] [PubMed]
42. Bischoff, A.; Perneger, T.V.; Bovier, P.A.; Loutan, L.; Stalder, H. Improving communication between physicians and patients who speak a foreign language. *Br. J. Gen. Pract.* **2003**, *53*, 541–546. [PubMed]
43. Hatch, M. *Common Threads: The Sexual and Reproductive Health Experiences of Immigrant and Refugee Women in Australia*; MCWH: Melbourne, Australia, 2012.

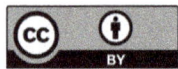

© 2018 by the authors. Licensee MDPI, Basel, Switzerland. This article is an open access article distributed under the terms and conditions of the Creative Commons Attribution (CC BY) license (http://creativecommons.org/licenses/by/4.0/).

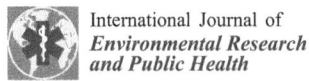

Commentary

Strengthening Emergency Care Systems to Mitigate Public Health Challenges Arising from Influxes of Individuals with Different Socio-Cultural Backgrounds to a Level One Emergency Center in South East Europe

Michèle Twomey [1,*], Ana Šijački [2], Gert Krummrey [3], Tyson Welzel [1,3], Aristomenis K. Exadaktylos [1,3] and Marko Ercegovac [2]

1. Centre of Excellence in Emergency Medicine, Cape Town 7700, South Africa; twelzel@earthling.net (T.W.); aristomenis.exadaktylos@insel.ch (A.K.E.)
2. Department of Emergency Medicine, Clinical Centre of Serbia, 11000 Belgrade, Serbia; asijacki@gmail.com (A.Š.); ercegovacmarko@gmail.com (M.E.)
3. Department of Emergency Medicine, Inselspital, University Hospital Bern, 3010 Bern, Switzerland; Gert.Krummrey@insel.ch
* Correspondence: micheletwomey@gmail.com; Tel.: +49-170-400-0501

Received: 29 December 2017; Accepted: 2 March 2018; Published: 12 March 2018

Abstract: Emergency center visits are mostly unscheduled, undifferentiated, and unpredictable. A standardized triage process is an opportunity to obtain real-time data that paints a picture of the variation in acuity found in emergency centers. This is particularly pertinent as the influx of people seeking asylum or in transit mostly present with emergency care needs or first seek help at an emergency center. Triage not only reduces the risk of missing or losing a patient that may be deteriorating in the waiting room but also enables a time-critical response in the emergency care service provision. As part of a joint emergency care system strengthening and patient safety initiative, the Serbian Ministry of Health in collaboration with the Centre of Excellence in Emergency Medicine (CEEM) introduced a standardized triage process at the Clinical Centre of Serbia (CCS). This paper describes four crucial stages that were considered for the integration of a standardized triage process into acute care pathways.

Keywords: emergency care; triage; healthcare system strengthening; migrant health

1. Introduction

"Emergencies occur everywhere, and each day they consume resources regardless of whether there are systems capable of achieving good outcomes" [1].

Emergency care is a critical part of a country's healthcare system and is transversal in nature moving across different levels of care, from a community bystander response or primary care mobile clinic to tertiary specialized interventions. In a healthcare system that has fully embraced and integrated emergency care as an essential component, emergency care is everyone's business. Health practitioners at all levels including doctors, nurses, paramedics, and first responders attend to emergencies (i.e., undifferentiated, unscheduled patients) not in the order in which they arrive but in order of acuity. Acuity goes beyond severity of illness/injury in that it includes the urgency for intervention that potentially leads to stabilization or improvement. Triage refers to the standardized prioritization process that determines a patient's acuity [1].

In contexts where the demand exceeds the capacity to match that demand the process of triage, if appropriately developed and comprehensively integrated into acute care pathways, has shown to utilize resources more efficiently and predict mortality [2]. The World Health Organization (WHO) in a systematic review of 59 low- and middle- income countries emphasizes the ongoing need to strengthen triage as a crucial requirement for efficient resource allocation and effective emergency intervention [3]. In upper middle-income countries such as Serbia, Bosnia, Herzegovina, and the former Yugoslav Republic of Macedonia (FYROM), the demand for emergency care has been growing, and the need for continuous strengthening of emergency care systems has been recognized [4–6]. The Clinical Centre of Serbia (CCS) located in Belgrade is a 3500-bed medical university center that serves the population of Belgrade and larger Serbia. It is considered the largest hospital complex in Europe treating more than 1 million patients every year with a 308-bed emergency center that was established in December 1987 [7]. More than 20,000 patients enter the emergency center on a monthly basis requiring time-critical initial assessment, investigation, and intervention, including resuscitation and stabilization.

In June and August 2015, the Ministry of Health of Serbia and the WHO Regional Office for Europe conducted a joint assessment of the preparedness and capacity of the Serbian health system to manage sudden large influxes of people seeking asylum or who were in transit. The report of this joint assessment highlights the need to systematically develop both local and national policies to include migrant health needs in all levels of health planning [8]. Another independent assessment of the needs of young refugees arriving in Europe identified that physical health issues predominate upon arrival and pose significant challenges to the national healthcare system [9]. While asylum centers are set up to provide primary care and limited emergency medical procedures, the majority of people are not resident in these centers and thus mostly enter the Serbian healthcare system at a tertiary acute care level through the emergency center [8]. As such, a standardized prioritization process based on a combination of clinical discriminators and a composite early warning score was determined as relevant and appropriate for a varied acuity distribution from emergent to non-urgent, thus covering a wide variety of conditions by not being specific to only certain conditions.

Emergency medicine as a specialty is becoming more established in Serbia and emergency care has been recognized as a critical component in a transversal approach to improving population health. From September 2016 to August 2017, as part of a larger emergency care improvement and patient safety effort, the Serbian Ministry of Health in collaboration with CEEM introduced a standardized triage process at the CCS. This paper outlines four stages that were considered crucial for the integration of a standardized triage process into acute care pathways and is intended as a high level commentary to inform policy makers.

2. Standardize Information Gathered, Make Data Visible, and Use It to Drive Decision-Making

By gathering baseline data and making it visible, the CCS's leadership team gained clarity on demand patterns, caseload, and current acute care pathways through the emergency center. Data collected via the hospital's electronic patient record system (InfoMedis) was also taken into account. Initial challenges that emerged during this stage related to how the current system was set up to capture data. To obtain a baseline snapshot, a core data team consisting of four nurses and two doctors was responsible for gathering information prospectively. This allowed for the inclusion of relevant indicators relating to real-time tracking of acuity distribution of patients on or shortly after arrival, as well as value-adding information during their acute care pathway. The indicators included mode and time of arrival, age of patient, presenting complaint, vital signs, special investigations, diagnosis, treatment, and disposition. In addition, an overview of available capacity was established (number and level of skilled human resources, spaces, structures, and equipment). All information available on demand and capacity was displayed visually. This was not only essential to inform future decision-making regarding healthcare organization but also to determine how to configure and standardize a triage process that is contextually appropriate for integration into the acute care pathways. A panel of four content experts reviewed the prospectively gathered data and annual statistics from InfoMedis during three discussion rounds after which a consensus was reached on the most prevalent clinical discriminators to be included. This process informed the modifications of the triage tool for use within the local context.

3. Contextually Configure and Standardize the Triage Process

The literature describes many different triage tools, models, and interpretations for the emergency center setting. Some of the triage scales that are used globally include the Australasian Triage Scale (ATS) [10], the Canadian Emergency Department Triage and Acuity Scale (CTAS) [11], the Emergency Severity Index (ESI) [12], and the South African Triage Scale (SATS) [13].

The details of how the triage process manifests itself depend on the context. The most useful aspects for distinguishing different contexts for this purpose are demand and capacity, which in turn determine (i) the choice of most appropriate triage tool; (ii) the training, experience, and level of staff required; (iii) how other processes are linked to triage; and (iv) the need for task-shifting and parallel processing [14].

Most triage tools are based on a list of clinical discriminators; some include individual vital signs, while others include early warning scores (EWSs) or symptom-based algorithms. Individual vital signs considered in isolation from each other are known to be poor predictors of life-threatening conditions in patients. EWSs are known for their ability to detect physiological changes relating to vital signs [15]. Combining various standardized physiological parameters into a composite EWS has been recognized as a powerful tool in initiating appropriate responses from the initial contact at triage [16]. The benefits of an EWS include its objectivity and the fact that an aggregated score is a stronger predictor than individual vital signs and reliance on routinely recorded vital signs [17].

The CCS's leadership team reviewed available triage instruments and chose to configure their triage process based on a modified version of SATS for three reasons: (i) comprehensiveness and safety in combining clinical discriminators and an EWS [18,19]; (ii) clarity and ease of use, which enables standardized training and reliable use [20]; (iii) evidence of widespread global adaptation and adoption from low- and middle- income countries such as Ghana [21] and Botswana [22] to high- income countries such as Norway and parts of Sweden [23]. A core training team of six doctors and three nurses was formed once a consensual adaptation process had been completed. All training material was made available in Serbian and an open-source mobile android decision support application was developed to aid the standardized training modules as well as the actual triage process for future routine use. Thus far, 30 nurse technicians have been trained in the standardized triage process, and further training is planned to cover the rest of the staff at the CCS.

4. Reorganize and Restructure Available Resources

A standardized triage process should ideally take place on arrival or within minutes of arrival at the emergency center in order to prioritize and stream patients into the appropriate care pathways. To introduce, integrate, and improve a standardized triage process, the necessary staff with appropriate experience and level of training, equipment, space, and decision support tools are vital prerequisites. The respective care pathways that follow the triage process are organized based on the available resources (i.e., training, experience and level of staff available as well as infrastructure, medical equipment, and supplies available) [10].

Adequate space for triage on arrival at the CCS was limited. After permission was granted for minor renovations, previously unused storage space became available and the triage station was doubled to accommodate two workstations with desk and chairs, eight stretcher patients, and eight seated patients. There are currently no emergency-medicine-trained physicians at the CCS that would be able to assist in the initial stabilization, work-up, and transfer of patients to appropriate definitive care. Therefore, the CCS's leadership team motivated and made urgent requests for eight additional doctors with Basic Life Support (BLS) or Advanced Trauma Life Support (ATLS) training. Thus far, two doctors with some BLS training have been appointed.

5. Redesigning Care Pathways to Integrate Standardized Triage

Currently nurse technicians are responsible for sorting patients on arrival. Previously, patients were sent to one of four specialist-assessment areas based on the presenting complaint (i.e., neurology, internal medicine, surgery, or cardiology). The specialist assessment was performed in order of arrival and not based on the patient's acuity. During busy periods, patients experienced long waiting times in the corridor before being seen by a specialist for assessment. This presented an increased risk for patients that were deteriorating rapidly and could not safely wait.

The target condition in redesigned care pathways is to fully integrate a standardized triage process on arrival where triage-trained nurse technicians document the crucial information gathered using a mobile android triage application. Further developments are required to link the mobile triage application to the electronic patient record system (InfoMedis). This information from the triage then determines the patient's acuity and enables the nurse technician to decide whether the patient needs to receive time-critical intervention or can safely wait to be seen. Dangerous situations of very sick patients deteriorating, while waiting for a specialist assessment are thus kept to a minimum. The standardized process of triage and its crucial link to other functions and care pathways is described in a local triage protocol and policy document. Both guiding and supporting documents are endorsed by the Head of Department, the triage team, and the Minister of Health and intended for regular review in the future.

6. Conclusions

All improvement initiatives take time to reach full adoption and integration. The amount of time needed and the extent to which integration occurs depends on the political will, the resources invested, the collective leadership, and the organizational learning culture. This emergency care improvement initiative is the start of a continuous quality improvement and patient safety approach that requires on-going review and numerous iterations over time.

While the collection and collation of some indicators may not yet be routine daily practice at the CCS, the target condition is to achieve real-time data collection to allow data-driven decision-making, time-critical response, and adjustment of emergency care services for all types of unpredictable fluctuations in caseload, whether they are related to an influx in health needs of migrants or to other situational or contextual changes. The initiation of a standardized triage process is an opportunity to move toward this target while simultaneously reducing the risk of missing or losing patients with life-threatening conditions in emergency waiting rooms.

Acknowledgments: We would like to acknowledge the support of the Ministry of Health of the Republic of Serbia, the Centre of Excellence in Emergency Medicine (www.ceem.info), and the embassy of the Republic of Serbia in Switzerland.

Author Contributions: Michèle Twomey wrote the first draft. Aristomenis K. Exadaktylos, Ana Šijački, and Marko Ercegovac contributed to subsequent versions of the article. Gert Krummrey and Tyson Welzel were part of the initial conceptual planning and development of the Serbian project and drafted of the paper.

Conflicts of Interest: The authors declare no conflict of interest.

References

1. Kobusingye, O.C.; Hyder, A.A.; Bishai, D.; Hicks, E.R.; Mock, C.; Joshipura, M. Emergency medical systems in low- and middle-income countries: Recommendations for action. *Bull. World Health Organ.* **2005**, *83*, 626–631. [PubMed]
2. Massaut, J.; Valles, P.; Ghismonde, A.; Jacques, C.J.; Louis, L.P.; Zakir, A.; Van den Bergh, R.; Santiague, L.; Massenat, R.B.; Edema, N. The modified South African Triage Scale system for mortality prediction in resource-constrained emergency surgical centers: A retrospective cohort study. *BMC Health Serv. Res.* **2017**, *17*, 594. [CrossRef] [PubMed]

3. Obermeyer, Z.; Abujaber, S.; Makar, M.; Stoll, S.; Kayden, S.R.; Wallis, L.A.; Reynolds, T.A. Emergency care in 59 low- and middle-income countries: A systematic review. *Bull. World Health Organ.* **2015**, *93*, 314–319. [CrossRef] [PubMed]
4. Nelson, B.D.; Dierberg, K.; Šćepanović, M.; Mitrović, M.; Vuksanović, M.; Milić, L.; VanRooyen, M.J. Integrating quantitative and qualitative methodologies for the assessment of health care systems: Emergency medicine in post-conflict Serbia. *BMC Health Serv. Res.* **2005**, *5*, 14. [CrossRef] [PubMed]
5. Nicks, B.; Spasov, M.; Watkins, C. The state and future of emergency medicine in Macedonia. *World J. Emerg. Med.* **2016**, *7*, 245–249. [CrossRef] [PubMed]
6. Salihefendic, N.; Zildzic, M.; Masic, I.; Hadziahmetovic, Z.; Vasic, D. Development of Emergency Medicine as Academic and Distinct Clinical Discipline in Bosnia and Herzegovina. *Med. Arch.* **2011**, *65*, 46–51. [CrossRef]
7. Tanjug. 25 Years Anniversary of the Emergency Centre Has Been Marked. Available online: http://www.zdravlje.gov.rs/showelement.php?id=5109 (accessed on 12 May 2012).
8. World Health Organisation. *Serbia: Assessing Health-System Capacity to Manage Sudden Large Influxes of Migrants*; Joint Report on a Mission of the Ministry of Health of Serbia and the WHO Regional Office for Europe with the Collaboration of the International Organisation for Migration; WHO Regional Office for Europe: Copenhagen, Denmark, 2015.
9. Hebebrand, J.; Anagnostopoulos, D.; Eliez, S.; Linse, H.; Pejovic-Milovancevic, M.; Klasen, H. A first assessment of the needs of young refugees arriving in Europe: What mental health professionals need to know. *Eur. Child Adolesc. Psychiatry* **2016**, *25*, 1–6. [CrossRef] [PubMed]
10. Australasian College for Emergency Medicine. Guidelines on the Implementation of the Australasian Triage Scale in Emergency Departments. 2000. Available online: http://www.acem.org.au/media/policies_and_guidelines/G24_Implementation__ATS.pdf (accessed on 13 November 2010).
11. Canadian Association of Emergency Physicians and National Emergency Nurses Affiliation of Canada. Implementation Guidelines for the Canadian Emergency Department Triage and Acuity Scale (CTAS). 1998. Available online: http://www.caep.ca/template.asp?id=B795164082374289BBD9C1C2BF4B8D32#guidelines (accessed on 10 November 2010).
12. Gilboy, N.; Tanabe, P.; Travers, D.A.; Rosenau, A.M.; Eitel, D.R. *Emergency Severity Index, Version 4: Implementation Handbook*; AHRQ Publication No. 05-0046-2; Agency for Healthcare Research and Quality: Rockville, MD, USA, 2005.
13. Twomey, M.; Wallis, L.A.; Thomson, M.L.; Myers, J.E. The South African triage scale (adult version) provides valid ratings when used by doctors and enrolled nursing assistants. *Afr. J. Emerg. Med.* **2012**, *2*, 3–12. [CrossRef]
14. Tuffin, H.; Twomey, M. Triage in emergency care: Concepts and context. *Recent Adv. Paediatr.* **2015**, *26*, 26–28.
15. Subbe, C.P.; Slater, A.; Menon, D.; Gemmell, L. Validation of physiological scoring systems in the accident and emergency department. *Emerg. Med. J.* **2006**, *23*, 841–845. [CrossRef] [PubMed]
16. Hancock, A.; Hulse, C. Recognizing and responding to acute illness: Using early warning scores. *Br. J. Midwifery* **2009**, *17*, 111–117. [CrossRef]
17. Day, A.; Oldroyd, C. The use of early warning scores in the emergency department. *J. Emerg. Nurs.* **2010**, *36*, 154–155. [CrossRef] [PubMed]
18. Twomey, M.; Cheema, B.; Buys, H.; Cohen, K.; de Sá, A.; Louw, P.; Ismail, M.; Finlayson, H.; Cunningham, C.; Westwood, A. Vital signs for children at triage: A multicentre validation of the revised South African Triage Scale (SATS) for children. *S. Afr. Med. J.* **2013**, *103*, 304–308. [CrossRef] [PubMed]
19. Dalwai, M.; Valles, P.; Twomey, M.; Nzomukunda, Y.; Jonjo, P.; Sasikumar, M.; Nasim, M.; Razaaq, A.; Gayraud, O.; Jecrois, P.R.; et al. Is the South African Triage Scale valid for use in Afghanistan, Haiti and Sierra Leone. *BMJ Glob. Health* **2017**, *2*. [CrossRef] [PubMed]
20. Dalwai, M.; Twomey, M.; Maikere, J.; Said, S.; Wakee, M.; Jemmy, J.P.; Valles, P.; Tayler-Smith, K.; Wallis, L.; ZachariahI, R. Reliability and accuracy of the South African Triage Scale when used by nurses in the emergency department of Timergara Hospital, Pakistan. *S. Afr. Med. J.* **2014**, *104*, 372–375. [CrossRef] [PubMed]
21. Gyedu, A.; Agbedinu, K.; Dalwai, M.; Osei-Ampofo, M.; Nakua, E.K.; Oteng, R.; Stewart, B. Triage capabilities of medical trainees in Ghana using the South African Triage Scale: An opportunity to improve emergency care. *Pan Afr. Med. J.* **2016**, *24*, 294. [CrossRef] [PubMed]

22. Mullan, P.; Torrey, S.B.; Chandra, A.; Caruso, N.; Kestler, A. Reduced overtriage and undertriage with a new triage system in an urban accident and emergency department in Botswana: A cohort study. *Emerg. Med. J.* **2014**, *31*, 356–360. [CrossRef] [PubMed]
23. Brevik, H.; Eide, M.; Engan, M.; Aalvik, R. SATS-N. Standardised Emergency Medicine Assessment and Prioritisation (Triage) Tool. User Manual 3.02. Available online: https://helse-bergen.no/seksjon/mottaksklinikken/PublishingImages/2017.03.20%20SATS-N%20users%20manual%20version%203.02.pdf (accessed on 20 March 2017).

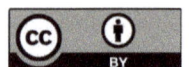

© 2018 by the authors. Licensee MDPI, Basel, Switzerland. This article is an open access article distributed under the terms and conditions of the Creative Commons Attribution (CC BY) license (http://creativecommons.org/licenses/by/4.0/).

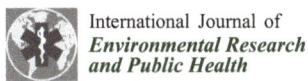

Article

Trauma and Depression among North Korean Refugees: The Mediating Effect of Negative Cognition

Subin Park [1], Yeeun Lee [1] and Jin Yong Jun [2,*]

[1] Department of Research Planning, Mental Health Research Institute, National Center for Mental Health, Seoul 04933, Korea; subin-21@hanmail.net (S.P.); tasarang1010@korea.ac.kr (Y.L.)
[2] Department of Social Psychiatry and Rehabilitation, National Center for Mental Health, Seoul 04933, Korea
* Correspondence: jjy826@naver.com; Tel.: +822-2204-0151; Fax: +822-2204-0393

Received: 24 January 2018; Accepted: 19 March 2018; Published: 25 March 2018

Abstract: North Korean refugees experience adaptation difficulties, along with a wide range of psychological problems. Accordingly, this study examined the associations between early traumatic experiences, negative automatic thoughts, and depression among young North Korean refugees living in South Korea. Specifically, we examined how different factors of negative automatic thoughts would mediate the relationship between early trauma and depressive symptoms. A total of 109 North Korean refugees aged 13–29 years were recruited from two alternative schools. Our path analysis indicated that early trauma was positively linked with thoughts of personal failure, physical threat, and hostility, but not with thoughts of social threat. The link with depressive symptoms was only significant for thoughts of personal failure. After removing all non-significant pathways, the model revealed that early traumatic experiences were positively associated with depressive symptoms (ß = 0.61, 95% CI = 0.48–0.73) via thoughts of personal failure (ß = 0.17, 95% CI = 0.08–0.28), as well as directly (ß = 0.44, 95% CI = 0.27–0.59). Interventions that target negative cognitions of personal failure may be helpful for North Korean refugees at risk of depression.

Keywords: North Korean refugees; depression; early trauma; negative automatic thoughts; path analysis

1. Introduction

Many North Korean refugees often report having experienced traumatic events in North Korea, especially during their escape from North Korea [1] and after settling in South Korea [2]. In particular, research has found that 49.3% of adult North Korean refugees have experienced or witnessed life-threatening events [3]. Among young North Korean refugees, 71% reported having experienced traumatic incidents in the past, such as the death or arrest of family members or hearing about these events, as well as being physically abused by family members or acquaintances [4]. As a result of having experienced such traumatic events, North Korean refugees represent a mentally vulnerable population. Indeed, these traumatic experiences have been consistently found to be associated with psychiatric problems and low life satisfaction among North Korean refugees. In general, the frequency and severity of traumatic experiences have been found to predict post-traumatic stress disorder, anxiety, and depression [4–9]. Indeed, depression is the most frequently reported mental health problem among adult North Korean refugees, with the prevalence of depression ranging from 29% [9] to 49% [10].

One possible mechanism through which traumatic experiences contribute to the affective symptoms of traumatized refugees may be the development and maintenance of negative cognitions. The cognitive theory of depression posits that repeated exposure to uncontrollable negative events that an individual fails to escape may alter how an individual perceives and interprets their own life events [11–13]. Specifically, when individuals experience a negative event, they attempt to understand and explain its causes. If negative events happen repeatedly and pervasively, they begin to interpret negative events as the consequences of their own actions and perceive them as unchangeable and generalizable to other domains (i.e., an internal, stable, and global attributional explanation) [13,14]. The frequently employed attributional explanations can negatively bias the victim's general beliefs about themselves and about the world [14,15], from which automatic thoughts with negative themes arises, so-called "streams of consciousness cognitions" [16] (e.g., I will have an accident; I've failed my life). In particular, negative events that happened early in an individual's life can crystallize more stable negative cognitions [14]. The negative cognition, in turn, acts as a cognitive vulnerability to the onset and persistence of affective disorders when facing prospective negative stressors [17,18], disenabling the person's active coping with stressful situations with hopelessness [11,12].

Cognitive theorists have further proposed the cognitive content-specificity hypothesis, which proposes the distinctiveness of cognitive contents underlying different types of psychiatric problems [19]. For instance, depression can be linked more with thoughts of personal loss and failure in the past tense, while anxiety is more related to future-oriented danger themes such as physical, psychological, or social threats [19,20]. Empirical data also supported the idea that the different contents of automatic thoughts are uniquely associated with each affective symptom, such as with anxiety and depression [16,21,22]. In this vein, there have been efforts to organize the structure of cognitions according to similarity in themes, such as danger, loss, and failure [23,24]. In such efforts, Schneiering and Rapee [25] found four distinct cognitive factors among frequent negative automatic thoughts—cognitions of social threat, physical threat, personal failure, and hostility. The factor structure was found to be consistent across age and gender, supporting the stable latent structure of automatic thoughts.

There is a paucity of research examining the pathway through which early traumatic experiences influence the mental health outcomes of North Korean refugees. North Korean refugees settling in South Korea are unique in that they share the same ethnicity, language, historical backgrounds, and physical features with the host people (i.e., South Koreans). Thus, they undertake very high risks, including the risk of forced repatriation, and a long flight process through third countries [26], with the expectation of entering a new society that they will seamlessly join. However, North Korean refugees are often faced with unexpected cultural gaps and social discrimination for their origin in North Korea [26]. These unexpected difficulties may reduce their ability to recover from early traumatization [27], presumably through reactivating negative cognitive contents developed throughout past trauma in early years. Identifying the cognitive mechanisms underlying psychological sequelae of the widespread adversities that North Korean refugees undergo would give insights into the core psychological factor to intervene to decrease the risk of developing adverse affective symptoms in this high-risk group. Therefore, this study analyzed a model linking early trauma with depressive symptoms via negative cognitions in young North Korean refugees. We specifically tested how different types of negative automatic thoughts according to the ideational contents would mediate the relationship.

2. Materials and Methods

2.1. Participants

Participants were recruited from two schools for North Korean refugees designed to prepare students for the national qualification examinations for middle- or high-school graduation. Two schools, both located in Seoul, South Korea, volunteered to participate in this study. Of the 114 students who attended these schools, five students declined to participate, resulting in a total of 109 students who were ultimately enrolled in the study. After obtaining approval from the school principal regarding the research protocol, the investigators visited each school, explained the purpose of the study, and obtained informed consent from the participants. This study was approved by the human subjects institutional review board at the National Center for Mental Health (no. 2015-17 and no. 116271-2017-22).

2.2. Measures

The socio-demographic variables assessed were sex, age, and perceived family economic status. Participants' perceived family social economic status (SES) was assessed using a five-point Likert scale (low = 1, low-middle = 2, middle = 3, high-middle= 4, and high = 5).

The Korean version of the Early Trauma Inventory Self Report-Short Form (ETISR-SF) [28,29] was used to assess the four domains of general experiences of traumatic events (11 items), as well as physical (5 items), emotional (5 items), and sexual abuse (6 items). The ETISR-SF consists of 27 items asking the experience of certain traumatic events that occurred before the age of 18 [28,29]. The presence of each traumatic experience was scored 1 (yes) or 0 (no), with total scores ranging from 0 to 27 (Cronbach's alpha = 0.86). To examine the link between variations in early trauma and depressive symptoms, we used early trauma sum scores by counting up the number of events that had ever occurred to the individual based on the scoring method created by the developers of this scale [28]. By comparing the validity of different methods for obtaining scores, Bremner et al. [28] concluded that the most parsimonious and easiest method is to count up the number of events that had ever occurred.

The Korean version of the Children's Automatic Thoughts Scale (CATS) [24,30] was used to assess a wide range of negative self-statements. The CATS consists of four cognitive content subscales, including physical threat (6 items; e.g., "I'm going to have an accident"; Cronbach's alpha = 0.947), social threat (10 items; e.g., "I'm worried that I'm going to get teased"; Cronbach's alpha = 0.828), personal failure (10 items; e.g., "I've made such a mess of my life"; Cronbach's alpha = 0.933), and hostility (6 items; e.g., "If someone hurts me, I have the right to hurt them back"; Cronbach's alpha = 0.915). Although the original version of the CATS contains 40 items, the Korean version only contains 32 items, as 8 items were excluded that showed low explanatory and discriminative power. Items are rated on a five-point Likert scale, with responses ranging from 0 (strongly disagree) to 4 (strongly agree), with higher scores reflecting a higher level of negative automatic thoughts [24,30].

The Korean version of the Center for Epidemiologic Studies-Depression Scale (CES-D) [31–33] was used to measure depression. The CES-D consists of 20 items rated on a four-point Likert scale, with responses ranging from 0 (rarely or never) to 3 (mostly or always), and total scores ranging from 0 to 60. A cutoff score of ≥ 21 is recommended in community settings to screen for individuals with depressive symptoms, and a cutoff score of ≥ 25 is recommended for a clinical diagnosis of depression in Korean populations [31,32]. This study used a cutoff score of ≥ 21 to classify participants with significant depressive symptoms.

2.3. Statistical Analysis

Descriptive statistics were first calculated for all socio-demographic and psychological variables for the entire sample. Correlation analysis was first conducted to test inter-relationships between psychological variables, including early trauma, depressive symptoms, and four factors of negative automatic thoughts. Path analysis was initially conducted on early trauma, depressive symptoms, and four factors of negative automatic thoughts (i.e., personal failure, physical threat, social threat, and hostility) to test which type of negative automatic thoughts could mediate the relationship between early traumatic experiences and depressive symptoms in North Korean refugees. Considering the significant effects on mental health of sex, age, and socioeconomic status noted in previous studies of North Korean refugees (for a review, see [26]), we adjusted for such sociodemographic variables as covariates in our model. The categorical variable (i.e., sex) was converted to a dummy variable in the model (i.e., female = 0, male = 1). To make our final model more parsimonious, the final path analysis was conducted after removing non-significant pathways and parameters that do not contribute to the outcome variable of interest (i.e., depressive symptoms) in a significant way [34]. All analyses were conducted using SPSS software Version 22.0 (SPSS Inc., Chicago, IL, USA) and AMOS Version 24.0 (SPSS Inc., Chicago, IL, USA). For all statistical analyses, $p < 0.05$ was considered significant.

3. Results

Of the 109 participants (68 females, 41 males; mean age = 19.52, SD = 3.28 years; 16 with low SES, 19 with low-middle SES, 49 with middle SES, 17 with high-middle SES, and 8 with high SES), 52 (47.7%) had significant depressive symptoms (CES-D $\geq$ 21). Table 1 presents the frequency of endorsement for different types of early traumatic events and each of the four domains. Among the respondents, 90.8% were endorsed for at least one early traumatic event and they reported, on average, 6.0 (SD 5.0) traumatic events. The most frequent early traumatic events included physical abuse (76.1%; M = 2.1, SD = 1.7), notably being slapped in the face (49.5%), punched or kicked (47.7%), hit with a thrown object (41.3%), and general traumatic events (76.1%; M = 2.1, SD = 2.1), notably, separation of parents (43.1%).

Table 1. Frequency of endorsement for the early trauma inventory item (N = 109).

Item	Frequency (%)
General trauma	76.1
T1. Natural disaster	10.1
T2. Serious accident	20.2
T3. Serious personal injury	27.5
T4. Serious injury/ illness of parent	22.0
T5. Separation of parents	43.1
T6. Serious illness/injury of sibling	10.1
T7. Serious injury of friend	14.7
T8. Witnessing violence	34.9
T9. Family mental illness	11.0
T10. Alcoholic parents	9.2
T11. Seeing someone murdered	10.1
Physical abuse	76.1
P1. Slapped in the face	49.5
P2. Burned with cigarette	34.9
P3. Punched or kicked	47.7
P4. Hit with thrown object	41.3
P5. Pushed or shoved	37.6
Emotional abuse	57.8
E1. Often put down or ridiculed	23.9
E2. Often ignored or made to feel you didn't count	37.6
E3. Often told you are no good	20.2
E4. Most of the time treated in cold or uncaring way	30.3
E5. Parents fail to understand your needs	27.5
Sexual abuse	18.3
S1. Touched in intimate parts in way that was uncomfortable	13.8
S2. Someone rubbing genitals against you	4.6
S3. Forced to touch intimate parts	5.5
S4. Someone had genital sex against your will	6.4
S5. Forced to perform oral sex	2.8
S6. Forced to kiss someone in sexual way	2.8

Table 2 presents correlations between early trauma and psychological variables. All main variables were significantly correlated with each other, with the exception of the correlation between early trauma and thoughts of social threat (r = 0.139, p = 0.149).

Table 2. Correlations among main variables.

Variable	1	2	3	4	5	6
1. CES-D	1					
2. ETI total	0.60 **	1				
3. CATS-Personal failure	0.61 **	0.40 **	1			
4. CATS-Social threat	0.20 *	0.14	0.33 **	1		
5. CATS-Physical threat	0.61 **	0.45 **	0.72 **	0.21 *	1	
6. CATS-Hostility	0.53 **	0.43 **	0.67 **	0.22 *	0.75 **	1
Mean	21.3	6.0	7.1	11.3	6.3	3.6
Standard deviation	10.9	5.0	8.6	5.6	8.1	5.3

CES-D, Center for Epidemiologic Studies-Depression Scale; ETI, Early Trauma Inventory; CATS, Children's Autonomic Thoughts Scale. * $p < 0.05$, ** $p < 0.01$.

Our first model (Figure 1) revealed that early trauma was positively associated with depressive symptoms (ß = 0.63; 95% CI = 0.50–0.74; $p = 0.01$). The links between early trauma and negative automatic thoughts were all significant with the exception of thoughts of social threat (ß = 0.15; 95% CI = −0.05–0.32; $p = 0.162$). The association of depressive symptoms with negative automatic thoughts was significant only with those of personal failure (ß = 0.28; 95% CI = 0.08–0.48; $p = 0.01$), but not with those of physical threat (ß = 0.24; 95% CI = −0.04–0.47; $p = 0.097$), social threat (ß = −0.01; 95% CI = −0.13–0.15; $p = 0.985$), or hostility (ß = 0.02; 95% CI = −0.16–0.25; $p = 0.971$) at a $p < 0.05$ significance level. These results indicate that only thoughts of personal failure may be a potential mediator of the association between early trauma and depressive symptoms.

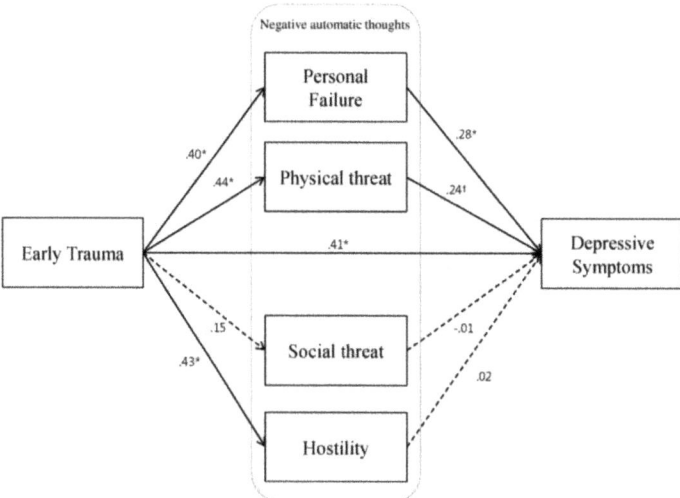

Figure 1. Path diagram illustrating the direct and indirect relationships between traumatic experiences, four types of negative automatic thoughts, and depressive symptoms, adjusting for sex, age, and family social economics status (Model 1). Standardized path coefficients (β) are reported in the model. Solid lines indicate significant associations and dotted lines indicate non-significant associations. † $p < 0.10$, * $p < 0.05$.

Accordingly, our final path analysis (Figure 2) was conducted to test the mediating role of the thoughts of personal failure in the association between early trauma and depressive symptoms (Figure 2), with the thoughts of physical threat, social threat, and hostility removed from the initial model. The path analysis consistently showed that early trauma events were positively associated with depressive symptoms (ß = 0.61; 95% CI = 0.48–0.73; p = 0.01) via thoughts of personal failure (ß = 0.17; 95% CI = 0.08–0.28; p = 0.01) as well as directly (ß = 0.44; 95% CI = 0.27–0.59; p = 0.01). These results indicated partial mediation effects of cognition of personal failure. Fit indices indicated that the model had a moderately good fit to the data (GFI = 0.97, NFI = 0.91, CFI = 0.96, RMSEA = 0.09).

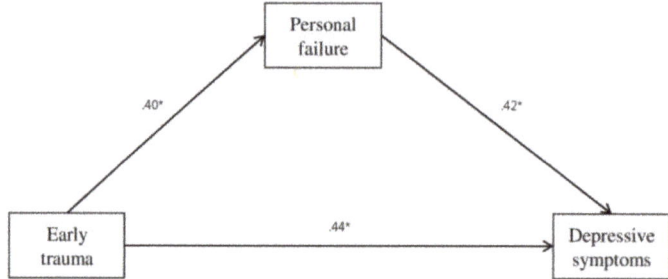

Figure 2. Path diagram illustrating the direct and indirect relationships between traumatic experiences, thoughts of personal failure, and depressive symptoms, adjusting for sex, age, and family social economics status (Model 2). Standardized path coefficients are reported in the model. Solid lines indicate significant associations. * p < 0.05. (as above mentioned)

4. Discussion

The prevalence of significant depressive symptoms of North Korean refugees in our study (47.7%) was as high as that of previous reports that used the same CES-D cut-off score of 21 or above [10,35,36]. The results of the present study indicated that early traumatic experiences were positively associated with depressive symptoms in a sample of North Korean refugees, which is consistent with prior studies that have found an association between childhood trauma and depression in other community populations [37,38].

Consistent with prior findings on the high prevalence of traumatic experiences in refugee populations [39,40], and specifically among North Korean refugees (for a review, [26]), our findings showed a high frequency of early traumatic experiences among North Korean adolescents and young adults. In comparison with healthy South Korean adolescent and adult samples from previous studies [29,41], young North Korean refugees in this study had a generally higher number of early traumatic events that had ever occurred (5.99 vs. 2.33–3.65). Specifically, the average number of general traumatic events and experiences of sexual abuse they had experienced (2.13, 0.36 respectively) was more than twice higher than that of Korean adolescents and adults (0.86–0.96, 0.13–0.17, respectively) and the number of instances of physical abuse and emotional abuse they had ever experienced (2.11, 1.39, respectively) also tends to be higher than that in the Korean samples (0.80–1.79, 0.54–0.74, respectively). The relatively greater number of endorsements for different types of traumatic events in our young North Korean refugee sample suggests widespread traumatic experiences and childhood maltreatment during their early years.

Furthermore, this study extends the understanding of the close link between early traumatic events and later depressive symptoms in North Korea refugees [7,8,42] by elucidating its underlying cognitive mechanisms. As hypothesized, in general, negative automatic thoughts partially mediated the association between early trauma and depressive symptoms, regardless of participants' sex, age, and socioeconomic status. The findings support cognitive theory of depression, which emphasizes the role of negative cognitions in linking past negative experiences, particularly in one's early years, with affective symptoms [11–13]. Our findings are also consistent with empirical data that has shown robust association of childhood trauma caused both by family and non-family perpetrators with negative cognitive style [14], as well as with adult depression [38].

This study further demonstrates the differential mediating roles of negative cognitions depending upon their themes. More specifically, the links between early trauma of North Korean refugees and their depressive symptoms were partially mediated by thoughts of personal failure, but not by thoughts of physical and social threat or hostility. In general, the findings support cognitive specificity theory, which proposes that different themes of cognitions are uniquely linked with each psychopathology [19]. This is in line with the fundamental assumptions of cognitive theorists, which argue that personal failure can be more linked with depression than with anxiety or anger [19,20].

While being subjected to the accumulated adversities in North Korea or during their escape, North Korean refugees may develop the inclination to attribute negative events to one's personal characteristics, such as ability, dispositions, or efforts, rather than to outside forces (i.e., internal attribution [13]), and this may cause them to engender the negative beliefs about the self and one's failure. These negative cognitive contents can be reactivated, especially when the refugees are faced with unexpected stressors after resettlement in South Korea [17], including acculturative stress, social discrimination, and isolation [43]. The reactivated negative cognitions may create helplessness in the face of actively coping with new adversities and, consequently, may hinder successful psychosocial adaptations in the host country. This can, in turn, reaffirm negative cognitions of the self. Such a vicious cycle could be applied to other refugee groups, with exposure to a wide array of traumatic experiences in their home country and during their flight, in addition to acculturative stress in their host country [40].

Our analysis also showed that North Korean refugees' early trauma was linked with activated thoughts of physical threat and hostility. Although these thoughts were not independently linked to depressive symptoms in our analysis, they may be linked to other psychological problems. Specifically, thoughts of physical threats can be linked with anxiety symptoms [19], whereas thoughts of hostility may be linked with anger and aggression by providing justification for such behaviors [44]. Future studies on the roles of the different contents of automatic thoughts in mediating early trauma and other psychiatric symptoms could extend the understanding of the cognitive mechanisms that underlie diverse psychological consequences of widespread trauma in refugee populations.

These findings also extend prior studies that have examined mediators and moderators of the association between traumatic events and psychiatric symptoms. For example, Kim [45] found that post-traumatic stress disorder (PTSD) symptoms mediated the negative effect of past interpersonal traumatic events on other mental health comorbidities, such as depression and anxiety. In a moderator analysis, Park et al. [6] found that the relationship between the number of past traumas and PTSD symptoms was stronger for those with alexithymia. Our findings further highlight the mediating role of the negative cognitive processes in psychological sequelae of early trauma. It should be noted that maladaptive cognitive patterns characterized by negative views of the self, future, and the world predict the persistence of depression in later years (for a review, [17]). In this vein, our findings suggest that, in order to alleviate and prevent later depressive symptoms, it is necessary to develop interventions that target negative cognitions for North Korean refugees with early trauma.

The present study has several limitations. First, given that this study was cross-sectional in nature, the temporal relationship among early traumatic experiences, negative cognition, and depressive symptoms could not be determined. It should be noted that mediation analyses are conditional on the validity of the path model being tested and cannot confirm causal model [46]. However, our model is a theoretically driven top-down model, which makes our mediation analysis more logically valid. Finally, given that schools volunteered to participate in this study, participants in the current study may not be representative of the larger population of young North Korean refugees.

5. Conclusions

Our data revealed that early traumatic experiences influence depressive symptoms, both directly and indirectly, via negative cognitions among young North Korean refugees. Given the high prevalence of depression as well as early trauma in this population, early depression screening is advisable for

North Korean refugees with severe traumatic experiences. In particular, our findings suggest that interventions for North Korean refugees with a high susceptibility to depression should aim to correct negative cognitive processes, especially cognitions regarding personal failure.

Acknowledgments: This work was supported by a National Research Foundation of Korea (NRF) grant funded by the Korean Government (NRF-2016R1D1A1B03931297).

Author Contributions: Subin Park and Jin Yong Jun conceived and designed the experiments; Jin Yong Jun collected the data; Subin Park analyzed the data and wrote the paper; Yeeun Lee helped to write the paper.

Conflicts of Interest: The authors declare no conflict of interest.

References

1. Jeon, W.T.; Yu, S.E.; Cho, Y.A.; Eom, J.S. Traumatic experiences and mental health of North Korean refugees in South Korea. *Psychiatry Investig.* **2008**, *5*, 213–220. [CrossRef] [PubMed]
2. Jeon, W.; Min, S.; Lee, M.; Lee, E. A study on adaptation of North Koreans in South Korea. *J. Korean Neuropsychiatr. Assoc.* **1997**, *36*, 145–161.
3. Nam, B.; Kim, J.Y.; DeVylder, J.E.; Song, A. Family functioning, resilience, and depression among North Korean refugees. *Psychiatry Res.* **2016**, *245*, 451–457. [CrossRef] [PubMed]
4. Kim, Y.-H. Predictors for mental health problems among young North Korean refugees in South Korea. *Contemp. Soc. Multicul.* **2013**, *3*, 264–285.
5. Choi, Y.; Lim, S.Y.; Jun, J.Y.; Lee, S.H.; Yoo, S.Y.; Kim, S.; Gwak, A.R.; Kim, J.-C.; Lee, Y.J.; Kim, S.J. The effect of traumatic experiences and psychiatric symptoms on the life satisfaction of North Korean refugees. *Psychopathology* **2017**, *50*, 203–210. [CrossRef] [PubMed]
6. Park, J.; Jun, J.Y.; Lee, Y.J.; Kim, S.; Lee, S.H.; Yoo, S.Y.; Kim, S.J. The association between alexithymia and posttraumatic stress symptoms following multiple exposures to traumatic events in North Korean refugees. *J. Psychosom. Res.* **2015**, *78*, 77–81. [CrossRef] [PubMed]
7. Kim, Y.J.; Cho, Y.A.; Kim, H.A. A mediation effect of ego resiliency between stresses and mental health of North Korean refugee youth in South Korea. *Child Adolesc. Soc. Work J.* **2015**, *32*, 481–490. [CrossRef]
8. Emery, C.R.; Lee, J.Y.; Kang, C. Life after the pan and the fire: Depression, order, attachment, and the legacy of abuse among North Korean refugee youth and adolescent children of North Korean refugees. *Child Abuse Negl.* **2015**, *45*, 90–100. [CrossRef] [PubMed]
9. Han, I.Y. Depressive traits of North Korean defectors. *Ment. Health Soc. Work* **2001**, *11*, 78–94.
10. Kim, H.H.; Lee, Y.J.; Kim, H.K.; Kim, J.E.; Kim, S.J.; Bae, S.-M.; Cho, S.-J. Prevalence and correlates of psychiatric symptoms in North Korean defectors. *Psychiatry Investig.* **2011**, *8*, 179–185. [CrossRef] [PubMed]
11. Beck, A.T. Cognitive models of depression. *J. Cogn. Psychother.* **1987**, *1*, 5–37.
12. Seligman, M.E.P. Learned helplessness. *Annu. Rev. Med.* **1972**, *23*, 407–412. [CrossRef] [PubMed]
13. Rose, D.T.; Abramson, L. Developmental predictors of depressive cognitive style: Research and theory. *Dev. Perspect. Depress.* **1992**, *4*, 323.
14. Gibb, B.E. Childhood maltreatment and negative cognitive styles: A quantitative and qualitative review. *Clin. Psychol. Rev.* **2002**, *22*, 223–246. [CrossRef]
15. Janoff-Bulman, R. Assumptive worlds and the stress of traumatic events: Applications of the schema construct. *Soc. Cogn.* **1989**, *7*, 113–136. [CrossRef]
16. Beck, A.T.; Brown, B.; Steer, R.A.; Eidelson, J.I.; Riskind, J.H. Differentiating anxiety and depression utilizing the Cognition Checklist. *J. Abnorm. Psychol.* **1987**, *96*, 179–183. [CrossRef] [PubMed]
17. Teasdale, J.D. Cognitive vulnerability to persistent depression. *Cogn. Emotion.* **1988**, *2*, 247–274. [CrossRef]
18. Mathews, A.; MacLeod, C. Cognitive vulnerability to emotional disorders. *Ann. Rev. Clin. Psychol.* **2005**, *1*, 167–195. [CrossRef] [PubMed]
19. Beck, A.T. *Cognitive Therapy of the Emotional Disorders*; New York American Library: New York, NY, USA, 1976.
20. Beck, A.T.; Clark, D.A. Anxiety and depression: An information processing perspective. *Anxiety Res.* **1988**, *1*, 23–36. [CrossRef]
21. Jolly, J.B.; Dyck, M.J.; Kramer, T.A.; Wherry, J.N. Integration of positive and negative affectivity and cognitive content-specificity: Improved discrimination of anxious and depressive symptoms. *J. Abnorm. Psychol.* **1994**, *103*, 544–552. [CrossRef] [PubMed]

22. Clark, D.A.; Beck, A.T.; Brown, G. Cognitive mediation in general psychiatric outpatients: A test of the content-specificity hypothesis. *J. Pers. Soc. Psychol.* **1989**, *56*, 958–964. [CrossRef] [PubMed]
23. Safren, S.A.; Heimberg, R.G.; Lerner, J.; Henin, A.; Warman, M.; Kendall, P.C. Differentiating anxious and depressive self-statements: Combined factor structure of the anxious self-statements questionnaire and the automatic thoughts questionnaire-revised. *Cogn. Ther. Res.* **2000**, *24*, 327–344. [CrossRef]
24. Schniering, C.A.; Rapee, R.M. Development and validation of a measure of children's automatic thoughts: The children's automatic thoughts scale. *Behav. Res. Ther.* **2002**, *40*, 1091–1109. [CrossRef]
25. Schniering, C.A.; Rapee, R.M. The structure of negative self-statements in children and adolescents: A confirmatory factor-analytic approach. *J. Abnorm. Child Psychol.* **2004**, *32*, 95–109. [CrossRef] [PubMed]
26. Lee, Y.; Lee, M.; Park, S. Mental health status of North Korean refugees in South Korea and risk and protective factors: A 10-year review of the literature. *Eur. J. Psychotraumatol.* **2017**, *8*, 1369833. [CrossRef] [PubMed]
27. Montgomery, E. Trauma, exile and mental health in young refugees. *Acta Psychiatr. Scand.* **2011**, *124*, 1–46. [CrossRef] [PubMed]
28. Bremner, J.D.; Bolus, R.; Mayer, E.A. Psychometric properties of the Early Trauma Inventory-Self Report. *J. Nerv. Ment. Dis.* **2007**, *195*, 211–218. [CrossRef] [PubMed]
29. Jeon, J.R.; Lee, E.H.; Lee, S.W.; Jeong, E.G.; Kim, J.H.; Lee, D.; Jeon, H.J. The early trauma inventory self report-short form: Psychometric properties of the Korean version. *Psychiatry Investig.* **2012**, *9*, 229–235. [CrossRef] [PubMed]
30. Moon, H.; Oh, K.; Moon, H. Validation study of Korean Children's Automatic Thoughts Scale. *Korean J. Clin. Psychol.* **2002**, *21*, 955–963.
31. Cho, M.J.; Kim, K.H. Diagnostic validity of the CES-D (Korean version) in the assessment of DSM-III-R major depression. *J. Korean Neuropsychiatr. Assoc.* **1993**, *32*, 381–399.
32. Cho, M.J.; Kim, K.H. Use of the Center for Epidemiologic Studies Depression (CES-D) Scale in Korea. *J. Nerv. Ment. Dis.* **1998**, *186*, 304–310. [CrossRef] [PubMed]
33. Radloff, L.S. The CES-D scale: A self-report depression scale for research in the general population. *Appl. Psychol. Meas.* **1977**, *1*, 385–401. [CrossRef]
34. Olobatuyi, M.E. *A User's Guide to Path Analysis*; University Press of America: Lanham, MD, USA, 2006; p. 40.
35. Lee, Y.-J.G.; Jun, J.Y.; Lee, Y.J.; Park, J.; Kim, S.; Lee, S.H.; Yu, S.Y.; Kim, S.J. Insomnia in North Korean refugees: Association with depression and post-traumatic stress symptoms. *Psychiatry Investig.* **2016**, *13*, 67–73. [CrossRef] [PubMed]
36. Jeon, B.-H.; Kim, M.-D.; Hong, S.-C.; Kim, N.-R.; Lee, C.-I.; Kwak, Y.-S.; Park, J.-H.; Chung, J.; Chong, H.; Jwa, E.-K.; et al. Prevalence and correlates of depressive symptoms among North Korean defectors living in South Korea for more than one year. *Psychiatry Investig.* **2009**, *6*, 122–130. [CrossRef] [PubMed]
37. Li, M.; D'Arcy, C.; Meng, X. Maltreatment in childhood substantially increases the risk of adult depression and anxiety in prospective cohort studies: Systematic review, meta-analysis, and proportional attributable fractions. *Psychol. Med.* **2015**, *46*, 717–730. [CrossRef] [PubMed]
38. Nelson, J.; Klumparendt, A.; Doebler, P.; Ehring, T. Childhood maltreatment and characteristics of adult depression: Meta-analysis. *Br. J. Psychiatry* **2016**. [CrossRef] [PubMed]
39. Porter, M.; Haslam, N. Predisplacement and postdisplacement factors associated with mental health of refugees and internally displaced persons: A meta-analysis. *JAMA* **2005**, *294*, 602–612. [CrossRef] [PubMed]
40. Steel, Z.; Chey, T.; Silove, D.; Marnane, C.; Bryant, R.A.; van Ommeren, M. Association of torture and other potentially traumatic events with mental health outcomes among populations exposed to mass conflict and displacement. *JAMA* **2009**, *302*, 537–549. [CrossRef] [PubMed]
41. Park, S. Reliability and validity of the early trauma inventory self report-short form among Korean adolescents. *J. Korean Acad. Child Adolesc. Psychiatry* **2018**, *29*, 2–6. [CrossRef]
42. Cho, Y.A.; Jeon, W.; Yu, J.J.; Um, J.-S. Predictors of depression among North Korean defectors: A 3-year follow-up study. *Korean J. Couns. Psychother.* **2005**, *17*, 467–484.
43. Korea Hana Foundation. *Survey on Social Integration of North Korean Defectors*; Korea Hana Foundation: Seoul, Korea, 2017.
44. Beck, A.T. *Prisoners of Hate: The Cognitive Basis of Anger, Hostility, and Violence*; HarperCollins: New York, NY, USA, 1999.

45. Kim, Y. Posttraumatic stress disorder as a mediator between trauma exposure and comorbid mental health conditions in North Korean refugee youth resettled in South Korea. *J. Interpers. Violence* **2014**, *31*, 425–443. [CrossRef] [PubMed]
46. Fiedler, K.; Harris, C.; Schott, M. Unwarranted inferences from statistical mediation tests—An analysis of articles published in 2015. *J. Exp. Soc. Psychol.* **2018**, *75*, 95–102. [CrossRef]

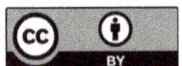

© 2018 by the authors. Licensee MDPI, Basel, Switzerland. This article is an open access article distributed under the terms and conditions of the Creative Commons Attribution (CC BY) license (http://creativecommons.org/licenses/by/4.0/).

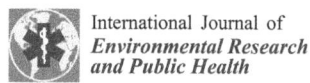

Commentary

The Emergency Medical System in Greece: Opening Aeolus' Bag of Winds

Ourania S. Kotsiou [1,*], David S. Srivastava [2], Panagiotis Kotsios [3], Aristomenis K. Exadaktylos [2] and Konstantinos I. Gourgoulianis [1]

1. Respiratory Medicine Department, Faculty of Medicine, University of Thessaly, Biopolis, 41500 Larissa, Greece; kgourg@med.uth.gr
2. Inselspital, University Hospital Bern, 3010 Bern, Switzerland; DavidShiva.Srivastava@insel.ch (D.S.S.); Aristomenis.Exadaktylos@insel.ch (A.K.E.)
3. International Business Department, Perrotis College, 57001 Thessaloniki, Greece; panagiotiskotsios@gmail.com
* Correspondence: raniakotsiou@gmail.com; Tel.: +30-2413-502812

Received: 21 March 2018; Accepted: 10 April 2018; Published: 13 April 2018

Abstract: An Emergency Medical Service (EMS) system must encompass a spectrum of care, with dedicated pre-hospital and in-hospital medical facilities. It has to be organised in such a way as to include all necessary services—such as triage accurate initial assessment, prompt resuscitation, efficient management of emergency cases, and transport to definitive care. The global economic downturn has had a direct effect on the health sector and poses additional threats to the healthcare system. Greece is one of the hardest-hit countries. This manuscript aims to present the structure of the Greek EMS system and the impact of the current economic recession on it. Nowadays, primary care suffers major shortages in crucial equipment, unmet health needs, and ineffective central coordination. Patients are also facing economic limitations that lead to difficulties in using healthcare services. The multi-factorial problem of in-hospital EMS overcrowding is also evident and has been linked with potentially poorer clinical outcomes. Furthermore, the ongoing refugee crisis challenges the national EMS. Adoption of a triage scale, expansion of the primary care network, and an effective primary–hospital continuum of care are urgently needed in Greece to provide comprehensive, culturally competent, and high-quality health care.

Keywords: ambulance; economic recession; emergency medical service; Greece; primary healthcare system; refugee; triage

1. Introduction

Emergency Medical Services (EMS) have been described as "a comprehensive system which provides the arrangements of personnel, facilities, and equipment for the effective, coordinated, and timely delivery of health and adequate and specialized services to victims of sudden illness or injury" [1]. High-quality EMS is a major factor in any healthcare system.

An EMS system encompasses a spectrum of care characterised by dedicated medical facilities at the pre-hospital and in-hospital levels. It has to be organised in such a way as to include all necessary services—such as triage accurate initial assessment, prompt resuscitation, efficient and effective medical management, and transport of emergency cases to definitive care [1].

However, recent estimates have shown that 24 million patients die each year in low- and middle-income countries due to unprepared pre-hospital and in-hospital medical systems [2]. In detail, it has been previously reported that, in high-income settings, 59% of trauma deaths that occurred at the pre-hospital level were deemed as preventable [3]. The rates increased further in the middle- and low-income prehospital environments (72% and 81%, respectively) [3,4]. On the other hand, globally, the prevalence and mortality of emergency conditions remain high [2–5]. The burden of disease that requires emergency management is higher in low-income countries [5]. Analytically, the median disability-adjusted life years (DALYs) burden has been estimated at 48,000, 25,000, and 16,000 per 100,000 people for low-, middle- and high-income countries respectively [5].

It is widely accepted that an economic recession may have a severe impact on the psychological well-being of the patient population and may act as a precipitator for suicide risk [6]. Furthermore, it can increase the burden of chronic diseases, for instance in case of chronic obstructive pulmonary disease [6]. An economic crisis may also impair the coronary health of vulnerable individuals [6]. Notably, it has been argued that an economic recession could pose negative consequences for both quality of care and patients' outcomes [6]. It should be emphasised that emergency departments (EDs) are where society's problems first show up, from drug abuse and domestic violence to the health problems of the poor and uninsured [7]. When the 2007 global economic downturn began, it spread to Europe rapidly and Greece was one of the hardest-hit countries. This manuscript aims to present the structure of the Greek pre-hospital and in-hospital emergency care and summarize the consequences of the current economic recession on the Greek EMS system. A computer-based search of the English literature was performed in PubMed and Scopus. The considerable body of information examined in this article includes data that are to a large extent, but not exclusively, presented in Greek studies.

2. Greek EMS Structure

2.1. Greek Pre-Hospital EMS Structure: Past and Present

Since the 1970s, prehospital emergency health care can mainly be divided into two distinct models. These are the "load and go" Anglo-American model versus the "delay and treat" Franco-German model [1]. Another EMS delivery system has attracted attention in the United Kingdom. According to this, the role of primary health care is strengthened, thus, increasing the percentage of patients who are treated in a pre-hospital community setting or at the scene of an incident [1]. These categorical distinctions were accurate until the end of the 20th century [1]. Today, most EMS systems around the world partially share features of all aforementioned models [1].

The Greek health system is cure-oriented. Anglo-American EMS principles are mainly applied in Greece. Before 1985, the Greek Red Cross and the Samaritans were responsible for rendering healthcare services, otherwise medical care was provided privately. The creation of the national healthcare system (ESY, NHS) in 1983 constituted a milestone in establishing a Greek healthcare system [8].

In 1915, Greek EMS began with the creation of the first aid station, funded by "Sotir" (Saviour), a non-profit organization [8]. From 1932 to 1988, the Samaritans founded several emergency stations in Athens, Thessaloniki, and Patras and equipped them with some ambulances [8]. In 1965, primary health care expanded into four major stations in Athens, Piraeus, Thessaloniki, and Patras, founded by the Social Insurance Institute (IKA). These stations were equipped with four additional ambulances [8]. In 1987, the two previous providers of EMS in Greece, the Hellenic Red Cross and IKA, merged to become the Hellenic EMS (EKAB) [8]. This process also established "166" as the national emergency number. Since then, Greek EMS has been exclusively handled by EKAB, which is entirely funded by the government [8].

2.2. Structure of Pre-Hospital EMS in Greece

Pre-hospital EMS is composed of different services ranging from healthcare positions attended by active medical personnel to call centres (dispatch centres) attended by professionals that can determine and handle urgency, to offer medical advice and to urgently dispatch a mobile medical unit [8].

2.2.1. EMS Dispatch System in Greece

Today, EMS is managed via 12 EKAB stations in the major Greek cities (Figure 1) [8]. Several substations in smaller cities are controlled by a central station, so that a larger area can be supervised.

Together this network covers 96.2% of the urban areas [8]. A local hospital coordinates and cooperates with local healthcare stations. It plays a crucial role in supporting primary care and acts as a gateway to more specialized care [8]. The EMS system supervises and provides advice to the EKAB stations [8].

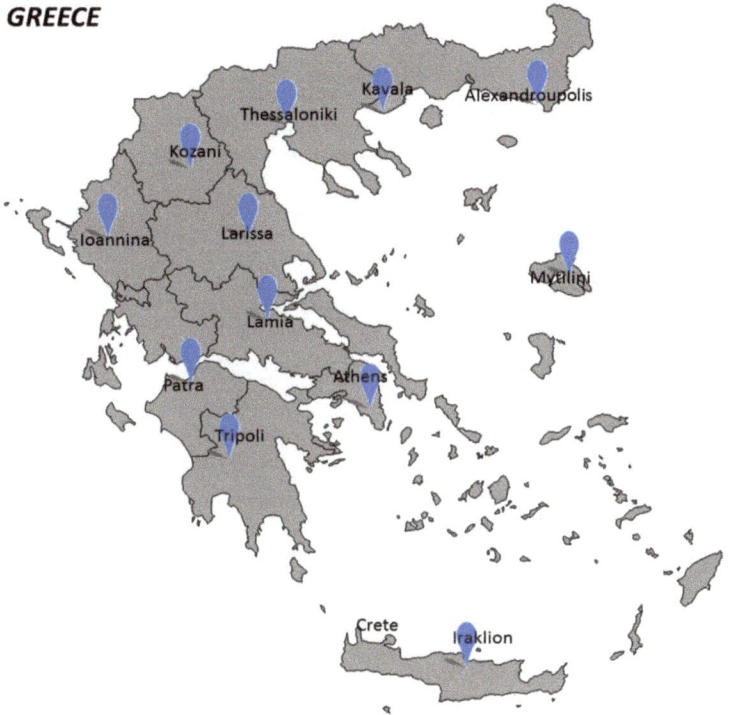

Figure 1. National Centres for Emergency Care (EKAB stations) in Greece. There are 12 EKAB stations in the major Greek cities: Athens, Thessaloniki, Patra, Iraklion (Crete), Larissa, Kavala, Ioannina, Alexandroupolis, Lamia, Mytilini, Tripoli, Kozani. Adapted from: https://www.ekab.gr/chorotaxiki-katanomi/ [9].

Accordingly, EKAB stations and substations have their medical staff administrators and call centre [8]. Healthcare functions are traditionally carried out by physicians and emergency medical technicians (EMTs) [8]. Further, each station has its ambulances and medical equipment [8]. The EKAB possesses 740 basic life support ambulances, of which 502 are used by EKAB stations and 238 by hospitals and primary healthcare stations. Moreover, it holds 174 Mobile Intensive Care Units (MICUs), along with 25 motorcycles, 4 small vehicles for minor roads (smart, fast, saxos), three helicopters, 2 traffic coordination centres, and 2 vehicles modified for disaster recovery (Figure 2) [8].

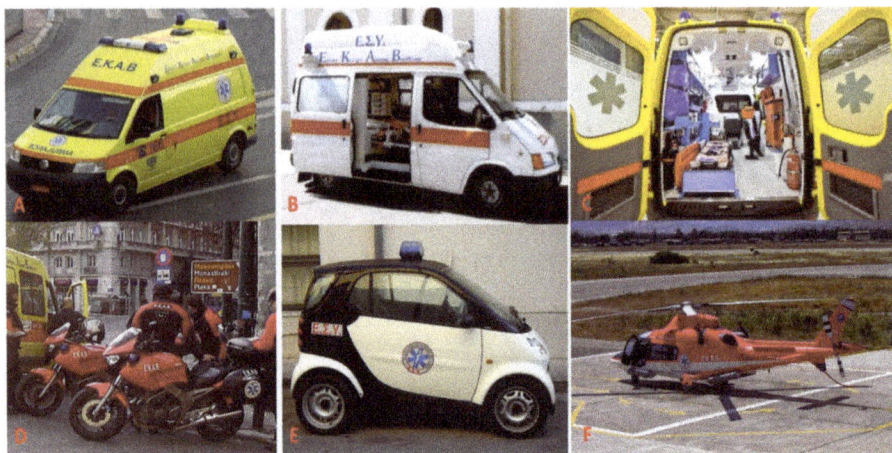

Figure 2. Types of EKAB ambulances. (**A,B**) Basic type of Ambulance; (**C**) Mobile Intensive Care Units; (**D**) Motorcycle ambulances; (**E**) Small vehicles for minor roads; (**F**) Helicopters.

Two types of ambulances are staffed by emergency personnel and are used for emergency transportations [8]. One type is the basic ambulance (Figure 2A,B) which has standard medical equipment for primary airway management procedures and oxygen delivery such as bag-mask ventilation, oxygen supplements, and a portable suction. Furthermore, it is equipped with an automated external defibrillator (AED), first aid wound care supplies, intravenous access kits, and immobilisation equipment. All ambulances are crewed by EMTs. This type of ambulance is the most commonly used [8].

The second type consists of MICUs (Figure 2C). These ambulances are equipped with more advanced equipment for skillful cardiopulmonary resuscitation, airway management, and adequate oxygenation, such as ventilators, pulse oximeters, a non-invasive transcutaneous pacemaker, a cardiac monitor, and defibrillators with (3-lead)-ECG-monitoring. MICUs are also fitted with intravenous access equipment, various devices for immobilization, as well as fluid replacement therapies in cases of hypovolemic shock and several drugs [8]. These units are mainly used in large cities like Athens and Thessaloniki and are staffed by a sole paramedic and an anesthesiologist [8]. Due to the heavy traffic conditions, these units can provide advanced life support much faster than an ambulance [8]. They initiate prehospital emergency care on the spot while waiting for the transport ambulance to arrive, thus saving valuable time when treating trauma patients [8].

The MICUs in Thessaloniki are also equipped with non-invasive positive pressure ventilation (Boussignac CPAP). They are certified to provide chest tube insertion and drainage as well as qualified management of difficult airways demanding intubation. Similarly, they are staffed both by a physician and EMTs [8].

Furthermore, in the five major cities (Athens, Thessaloniki, Patras, Larissa, and Iraklion), motorcycle ambulances are either single- or double-crewed. Specifically, they carry a solo paramedic (in Thessaloniki), or there is one physician with paramedic coverage (in Athens, Patras, Iraklion and Ioannina), respectively, to achieve a rapid response in the provision of medical care (Figure 2D) [8].

EKAB is also a significant aeromedical transportation provider, being the owner of three helicopters (Augusta A-109 Power) (Figure 2E) [8]. It has been recently estimated that approximately 500,000 patients are transported by EKAB per year. Furthermore, 2000 to 2500 medical flights were conducted per year [8].

Emergency medical support (EKAB) is accessible throughout the country firstly by the universal emergency phone number "112" as well as by the toll-free "166" (Figure 3) [8].

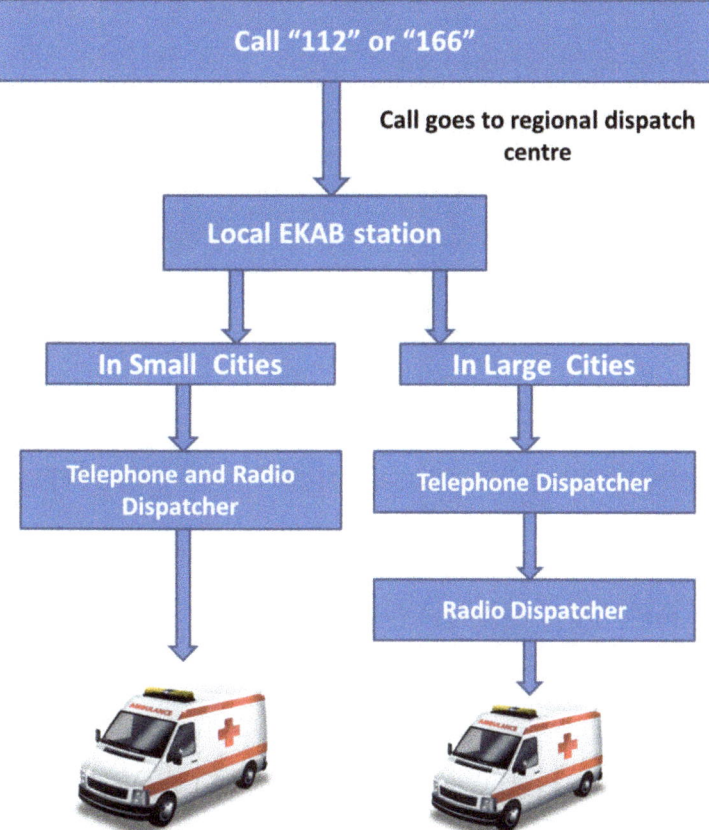

Figure 3. Dispatch process flowchart for Greece. All EKAB stations have their dispatch centres. EKAB is accessible throughout the country firstly by the European emergency phone number "112" as well as by the toll-free, easy to remember "166". The call goes to the regional dispatch centre. A telephone dispatcher receives various calls and prioritises them according to importance or urgency. In large cities, telephone dispatchers mobilize the appropriate number of nearest available mobile ambulances or Mobile Intensive Care Units (MICUs) via radio communications and provide directions to arrive at the scene of the incident. On the contrary, in small cities, the dispatcher telephones the nearest ambulance station or else passes mobilization instructions to the radio operator if an ambulance is already mobile. Adapted from: Page C et al. [10].

The dispatch centres consist of experienced operators (dispatchers) who triage phone calls; a complete telephone and radio recording system; and a computer network for data throughput, storage, and processing [10]. A properly implemented EMS telemedicine system is used for the guidance of aeromedical transportation [8]. EKAB dispatcher control stations handle emergency calls via telephone or radio communications [8,10]. The dispatchers receive calls from individuals, pre-hospital or in-hospital healthcare facilities, and other emergency agencies such as police or fire brigades [8]. They prioritize the urgency and decide where the case should be transferred. Besides, there is direct communication between the transferring and receiving facilities [8]. All dispatch centres are composed of physicians [8]. In case of a catastrophe, one of the major priorities of the dispatch centre is to coordinate healthcare institutes with other rescue services, such as the military, the police, and the firefighters [8]. Moreover, although the improvement of telemedicine systems has allowed wireless data transmission from moving vehicles, these technologies still are not widely used in Greek EMS system [1].

Remarkably, emergency medicine is not yet a recognised specialty in Greece. However, a Greek Society for Emergency Medicine was established in 2007 [8].

Furthermore, education and training centres were established in almost all EKAB stations in 1987 [8]. By 1989, all EMTs had received a 40 h training course [8]. In 1989, the Ministry of Health introduced a basic EMT training program [8]. Since 1995, four EKAB education centres have been founded in the biggest Greek cities (Athens, Thessaloniki, Patras, and Iraklion) and offered physicians a one-year course, comprising 400 h of training, 75 h of classroom-based training, 25 h of workshops, and 300 h of skills training. The training program is performed at EDs, Departments of Anesthesiology, adult and Neonatal Intensive Care Units, Cardiac Intensive Care Units and in the MICUs [8]. Currently, courses are organised into subjects that cover assessment of the critical illness and triage, airway skills, basic and advanced life support (BLS, ALS), resuscitation and advanced trauma life support (immobilization of injured bones and wound management) [8].

In 2000, a more advanced educational program was developed, establishing and developing a professional body recognised by national law [8]. This free of charge, two-year program offers extensive theoretical knowledge and practical experience through 1400 h of technical training, divided into 800 h of theoretical training and 600 h of clinical practice in hospitals and ambulances [8]. Furthermore, these programs offer courses in anatomy, physiology, pharmacology, pathology, ECG-monitoring, as well as training in methods of venous access, disaster management, established guidelines, safe driving, the English language, communication systems, and technologies and computer training [8]. Lastly, two semester-length training courses have been recently approved by the National Organization for the Certification of Qualifications and Vocational Guidance (EOPPEP), a national authority responsible for lifelong learning services [8]. After having completed each of the aforementioned courses, recipients obtain the diploma of "Adequacy in Prehospital Emergency Medicine" [8]. More anesthetists and fewer cardiologists were among the first physicians who were employed by EKAB services and National Health System [8].

2.2.2. Primary Healthcare Services in Greece

The Greek NHS consists of 201 rural and 3 urban primary healthcare centres, 1478 positions in rural medicine and many outpatient departments in 140 public hospitals [11]. Primary health centres are composed of 1787 full-time salaried doctors (mainly general practitioners (GPs), specialists in internal medicine, paediatricians and dentists) and approximately 2414 other health professionals, most of them enjoying permanent tenure [11]. Thus, many small medical centres are often staffed by medical doctors without a specialty [11]. Significantly, only recently, young and inexperienced doctors have been gradually replaced by general practitioners, according to the national law 2519/97, which, however, was passed in 1997 [11].

From 1994 to 2009, several reform proposals were aimed at encouraging patients' freedom of choice in health care, at introducing the family physician as the cornerstone of primary care system's structure, and unifying primary care services [11], but eventually none were implemented [11].

Consequently, the approaching obstacles faced by patients in rural areas forcing them to seek quality healthcare services in urban areas, private practice, and EDs [11].

Furthermore, some of the main reasons for the high primary healthcare costs are, firstly, that most GPs, although they work for the NHS, are also private practitioners, and, secondly, the repetition of tests and prescriptions due to poor electronic medical record systems [11–13]. The latter is perhaps the most critical factor demonstrating the ineffectiveness of the existing control mechanisms of health insurance funds [11–13].

2.3. In-Hospital EMS in Greece

An ED may be considered the benchmark, by which the quality of a healthcare system is estimated [1]. EDs constitute the vital link between pre-hospital and in-hospital medical care that provides professional care at any time [14].

The most basics components of a well-functioning control ED are the presence of triage, supported by national clinical guidelines to help state EMS systems to standardise their patient care [1,5]. Overcrowding and misuse of EDs have established the need for development and introduction of triage protocols throughout the whole EMS system, to achieve appropriate emergency care for patients [14]. Although almost all European Members (24/27) record triage protocol compliance in their hospital, only 19 countries claim that triage protocols are used by physicians [14–16]. Furthermore, only 9/27 and 10/27 European Member States have approved guidelines standardised by national standards or electronic recording, respectively [14–16].

In Greece, the majority of in-hospital EMS settings use triage systems to prioritise incoming patients rapidly. The aforementioned systems are standardised at a national level. However, the networks of clinical information are underdeveloped [16] and triage protocols are often not used by physicians [14–16]. In most cases, patients presenting to an ED have typically first been assessed by a nurse [15,16]. Hence, the nurse is allowed to assign the patient to a queueing system [15,16]. The emergency cases in Greece are usually sorted into surgical or medical emergencies and appropriately treated by specialists. Most of the subspecialties are forced to make disposition decisions, based mainly on their expertise and intuition, unfortunately without the presence of a standardized set of uniform codes and guidelines [14,15]. In life-threatening situations, anesthetists are involved [14,15]. Usually, the anesthetists manage the in-hospital emergencies or act as part of the resuscitation team [14,15]. In 2003, a law was promulgated governing the EDs' development and operation in public hospitals with more than 200 beds. In 2004, the Olympic Games emerged as an important tool of EDs' renewal [8].

3. Does Economic Recession Lead to Healthcare Crisis? What the Numbers Tell Us

According to the latest census by the Hellenic Statistical Authority (2011), Greece has a population of 10,816,286 [17]. The Greek population is equivalent to 0.15% of the total world population [17]. 78.7% of the population is urban (8,764,013 people in 2018) and they often have difficulties in accessing healthcare services [17]. Greece is one of the countries hardest hit by the economic crisis that began in 2009, and which has forced millions into poverty [18,19]. According to estimates made by Eurostat in 2015, 35.7% of the population are at risk of poverty or social exclusion [18,19].

The economic recession had a particularly significant negative impact on the gross domestic product (GDP) in Greece, as well as on annual healthcare spending growth. The country's GDP fell from 236 billion € in 2008 to 184 billion € in 2016, a value loss of 22% [18].

Before the crisis, total health expenditure was estimated at 8.6% of GDP in 2003. It rose further in 2009 reaching 9.9%, of which 5.3% and 4.5% was of public and private origin, respectively [19]. Notably, total health expenditure as a percentage of GDP was in line with the European average, but has decreased substantially since the crisis started [18]. The mean per capita expenditure on health services in Greece was about threefold lower than the mean amount for European Union (EU) (€26.2 vs. €75.8) in 2009 [18] and dropped further by 13% in the coming years (€23.1 in 2012). Additionally, the mean per capita healthcare expenditure suffered a decline from €2977 in 2009 to €1663 in 2015 with an overall decrease of 6.6% since 2009 [13,19,20].

For Greece, this drop signaled a fall in health spending [18]. According to Eurostat, the Greek healthcare system was allocated €8.5 billion in 2016, or 4.9% of GDP [21].

Total (outpatient) pharmaceutical expenditure has been estimated to have decreased by 32% (€2.1 billion), but this was to the benefit of the Social Health Insurance funds which are the main funders of these expenditures [19]. The largest reduction was in public pharmaceutical expenditure (and other non-medical durables), at 43.2%—from €5.2 billion (roughly 2.25% of GDP) in 2009 to

€2.95 billion (or 1.53% of GDP) in 2012 [19]. According to the terms laid down by the Memorandum of Understanding (MoUs) that designate the country's fiscal policies and which was signed in 2009 by the Greek governments, the International Monetary Fund (IMF), the European Central Bank (ECB), and the European Commission (EC), pharmaceutical expenditure should not have exceeded €2.44 billion in 2013 and €2 billion in 2014 [20]. If these thresholds were exceeded, clawbacks from the pharmaceutical companies would be used to balance the budget [20]. Moreover, out-of-pocket pharmaceutical expenditure increased as a percentage of total health expenditure—from 27.6% in 2009 to 28.8% in 2012 [19,22].

It is also accepted that the frequency with which patients access emergency care is usually more strongly associated with a country's burden of diseases than its gross national income [5]. In fact, the economic recession has negatively affected the health status of the population in Greece [6,18]. The leading causes of death in the country are cardiovascular diseases, malignancies, and external causes of injury (accidents) and poisoning (suicides and homicides), which are responsible for 72% of all deaths across the world, in 2015 [23]. Moreover, premature mortality rates, mainly from cardiovascular diseases, are higher in Greece than the European average [23]. Likewise, age-standardised mortality from all causes is higher in Greece than in other European countries, which can be explained by the excess mortality from diseases of the circulatory and respiratory system [23]. Moreover, the numbers of infant and maternal deaths, and suicides and homicides (for males only) have also increased [23].

4. Impact of the Economic Recession on EMS Function

4.1. Impact of the Economic Recession on Pre-Hospital EMS System

Though Greece's economic recession may be stealing the limelight, the National Health Service as well EMS has been majorly affected by austerity [24]. The major problems that emergency service providers face today are the following: unbalanced distribution of primary healthcare centres according to population densities, inadequate training of primary healthcare staff, inefficient communication and transfer protocols, understaffing of ambulance services and unpaid overtime, and unrepaired vehicles due to budget problems [24]. There are reports documenting that some of Athens's ambulances have many hundreds of thousands kilometers on the clock, and many are temporally out of use as a result of a lack of spare parts. It has also been reported that, at night, only a few vehicles cover the needs of a high-density population of more than 4 million. The problem of inadequate ambulance services becomes more evident in some islands and remote rural areas (mountain villages). In these cases, private ambulances, EKAV helicopters, and taxis may be legitimate alternatives, depending on the severity and urgency of the disease [8]. Since the beginning of the economic recession, spending on health care has been deeply cut, taxes have been hiked, and pensions have been in a steady decline. The shortages of critical medical supplies reveal the true extent of the crisis [24,25]. In particular, healthcare expenditure fell by 25% since 2009, thus leading to significant healthcare equipment deficits [6,25]. A Greek study conducted at the beginning of economic recession revealed the scarcity of crucial items of equipment such as spirometers in rural primary care [12,24,25]. Specifically, only 4.6% of rural doctors had spirometers that were considered adequate for clinical use [12,24,25]. Furthermore, during the last decade, state-funded pensions have suffered significant reductions; wages have been lowered by 20% and higher co-payments—up to 25% of a drug's purchase price—have led to patients struggling to pay for medications [6,11,13]. Crucially, treatment non-adherence has been associated with more exacerbations and hospitalisations annually. Hence, the burden of many chronic diseases seems to be affected by an economic recession [6].

Primary health care suffers from many weaknesses, including unmet health needs in parallel with unnecessary overuse of curative treatments and diagnostic services. Overall, according to Filippidis et al., the prevalence of unmet need for health care has significantly increased from 10.0% in 2010 to 21.9% in 2015 [22]. Moreover, some ethics-related issues come to the surface. Data support the contention that primary care doctors do not declare all private practice [11]. Interestingly, it has been documented that the private primary care sector in Greece absorbs more than 65% of total private health expenditure and private diagnostic centres generate substantial earnings [11].

According to a study by Karakolias et al., nowadays, most doctors consider that their salary is unfairly low and that were paid less than private sector counterparts [26]. Younger respondents highlighted the fact that current low salaries favour dual employment and claiming informal fees from patients [26]. Older respondents underlined the negative impact of low wages on productivity and quality of services [26]. Greek primary care doctors are dissatisfied with the current remuneration scheme [26]. Consequently, many doctors have left Greece since 2010, ending up in countries, where Europe's economic turmoil has had less impact.

4.2. Impact of the Economic Recession on In-Hospital EMS System

4.2.1. Overcrowding

EDs offer whole-day, free of charge, preventive, curative services responsive to emergencies as well as rehabilitation services—mainly to urban and semi-urban populations [27]. On the other hand, in primary care facilities, uninsured patients have to pay their medical bills for most care visits. The only exception to this rule is an expat employed in Greece, with a social security card (known as an AMKA), who pays for public health insurance. In 2016, the Greek government extended health coverage to uninsured people who are registered as unemployed as well as to refugees. Specifically, those who have less than 2400 euro per year of earned income are entitled to free health care, with the threshold rising according to the number of children in families.

In the years of crisis there has been a shift from the private to the public healthcare sector, as shown by an increase of 24% in the number of admissions to public hospitals from the very beginning of the crisis (from 2009 to 2010), that continued to rise in the first half of 2011 by 8% [11]. Conversely, it has also been documented that there was a decrease in admissions to private hospitals in the period 2009–2010 [10]. Out-of-pocket payments are high in care provided by the private sector. The reductions in health budgets—imposed after 2009—were accompanied by increases in the numbers of persons unable to access health care, particularly and vulnerable groups [28].

During the past few decades, a continuous rise in the rate of ED visits has been observed globally [14]. Emergency room (ER) crowding has become a widespread problem worldwide [29]. Crowding is defined as a situation in which the identified need for emergency services exceeds available resources for patient care in the ED, hospital, or both [29]. This increase is exacerbated by a hospital's organisational problems, for instance, shortages of staff, laboratory, and admission delays. Accordingly, an ED becomes overcrowded, with inevitable consequences [14,27,30]. However, the extent of the workload currently has not been thoroughly evaluated in Greece, as patient data are not regularly recorded.

It has been reported that EDs accepted more than 5,000,000 patients per year [30]. This corresponds to the 40% of the total of patients who visit public hospitals. The body of aggregated literature strongly argues that ED overcrowding is associated with potentially poorer clinical outcomes, including mortality [29]. A primary factor that may cause crowding in Greek EDs is the inadequate staffing [23]. The Greek EMS system is characterised by a low density of nurses as well as high hospitalisation rates [23]. However, it is striking that Greece has one of the highest number of physicians (6.17 physicians per 1000 people, in 2013) in the world [23]. This number has increased after the crisis began, as in 2004 the figure was only 4.38 per 1000 people [11]. Although the density of physicians is one of the highest in Europe, high unemployment rates forced many doctors to seek work abroad. Without a doubt, the stress of this unsupportive work environment leads doctors to emotional burnout and depression [24].

At the begging of the economic recession, 48 hospital beds per 10,000 people were recorded [23]. This rate was higher than in other advanced countries such as the United Kingdom (39 beds), Italy (39 beds) and Spain (34 beds) [22,23]. Notably, to serve unexpected inpatient care, Greek public hospitals present a 14% excess bed capacity [31]. In 2011, the Ministry for Health and Social Solidarity announced its intention to reduce public hospitals and the proportion of beds available for general purposes in the country [8]. Hence, the number of public facilities and hospital beds has been declining over the last years, from 140 hospitals with 36,400 beds to 83 hospitals with 33,000 beds [8]. Taking into consideration that hospital bed shortages are factors that affect crowding, the future may be much worse than the past over time. In short, cutting the health workforce's salaries, limiting recruitment of health personnel, and reducing procurement of medical supplies constitute a triple threat to the population's health and well-being [24].

The ageing of the population as well as the upcoming economic and social implications of the aging process, raise concerns in all western countries, as they seem to have a considerable effect on healthcare systems leading to overcrowding. In Greece, the population aged over 65 will exceed 3.5 million in 2060, compared to 2.1 million in 2008 [23]. In other words, an impressive increase of 68% in the ageing population is expected, alongside with a 10% and 18% decrease in the young, aged 1–14, and productive people, aged 15–64, respectively [23].

4.2.2. Effects of the Economic Recession on Cardiovascular Disease

With all Greece's problems, raising taxes and cutting government spending has led to a sharp economic slowdown and higher unemployment. The unemployment rate in Greece the highest among the European countries, reaching 27% in 2014, and fell to 23.5% in 2016 [17].

Harm in coronary health cannot be ruled out during an economic recession and cardiovascular disease may be partly attributable to the consequences of unemployment. Remarkably, it has been reported that death rates by diseases of the circulatory system declined more slowly after the onset of the crisis than before [32]. Besides, coronary artery diseases are the most common cause of high death rates in emergency or home cases, since still two-thirds of all patients die before reaching the ED [33]. This impression is based on studies more than a decade old which found that among patient older than 55 years who died from cardiac arrest, 91% did so outside hospital [33]. In fact, when thrombolysis is required, survival is related to the "call to needle" time, which should be less than 60 min [33].

Likewise, the incidence of stroke in Greece is among the highest in the western world, with a very low proportion of surviving patients [34]. Stroke deaths in Greece reached 20,662 or 21.86% of total deaths [35]. These data rank Greece as 101th (highest mortality per capita) globally. Stroke mortality is as high as 130 per 100,000 in the general population [34,35]. According to data from the ViewCronos database, mortality for stroke in Greece is 50% higher than the mean mortality rates of the EU [34,35]. There are 3 different types of settings where a patient with stroke can be admitted to a Greek state hospital [34,35]. These include a medical ward (MW), a neurology ward (NW), and a specialised stroke bay (SB). The SB is a designated area for stroke care attached to an NW [34,35]. Nonetheless, currently, Greece has only 2 designated SBs, one in the capital of Athens and another in the co-capital, Thessaloniki [34,35]. The staffing ratio is approximately 8 to 10 patients to each nurse on all of the MWs and NWs, and the ratio is 6:1 on the SB unit [33,34]. The long-standing economic recession in Greece has resulted in "skeleton staff" throughout public hospitals where new job opportunities are scarce [34,35]. Additionally, there are no graduate stroke programs [34,35]. Greek nurses in general, and those working in stroke care individually are in need of greater educational support because stroke is not viewed as a high priority by healthcare policy makers [34,35]. Gioldasis et al., estimated that the in-hospital cost of stroke is characteristically dependant on the type of stroke [36]. The average cost of an ischaemic stroke calculated to be $3908 [36]. Patients with intracerebral hemorrhage incurred the highest costs of care, at roughly $5583 on average [35]. In contrast, patients with a lacunar stroke were the least costly, at approximately $2423 on average [36]. The cost of treatment has been reported to account for approximately 10% of bed-day expenses [36].

4.2.3. Effects of the Economic Recession on the Prevalence of Accidents

Greece has the third highest rate of death due to car accidents. 77.4% of the 2500 fatal injuries due to car crashes happen far away from any healthcare institution, thus resulting in longer response times. Notably, the 66% of injured patients die during the first 24 h [37]. It has been recognized that Greece has the highest number of deaths from single vehicle road collisions in the EU [23]. This is a sobering thought, given that road accidents of this type accounted for 42% of road fatalities. However, some results also supported the idea that an economic recession led to a healthier lifestyle [6,32]. Laliotis et al., documented that deaths from vehicular accidents declined faster after the onset of the crisis, especially among men between the ages of 20 and 34 [32]. The continually increasing costs of fuel, taxation in combination with the rising costs of vehicle insurances, services, and toll fees forced many drivers to shift to cheaper means of transportation [38,39]. The recorded alcohol consumption per capita for the adult population in Greece decreased over the last three decades to a record low of 7.9 L per capita in 2010 [23].

Moreover, according to Pouliakas and Theodosiou, there seems to be a correlation between occupational accidents with factors such as low educational level, long hours at work, low family income, long-lasting unemployment, monotony, employees' lack of satisfaction, and non-creative work in general [37]. In periods of prolonged economic downturn and weak financial performance, there is an increase in the frequency of occupational injuries [37]. The causes are found in the increased workload, pressing working conditions, employment insecurity, reduced investment for the decrease and elimination of occupational hazards, work-related stress, increased average age of employees, as well as the increased participation of migrants in the final product [37].

Furthermore, the incidence of fractures due to interpersonal violence increased during the period of the severe economic [39]. Moreover, a significant concern is the lack of appropriate equipment for surgical innervations, resulting in problematic curative healthcare services [29]. Consequently, the crisis directed surgical patients to the public healthcare sector only in cases of severe diseases [29].

5. The Refugee Crisis Challenges Greek EMS System

The unprecedented flow of migrants arriving in Europe over the last three years has caused major health consequences. Specifically, in June 2015, 124,000 migrants and refugees had arrived in Greece. This represents a 750% increase compared to 2014 [40]. The Greek Government on 1st March 2016 was forced to request emergency funds from the EU to provide shelter for the unexpected wave of refugees. The amount needed has been estimated at 480 million euros [39]. Additionally, it has been argued that more than 60,000 asylum seekers were trapped in Greece due to closed European borders [40]. Therefore, it is essential the country identifies practical long-term solutions to hosting approximately 40,000–60,000 refugees [41]. Overall, the dramatic increase in the number of asylum seekers and migrants entering the country resulted in major political, economic, social, and health dimensions [40,41]. Specifically, this influx created significant challenges for all national healthcare systems across Europe, and consequently in Greece [40,41].

In fact, hospitals are struggling to respond to the needs and demands of both local people and migrants, mainly due to a lack of resources as previously mentioned [40,41]. Whilst they theoretically have access to the treatment in public hospitals, in reality, access is difficult due to a general lack of medical and human resources [40,41]. Moreover, lack of precise mechanisms for coordination creates significant difficulties in the implementation of national health policy. Despite the fact that the Greek Social Security System is thought to cover unemployed or uninsured people it seems extremely difficult to cover any additional care expenses burden amid economic crisis [40,41]. This means that the vast majority of immigrants will seek medical help in the public sector only in emergency settings and for advanced illness [40,41]. To address these needs, healthcare providers should also be trained in applying integrated and culturally competent health care [40,41].

6. Conclusions and Future Directions

The Greek EMS system has been profoundly affected by the economic recession. As per capita health spending growth has slowed significantly since 2009, all major health spending categories have been affected to varying degrees. The primary healthcare network is characterised by inconsistency in the availability, accessibility, and quality of primary healthcare services between urban and rural areas. Reductions in health expenditure have led to inadequate health promotion services. Furthermore, the multi-factorial problem of in-hospital EMS overcrowding has rapidly deteriorated and resulted in severe safety issues for patients. There is also evidence that the economic crisis has substantially affected chronic patients' access to healthcare services, jeopardising patients' well-being. The current economic framework poses additional threats to the healthcare system and its sustainability.

Future Directions

Nevertheless, it is generally accepted that there are no "quick fixes". Innovative operational and workforce models of care within EDs constitute a real solution. Urgent needs include the expansion of the primary medical network and outpatient departments, the development of the independent specialization or specialty of emergency medicine—highly trained physicians who will reduce the ED's workload—and the adoption of a triage scale in all hospitals. The quality and efficiency of primary care could be empowered by introducing quality indicators, as well as the distribution of practice guidelines and clinical protocols for the most common diseases and health problems. Furthermore, development of an electronic file for recording patient data would automate EMS processes. Continuing medical education (CME) as a useful method of assessment is a valuable tool to improve guideline adherence and implementation in many diseases. Quality assessment and management systems should also be developed to monitor the changes. Effective enforcement of the aforementioned concerns is expected to have a favourable effect on the Greek primary healthcare system, and such proposals may be a first attempt to improve the current EMS system.

Author Contributions: O.S.K. developed the layout of the manuscript, provided literature review, and edited content. D.S.S., A.K.E. and K.I.G. critically evaluated the draft of the manuscript. P.K. critically evaluated the topics in the areas of economics.

Conflicts of Interest: The authors declare no conflict of interest.

References

1. Al-Shaqsi, S. Models of International Emergency Medical Service (EMS) Systems. *Oman Med. J.* **2010**, *25*, 320–323. [CrossRef] [PubMed]
2. Hsia, R.Y.; Thind, A.; Zakariah, A.; Hicks, E.R.; Mock, C. Prehospital and Emergency Care: Updates from the Disease Control Priorities, Version 3. *World J. Surg.* **2015**, *39*, 2161–2167. [CrossRef] [PubMed]
3. Sakran, J.V.; Greer, S.E.; Werlin, E.; McCunn, M. Care of the injured worldwide: Trauma still the neglected disease of modern society. *Scand. J. Trauma Resusc. Emerg. Med.* **2012**, *20*, 64. [CrossRef] [PubMed]
4. Lozano, R.; Naghavi, M.; Foreman, K.; Lim, S.; Shibuya, K.; Aboyans, V.; Abraham, J.; Adair, T.; Aggarwal, R.; Ahn, S.Y.; et al. Global and regional mortality from 235 causes of death for 20 age groups in 1990 and 2010: A systematic analysis for the global burden of disease study 2010. *Lancet* **2012**, *380*, 2095–2128. [CrossRef]
5. Chang, C.Y.; Abujaber, S.; Reynolds, T.A.; Camargo, C.A., Jr.; Obermeyer, Z. Burden of emergency conditions and emergency care usage: New estimates from 40 countries. *Emerg. Med. J.* **2016**, *33*, 794–800. [CrossRef] [PubMed]
6. Kotsiou, O.S.; Zouridis, Z.; Kosmopoulos, M.; Gourgoulianis, K.I. Impact of the financial crisis on COPD burden: Greece as a case study. *Eur. Respir. Rev.* **2018**, *27*, 170106. [CrossRef] [PubMed]
7. Morganti, K.G.; Bauhoff, S.; Blanchard, J.C.; Abir, M.; Iyer, N.; Smith, A.; Vesely, J.V.; Okeke, E.N.; Kellermann, A.L. The Evolving Role of Emergency Departments in the United States. *Rand Health Q.* **2013**, *3*, 3. [PubMed]
8. Papaspyrou, E.; Setzis, D.; Grosomanidis, V.; Manikis, D.; Boutlis, D.; Ressos, C. International EMS systems: Greece. *Resuscitation* **2004**, *63*, 255–259. [CrossRef] [PubMed]

9. Εθνικό Κέντρο Άμεσης Βοήθειας. Available online: https://www.ekab.gr/chorotaxiki-katanomi/ (accessed on 13 April 2018).
10. Page, C.; Sbat, M.; Vazquez, K.; Yalcin, Z.D. Analysis of Emergency Medical System across the world, Project No: MQF-IQP 2809, Worcester Polytechnic Institute. 2013. Available online: https://web.wpi.edu/Pubs/Eproject/Available/E-project042413092332/unrestricted/MQFIQP2809.pdf (accessed on 15 March 2018).
11. Kondilis, E.; Smyrnakis, E.; Gavana, M.; Giannakopoulos, S.; Zdoukos, T.; Iliffe, S.; Benos, A. Economic crisis and primary care reform in Greece: Driving the wrong way? *Br. J. Gen. Pract.* **2012**, *62*, 264–265. [CrossRef] [PubMed]
12. Lionis, C.; Symvoulakis, E.K.; Markaki, A.; Vardavas, C.; Papadakaki, M.; Daniilidou, N.; Souliotis, K.; Kyriopoulos, I. Integrated primary health care in Greece, a missing issue in the current health policy agenda: A systematic review. *Int. J. Integr. Care* **2009**, *9*, e88. [CrossRef] [PubMed]
13. Stafyla, E.; Kotsiou, O.S.; Deskata, K.; Gourgoulianis, K.I. Missed diagnosis and overtreatment of COPD among smoking primary care population in Central Greece: Old problems persist. *Int. J. Chron. Obstruct. Pulmon. Dis.* **2018**, *13*, 487–498. [CrossRef] [PubMed]
14. Imperato, J.; Morris, D.S.; Binder, D.; Fischer, C.; Patrick, J.; Sanchez, L.D.; Setnik, G. Physician in triage improves emergency department patient throughput. *Intern. Emerg. Med.* **2012**, *7*, 457–462. [CrossRef] [PubMed]
15. Agouridakis, P.; Hatzakis, K.; Chatzimichali, K.; Psaromichalaki, M.; Askitopoulou, H. Workload and case-mix in a Greek emergency department. *Eur. J. Emerg. Med.* **2004**, *11*, 81–85. [CrossRef] [PubMed]
16. World Health Organization. Emergency Medical Services Systems in the European Union. Available online: http://www.euro.who.int/__data/assets/pdf_file/0016/114406/E92038.pdf (accessed on 15 March 2018).
17. Hellenic Statistical Authority. Greece in Figures July–September 2017. Available online: http://www.statistics.gr/en/greece-in-figures (accessed on 15 March 2018).
18. OECD (2018). Poverty Rate (Indicator). Available online: http://dx.doi.org/10.1787/0fe1315d-en (accessed on 15 March 2018).
19. Eurostat. People at Risk of Poverty or Social Exclusion. Available online: http://ec.europa.eu/eurostat/statistics-explained/index.php/People_at_risk_of_poverty_or_social_exclusion (accessed on March 2018).
20. Economou, C.; Kaitelidou, D.; Kentikelenis, A.; Maresso, A.; Sisouras, A. The impact of the crisis on the health system and health in Greece. In *Economic Crisis, Health Systems and Health in Europe. Country Experience*; Maresso, A., Mladovsky, P., Thomson, S., Sagan, A., Karanikolos, M., Richardson, E., Cylus, J., Evetovits, T., Jowett, M., Figueras, J., et al., Eds.; Observatory Studies Series No. 41; WHO Regional Office for Europe: Copenhagen, Denmark, 2015. Available online: http://www.euro.who.int/__data/assets/pdf_file/0010/279820/Web-economic-crisis-health-systems-and-health-web.pdf?ua=1 (accessed on 15 March 2016).
21. OECD. Health at a Glance: Europe 2016. Available online: http://www.oecd.org/health/health-at-a-glance-europe-23056088.htm (accessed on 15 March 2018).
22. Filippidis, F.T.; Gerovasili, V.; Millett, C.; Tountas, Y. Medium-term impact of the economic crisis on mortality, health-related behaviours and access to healthcare in Greece. *Sci. Rep.* **2017**, *7*, 46423. [CrossRef] [PubMed]
23. World Health Organization. Greece Profile of Health and Well-Being. 2016. Available online: http://www.euro.who.int/__data/assets/pdf_file/0010/308836/Profile-Health-Well-being-Greece.pdf?ua=12003:170--177 (accessed on 15 March 2018).
24. Rachiotis, G.; Kourousis, C.; Kamilaraki, M.; Symvoulakis, E.K.; Dounias, G.; Hadjichristodoulou, C. Medical supplies shortages and burnout among Greek health care workers during economic crisis: A pilot Study. *Int. J. Med. Sci.* **2014**, *11*, 442–447. [CrossRef] [PubMed]
25. Oikonomidou, E.; Anastasiou, F.; Dervas, D.; Patri, F.; Karaklidis, D.; Moustakas, P.; Andreadou, N.; Mantzanas, E.; Merkouris, B. Rural primary care in Greece: Working under limited resources. *Int. J. Qual. Health Care* **2010**, *22*, 333–337. [CrossRef] [PubMed]
26. Karakolias, S.; Kastanioti, C.; Theodorou, M.; Polyzos, N. Primary Care Doctors' Assessment of and Preferences on Their Remuneration. *Inquiry* **2017**, *54*, 46958017692274. [CrossRef] [PubMed]
27. Kontos, M.; Moris, D.; Davakis, S.; Schizas, D.; Pikoulis, E.; Liakakos, T. The effect of financial crisis on the profile of the patients examined at the surgical emergencies of an academic institution in Greece. *Ann. Transl. Med.* **2017**, *5*, 99. [CrossRef] [PubMed]
28. Simou, E.; Koutsogeorgou, E. Effects of the economic crisis on health and healthcare in Greece in the literature from 2009 to 2013: A systematic review. *Health Policy* **2014**, *115*, 111–119. [CrossRef] [PubMed]

29. Sun, B.C.; Hsia, R.Y.; Weiss, R.E.; Zingmond, D.; Liang, L.J.; Han, W.; McCreath, H.; Asch, S.M. Effect of emergency department crowding on outcomes of admitted patients. *Ann. Emerg. Med.* **2013**, *61*, 605–611. [CrossRef] [PubMed]
30. Vourvahakis, D.; Chronaki, C.E.; Kontoyiannis, V.; Panagopoulos, D.; Stergiopoulos, S. Traffic Accidents in Crete (1996–2006): The Role of the Emergency Coordination Center. *Stud. Health Technol. Inform.* **2010**, *160*, 505–509. [PubMed]
31. Knox Lovell, C.A.; Rodriguez-Alvarez, A.; Wall, A. The effects of stochastic demand and expense preference behavior on public hospital costs and excess capacity. *Health Econ.* **2008**, *18*, 227–235. [CrossRef] [PubMed]
32. Laliotis, I.; Ioannidis, J.P.; Stavropoulou, C. Total and cause-specific mortality before and after the onset of the Greek economic crisis: An interrupted time-series analysis. *Lancet Public Health* **2016**, *1*, e56–e65. [CrossRef]
33. Zagożdżon, P.; Parszuto, J.; Wrotkowska, M.; Dydjow-Bendek, D. Effect of unemployment on cardiovascular risk factors and mental health. *Occup. Med.* **2014**, *64*, 436–441. [CrossRef] [PubMed]
34. Theofanidis, D.; Fountouki, A. An Overview of Stroke Infrastructure, Network, and Nursing Services in Contemporary Greece. *J. Neurosci. Nurs.* **2017**, *49*, 247–250. [CrossRef] [PubMed]
35. Vasiliadis, A.V.; Ziki, M. Current status of stroke epidemiology in Greece: A panorama. *Neurol. Neurochir. Pol.* **2014**, *48*, 449–457. [CrossRef] [PubMed]
36. Gioldasis, G.; Talelli, P.; Chroni, E.; Daouli, J.; Papapetropoulos, T.; Ellul, J. In-hospital direct cost of acute ischemic and hemorrhagic stroke in Greece. *Acta. Neurol. Scand.* **2008**, *118*, 268–274. [CrossRef] [PubMed]
37. Pouliakas, K.; Theodossiou, I. The Economics of Health and Safety at Work: An Interdisciplinary Review of the Theory and Policy. *J. Econ. Surv.* **2013**, *27*, 167–208. [CrossRef]
38. Michas, G. Road traffic fatalities in Greece have continued to fall during the financial crisis. *BMJ* **2015**, *350*, 3081. [CrossRef] [PubMed]
39. Rallis, G.; Igoumenakis, D.; Krasadakis, C.; Stathopoulos, P. Impact of the economic recession on the etiology of maxillofacial fractures in Greece. *Oral Surg. Oral Med. Oral Pathol. Oral Radiol.* **2015**, *119*, 32–34. [CrossRef] [PubMed]
40. Moris, D.; Kousoulis, A. Refugee crisis in Greece: Healthcare and integration as current challenges. *Perspect. Public Health* **2017**, *137*, 309–310. [CrossRef] [PubMed]
41. De Paoli, L. Access to health services for the refugee community in Greece: Lessons learned. *Public Health* **2018**, *157*, 104–106. [CrossRef] [PubMed]

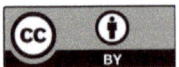 © 2018 by the authors. Licensee MDPI, Basel, Switzerland. This article is an open access article distributed under the terms and conditions of the Creative Commons Attribution (CC BY) license (http://creativecommons.org/licenses/by/4.0/).

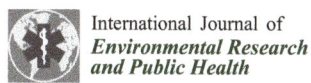

Article

Impact of the Introduction of the Electronic Health Insurance Card on the Use of Medical Services by Asylum Seekers in Germany

Kevin Claassen [1] and Pia Jäger [2],*

[1] Faculty of Social Sciences, Ruhr-University Bochum, Universitätsstr. 150, 44801 Bochum, Germany; kevin.claassen@rub.de
[2] Department of Psychiatry Psychotherapy and Preventative Medicine, Faculty of Medicine, LWL-University Hospital, Ruhr-University Bochum, Universitätsstr. 150, 44801 Bochum, Germany
* Correspondence: pia.jaeger@rub.de; Tel.: +49-234-32-28971

Received: 17 March 2018; Accepted: 23 April 2018; Published: 25 April 2018

Abstract: **Objectives:** Asylum seekers in Germany represent a highly vulnerable group from a health perspective. Furthermore, their access to healthcare is restricted. While the introduction of the Electronic Health Insurance Card (EHIC) for asylum seekers instead of healthcare-vouchers is discussed controversially using politico-economic reasons, there is hardly any empirical evidence regarding its actual impact on the use of medical services. The aim of the study is to examine this impact on the use of medical services by asylum seekers as measured by their consultation rate of ambulant physicians (CR). **Study Design:** For this purpose, a standardized survey was conducted with 260 asylum seekers in different municipalities, some of which have introduced the EHIC for asylum seekers, while others have not. **Methods:** The period prevalence was compared between the groups "with EHIC" and "without EHIC" using a two-sided t-test. Multivariate analysis was done using a linear OLS regression model. **Results:** Asylum seekers in possession of the EHIC are significantly more likely to seek ambulant medical care than those receiving healthcare-vouchers. **Conclusions:** The results of this study suggest that having to ask for healthcare-vouchers at the social security office could be a relevant barrier for asylum seekers.

Keywords: public health; asylum seeker; Electronic Health Insurance Card; refugee; Germany

---

1. Introduction

Worldwide there are 65.3 million people fleeing from war, violence and persecution [1]. In 2015 and 2016, a total of 1,222,194 refugees submitted a request for asylum in Germany. The German Federal Office for Migration and Refugees made 978,459 decisions about applications. The average operation time was 5.4 months [2,3]. A total of 21.21% of the asylum seekers were allocated to North Rhine-Westphalia in 2016 [4].

Overall, there is a complex relationship between flight and health, wherein there are many mutually influential factors [5]. While morbidity and mortality of migrants, which are similar to those of the majority population, are discussed as "healthy migrant effects", there are some peculiarities among asylum seekers [6]. Among other things, there are increased rates of infectious diseases such as tuberculosis, HIV or hepatitis, scabies or measles [7–9].

Of particular relevance is the occurrence of mental illnesses and psychosocial stress. First, both the flight itself and its causes are linked to mental stress and disturbance patterns that may include risk factors, and secondly, they are particularly difficult to detect in this population [10–12]. Refugees were often exposed to traumatic experiences such as violence and loss of relatives [13]. During flight and in refugee camps, the risk factors accumulate and are reinforced by constant stress such as malnutrition and sleep deprivation [14]. Over the post-migration phase, refugees are burdened with additional challenges, including loss of social status, discrimination, language barriers, and a foreign culture [15]. Especially frequent is the occurrence of trauma sequelae such as post-traumatic stress disorders (PTSD), and depressions or anxiety disorders [10]. Accurate data on the prevalence of these vary widely, including rates of 5% for post-traumatic stress disorders up to 40% with evidence for psychiatric comorbidity [16,17].

At the same time, preventive and early detection examinations of asylum seekers and their children are less frequently used in Germany, while multifaceted barriers to access to healthcare are described [18].

Asylum seekers and those with a permit of residence, according to §§ 23 to 25 of the Residence Act, receive benefits according to the Asylum Seekers' Benefits Act ("*Asylbewerberleistungsgesetz*", AsylbLG) [19]. Their access to healthcare is restricted as compared to the majority population. Healthcare benefits for asylum seekers are based on §§ 4 and 6, which state that there is only acute and emergency care, treatment of pain, pregnancy- and birth care plus "necessary preventive measure" to grant [7]. Asylum seekers have to visit their social security office in order to obtain a healthcare-voucher which can be used to visit a doctor. Social security offices have been criticized for a lack of sufficient medical competence to decide about the need for medical treatment of a highly vulnerable group [20].

While an increase of visits to the doctor would lead to higher expenditures in the short run, it can also be viewed as one preventive part of health-related behavior regarding this population [21]. For this reason, it could lead to a decrease of expenditures in the long run, because chronification of diseases might be avoided.

At the end of 15 months, asylum seekers are granted benefits according to the twelfth Social Security Code. The § 2 AsylbLG was changed in 2014, so that asylum seekers now have to wait 15 months instead of 48 months in order to receive an Electronic Health Insurance Card (EHIC) which allows them to visit a doctor without being forced to show a healthcare-voucher [19].

Since 2015, each federal state of Germany can decide whether to hand out the EHIC to asylum seekers, right from the beginning of their stay. Therefore, they have to reach a framework agreement in negotiations with the states' associations of health insurers [22].

By the end of 2017, except for Bavaria and Saxony, the German federal states have either decided for the introduction of the EHIC for asylum seekers or are currently in consultations. In North Rhine-Westphalia the municipalities are free to decide whether to introduce the EHIC for asylum seekers or not. Initially 16 municipalities including Bochum have introduced it by January 2016. The close-by cities Herne and Datteln still have not established it. This enables the comparison used in the study at hand.

North Rhine-Westphalia has to pay the health insurers a fixed rate of 8% a month per asylum seeker for the new incurred administration costs with 10 Euro being the minimum fee in any case. In return the health insurer has to inform the asylum seekers about the usage of the EHIC. Supporters argue that administration costs will decrease due to the disappearance of the obligation to decide about applications for healthcare-vouchers by asylum seekers at social security offices [23].

The number of benefits is still guided by §§ 4 and 6 AsylbLG. The criterion of deferability is not examined anymore, so that the treatment is now primarily indicated by the treating physicians, rather than employees of the social office. Instead, preventive cures, dentures, domestic aid, artificial insemination and sterilization, chronic disease management programs, selective tariffs as well as benefits abroad are explicitly excluded [24].

Critics argue that there is another incentive for migrating to Germany [25]. Further, an unregulated increase of healthcare costs is expected as a consequence of the fact that there is no incentive for the health insurers to reject benefits due to their own financial interest. Otherwise there is an incentive for healthcare providers to bill additional benefits when they already reached their Volume of Standard Benefits (*Regelleistungsvolumen*). Thus, the regular treatment of asylum seekers is not liable to budget restrictions [23].

Apart from that, the benefits are billed according to Uniform Assessment Standard (*Einheitlicher Bewertungsmaßstab*) instead of Medical Fee Schedule (*Gebührenordnung für Ärzte*). This means that the treatment of asylum seekers is controlled by Statutory Health Insurance and not viewed as a quasi-private service any longer [20].

As it is unknown in which direction an increase of the frequency of visits to the doctor by asylum seekers given the EHIC compared to a system of healthcare-vouchers affects overall healthcare costs, the study at hand aims to examine whether the mentioned increase is to be expected at all.

2. Study-Design & Methods

Due to a lack of available public data at this stage, asylum seekers themselves were asked in order to examine whether there is a difference in terms of ambulant visits to the doctor between asylum seekers with and without regular access to the German healthcare system. Null hypothesis states that there is no difference.

The study at hand used an ex-post-facto design via surveying 260 asylum seekers in the three municipalities Bochum, Datteln and Herne in North Rhine Westphalia, Germany. These were chosen due to Bochum being one of the municipalities which have introduced the EHIC for asylum seekers as soon as possible. Existing cooperation with Datteln and Herne simplified the access to the field in close-by municipalities. Ex-ante, it had been calculated that a minimum sample size of 210 cases would be sufficient to detect a medium effect size (d = 0.5), given a two-sided rejection region with a significance level of $\alpha = 0.05$ and a statistical power of 95% if the two analyzed groups (with and without EHIC) are equally large [26]. The interviews were conducted in October 2016 and October 2017 using a standardized questionnaire in German, English, French, Arabic and Farsi with the support of interpreters. The survey was conducted on the respondents' voluntary basis. All participants provided informed consent. They were approached by social workers, students or interpreters under supervision of the researchers. The questionnaire was processed independently and anonymously. In individual cases, comprehension questions were answered. At the time of the survey, the respondents lived in fourteen different community camps or urban facilities different from the reception centers of North Rhine-Westphalia.

Here, the count of visits to the doctor was inquired. Alongside the length of the stay in Germany up to the point of the survey, the period in which the respondents had been in possession of the EHIC was also asked for. Thus, the period prevalence can be determined for different doctor contacts, so that the monthly consultation rate of ambulant physicians (CR) acts as the main outcome. A total of 93 asylum seekers, who had used both healthcare-vouchers and the EHIC in order to see a physician, were treated as different cases who were in each system for a certain amount of time. Consequently, they have been taken into account in both groups. The CR was compared between the groups "with EHIC" and "without EHIC" by using a two-sided *t*-test with Welch-approximation due to the possibility of different variances [27]. It was assumed that the difference in population follows a t-distribution. Intraindividual differences were tested for within the group of 93 asylum seekers who had used both healthcare-vouchers and the EHIC over time. If only the count of healthcare-vouchers was remembered, the average count of visits to the doctor per healthcare-voucher was inputted.

Various other variables may represent a confounder in the comprehension of the physician contacts. So therefore, the presence of chronic diseases—whereby the most common chronic diseases are covered [28]—in the community, the months in Germany at the time of the survey, German language skills, age, sex, education and currently being on medication along with the date of the survey, country of origin and visits to the hospital or volunteering doctors were all factors especially considered and included as potential disturbers. In addition, the respondents rated their language skills by themselves using a scale from one ("very bad") to five ("very good"). Education was measured as an ordinally scaled variable, ranging from one for no educational degree to five for a university degree. The date of the survey was also taken into account.

Those of the variables that show a Pearson correlation coefficient greater than 0.1 either with the count of visits to the doctor or with the ownership of the EHIC were controlled for using a linear OLS-regression model.

Goodness of fit was assessed by the adjusted coefficient of determination. Multicollinearity was tested for using variation inflation factors (VIF) assuming that those with values smaller than four were without problems [29]. Residual analysis was done by testing the assumptions of normal distribution and homoscedasticity using Shapiro–Wilk- and Breusch–Pagan-test. It was assumed that the residuals follow a normal distribution with constant variance [30].

Ex-ante, three observations were omitted completely for several values being either unrealistic or inconsistent. Item nonresponse was handled by mean imputation. Asylum seekers who used both healthcare-vouchers and the EHIC in order to see a physician were treated in the calculation of the period prevalence as different cases who were in each system for a certain amount of time.

3. Results

In total, 260 asylum seekers were interviewed in this study. A total of 137 of these persons were in possession of the EHIC. A total of 216 of the respondents were at least temporarily provided with healthcare-vouchers. Thus, 93 asylum seekers had been able to collect experiences with healthcare-vouchers as well as with the EHIC, because during their stay they first had been treated with healthcare-vouchers and after some time they received the EHIC.

The observation period of the group "with EHIC" thus consists of 2602.86 months. In contrast, the group without EHIC" shows an observation period of 2453.76 months.

The respondents were 31.12 years old on average with a range of 18 to 66 years if asylum seekers who had used both healthcare-vouchers and the EHIC are treated as different cases (pre and post EHIC). At 80%, the majority of them was male. With a total of 54%, Syria, Iraq and Afghanistan were the most frequently mentioned countries of origin. A total of 17% said they received a college degree, 5% vocational training and 25% the general qualification for university entrance. A total of 37% had not graduated from school. Further characteristics can be found in Table 1.

Table 1. Description of the main characteristics of the analyzed sample (n = 353; rounded percentages).

Characteristic	Percentage
Age in years (mean ± SD)	31.12 ± 9.49
Sex	
Male	80%
Country of origin	
Syria	30%
Iraq	14%
Afghanistan	10%
Iran	7%
Albania	1%
Eritrea	5%
Pakistan	2%
Serbia	1%
Other	30%
Family status	
Single	56%
Married	39%
Divorced	3%
Widowed	2%

Table 1. Cont.

Characteristic	Percentage
Education	
College degree	17%
General qualification for university entrance	25%
Vocational training	5%
Other	16%
No educational degree	37%
Children	
None	60%
One child	9%
Two children	12%
More than two children	19%
Municipality	
Bochum	72%
Datteln	23%
Herne	5%
Point of the Survey	
2016	39%
2017	61%
Months in Germany (mean ± SD)	14.32 ± 10.54
German language skills	
1—very bad	18%
2—bad	23%
3—average	33%
4—good	21%
5—very good	4%
Currently on medication	
Yes	23%
Missing information	4%
Chronic Disease	
Yes	60%
Missing information	1%
Diseases	
Heart disease	5%
Psychiatric disorder	17%
Joint disease	7%
Diabetes	4%
Back pain	12%
Cancer	1%
Thyroid disease	3%
Other	20%
Electronic Health Insurance Card (EHIC)	
Yes	57%
Consultation rate of ambulant physicians (CR; visits to the doctor per month) (mean + SD)	0.32 ± 0.49
Contacts to further physicians	
Hospital	35%
Volunteers (e.g., in camp)	9%

The mean CR was 0.32 ± 0.49 doctor contacts per month over all groups. As seen in Figure 1 owners of the EHIC showed a mean of 0.49 ± 0.65, while the mean of those who had to ask for healthcare-vouchers was 0.21 ± 0.39. The t-distributed mean difference of 0.28 is significant at $p < 0.01$.

The 95% confidence interval includes mean differences between 0.14 and 0.41. The Pearson correlation coefficient was 0.25.

Within the group of asylum seekers who had used both the EHIC and healthcare-vouchers ($n = 93$), it was found that after receiving the EHIC, there was also a significant intra-individual increase of the CR ($\Delta = 0.27$, $p < 0.01$).

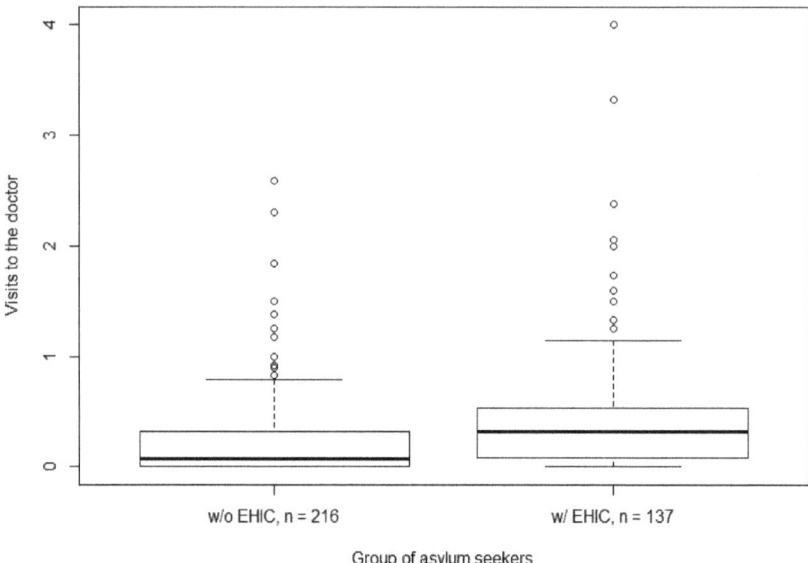

Figure 1. Consultation rate of ambulant physicians per month among a sample of asylum seekers in Germany stratified for ownership of the Electronic Health Insurance Card (EHIC) (with EHIC: $n = 137$, without EHIC: $n = 216$).

Several chronic diseases, age, sex as well as the respondent's level of education and country of origin as well as contacts to hospital and volunteering physicians showed a correlation smaller than 0.1 with the count of visits to the doctor and the ownership of the EHIC. They were omitted in the linear regression model.

A total of 71.95% were asked in Bochum, 23.23% in Datteln and 4.82% in Herne. The highest correlation ($r = 0.29$) was found between Bochum and the EHIC. At the same time, the CR was not affected by the municipality following correlations each smaller than 0.1.

Being on medication was positively associated with the CR ($r = 0.25$), whereas it was not associated with the ownership of the EHIC. At the time of the interview, 23.23% of the respondents were on medication, 73.94% were not; 0.04% did not answer the question. A total of 4.53% suffered from heart or other cardiovascular diseases. Cardiovascular diseases were correlated with the CR ($r = 0.21$), but not with the EHIC. The outcome's correlation with cardiovascular diseases was outperformed by its correlation with psychiatric disorders ($r = 0.24$), from which 17% were suffering. A weaker association was discovered between the CR and joint diseases, from which 6.52% were suffering ($r = 0.12$).

Months being in Germany up to the point of survey correlated with the ownership of the EHIC ($r = 0.35$), but not with the CR. German language skills were slightly correlated with the ownership of the EHIC ($r = 0.11$) and were thus entered into the regression model. The date of the survey was slightly correlated with the count of visits to the doctor ($r = 0.12$). A total of 39.09% of the respondents were asked in October 2016, and 60.91% in October 2017.

A linear regression of the CR, the results of which can be found in Table 2, was done on the aforementioned predictors with correlations greater than 0.1. A proportion of 0.21 of the variance of the CR can be explained by the variance of the predicting variables. The adjusted R-Squared equals 0.19. The impact of the EHIC, psychiatric disorders and belonging to the municipality of Herne was positive and highly significant ($p < 0.01$). Ownership of the EHIC directly increased the CR by approximately 0.31 doctor contacts per month. The value of this regression coefficient exceeded the mean difference, which suggests that there is a mild suppression of the relationship of interest by the controlled for confounders. The positive effects of medication and cardiovascular diseases as well as the negative effect of being asked in 2017 were still significant on the 5% level.

The VIF ranged from 1.22 to 1.78, indicating that there was no severe multicollinearity. The Shapiro–Wilk-test signals that null hypothesis of normal distribution of residuals is to be rejected ($p < 0.01$). Moreover, the Breusch–Pagan-test suggests that there is heteroscedasticity ($p < 0.01$). Eliminating 25 cases with values of Cook greater than 4/n did not lead to the Breusch–Pagan null hypothesis being tenable [29]. These limitations of the statistical analysis must be taken into consideration regarding the interpretation of the results.

Table 2. Factors associated with the consultation rate of ambulant physicians per month among a sample of asylum seekers in Germany (with EHIC: $n = 137$, without EHIC: $n = 216$).

Characteristic	Coefficient (Standard Error)	P-Value
Health system related variables		
Electronic Health Insurance Card (yes vs. no)	0.31 (0.06)	0.00
Medication (yes vs. no)	0.14 (0.06)	0.02
Language skills		
German (per increase on a scale from 1 to 5)	0.02 (0.02)	0.50
Diseases		
Heart disease (yes vs. no)	0.25 (0.13)	0.05
Psychiatric disorders (yes vs. no)	0.30 (0.07)	0.00
Joint disease (yes vs. no)	−0.03 (0.11)	0.81
Municipality		
Datteln (yes vs. no, compared to Bochum)	0.10 (0.07)	0.18
Herne (yes vs. no, compared to Bochum)	0.45 (0.12)	0.00
Time variables		
Point of the survey (2017, compared to 2016)	−0.16 (0.06)	0.01
Months in Germany (per additional month)	0.00 (0.00)	0.25

All in all, the availability of the EHIC presented itself as an independent predictor of the use of outpatient healthcare, because the CR was significantly lower in the group of patients "without EHIC" than in the group "with EHIC".

4. Discussion

Those asylum seekers in Germany who were in possession of the EHIC due to living in Bochum or after 15 months of residence, visited their ambulant doctors significantly more often, as compared to the rest of the asylum seekers who had to ask the social security office for healthcare-vouchers.

Controlling for third variables indicates that the impact of the EHIC exists independent of the presence of chronic diseases, the municipality, months being in Germany up to the point of the survey, German language skills, age, sex, level of education, currently being on medication, the date of the survey, country of origin and visits to the hospital or voluntary doctors.

The study at hand is to be credited for its confirmation of the hypothesis that the introduction of the EHIC for asylum seekers nearly from the beginning of their residence does increase their monthly CR of ambulant physicians.

Nevertheless, the resulted sample of EHIC owning asylum seekers matches the Germans' CR on average when the structure of age and sex is taken into consideration. The average German sees his/her ambulant doctors 9.2 times per year. Women visit their doctors 1.5 times per year more often on average than men. The relevant age group from 30 up to and including 39 shows a frequency of 7.7. If only men in this age group are viewed, their value is 5.7 which is equivalent to 0.48 visits per month, which does not significantly differ from the asylum seekers with EHIC [31].

Therefore, the results for unrestricted access are in line with previous research regarding the majority population, indicating that there is no significant difference between asylum seekers and the age-corrected autochthonous population in Germany in terms of visits to the doctor. In spite of that, it could be shown that the non-possession of the EHIC leads to a significantly lower use of the healthcare system among asylum seekers. Consequently, healthcare-vouchers can be viewed as a major obstacle in the medical care of this group.

Simultaneously, data on doctoral contacts by asylum seekers in Germany is scarce. Sönmez et al. interviewed 660 women in their "study on female refugees" in five German federal states. Only 16% of these women indicated that they have access to general medical care [32]. This can be interpreted as further evidence that there are systematic barriers to healthcare for asylum seekers in Germany.

Although the distribution of asylum seekers to the federal states, and further to the municipalities, takes place largely independent of person-specific characteristics, it has to be recognized that the results of the present study are limited locally and quantitatively. The clustered sample of the given number of cases, does not allow for drawing conclusions about the whole population of asylum seekers in Germany. However, an obvious trend can nonetheless be seen.

The central model explains a small amount of the overall variation of the outcome, while residuals do not scatter randomly. This could be due to decisive variables that were missing in the survey. In addition, there could have been interference effects, such as selection bias, e.g., absence due to parallel language courses, or that the mother tongue of the interviewed could not be covered by interpreters, or due to memory gaps.

What the survey does not provide is an educated guess about the actual costs of the increase of visits to the doctor. Although the EHIC for asylum seekers seems to remove barriers, it has to be detected in future research, whether the increase translates into higher overall costs. It can be supposed that, while healthcare costs will be increased in the short run, they will decrease in the long run due to the prevention and early treatment of possibly chronic diseases.

Fewer visits to the doctor for prevention or in the presence of mild to moderate symptoms may result in adverse health consequences for those affected, that would not only burden the people, but could also lead to significantly higher follow-up costs. Specifically, regarding the existing difficulties in the treatment of mental illnesses, such as PTSD, the occurrence of comorbidities (e.g., depression and addiction disorders) as a result of complications has to be expected due to a lack of adequate early treatment [33]. Their psychosocial effects can also lead to negative consequences for the social environment and society as a whole, i.e., in terms of integration by means of alienating a social group. In order to avoid medium- to long-term health consequences for asylum seekers as well as possible additional expenditures and adverse societal effects, it is worthwhile to provide an unrestricted access to healthcare.

This claim can be reinforced by the fact that, since the introduction of the EHIC for asylum seekers in Hamburg in 2012, the benefits remained constant while the administration costs could be decreased [34]. Moreover Bozorgmehr/Razum found out, by analyzing data from German Federal Statistical Office from 1994 to 2013, that restricting healthcare access of asylum seekers has generated additional costs in the average amount of 375.80 Euro per capita that lead to additional costs of 1.56 billion Euro for the whole period of time [35].

5. Conclusions

In this study, it could be shown that asylum seekers in possession of the EHIC are significantly more likely to seek ambulant medical care than those receiving healthcare-vouchers. Their CR, however, does not significantly differ from the age-corrected CR of the autochthonous population, as mentioned in the discussion section. Taking into account relevant covariables, the possession of the EHIC can be viewed as an independent influencing factor on the asylum seekers' use of medical care. These results suggest that having to ask for healthcare-vouchers at the social security office could be a relevant barrier for asylum seekers. This could result in a lack of necessary treatment or precautionary measures, possibly resulting in complications or chronification. On the other hand, the ownership of the EHIC does not seem to lead to a more frequent use of medical services by the asylum seekers interviewed in the context of the study at hand if their count of visits to the doctor is compared to data of the German age-corrected total population. Further research from a health economical perspective—also with greater regional coverage—as well as the development of practice-oriented care approaches in order to reduce access barriers is therefore desirable.

Author Contributions: Kevin Claassen was responsible for the design of the study, data collection, analysis and interpretation as well as manuscript development. Pia Jäger was responsible for the design of the study, data collection and contribution to the manuscript.

Acknowledgments: We would like to thank Winter and the employees of the city in Bochum, Dora and his staff as well as the employees of the social security office in Herne. Because of their commitment and their active support, it was possible to carry out this study at all. In addition, we want to thank the students Heike-Christine Rothe, Charlotte Otterbach, Katharina Jäger, Milan Vollack, Robin Maler and Felix-Pascal Joswig for participating in the study as a part of their research module. For the many helpful comments and for the support issuing the manuscript we would like to cordially thank our mentors N. Ott and G. Juckel. The costs to publish in open access are largely covered by the publication fund of the Ruhr-University Bochum.

Ethical Approval: Ethical approval for this study was provided by the Bochum ethical review committee, reference number 16-5920. All participants in the study provided informed consent.

Conflicts of Interest: The authors declare no conflict of interest as well as no external funding.

Abbreviations

The following abbreviations are used in this manuscript:

EHIC	Electronic Health Insurance Card
CR	Consultation Rate of Ambulant Physicians
VIF	Variation Inflation Factors
PTSD	Post-Traumatic Stress Disorder

References

1. UNHCR. UNHCR Global Trends-Forced Displacement in 2016. Available online: http://www.unhcr.org/globaltrends2016/ (accessed on 29 December 2017).
2. Bundesamt für Migration und Flüchtlinge. Aktuelle Zahlen zu Asyl 2017. Available online: http://www.bamf.de/SharedDocs/Anlagen/DE/Downloads/Infothek/Statistik/Asyl/aktuelle-zahlen-zu-asyl-januar-2017.pdf?__blob=publicationFile (accessed on 15 January 2018).
3. Sachverständigenrat deutscher Stiftungen für Integration und Migration. *Fakten zur Asylpolitik*; Sachverständigenrat deutscher Stiftungen für Integration und Migration: Berlin, Germany, 2017.
4. BAMF-Bundesamt für Migration und Flüchtlinge Asyl und Flüchtlingsschutz. Available online: http://www.bamf.de/DE/Fluechtlingsschutz/fluechtlingsschutz-node.html (accessed on 19 January 2018).
5. Schenk, L. *Migrationssensible Gesundheitsforschung*; Freie Universität Berlin: Berlin, Germany, 2016.
6. Razum, O.; Zeeb, H.; Rohrmann, S. The "healthy migrant effect"–not merely a fallacy of inaccurate denominator figures. *Int. J. Epidemiol.* **2000**, *29*, 191–192. [CrossRef] [PubMed]
7. van Burg, J.L.; Verver, S.; Borgdorff, M.W. The epidemiology of tuberculosis among asylum seekers in the Netherlands: Implications for screening. *Int. J. Tuberc. Lung Dis.* **2003**, *7*, 139–144. [PubMed]

8. Clark, R.C.; Mytton, J. Estimating infectious disease in UK asylum seekers and refugees: A systematic review of prevalence studies. *J. Public Health* **2007**, *29*, 420–428. [CrossRef] [PubMed]
9. Seilmaier, M.; Guggemos, W.; Alberer, M.; Wendtner, C.M.; Spinner, C.D. Infektionen bei Flüchtlingen. *Notf. Rettungsmedizin* **2017**, *20*, 216–227. [CrossRef]
10. Silove, D.; Sinnerbrink, I.; Field, A.; Manicavasagar, V.; Steel, Z. Anxiety, depression and PTSD in asylum-seekers: Assocations with pre-migration trauma and post-migration stressors. *Br. J. Psychiatry* **1997**, *170*, 351–357. [CrossRef] [PubMed]
11. Crumlish, N.; O'Rourke, K. A Systematic Review of Treatments for Post-Traumatic Stress Disorder among Refugees and Asylum-Seekers. *J. Nerv. Ment. Dis.* **2010**, *198*, 237. [CrossRef] [PubMed]
12. Frank, L.; Yesil-Jürgens, R.; Razum, O.; Bozorgmehr, K.; Schenk, L.; Gilsdorf, A.; Rommel, A.; Lampert, T. Health and healthcare provision to asylum seekers and refugees in Germany. *J. Health Monit.* **2017**, *21*, 22–41. [CrossRef]
13. Gavranidou, M.; Niemiec, B.; Magg, B.; Rosner, R. Traumatische Erfahrungen, aktuelle Lebensbedingungen im Exil und psychische Belastung junger Flüchtlinge. *Kindh. Entwickl.* **2008**, *17*, 224–231. [CrossRef]
14. Izutsu, T.; Tsutsumi, A.; Sato, T.; Naqibullah, Z.; Wakai, S.; Kurita, H. Nutritional and Mental Health Status of Afghan Refugee Children in Peshawar, Pakistan: A Descriptive Study. *Asia Pac. J. Public Health* **2005**, *17*, 93–98. [CrossRef] [PubMed]
15. Ellison, C.G.; Boardman, J.D.; Williams, D.R.; Jackson, J.S. Religious Involvement, Stress, and Mental Health: Findings from the 1995 Detroit Area Study. *Soc. Forces* **2001**, *80*, 215–249. [CrossRef]
16. Gäbel, U.; Ruf, M.; Schauer, M.; Odenwald, M.; Neuner, F. Prävalenz der Posttraumatischen Belastungsstörung (PTSD) und Möglichkeiten der Ermittlung in der Asylverfahrenspraxis. *Z. Klin. Psychol. Psychother.* **2006**, *35*, 12–20. [CrossRef]
17. Fazel, M.; Wheeler, J.; Danesh, J. Prevalence of serious mental disorder in 7000 refugees resettled in western countries: A systematic review. *Lancet* **2005**, *365*, 1309–1314. [CrossRef]
18. Robert-Koch-Institut. RKI-Pressemitteilungen-Schwerpunktthema Gesundheit von Migranten und Geflüchteten. Available online: https://www.rki.de/DE/Content/Service/Presse/Pressemitteilungen/2016/08_2016.html (accessed on 22 July 2017).
19. Bundesministerium der Justiz und für Verbraucherschutz Asylbewerberleistungsgesetz in der Fassung der Bekanntmachung vom 5. August 1997 (BGBl. I S. 2022), das zuletzt durch Artikel 4 des Gesetzes vom 17. Juli 2017 (BGBl. I S. 2541) geändert worden ist, 5 August 1997.
20. Epping, B. Medizinische Versorgung von Flüchtlingen: Teure Hürden. *Z. Orthop. Unfallchirurgie* **2017**, *155*, 129–134. [CrossRef] [PubMed]
21. Kasl, S.V.; Cobb, S. Health Behavior, Illness Behavior and Sick Role behavior: I. Health and Illness Behavior. *Arch. Environ. Health Int. J.* **1966**, *12*, 246–266. [CrossRef]
22. § 264 SGB V, Übernahme der Krankenbehandlung für nicht Versi...—Gesetze des Bundes und der Länder. Available online: http://www.lexsoft.de/cgi-bin/lexsoft/justizportal_nrw.cgi?xid=137489,351 (accessed on 19 January 2018).
23. Wächter-Raquet, M. Einführung der Gesundheitskarte für Asylsuchende und Flüchtlinge. 2016, Gütersloh, Bertelsmann Stiftung. Available online: https://www.bertelsmann-stiftung.de/fileadmin/files/BSt/Publikationen/GrauePublikationen/Studie_VV_Gesundheitskarte_Fluechtlinge_2016.pdf (accessed on 20 December 2017).
24. Ministerium für Gesundheit, Emanzipation, Pflege und Alter des Landes Nordrhein-Westfalen (MGEPA). Rahmenvereinbarung zur Übernahme der Gesundheitsversorgung für nicht Versicherungspflichtige gegen Kostenerstattung nach § 264 Absatz 1 SGB V in Verbindung mit §§ 1,1a Asylbewerberleistungsgesetz in Nordrhein-Westfalen. p. 27.05.2017. Available online: https://www.mhkbg.nrw/mediapool/pdf/gesundheit/Gesundheitskarte_Fluechtlinge/Rahmenvereinbarung_Online.pdf (accessed on 25 December 2017).
25. Deutsche Ärztezeitung Flüchtlinge: Union gegen E-Card für Asylbewerber. Available online: http://www.aerztezeitung.de/politik_gesellschaft/gp_specials/fluechtlinge/article/893399/fluechtlinge-union-e-card-asylbewerber.html (accessed on 20 January 2018).
26. Faul, F.; Erdfelder, E.; Lang, A.G.; Buchner, A. G*Power 3: A flexible statistical power analysis program for the social, behavioral, and biomedical sciences. *Behav. Res. Methods* **2007**, *39*, 175–191. [CrossRef] [PubMed]

27. Ruxton, G.D. The unequal variance *t*-test is an underused alternative to Student's *t*-test and the Mann–Whitney U test. *Behav. Ecol.* **2006**, *17*, 688–690. [CrossRef]
28. GBD 2016 Disease and Injury Incidence and Prevalence Collaborators. Global, regional, and national incidence, prevalence, and years lived with disability for 328 diseases and injuries for 195 countries, 1990–2016: A systematic analysis for the Global Burden of Disease Study 2016. *Lancet* **2017**, *390*, 1211–1259. [CrossRef]
29. Wollschläger, D. *R Kompakt*; Springer: Berlin/Heidelberg, Germany, 2016; ISBN 978-3-662-49101-0.
30. Ohr, D. Lineare Regression: Modellannahmen und Regressionsdiagnostik. In *Handbuch der Sozialwissenschaftlichen Datenanalyse*; Wolf, C., Best, H., Eds.; VS Verlag für Sozialwissenschaften: Wiesbaden, Germany, 2010; pp. 639–675, ISBN 978-3-531-16339-0.
31. Rattay, P.; Butschalowsky, H.; Rommel, A.; Prütz, F.; Jordan, S.; Nowossadeck, E.; Domanska, O.; Kamtsiuris, P. Inanspruchnahme der ambulanten und stationären medizinischen Versorgung in Deutschland: Ergebnisse der Studie zur Gesundheit Erwachsener in Deutschland (DEGS1). *Bundesgesundheitsblatt-Gesundheitsforschung-Gesundheitsschutz* **2013**, *56*, 832–844. [CrossRef] [PubMed]
32. Sönmez, E.; Jesuthasan, J.; Abels, I.; Nassar, R.; Kurmeyer, C.; Schouler-Ocak, M. Study on female refugees–A representative research study on refugee women in Germany. *Eur. Psychiatry* **2017**, *41*, 251. [CrossRef]
33. Flatten, G.; Gast, U.; Hofmann, A.; Knaevelsrud, C.; Lampe, A.; Liebermann, P.; Maercker, A.; Reddemann, L.; Wöller, W. S3—Leitlinie Posttraumatische Belastungsstörung. *Trauma und Gewalt* **2011**, *3*, 202–210.
34. Burmester, F. *Auswirkungen der Zusammenarbeit mit der AOK Bremen/Bremerhaven aus Sicht der Behörde für Arbeit, Soziales, Familie und Integration*; Behörde für Arbeit, Soziales, Familie und Integration Hamburg: Hamburg, Germany, 2014.
35. Bozorgmehr, K.; Razum, O. Effect of Restricting Access to Health Care on Health Expenditures among Asylum-Seekers and Refugees: A Quasi-Experimental Study in Germany, 1994–2013. *PLoS ONE* **2015**, *10*, e0131483. [CrossRef] [PubMed]

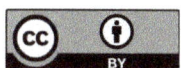

© 2018 by the authors. Licensee MDPI, Basel, Switzerland. This article is an open access article distributed under the terms and conditions of the Creative Commons Attribution (CC BY) license (http://creativecommons.org/licenses/by/4.0/).

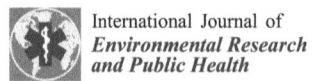 International Journal of
Environmental Research and Public Health

Article

Immunization Offer Targeting Migrants: Policies and Practices in Italy

Teresa Dalla Zuanna [1], Martina Del Manso [2], Cristina Giambi [2], Flavia Riccardo [2], Antonino Bella [2], Maria Grazia Caporali [2], Maria Grazia Dente [2], Silvia Declich [2,*] and The Italian Survey CARE Working Group [†]

1. Department of Cardiac, Thoracic and Vascular Sciences, and Public Health, University of Padova, 35122 Padova, Italy; teresadallazuanna@gmail.com
2. National Institute of Health (Istituto Superiore di Sanità, ISS), viale Regina Elena, 299-00161 Rome, Italy; martina.delmanso@iss.it (M.D.M.); cristina.giambi@iss.it (C.G.); flavia.riccardo@iss.it (F.R.); antonino.bella@iss.it (A.B.); mariagrazia.caporali@iss.it (M.G.C.); mariagrazia.dente@iss.it (M.G.D.)

* Correspondence: silvia.declich@iss.it; Tel.: +39-06-4990-4007
† Italian survey CARE Working Group: Stefania Iannazzo (Ministery of Health), Anna Domenica Mignuoli (Calabria Region), Anna Tosti (Umbria Region), Lorenza Ferrara (Local Health Unit of Alessandria, Piemonte Region), Maria Grazia Pascucci and Roberto Cagarelli (Emilia Romagna Region), Maria Grazia Zuccali (Trento Autonomous Province), Maria José Caldés (Global Health Center, Toscania Region), Martina Bortoletto (Veneto Region), Monica Bevilacqua (Bolzano Autonomous Province), Patrizia Carletti (Observatory on Health Inequalities, Marche Region), Pierina Tanchis (Sardegna Region), Rosa Prato and Maria Giovanna Cappelli (University of Foggia, Puglia Region), Maria Serena Gallone (University of Bari, Puglia Region), Sabrina Senatore (Lombardia Region), Valentina Brussi (Local Health Unit of Udine, Friuli Venezia Giulia Region), Tolinda Gallo (Friuli Venezia Giulia Region), Mario Palermo (Sicilia Region); careproject@iss.it

Received: 12 April 2018; Accepted: 7 May 2018; Published: 12 May 2018

Abstract: The unprecedented flow of migrants over the last three years places Italy in front of new issues regarding medical care from the rescue phase up to the integration into the national health services, including preventive actions. We used online questionnaires to investigate the Italian national and regional policies for immunization offer targeting asylum seekers, refugees, irregular migrants and unaccompanied minors. Another questionnaire was used to assess how these policies are translated into practice in migrant reception centres and community health services. Questionnaires were filled out at the national level, in 14 out of 21 Regions/Autonomous Provinces, and in 36 community health services and 28 migrant reception centres. Almost all responders stated that all vaccinations included in the National Immunization Plan are offered to migrant children and adolescents. The situation concerning adults is fragmented, with most of the Regions and local centres offering more vaccines than the national offer—which include polio, tetanus and measles–mumps–rubella. Data on immunized immigrants is archived at the regional/local level with different methods and not available at the national level. Further efforts to ensure consistency in vaccine provision and adequate mechanisms of exchanging data are needed to guarantee a complete vaccination offer and avoid unnecessary health actions, including unnecessary re-vaccination.

Keywords: refugee health; asylum seekers; migrants; infectious diseases; vaccination; Italy

1. Introduction

During 2016, 511,371 people have travelled to Europe from Africa and Asia [1]. Compared with previous years, the proportion of migrants that arrived in Italy increased due to the closure of the Balkan route in March 2016. By the end of the year, 181,436 people had crossed the Mediterranean reaching the Italian coast, approximately 30,000 more than in 2015 [2].

In Italy, all incoming migrants were hosted upon arrival in hotspots located near borders, where they were expected to stay 24 to 48 h. Here, migrants would receive a medical consultation and emergency care if in need. Migrants who did not ask for asylum were then relocated in secure governmental Centres for Identification and Expulsion (CIE), waiting to be accompanied back to their country of origin [3]. Conversely, when migrants wished to seek asylum in Italy, they were sent to the first reception centres, also known as "hubs", non-secure large centres for asylum seekers, located throughout the Italian territory. Here, they were expected to stay for a maximum of 30 days while their asylum claim was being placed [4].

After leaving hubs, migrants seeking asylum or recognized as refugees were taken under the responsibility of a specific system designed for the protection of asylum seekers and refugees (SPRAR system). The SPRAR system offers a set of accommodation and integration services aimed at guaranteeing the protection of asylum seekers and refugees and at facilitating integrated reception at the community level [5]. The increasing number of migrants coming to Italy in the last years has made this system's reception capacity insufficient. For this reason, since 2015, additional highly diverse accommodation structures have been authorized. These structures have been called "extraordinary holding centres" (CAS). Their aim was to reduce delays in the relocation of migrants from hubs to the SPRAR system. The migratory pressure, however, has not decreased and in 2016 there were about 3100 CAS structures that hosted more than 70% of all asylum seekers, while only 7% were in hubs, and less than 20% were hosted through the SPRAR system [6].

Migrants may experience a number of health issues caused by the living conditions faced during the migratory journey and once in migrant reception centres; overcrowding could also favour the occurrence of outbreaks. For vaccine preventable diseases (VPD), these could be fuelled by low immunization coverage among the hosted populations [7–11]. In November 2015, the Joint Statement of the World Health Organization (WHO), the United Nations High Commissioner for Refugees (UNHCR) and the United Nations Children's Fund (UNICEF) [12] and the technical document issued by the European Centre for Disease, Prevention and Control (ECDC) [13] supported the implementation of a comprehensive vaccination offer targeting newly arrived migrants and stated some principles to guide this process.

Migrants residing in the Italian territory have the right to access the same community health services that are available for Italian citizens, while irregular migrants are provided with a temporary health code (STP code) to access, free of charge, 'urgent' or 'essential' care, including some preventive care [14]. The Italian National Health System (NHS) universally offers vaccinations largely free of charge [15]. According to National Immunization Plan (NIP) 2012–2014, in force in 2016, in the first 15 months of age, all children should receive the complete vaccination courses for diphtheria, tetanus, pertussis (DTP), poliomyelitis (IPV), measles-mumps-rubella (MMR), hepatitis B (HBV), haemophilus influentiae type b (HiB), pneumococcus (PCV), meningococcus C (MenC). From 6 to 15 years, children should receive booster doses for DTP, IPV, MMR, a dose of MenC if not immunized before, varicella if susceptible and at 12 years the vaccine against papilloma virus (HPV) for girls only. Adults should receive a booster dose for DTP each 10 years, MMR if susceptible and vaccination against influenza from 65 years. Additional vaccinations are provided depending on risk conditions and epidemiological situations [16].

The responsibility for the provision of health services in Italy has been gradually decentralized at sub-national level to 19 Regions and two Autonomous Provinces (AA.PP.) [17,18]. In each Region/A.P., geographically based local health units (LHU) directly deliver community health services and primary care, including vaccines in public immunization services [15]. In some cases, they are administered by paediatricians/general practitioners (GPs). Due to decentralization, some variations in the vaccination offered across the Regions/AA.PP. are possible both for Italian citizens and for migrants.

Previous studies have assessed immunization policies targeting asylum seekers, refugees, irregular migrants and unaccompanied minors among different Mediterranean countries [19,20] and few studies within specific local settings in Italy [21–23], but, to the best of our knowledge, nobody has explored policies and practices within the Italian territory.

The aim of this paper is to describe national and regional immunization policies targeting asylum seekers, refugees and irregular migrants in Italy and their local application in migrant reception centres and community health services.

2. Materials and Methods

This cross-sectional survey was part of a wider study conducted in six European countries, in the frame of the CARE project (Common Approach for Refugees' and migrants' health) [24].

In Italy, the survey was conducted with two questionnaires to collect data on immunization policies targeting asylum seekers, refugees, irregular migrants and unaccompanied minors at the national and regional level. A third questionnaire, to explore how national policies are applied at the local level, was developed in two versions: one for migrant reception centres and one for community health services. The questionnaires were tested by CARE project partners and modified accordingly.

The national and regional questionnaires were addressed to public health experts working in the field of infectious disease control and vaccination programmes, at the national or regional level, respectively. At the local level, we contacted migrant reception centres from a list provided by the Ministry of Interior and community health services in each Region/A.P. as suggested by the regional public health experts. For each centre/service, the request to fill in the questionnaire was addressed to either the person in charge of the centre/service or a health professional. Only centres with health professionals were asked to complete the survey and were included in the analysis.

The electronic questionnaires were developed using an online software, Survey Monkey [25], and a link to the online questionnaire was sent via email to the identified contact persons. Questions were closed-ended, with optional space for input of free text, and covered the following aspects:

i. legal framework/regulations supporting vaccination offer to asylum seekers, refugees, irregular migrants and unaccompanied minors;
ii. target groups for vaccination, assessment of immunization status and vaccination offered to migrants (children, adolescents and adults);
iii. place for vaccination delivery, availability of Standard Operating Procedures (SOPs) for migrants' immunization;
iv. recording and transmission of data on administered vaccines, and challenges.

For migration-related definitions, we refer to the International Organization for Migration (IOM) glossary of terms [26]. The legal framework/regulation is defined as a law, a recommendation or an immunization plan supporting migrants' vaccination. SOPs are procedures that are shaped from the legal framework and involve actions to achieve the goals set out in the strategy and imply an organization setting out the rules and monitoring their implementation [20].

The national survey was launched in October 2016, the regional and local surveys in November 2016. Data collection was completed in February 2017.

We carried out a descriptive analysis of the data collected at the national, regional and local level in Italy. We performed frequency analysis for all the categorical variables collected and the proportions of responses were summarized.

3. Results

3.1. Profile of the Responders

The national questionnaire was filled in by people in charge of the Infectious disease/VPD Unit at the Ministry of Health (MoH). We received the regional questionnaire from 14 out of 21 Regions/AA.PP.; it was filled in by the public health experts in charge of infectious diseases control at the regional level. At the local level, we received 64 questionnaires: 36 from community health services and 28 from migrant reception centres (Figure 1).

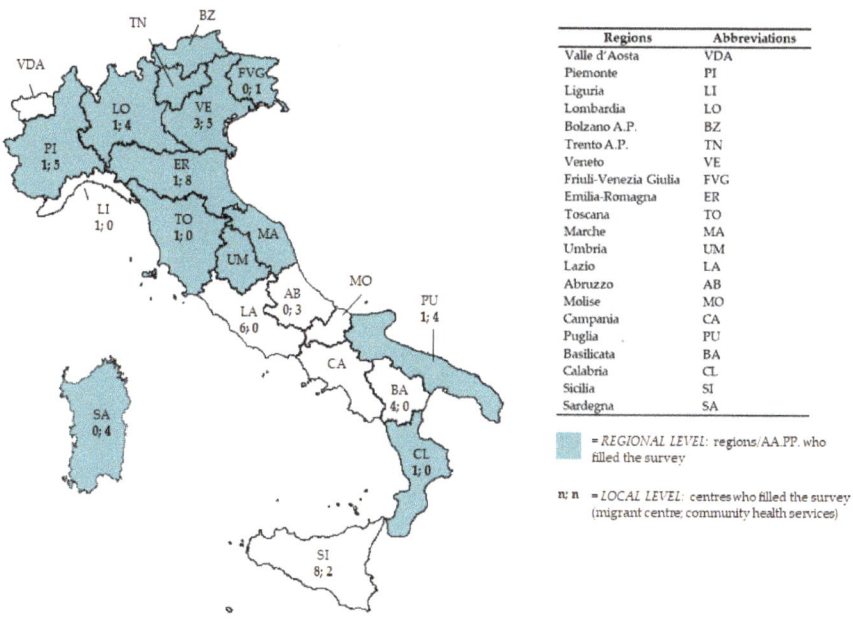

Figure 1. Regions/Autonomous Provinces and local centres/services responding to the questionnaire. Italy, 2017.

3.2. Vaccination Offer at National and Regional Levels

3.2.1. Legal Framework Supporting Vaccination Offers Targeting Asylum Seekers, Refugees, Irregular Migrants and Unaccompanied Minors

A national legal framework has been specifically established for asylum seekers, refugees, and irregular migrants' immunization, with several ministerial decrees since 1993 [27–30]. In addition, the National Plan for Elimination of Measles and congenital rubella 2010–2015 provided indications to increase coverage among "hard-to-reach" groups such as nomads and immigrants [31].

Eight Regions (Piemonte (PI), Bolzano A.P. (BZ), Veneto (VE), Friuli Venezia Giulia (FVG), Emilia Romagna (ER), Umbria (UM), Puglia (PU), Sicilia (SI)) reported having a regional regulation in place supporting migrants' immunization, while the other six (Lombardia (LO), Trento A.P. (TN), Toscana (TO), Marche (MA), Calabria (CL), Sardegna (SA)) just follow the national policy (Table 1).

Table 1. National and regional policies of immunization offer targeting migrants in Italy.

Question	National Level	N of Regions *	% **	Regions
Is there a regional regulation supporting immunization of migrants?				
None	-	6/14	43	LO, TN, TO, MA, CL, SA
Regional regulation specific for migrants ^	-	8/14	57	PI (2012) [1], BZ (2016), VE (2014), FVG (2016), ER (2014), UM (2015), PU (2009) SI (2011)
CHILDREN/ADOLESCENTS				
Which are the target groups for vaccination?				
Immigration status				
All (asylum seekers, refugees, irregular migrants, unaccompanied minors)	X	14/14	100	PI, LO, BZ, TN, VE, FVG, ER, TO, MA, UM, PU, CL, SI, SA
Age group (years)				
0–15		6/14	43	BZ, VE, UM, CL, SI, SA
0–18	X	8/14	57	PI, LO, TN, FVG, ER, TO, MA, PU
Risk conditions				
None	X	14/14	100	PI, LO, BZ, TN, VE, FVG, ER, TO, MA, UM, PU, CL, SI, SA
Is the immunization status verified through anamnesis or check of vaccination card?				
Yes	X	14/14	100	PI, LO, BZ, TN, VE, FVG, ER, TO, MA, UM, PU, CL, SI, SA
Use of laboratory test if migrant has no immunization card?				
Yes	X (HBV, tetanus)	9/13	69	PI (tetanus, measles, HBV), LO (tetanus, diphtheria), BZ (tetanus, diphtheria, HBV), TN (tetanus), FVG (tetanus, HBV, varicella), ER (tetanus, measles, rubella, HBV), UM [2], PU (IPV, MMR, varicella, HBV), SI [2]
Which vaccinations are offered to susceptible migrants?				
All vaccinations included in the NIP	X	13/14	93	PI, LO, BZ, VE, FVG, ER, TO, MA, UM, PU, CL, SI, SA
IPV, tetanus, diphtheria, MMR		1/14	7	TN
ADULTS				
Which are the target groups for vaccination?				
Immigration status				
All (asylum seekers, refugees, irregular migrants)	X	14/14	100	PI, LO, BZ, TN, VE, FVG, ER, TO, MA, UM, PU, CL, SI, SA
Age group (years)				
No limits other than those in the NIP	X	14/14	100	PI, LO, BZ, TN, VE, FVG, ER, TO, MA, UM, PU, CL, SI, SA
Risk conditions				
None	X [3]	13/14	93	PI, LO, BZ, TN, VE, FVG, ER, TO, MA, UM, PU, CL, SI
from polio endemic countries/countries at risk of polio reintroduction		1/14	7	SA
Is the immunization status verified through anamnesis or check of vaccination card in ADULTS?				
Yes	X (polio)	14/14	100	PI, LO, BZ, TN, VE, FVG, ER, TO, MA, UM, PU, CL, SI, SA
Use of laboratory test if migrant has no immunization card?				
Yes	X (HBV, tetanus)	4/14		BZ (tetanus, HBV), TN (tetanus), ER (tetanus, HBV, measles, rubella), CL (all included in the NIP, according to risks)
Informed consent before vaccinating (both for ADULTS and CHILDREN)?				
Yes, oral	n.a. [4]	5/11	45	PI, TN, VE, FVG, MA
Yes, written		6/11	55	LO, BZ, ER, TO, PU, CL
Sites for vaccination delivery (both for ADULTS and CHILDREN)?				
Holding level	X	6/14	43	TN, VE, FVG, TO, PU, SI
Vaccination services	X	13/14	93	PI, LO, BZ, TN, VE, FVG, ER, TO, MA, UM, CL, SI, SA
Primary health care (GP/Paediatricians)		3/14	21	TO, PU [5], CL

* In some cases the denominator is not 14, representing the number of regions responding to each question; ** In some cases column percentages do not add up to 100% because answers to some questions were not mutually exclusive; ^ the year of publication of the regional regulation is reported among brackets; [1] A regional regulation has been released after the closure of the survey; [2] UM and SI stated that they use laboratory test but did not specify for which VPDs; [3] Particular attention paid to migrants from polio endemic countries or countries at risk for polio reintroduction, and those with wounds at risk for tetanus; [4] Not available (n.a.): as the variability of procedures at the regional and local level, the Italian responder could not provide this information; [5] Influenza and PCV vaccinations for adults are administered by GPs. Abbreviations: present (X) Lombardia (LO), Trento A.P. (TN), Toscana (TO), Marche (MA), Calabria (CL), Sardegna (SA), Piemonte (PI), Bolzano A.P. (BZ), Veneto (VE), Friuli Venezia Giulia (FNG), Emilia Romagna (ER), Umbria (UM), Puglia (PU), Sicilia (SI), National Immunization Plan (NIP), poliomyelitis (IPV), measles-mumps-rubella (MMR), hepatitis B (HBV).

3.2.2. Vaccination Offer to Migrant Children and Adolescents

Both at national and regional levels, responders answered that vaccinations were offered to all migrant children/adolescents regardless of their legal status (asylum seekers, refugees, irregular migrants and unaccompanied children) and without setting any limit for risk condition other than those provided in the NIP. The upper age limit for vaccination offer targeting children/adolescent migrants was 15 years for Italy and VE, BZ, UM, CL, SI and SA, or 18 years for the remaining regions.

The responder at the national level and all Regions indicated that immunization status was checked though anamnesis or verification of the immunization cards. At the national level, the responder stated that laboratory tests of immunity for tetanus and HBV is planned, if the migrants have no immunization card. Most regions also used laboratory tests mainly for tetanus and HBV.

At the national level and 13/14 Regions, migrant children and adolescents susceptible or with undocumented status were offered all the vaccinations included in the NIP appropriate for age. TN offered to migrants only vaccinations against polio, tetanus, diphtheria and MMR (Table 1).

3.2.3. Vaccination Offer to Migrant Adults

At the national level, vaccinations were offered to adult migrants, regardless of their legal status and without age specification. As for ministerial decrees, particular attention was paid to migrants coming from polio endemic countries or from countries at risk of polio reintroduction, and to those with wounds at risk for tetanus infection. All 14 of the responding Regions offered immunization to adult migrants without any limit for age groups, although with differences across Regions. In addition, 13/14 Region/AA.PP. did not set any limit for any risk condition other than those provided in the NIP.

Also for adults, at national and regional levels, the immunization status was assessed through anamnesis or by verifying the immunization card. When the vaccination status was undocumented, laboratory testing was recommended at national level and performed in four Regions, mainly for tetanus and HBV (Table 1).

According to national policies, adult migrants susceptible or with an undocumented status were offered vaccinations against polio, tetanus (limited to people presenting risk conditions like exposed wounds) and MMR. Five regions reported that migrant adults received all the vaccinations included in the NIP appropriate for age, while the others indicated that only some vaccinations were offered to migrant adults (Table 2).

Table 2. Vaccination offer to adult migrants documented as susceptible or with an undocumented immunization status, Italy, regions and at local level.

Vaccine	ITALY	REGIONS													LOCAL LEVEL	
		PI	LO	BZ	TN	VE	FVG	ER	TO	MA	UM	PU	CL	SA	SI	Migrant Centres (3) [a]	Health Services (30) [a]
Polio	X	X	X	X	X	X	X	X	X	X	X	X	X	X	X		14
Tetanus	X [b]	X	X	X	X	X	X	X	X	X	X	X	X	X	X [b]	2 *	28
Diphtheria		X	X	X	X	X	X	X	X	X	X	X	X			2 *	27
Pertussis						X	X	X	X		X	X				? *	19
MMR	X			X		X	X	X	X	X	X	X	X			2 *	22
Varicella				X			X [c]									2 *	18
Hepatitis B						X	X	X *	X *		X *	X *				2 *	20 *,[d]
Hepatitis A							X *	X *	X *		X *	X *				2 *	16 *
BCG [e]																	
Influenza							X *	X *	X *		X *	X *				3 *	20 *
PCV				X			X *	X *	X *		X *	X *				2 *	16 *
Meningococcus C/ACWY							X *	X *	X *		X *	X *				2 *	15 *

[a] the number indicates the number of migrant centres and health services; [b] in case of exposed wounds; [c] To women in fertile age; [d] three centres specified that is performed only to people negative to immunization check through laboratory testing; [e] Bacillus Calmette-Guerin; * Four Regions, one migrant centre and 15 health services, limited this offer to population at-risk according to NIP. Abbreviations: present (X).

3.2.4. Vaccine Delivery

According to national policies, vaccinations should be delivered at holding level and community level for children and adults. Vaccines were routinely administered at community level in all Regions, for all age groups (vaccination centres or primary health care centres). In six regions (TN, VE, FVG, TO, CL, SI), vaccinations are delivered also at holding level (Table 1).

Informed consent was always required: verbally in five Regions and in written form in six Regions, among the 11 Regions/P.A. (Table 1).

The responder at the national level did not indicate the presence of SOPs for vaccine delivery for migrants, while seven Regions reported to have SOPs, available in the place of vaccination delivery (BZ, TN, VE, ER, TO, UM, PU). In some Regions, SOPs contained procedures for the facilitation of access to vaccination services for children/adolescents (BZ, VE, ER, TO, UM, PU) and for adults (VE, TO, UM, PU).

3.2.5. Recording of Information on Administered Vaccines and Practical Challenges

The national responder stated that there was not yet a national immunization electronic registry recording all vaccines administered to local population, nor to migrants. In addition, 10/14 Regions affirmed that data on immunised migrants were recorded in regional immunization registries, mostly in the same electronic (PI, LO, BZ, VE, FVG, ER, UM, PU) or paper based (CL, SA) registry for general population. TN and TO developed an electronic registry specifically for migrants. MA recorded the information only in individual immunization cards. In three Regions (BZ, VE, PI), methods for data recording varied by migration centre. Eight Regions made this information available: to Local Health Authorities (BZ, VE, TO, UM, PU), Regional Health Authorities-RHA (VE, FVG, ER, UM, PU), other centres where migrants were relocated (ER, TO) and to regional epidemiology centres (PI, PU).

The main practical challenges faced an immunization offer to migrants are listed in Table 3.

In addition, most Regions enlightened the difficulty of getting information on the immunization status from immunization cards because these are rarely available.

Table 3. Practical challenges in migrants' vaccination at national, regional and local level.

Challenges	ITALY	REGIONS	LOCAL LEVEL	
			Migrant Centres (28) [a]	Health Services (36) [a]
Scarcity of resources	X	PI, LO, TN, ER, TO, PU, CL, SA	6	17
Need of specific training of health care workers on migrant health	X	LO, TO, MA, SA	3	11
Lack of operating procedures	X	PI, MA, CL	4	8
Scarce collaboration within health institutions		PI, LO, MA, TO	7	5
Low compliance of migrants to vaccination		VE	5	7
Lack of health staff		BZ		
Logistic issues			4	2
Waiting time			1	
Difficulties due to the short time of staying of migrants and the frequency of relocation			1	1
Language barriers				3

[a] the number indicates the number of migrant centres and health services. Abbreviations: present (X).

3.3. Vaccination Offer at Local Level

3.3.1. General Information on Responding Centres

The 28 migrant reception centres that filled in the survey were 18 CAS, four centres for unaccompanied minors, five Hubs (with a capacity of 1246, 1200, 744, 496, 414 people) and one CIE (with a capacity of 219 people). Information was collected from 36 community health services from nine Regions. These centres were vaccination services (27), PHC centres (3), or centres of public health/prevention services (6). Characteristics of responding migrant and health services are summarized in Table 4.

Table 4. Characteristics of responding migrant reception centres and community health services.

Total No. of Responding Centres		Migrant Centres (28) [a]	Health Services (36) [a]
Dealing with children/adolescents		15 [b]	35
Dealing with adults		25	32
Performing Health assessment		23	23
Giving a personal health card to migrants		23	22
Available cultural mediators		28	13 [c]
Length of stay of migrants in the centre [d]	<6 months	6	
	6–12 months	12	
	>12 months	10	
Maximum capacity of the centre [d]	<50 people	9	
	51–150	11	
	151–300	1	
	>300	7	
Presence of an outpatient clinics inside the centre [d]		22	
Who provides health services? [d]	PHC services	22	
	NGOs	7	
	Staff of the centre	5	

[a] the number indicates the number of migrant centres and health services; [b] all Hubs were hosting minors; CIE wasn't; [c] four other centres explained that the staff of the migrant centres helped in translating; [d] these questions were addressed to migrant centres only.

3.3.2. Immunization Practices in Migrant Reception Centres

Of the 15 migrant centres hosting minors (including 5 Hubs), 10 indicated that there was a check of immunization status, for all vaccinations included in the NIP appropriate for age. Only five of these centres (including four Hubs) indicated that they offered vaccinations to children/adolescents, all of them providing all the vaccinations included in the NIP appropriate for age. Vaccines were available in two hub centres, while, in the other three centres, they were provided by the community health services and administered by internal health staff. Informed consent is always required (written or verbal) to migrants or to their parents.

Of the 25 centres accommodating adults, seven checked the immunization status and three of them offered vaccinations to migrant adults (three Hubs, also offering vaccination to minors). One administered all vaccinations according to the NIP to adults of all ages, another addressed the vaccination offer to groups at risk only, the third administered only influenza vaccine (Table 2). Vaccines were delivered by the staff of the institution who oversaw the centre in two cases, and by staff of the vaccination service in the third case, and written informed consent was required.

Six out of 10 centres not offering vaccines to children, and 11/22 not offering vaccines to adults reported that they informed migrants on their immunization needs. In addition, sometimes dedicated health staff facilitated migrants' access to vaccination services (in four centres for minors and five for adults), or the staff of the centre contacted the vaccination service to fix a date for the administration of vaccines (two cases), or informed the service through a systematic information flow on the number of migrants in the centre that needed to be vaccinated (three cases).

Six centres also highlighted the presence of formal agreements between the centre and the vaccination service for the provision of vaccines.

All five migrant centres that offered vaccines registered data on vaccine administration, and made them available for other institutions (Table 5). Practical challenges faced by migrant centres are listed in Table 3.

Table 5. Recording and transmission of information on administered vaccines, migrant reception centre and community health services.

	Migrant Reception Centres (5) *	Community Health Services (36) *
Is information on vaccine administration recorded?		
Yes (specify where, more than one answer possible)	5	35 [1]
Individual health record delivered to migrants	4	18
Electronic archive dedicated to migrants	2	9
Paper archives dedicated to migrants	3	8
General population electronic immunization registries	3	25
General population paper-based immunization registries	2	4
Is information on vaccine administration made available to other institutions?		
Yes (specify to whom, more than one answer possible)	5	30 [1]
It follows the same flow of the information on immunization of general population	-	18
To migrants' holding centres	-	15
To LHU vaccination services	4	9
To GPs and paediatricians	-	5
To holding centres where migrants are relocated	4	6
To local health authorities	1	3
To regional health authorities	-	7
To international institutions	1 (IOM)	-

* only migrant centres and community health services administering vaccines; [1] one health service did not answer to these questions.

3.3.3. Immunization Practices in Community Health Services

At the community level, in all 35 health services dealing with paediatric patients (the same offering vaccinations to native population), the immunization status was checked through anamnesis and vaccination card verification. Twenty-five centres reported also performing laboratory tests in case of unknown immunization status (22 for tetanus, 21 for HBV, six for MMR, six for diphtheria, five for varicella, one for the serogroups A, C, W and Y of Meningococcus and pertussis). All 35 centres also offered vaccinations to migrant children/adolescents. Thirty-three offered all vaccinations included in the NIP appropriate for age, one limited the offer to polio, diphtheria, tetanus, HBV, influenza, and MenC, the other to polio, DTP, HBV, Hib, PCV, and MMR. Informed consent was required in 34 out of 35 centres, written in 23 of them.

Twenty-six of the 32 health services dealing with adults reported verifying the immunization status of migrant adults, through anamnesis or by viewing the vaccination card. Twelve centres also provided laboratory testing, if necessary, for HBV (11), tetanus (5), MMR (3), and HAV (1). Thirty out of 32 centres indicated that they offered vaccinations to migrant adults, most of them without any limit related to age or to specific conditions (one specified that the offer was limited to adults from Afghanistan, Cameroon, Equatorial Guinea, Ethiopia, Iraq, Nigeria, Pakistan, Somalia, and Syria, one delivered vaccines to adults at risk only). Half of the centres provided all vaccinations included in the NIP appropriate for age, while others offered only some vaccinations (Table 2). Informed consent was always required, written (19) or verbal (11). Some health services also reported that the staff could conduct outreach vaccination activities in migrant centres (five for migrant children and eight for migrant adults), especially if the number of migrants that needed to be vaccinated was high.

Data on administered vaccines were recorded by 35 out of 36 health services, and the information was made available by 30 health services (Table 5). Practical challenges faced by health services are listed in Table 3.

4. Discussion

As stated by WHO-UNHCR-UNICEF, vaccination access is recommended as part of the health support offered to migrants and should be performed with a systematic, sustainable and non-stigmatizing approach [12]. To our knowledge, this is the first study conducted in Italy to explore national and regional immunization policies targeting migrants and to assess how policies are implemented at local level.

We found that while in case of children the vaccination offer is widespread across Italy, different immunization policies are in place in the Italian Regions for adults. Vaccination against poliomyelitis and tetanus is offered to adults in all the responding Regions as recommended at national level, but only some of them offer MMR vaccination, which is considered a priority by WHO and ECDC, together with vaccination against polio. Some Regions offer more vaccinations than those recommended at the national level, some even offer all vaccinations included in the NIP appropriated for age. In addition, most of the community health services offer a range of vaccinations wider than what is provided by the national policies. The overprovision of vaccinations at regional and local levels compared to the national policies may be explained by several reasons: (i) the attempt to favour the integration of migrants in the community, by offering them all the vaccinations offered to the native population; (ii) the fear that migrants coming from highly endemic countries and living in overcrowded settings are at a higher risk of epidemic outbreaks; (iii) the fear of health threats brought by the mass immigration as the spreading of communicable diseases to the general population whose vaccination coverage is sub-optimal [32]. The observed overprovision is in line with European indications. In fact, although MMR and polio vaccines are a priority [12], a recent review on the current scientific evidence on vaccination in migrants and refugees states that, along with these vaccines, priority should be given also to HBV, diphtheria, tetanus and pertussis [33]. Furthermore, in densely populated settings, vaccinations against meningococcal disease, varicella, pneumococcus, and influenza during the cold season are also recommended [34,35]. Recently, the Italian guidelines for health checks and protection pathways for migrants on arrival have been published [36]. Recommendations concerning vaccination practices include all vaccinations in the NIP appropriate for age for unvaccinated children or children with an undocumented status (0–14 years), while, for adults, polio, diphtheria-tetanus-pertussis, MMR and varicella (except pregnant women), and HBV (after laboratory test of immunity) are indicated [36].

Asylum seekers, refugees, irregular migrants and unaccompanied minors can be moved from one reception centre to another, also across different Regions, and once obtained the asylum seeking or refugee status, they are free to move within the country [37]. Therefore, the regional heterogeneity we observed could impact the type of vaccination offer that adult migrants receive. Sharing of common indications on vaccinations offered to migrants should be encouraged.

Stating current recommendations, the vaccination offer provided according to the national legal framework should be updated, and include vaccines that are already offered by most (but not all) Regions, taking in consideration the availability of human and economic resources. The publication of the Italian guidelines [36] could set the direction of the national regulation.

We found that, in the whole Italian territory, vaccinations are delivered at the community level, mainly through public vaccination services. This is in line with international and Italian recommendations [12,36], and with policies in most European and Mediterranean countries [19,20] that do not recommend immunization at border crossings unless there is an outbreak. In fact, considering that intervals of months can be required between doses, the follow up of immunization series would be hard if the cycle has started at the entry point [12].

Few of the participating Regions/AA.PP and migrant centres reported to have developed procedures to facilitate the access of migrants to the community immunization services, such as dedicated staff to favour the access and fix a date for vaccination, or a systematic flow of information about migrants that need to be vaccinated. It represents a crucial point because it is known that many migrants have limited access to healthcare services because of legal, linguistic, and cultural barriers [13,19]. The local implementation of migrant-friendly procedures to guarantee migrant immunization should be supported.

International guidelines [12] indicate that tracking immunization data of migrant populations and exchange data on administered vaccines would allow appropriately planning immunization series and avoiding duplication of vaccination. We found that mechanisms to record and transmit data on administered vaccines are highly heterogeneous across Regions and local centres. A fundamental instrument to improve the homogeneity and coordination of the vaccination offer in Italy would be a national immunization electronic registry for recording vaccination of immunized migrants. This is a longstanding problem in Italy, where there is no national immunization electronic registry, even for Italian citizens [38]. The new Italian NIP 2017–2019 identified it as a critical issue that should be quickly implemented [39].

Furthermore, considering that Italy is part of the Schengen area, diversity in vaccination offer and data recording makes it more complicated to track migrants across countries to guarantee that migrants complete their immunization schedules and avoid re-vaccination [40]. Synergies in vaccination offer and appropriate mechanisms to promote collaboration and sharing of good practices are therefore needed foremost at the national level but also among different countries [40].

Recurring practical challenges in delivering the vaccination offer were consistently identified at all levels. Along with the scarce collaboration within health institutions and lack of operating procedures that have been highlighted by the fragmentation of the vaccination offer, other problems were low resources and need of specific training of HCW on migrant health. At the local level, some problems were reported that were not indicated at the national–regional level: in particular, low compliance of migrants to vaccination, logistic aspects, language barriers, and very scarce availability of prior immunization individual cards. Similar challenges were identified at the European level and the provision of interpreters, cultural mediators and information in the languages of the migrants were suggested as useful interventions to address the existing barriers to vaccination delivery and utilization [40]. Investigating real world challenges at the local level is essential for addressing the more pressing issues, and to allocate human and financial resources to improve migrants' immunization offers.

Our survey presents several limitations. Firstly, it is not fully representative of the Italian situation. The absence of seven Regions may not give a complete picture of what happens in the Italian territory. Despite this, the responding Regions were well distributed in the Italian territory, covering areas of Northern, Central and Southern Italy and hosting 75% of the migrants arrived in Italy by the end of 2016 [2]. Health and migrant centres are also not representative. Even if contact points were identified in each Region, and all the governmental centres were contacted, participation in the survey was voluntary, and therefore some Regions are more represented than others. Furthermore, we could not stratify answers given at the local level by Region, given the small number.

5. Conclusions

This study provides an overview of immunization policies and practices targeting asylum seekers, refugees, irregular migrants and unaccompanied minors in Italy. The immunization provision for migrant children is guaranteed by national policies and is widespread at the local level. The national offer targeting adults is limited, but it is often increased by regional policies, although diversified.

Further efforts to ensure consistency in vaccine provision across Regions and local centres are needed to guarantee a complete vaccination offer and avoid unnecessary health actions, including unnecessary re-vaccination.

Fragmentation in data collection and recording has been documented at all levels. A national immunization electronic registry should be encouraged to record each vaccination administered, share data on vaccination coverage and monitor the immunization state.

Furthermore, difficulties that have been reported at the local level are not known at the central level. This gap should be bridged as these problems need to be addressed when considering national policies and resource allocations.

Author Contributions: All authors have contributed substantially to the conception of the work. C.G., M.D.M. and S.D. conceived and designed the study, C.G. and M.D.M. developed the questionnaires. M.D.M., C.G. and T.D.Z. collected the data with the survey tool and analyzed the data. T.D.Z. wrote the preliminary paper and M.D.M., C.G., F.R., A.B., M.G.C., M.G.D. and S.D. critically revised the preliminary paper. The CARE Italian survey working group filled out the questionnaires and critically revised the preliminary paper. All of the authors read and approved the final version of the manuscript.

Acknowledgments: The CARE survey on immunization offer targeting migrants was implemented in the framework of the project "717217/CARE" that received funding from the EU health Programme (2014–2020). We acknowledge the contribution and inputs of all Italian participants in the CARE Survey on immunization offer targeting migrants. In addition to the Italian Survey CARE Working Group, that includes the referents for the national and regional surveys, all persons from the Health Services and the Migrant Centres that filled in the questionnaire for the local survey.

Conflicts of Interest: The authors declare no conflict of interest.

References

1. FRONTEX. Migratory Routes Map. Available online: http://frontex.europa.eu/trends-and-routes/migratory-routes-map/ (accessed on 3 March 2017).
2. Italian Ministry of the Interior. Cruscotto Statistico Giornaliero. Available online: http://www.libertaciviliimmigrazione.dlci.interno.gov.it/it/documentazione/statistica/cruscotto-statistico-giornaliero (accessed on 10 July 2017).
3. Italian Ministry of Interior. Schema di Capitolato di Appalto per la Gestione dei Centri di Accoglienza per Immigrati. Available online: http://www1.interno.gov.it/mininterno/export/sites/default/it/assets/files/28_2014/2014_06_20_capitolato_appalto_approvato_D.M._21-11-2008.pdf (accessed on 13 July 2017).
4. Centro Studi e Ricerche IDOS. *Dossier Statistico Immigrazione*; IDOS, Ed.; IDOS: Rome, Italy, 2016; ISBN 9788864800462.
5. SPRAR-Manuale Operativo. Available online: http://www.meltingpot.org/IMG/pdf/sprar_-_manuale_operativo_2015-2.pdf (accessed on 16 July 2017).
6. Anci, Caritas Italiana, Cittalia, Fondazione Migrantes, Ministry of Interior-Sprar, with the Contribution of UNHCR: Rapporto Sulla Protezione Internazionale in Italia, 2016. Available online: http://www.anci.it/Contenuti/Allegati/Rapporto%20protezione%20internazionale%202016.pdf (accessed on 9 July 2017).
7. WHO Regional Office for Europe. Migration and Health: Key Issues. Available online: http://www.euro.who.int/en/health-topics/health-determinants/migration-and-health/migranthealth-in-the-european-region/migration-and-health-key-issues (accessed on 15 July 2017).
8. WHO Data on Immunization, Vaccines and Biologicals. Available online: http://www.who.int/immunization/monitoring_surveillance/data/en/ (accessed on 8 January 2018).
9. Napoli, C.; Riccardo, F.; Declich, S.; Dente, M.G.; Pompa, M.G.; Rizzo, C.; Rota, M.C.; Bella, A.; National Working Group. An early warning system based on syndromic surveillance to detect potential health emergencies among migrants: Results of a two-year experience in Italy. *Int. J. Environ. Res. Public Health* **2014**, *11*, 8529–8541. [CrossRef] [PubMed]
10. Castelli, F.; Sulis, G. Migration and infectious diseases. *Clin. Microbiol. Infect.* **2017**, *23*, 283–289. [CrossRef] [PubMed]
11. European Centre for Disease Prevention and Control. Handbook on Using the ECDC Preparedness Checklist Tool to Strengthen Preparedness against Communicable Disease Outbreaks at Migrant Reception/Detention Centres. Available online: http://ecdc.europa.eu/en/publications/Publications/preparedness-checklist-migrant-centres-tool.pdf (accessed on 3 July 2017).
12. WHO Regional Office per Europe. WHO-UNHCR-UNICEF Joint Technical Guidance: General Principles of Vaccination of Refugees, Asylum-Seekers and Migrants in the WHO European Region. Available online: http://www.euro.who.int/en/health-topics/disease-prevention/vaccines-and-immunization/news/news/2015/11/who,-unicef-and-unhcr-call-for-equitable-access-to-vaccines-for-refugees-and-migrants/who-unhcr-unicef-joint-technical-guidance-general-principles-of-vaccination-of-refugees,-asylumseekers-and-migrants-in-the-who-european-region (accessed on 16 July 2017).

13. ECDC Technical Document: Infectious Diseases of Specific Relevance to Newly-Arrived Migrants in the EU/EEA. Available online: https://ecdc.europa.eu/sites/portal/files/media/en/publications/Publications/Infectious-diseases-of-specific-relevance-to-newly-arrived-migrants-in-EU-EEA.pdf (accessed on 16 July 2017).
14. Italian National Law N. 40, 1998. Available online: http://www.camera.it/parlam/leggi/98040l.htm (accessed on 8 January 2018).
15. European Observatory on Health Systems and Policies. The Health Systems and Policy Monitor. Available online: http://www.hspm.org/searchandcompare.aspx (accessed on 3 March 2017).
16. Italian National Immunization Plan 2012–2014. Available online: http://www.salute.gov.it/imgs/C_17_pubblicazioni_1721_allegato.pdf (accessed on 19 November 2017).
17. Constitutional Law N. 3, 18 Oct 2001. Modifiche al Titolo V Della Parte Seconda Della Costituzione. Available online: http://www.parlamento.it/parlam/leggi/01003lc.htm (accessed on 8 May 2018).
18. Lo Scalzo, A.; Donatini, A.; Orzella, L.; Cicchetti, A.; Profi li, S.; Maresso, A. Italy: Health system review. *Health Syst. Transit.* **2009**, *11*, 1–216. Available online: http://www.euro.who.int/__data/assets/pdf_file/0006/87225/E93666.pdf (accessed on 3 March 2017).
19. Riccardo, F.; Dente, M.G.; Kojouharova, M.; Fabiani, M.; Alfonsi, V.; Kurchatova, A.; Vladimirova, N.; Declich, S. Migrant's access to immunization in Mediterranean Countries. *Health Policy* **2012**, *105*, 17–24. [CrossRef] [PubMed]
20. Giambi, C.; Del Manso, M.; Dente, M.G.; Napoli, C.; Montaño-Remacha, C.; Riccardo, F.; Declich, S. Immunization Strategies Targeting Newly Arrived Migrants in Non-EU Countries of the Mediterranean Basin and Black Sea. *Int. J. Environ. Res. Public Health* **2017**. [CrossRef] [PubMed]
21. Germinario, C.; Gallone, M.S.; Tafuri, S. Migrant health: The Apulian model. *Epidemiol. Prev.* **2015**, *39*, 76–80. [PubMed]
22. El-Hamad, I.; Pezzoli, M.C.; Chiari, E.; Scarcella, C.; Vassallo, F.; Puoti, M.; Ciccaglione, A.; Ciccozzi, M.; Scalzini, A.; Castelli, F. Point-of-Care Screening, Prevalence, and Risk Factors for Hepatitis B Infection Among 3728 Mainly Undocumented Migrants from Non-EU Countries in Northern Italy. *J. Travel Med.* **2015**, *22*, 78–86. [CrossRef] [PubMed]
23. Tornesello, M.; Cassese, R.; De Rosa, N.; Buonaguro, L.; Masucci, A.; Vallefuoco, G.; Palmieri, S.; Schiavone, V.; Piccoli, R.; Buonaguro, F.M. High Prevalence of Human Papillomavirus Infection in Eastern European and West African women immigrants in South Italy. *APMIS* **2011**, *119*, 701–709. [CrossRef] [PubMed]
24. CARE. "Common Approach for Refugees and Other Migrants' Health". Communicable Diseases Monitoring. Available online: http://careformigrants.eu/communicable-diseases-monitoring/ (accessed on 17 July 2017).
25. SurveyMonkey®. Available online: http://it.surveymonkey.com/home.aspx. (accessed on 2 February 2017).
26. International Organization for Migration (IOM), Glossary of Termis. Available online: http://www.iom.int/key-migration-terms (accessed on 15 December 2017).
27. Ministerial Circular, N. 8, 1993. Available online: http://www.trovanorme.salute.gov.it/norme/renderNormsanPdf?anno=0&codLeg=23605&parte=1%20&serie (accessed on 3 March 2017).
28. Operative Procedure, 2011. Available online: http://www.salute.gov.it/imgs/C_17_newsAree_1478_listaFile_itemName_1_file.pdf (accessed on 3 March 2017).
29. Ministerial Circular, 2014. Available online: http://www.seremi.it/sites/default/files/Ministero%20Salute%20-%20Aggiornamento%20delle%20raccomandazioni%20di%20immunoprofilassi%20virus%209%20maggio%202014.pdf (accessed on 3 March 2017).
30. Ministerial Circular, 2017. Available online: http://www.trovanorme.salute.gov.it/norme/renderNormsanPdf?anno=2017&codLeg=59725&parte=1%20&serie=null (accessed on 20 November 2017).
31. National Plan for Elimination of Measles and Congenital Rubella 2010–2015. G.U. Serie Generale n.297 of 23/12/2003. Available online: http://www.salute.gov.it/imgs/C_17_pubblicazioni_1519_allegato.pdf (accessed on 29 January 2018).
32. Italian Ministry of Health. Coperture Vaccinali Pediatriche, i Dati 2015 [Childhood Vaccination Coverage Data, 2015]. Available online: http://www.salute.gov.it/portale/news/p3_2_1_1_1.jsp?menu=notizie&p=dalministero&id=2718 (accessed on 17 July 2017).
33. Mipatrini, D.; Stefanelli, P.; Severoni, S.; Rezza, G. Vaccinations in migrants and refugees: A challenge for European health systems. A systematic review of current scientific evidence. *Pathog. Glob. Health* **2017**, *111*, 59–68. [CrossRef] [PubMed]

34. Clark, R.C.; Mytton, J. Estimating infectious disease in UK asylum seekers and refugees: A systematic review of prevalence studies. *J. Public Health* **2007**, *29*, 420–428. [CrossRef] [PubMed]
35. Cochrane, A.; Evlampidou, I.; Irish, C.; Ingle, S.M.; Hickman, M. Hepatitis B infection prevalence by country of birth in migrant populations in a large UK city. *J. Clin. Virol. Off. Publ. Pan Am. Soc. Clin. Virol.* **2015**, *68*, 79–82. [CrossRef] [PubMed]
36. Linee Guida Sulla Tutela Della Salute e L'assistenza Sociosanitaria Alle Popolazioni Migranti [Italian Guidelines for Migrants' Health]. Available online: http://www.inmp.it/index.php/ita/Pubblicazioni/Libri/Rassegna-di-revisioni-sistematiche-linee-guida-e-documenti-di-indirizzo-sulla-salute-degli-immigrati-Scarica-il-documento (accessed on 20 July 2017).
37. Italian Ministry of Interior. I Diritti Riconosciuti. Available online: http://www.integrazionemigranti.gov.it/Areetematiche/ProtezioneInternazionale/Pagine/I-diritti.aspx (accessed on 15 July 2017).
38. D'Ancona, F.; Gianfredi, V.; Riccardo, F.; Iannazzo, S. Immunization strategies at national level in Italy and the roadmap for a future Italian National Registry. *Ann. Ig.* **2018**, *30*, 77–85. [PubMed]
39. Piano Nazionale di Prevenzione Vaccinale (PNPV) 2017–2019 (National Immunization Plan). Available online: https://www.salute.gov.it/imgs/C_17_pubblicazioni_2571_allegato.pdf (accessed on 10 July 2017).
40. De Vito, E.; Parente, P.; de Waure, C.; Poscia, A.; Ricciardi, W. *A Review of Evidence on Equitable Delivery, Access and Utilization of Immunization Services for Migrants and Refugees in the WHO European Region*; Health Evidence Network Synthesis Report; WHO: Geneva, Switzerland, 2017; Volume 53.

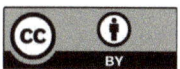

© 2018 by the authors. Licensee MDPI, Basel, Switzerland. This article is an open access article distributed under the terms and conditions of the Creative Commons Attribution (CC BY) license (http://creativecommons.org/licenses/by/4.0/).

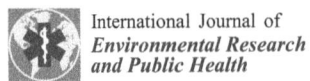

Commentary

Time to Rethink Refugee and Migrant Health in Europe: Moving from Emergency Response to Integrated and Individualized Health Care Provision for Migrants and Refugees

Karl Puchner, Evika Karamagioli *, Anastasia Pikouli, Costas Tsiamis, Athanasios Kalogeropoulos, Eleni Kakalou, Elena Pavlidou and Emmanouil Pikoulis

International Medicine—Health Crisis Management, Medical School, NKUA, Dilou1 & M. Asias, 11527 Athens, Greece; karl.puchner@gmx.de (K.P.); pikoulianastasia@gmail.com (A.P.); ctsiamis@med.uoa.gr (C.T.); kardamyla.chios@gmail.com (A.K.); ekakalou@yahoo.gr (E.K.); lenapvld@gmail.com (E.P.); mpikoul@med.uoa.gr (E.P.)
* Correspondence: karamagioli@gmail.com; Tel.: +30-210-7461455

Received: 15 April 2018; Accepted: 25 May 2018; Published: 28 May 2018

Abstract: In the last three years, the European Union (EU) is being confronted with the most significant influx of migrants and refugees since World War II. Although the dimensions of this influx—taking the global scale into account—might be regarded as modest, the institutional response to that phenomenon so far has been suboptimal, including the health sector. While inherent challenges of refugee and migrant (R&M) health are well established, it seems that the EU health response oversees, to a large extend, these aspects. A whole range of emergency-driven health measures have been implemented throughout Europe, yet they are failing to address adequately the changing health needs and specific vulnerabilities of the target population. With the gradual containment of the migratory and refugee waves, three years after the outbreak of the so-called 'refugee crisis', we are, more than ever, in need of a sustainable and comprehensive health approach that is aimed at the integration of all of migrants and refugees—that is, both the new and old population groups that are already residing in Europe—in the respective national health systems.

Keywords: refugee and migrant (R&M) health; refugee crisis; healthcare; European Union (EU)

1. Introduction

According to the World Health Organization (WHO), both at the global and national levels, the health policies and strategies to manage the health consequences of migration and displacement have failed to keep up with the speed and diversity of modern migration and displacement [1]. The approaches are frequently fragmented and costly, sometimes operating in parallel to national health systems, and may depend on external funding, which can lack sustainability. In addition to the systemic response deficiencies that have been observed, refugee and migrant (R&M) health as a field, exhibits significant inherent challenges as it is dealing with people that are in transit, with multiple vulnerabilities within an unstable sociopolitical context. Although often underestimated, the exposure to health risks during the transit phase is immense. Evidence from past refugee and migrant movements show that, depending on the context, up to more than 20% of the population on the move might die on the grounds of murder, illness, or accidents [2]. Apart from the disproportionally high mortality rate, R&M populations exhibit a series of specific vulnerabilities that pose further risks for their health status. Prolonged fear, chronic anxiety, low self-esteem, loss of control, and alienation are common emotional states among R&M—it is known that chronic exposure to these may have a detrimental effect on health [3]. However, the increased vulnerability of R&M is not only caused by adverse emotional states but also by the underlying structural factors influencing the basic social determinants of health. The major impact that social determinants may have on health status is widely recognized, with the WHO proclaiming action on social justice as a top health policy priority [4]. In particular, poor or insecure housing, higher exposure to and lesser protection from violence, barriers to employment, the legal, and the educational and the health system are potent morbidogenic conditions which R&Ms have often to endure in host countries [5,6]. Finally, it should not be forgotten that R&M movements occur in and/or trigger an unstable sociopolitical context and they are frequently also characterized by changing epidemiological patterns, depending on the transitional phase. Thus, while acute and pressing health problems, such as accidents and acute infections, typically dominate the epidemiology of first phase of transition, it is with provisional or permanent settlement that the full burden of chronic diseases and mental health illness unfolds [7].

This manuscript aims to assess the current R&M health response and discuss the necessity for an integrated and individualized health care provision model for migrants and refugees in the European context.

2. R&M Health in the European Context

For the first time after World War II, the country members of the European Union (EU) have been confronted with a significant influx of R&M. Contrary to the prior mass population movements that were unfolding in Europe, the current influx consists of a highly inhomogeneous population of third country nationals with diverse ethnical and social backgrounds, migration motives, and legal status, and on arrival, these people may have and/or can achieve in the respective host country based on international, national, and EU law (i.e., asylum seekers, refugee, migrants, and undocumented migrants). During the peak year of the R&M movements, in 2015, the UNHCR registered 1,015,078 sea arrivals on EU territory. However, within the context of the EU–Turkey deal and other bilateral agreements with neighboring states, which are aimed at containment of the R&M movements towards Europe, the arrivals had dropped to less than 171,000 in 2017 [8]. With more than 65 million forcibly displaced people living worldwide and a global migrant population of 258 million people [9], it becomes evident that the recent R&M wave that is reaching the EU is of a rather moderate scale. Given the substantial demographic and huge economic size of the EU—its share of the world GDP reaches 23%—it is highly unlikely that the recent R&M wave overstretches the immigration capacity of the member states [10]. Yet, surprisingly enough, the term 'refugee crisis', which emerged in 2015, has dominated ever since the public discourse and has substantially influenced the political landscape both at a European and national level. In line with this rather abrupt reaction of the public opinion, most of the policy response to the R&M wave has been emergency driven without any long-term scope, common vision, and/or acting among the EU-member states, which often results in desultory, uncoordinated, or even contradictory responses at all levels, including the field of R&M health.

A multitude of stakeholders, from (non-governmental organizations) NGOs to ministries and European authorities with various mandates and portfolios, have co-acted in financing and providing provisional health services to R&M during the past few years. Yet, the success of this mass mobilization of resources and manpower, in terms of health outcomes, is rather modest. With the extremely limited legal pathways that are offered to people seeking international protection by the EU, the unsafe trespassing of the Mediterranean Sea, was and remains, even three years after the peak of the recent R&M wave, the predominant entry route into Europe. The dangerous voyage, in combination with the indecisiveness of the EU and its member states to establish an effective sea rescue response mechanism, poses a life-threatening situation—it is estimated that more than 12,000 people have died or disappeared along the trespassing routes in the Mediterranean Sea since 2015 [8]. It should also be added that the lack of legal pathways and safe passage for people on the move favors a dependency on smuggler and trafficking networks, which automatically exacerbates their exposure to violence and insecurity [11]. Although, as in every R&M mass movement, the transit accommodation in camps and other types of mass accommodation often constitutes an inevitable interim solution, and little has been done in order to prevent health hazards that arise from overcrowding and prolonged stay under poor living conditions. Numerous reports on measles and varicella outbreaks in refugee camps throughout the EU are indicative of a deferred and/or delayed vaccination coverage of this vulnerable population, while the frequently observed scabies and sporadic Hepatitis A outbreaks are suggestive of the negligence of basic water, sanitation, and hygiene measures by the respective public health authorities [12–14]. These, by all means preventable, outbreaks sustain the common but ill-founded concern of R&M spreading infectious diseases. Prolonged or consecutive stays in camps and reception centers, were and still are routine practice in many member states, substantially aggravating the health status, particularly of the most vulnerable, that is, of the children, multimorbid patients, and people living with disabilities [15]. In addition, it becomes evident that the health authorities throughout the EU have grossly underestimated the importance of mental health services with protracted and grave psychiatric manifestations being currently a frequent phenomenon among the population that are under discussion [16,17]. Tailored interventions targeting systematically highly prevalent health problems among the R&M populations, such as exposure to sexual and gender based violence (SGBV) and post traumatic stress disorders (PTSD), are still rarely encountered in the EU context [18]. There is enough evidence showing that restricting access to health care for R&M is not only unfavorable for the health status of this population but it is also economically counterproductive for the health system of the host country [19]. Contrary to that evidence, the health policy for R&M in the EU remains predominantly restrictive. In particular, unconditional and free access to healthcare for undocumented migrants is restricted to emergency services in most of the EU member states, leading to a de facto exclusion of this population group from the majority of preventive healthcare services [20]. Furthermore, legislation reform for equalizing access to the health care of refugees/asylum seekers with the rest of the insured population is still pending in many countries, such as Germany, Denmark, and Belgium [21]. In this context, it is also worth mentioning that only 13 of the 28-member states offer free of charge interpreting services to patients, while none of the EU member states have, until now, an official health strategy targeting migrants [21,22].

3. The Need to Move from Emergency Response to Integrated and Individualized Health Care Provision for Migrants and Refugees

Three years after the peak influx of R&M in 2015 into the EU territory, the EU health response is still predominantly emergency-driven. Although the new arrivals are gradually contained, the policies and operations, including health, remain short-term financed, short-sighted, and essentially unharmonized with the international obligations of the EU. One of the most blatant examples of these failures is the current border management, which appeals to a prolonged 'emergency state', and primarily consists of policing, securitization, and off-shoring and out-sourcing of activities that are aimed at fending off immigrants. Thus, it is inherently in conflict with the human rights framework and the Health in All Policies (HiAP) approach, to which the EU is officially committed. Furthermore, it should be noted that the EU has recently made explicit commitments under the UN Sustainable Development Goals, which recognizes the positive contribution of refugees and migrants to have inclusive growth and sustainable development, and to promote universal health coverage of all people, irrespective of their legal status [23]. Notwithstanding the encouragement of developments at the policy level, such as the recent recast of the Reception Directive, which contains improvement and harmonization of the reception conditions throughout the EU [24], a further improvement of legislation, harmonization, and broadening of entitlement to free health care is urgently needed for both the new R&M and the majority of R&M that are already residing in Europe. Parallel to this, intensified efforts that are aimed at assessing and tackling huge public health problems of the R&M population, such as mental health impairment, vaccination coverage, and SGBV, are essential. These measures, although requiring substantial investments, can pave the path to full integration of the majority of the R&Ms in the respective country health system, significantly improving the health status of the general population and significantly reducing health expenditure in the long run.

In addition to the actions at the policy level, a comprehensive and tailored operational approach is needed in order to ensure a smooth integration of the individual patients into the respective health systems. A multidisciplinary assessment of social determinants, such as the housing situation, legal, employment, and insurance status, at the very first contact with the health system is key in order to start addressing the parallel health needs and pressing social issues that can significantly affect the health status of the individual. A timely linkage, after first contact with the health system to a primary health care unit with extended health, social, and interpretation services, will thus allow the prioritization of problems and coordinated referral, and could further enhance the integration of the individual patient in the respective health system, without overstretching the capacities of the secondary and tertiary health care level (Figure 1).

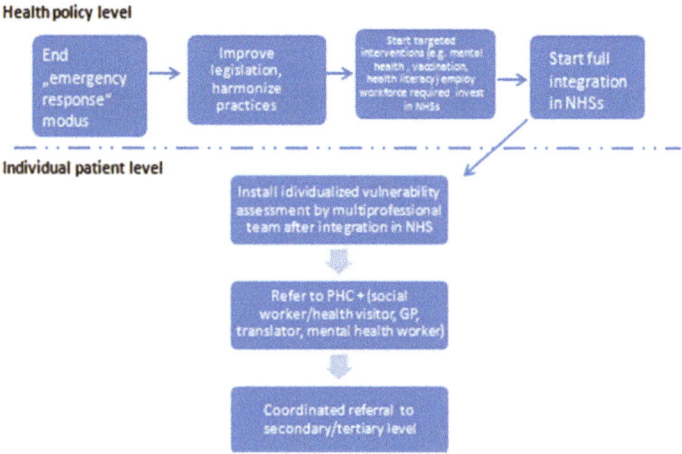

Figure 1. Integrated and individualized health care healthcare provision scheme.

4. Conclusions

In the face of the current situation, it is key to not only to deal with the short-term needs of the recently arrived R&M, but to also to integrate long-term R&M health responses in the respective health systems of the member states and thus strengthen the public health at the national and European level. Access to responsive, people-centered health systems is essential in order to ensure good quality health care for all refugees, asylum seekers, and migrants, not only during their migration journey but also after settlement in their respective host countries. This implies mainstreaming of R&M health in all European and national policies that are related to migration; reducing R&M specific vulnerabilities; overcoming formal and informal barriers to health care, such as language, administrative hurdles, or lack of information about health entitlements and meeting the needs of all of the R&Ms, irrespective of their legal status.

Author Contributions: Karl Puchner developed the layout of the manuscript, provided literature review, and edited the content. Evika Karamagioli, Anastasia Pikouli, Costas Tsiamis, Athanasios Kalogeropoulos, Eleni Kakalou, and Elena Pavlidou contributed to the subsequent versions of the article. Emmanouil Pikoulis critically evaluated the draft of the manuscript.

Conflicts of Interest: The authors declare no conflict of interest.

References

1. World Health Organization (WHO). *Promoting the Health of Refugees and Migrants—Draft Framework of Priorities and Guiding Principles to Promote the Health of Refugees and Migrants*; World Health Assembly, A70/24, Provisional Agenda Item 13.7; WHO: Geneva, Switzerland, 2017.
2. Keely, C.; Reed, H.; Waldman, R. Understanding Mortality Patterns in Complex Humanitarian Emergencies. In *Forced Migration & Mortality*; Reed, H.E., Keely, C.B., Eds.; Commission on Behavioral and Social Sciences and Education National Research Council; National Academy Press: Washington, DC, USA, 2001; pp. 1–51.
3. Levecque, K.; Lodewyckx, I.; Vranken, J. Depression and generalised anxiety in the general population in Belgium: A comparison between native and immigrant groups. *J. Affect. Disord.* **2007**, *97*, 229–239. [CrossRef] [PubMed]
4. World Health Organization. *Closing the Gap in a Generation: Health Equity through Action on the Social Determinants of Health*; Final Report of the Commission on Social Determinants of Health; WHO: Geneva, Switzerland, 2018.
5. Tinghog, P.; Hemmingsson, T.; Lundberg, I. To what extent may the association between immigrant status and mental illness be explained by socioeconomic factors? *Soc. Psychiatry Psychiatr. Epidemiol.* **2007**, *42*, 990–996. [CrossRef] [PubMed]
6. Fleischman, Y.; Willen, S.S.; Davidovitch, N.; Mor, Z. Migration as a social determinant of health for irregular migrants: Israel as case study. *Soc. Sci. Med.* **2015**, *147*, 89–97. [CrossRef] [PubMed]
7. Zimmerman, C.; Kiss, L.; Hossain, M. Migration and health: A framework for 21st century policy-making. *PLoS Med.* **2011**, *8*, e1001034. [CrossRef] [PubMed]
8. UNHCR. Mediterenean Situation Sea Arrivals. 2018. Available online: https://data2.unhcr.org/en/situations/mediterranean (accessed on 13 April 2018).
9. *United Nations DoEaSA, Population Division*; International Migration Report; United Nations: New York, NY, USA, 2017.
10. Strandell, H.; Wolff, P. *The EU in the World*, 2016 ed.; Eurostat: Brussels, Belgium, 2016; pp. 77–90.
11. Freedman, J. Sexual and gender-based violence against refugee women: A hidden aspect of the refugee "crisis". *Reprod. Health Matters* **2016**, *24*, 18–26. [CrossRef] [PubMed]
12. Jones, G.; Haeghebaert, S.; Merlin, B.; Antona, D.; Simon, N.; Elmouden, M.; Battist, F.; Janssens, M.; Wyndels, K.; Chaud, P. Measles outbreak in a refugee settlement in Calais, France: January to February 2016. *Euro Surveill.* **2016**, *21*, 30167. [CrossRef] [PubMed]
13. Mellou, K.; Chrisostomou, A.; Sideroglou, T.; Georgakopoulou, T.; Kyritsi, M.; Hadjichristodoulou, C.; Tsiodras, S. Hepatitis A among refugees, asylum seekers and migrants living in hosting facilities, Greece, April to December 2016. *Euro Surveill.* **2017**, *22*, 30448. [CrossRef] [PubMed]
14. Vairo, F.; Di Bari, V.; Panella, V.; Quintavalle, G.; Torchia, S.; Serra, M.C.; Sinopoli, M.T.; Lopalco, M.; Ceccarelli, G.; Ferraro, F.; et al. An outbreak of chickenpox in an asylum seeker centre in Italy: Outbreak investigation and validity of reported chickenpox history, December 2015–May 2016. *Euro Surveill.* **2017**, *22*. [CrossRef] [PubMed]
15. Blitz, B.K.; d'Angelo, A.; Kofman, E.; Montagna, N. Health Challenges in Refugee Reception: Dateline Europe 2016. *Int. J. Environ. Res. Public Health* **2017**, *14*, 1484. [CrossRef] [PubMed]
16. Anagnostopoulos, D.C.; Giannakopoulos, G.; Christodoulou, N.G. A Compounding Mental Health Crisis: Reflections from the Greek Experience with Syrian Refugees. *Am. J. Psychiatry* **2016**, *173*, 1081–1082. [CrossRef] [PubMed]
17. Jefee-Bahloul, H.; Bajbouj, M.; Alabdullah, J.; Hassan, G.; Barkil-Oteo, A. Mental health in Europe's Syrian refugee crisis. *Lancet Psychiatry* **2016**, *3*, 315–317. [CrossRef]
18. Sijbrandij, M.; Acarturk, C.; Bird, M.; Bryant, R.A.; Burchert, S.; Carswell, K.; de Jong, J.; Dinesen, C.; Dawson, K.S.; el Chammay, R.; et al. Strengthening mental health care systems for Syrian refugees in Europe and the Middle East: Integrating scalable psychological interventions in eight countries. *Eur. J. Psychotraumatol.* **2017**, *8*, 1388102. [CrossRef] [PubMed]
19. Bozorgmehr, K.; Razum, O. Effect of Restricting Access to Health Care on Health Expenditures among Asylum Seekers and Refugees: A Quasi Experimental Study in Germany, 1994–2013. *PLoS ONE* **2015**, *10*, e0131483. [CrossRef] [PubMed]

20. Gray, B.H.; van Ginneken, E. Health care for undocumented migrants: European approaches. *Issue Brief.* **2012**, *33*, 1–12. [PubMed]
21. Médecins du Monde. *European Network to Reduce Vulnerabilities in Health-Observatory Reports*; Legal Report on Access to Healthcare in 16 European Countries; Médecins du Monde: Paris, France, 2017.
22. EWSI Editorial Team EC. Migrant Health across Europe: Little Structural Policies, Many Encouraging Practices. 2018. Available online: https://ec.europa.eu/migrant-integration/feature/migrant-health-across-europe (accessed on 12 April 2018).
23. Eurostat Monitoring Report. How Has the EU Progressed towards the Sustainable Development Goals? 2017. Available online: http://ec.europa.eu/eurostat/documents/2995521/8462309/8-20112017-AP-EN.pdf/f5e04614-0595-47ce-b17f-0f87648ddcd5 (accessed on 20 November 2017).
24. European Commission. *Proposal for a Directive of the European Parliament and of the Council Laying Down Standards for the Reception of Applicants for International Protection (Recast) COM (2016) 465 Final*; European Commission: Brussels, Belgium, 2016.

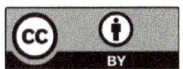

© 2018 by the authors. Licensee MDPI, Basel, Switzerland. This article is an open access article distributed under the terms and conditions of the Creative Commons Attribution (CC BY) license (http://creativecommons.org/licenses/by/4.0/).

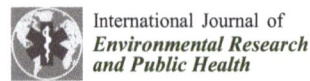

Review

Key Dimensions for the Prevention and Control of Communicable Diseases in Institutional Settings: A Scoping Review to Guide the Development of a Tool to Strengthen Preparedness at Migrant Holding Centres in the EU/EEA

Flavia Riccardo [1,2,*], Jonathan E. Suk [3], Laura Espinosa [3,4], Antonino Bella [2], Cristina Giambi [2], Martina Del Manso [2], Christian Napoli [2,5], Maria Grazia Dente [2], Gloria Nacca [2] and Silvia Declich [2]

1. European Programme for Intervention Epidemiology Training (EPIET), European Centre for Disease Prevention and Control, (ECDC), Solna 169 73, Sweden
2. Istituto Superiore di Sanità, Rome 00161, Italy; antonio.bella@iss.it (A.B.); cristina.giambi@iss.it (C.G.); martina.delmanso@iss.it (M.D.M.); christian.napoli@uniroma1.it (C.N.); mariagrazia.dente@iss.it (M.G.D.); gloria.nacca@iss.it (G.N.); silvia.declich@iss.it (S.D.)
3. European Centre for Disease Prevention and Control, (ECDC), Solna 169 73, Sweden; Jonathan.Suk@ecdc.europa.eu (J.E.S.); lau.espinosa.m@gmail.com (L.E.)
4. UCD School of Agriculture and Food Science, University College Dublin, Dublin D04 V1W8, Ireland
5. Department of Medical Surgical Sciences and Traslational Medicine, "Sapienza" University of Rome, Rome 00185, Italy
* Correspondence: flavia.riccardo@iss.it; Tel.: +39-06-4990-4322

Received: 4 April 2018; Accepted: 29 May 2018; Published: 30 May 2018

Abstract: Migrant centres, as other institutions hosting closed or semi-open communities, may face specific challenges in preventing and controlling communicable disease transmission, particularly during times of large sudden influx. However, there is dearth of evidence on how to prioritise investments in aspects such as human resources, medicines and vaccines, sanitation and disinfection, and physical infrastructures to prevent/control communicable disease outbreaks. We analysed frequent drivers of communicable disease transmission/issues for outbreak management in institutions hosting closed or semi-open communities, including migrant centres, and reviewed existing assessment tools to guide the development of a European Centre for Disease Prevention and Control (ECDC) checklist tool to strengthen preparedness against communicable disease outbreaks in migrant centres. Among articles/reports focusing specifically on migrant centres, outbreaks through multiple types of disease transmission were described as possible/occurred. Human resources and physical infrastructure were the dimensions most frequently identified as crucial for preventing and mitigating outbreaks. This review also recognised a lack of common agreed standards to guide and assess preparedness activities in migrant centres, thereby underscoring the need for a capacity-oriented ECDC preparedness checklist tool.

Keywords: migrant health; preparedness; communicable diseases

1. Introduction

Migration, one of the determinants of population change in the European Union (EU), is a continuous long-term reality [1] that has been described also as a driver for economic growth [2]. Notwithstanding, it is often addressed in a complex climate, where security, rather than health, drives management priorities [3]. In this context, EU public health authorities are asked to provide relevant, proportionate, and targeted action [4]. In 2015, Europe received over 1.2 million asylum seekers [5], placing considerable strain on the provision of health services [6].

Undocumented migrants entering continental Europe are often placed for a short period of time (hours–days) in temporary accommodation facilities. Here, they are identified, offered an initial medical assessment/screening [7], and provided medical care, if needed. Following this, depending on their legal status (asylum seekers vs irregular migrants), they can be transferred to medium term accommodation facilities, migrant reception or detention institutions (hereby migrant centres), where they can stay for a longer period of time (weeks–months).

Migrant centres in Europe are institutions that typically host semi-open (reception centres) and closed (detention centres) communities. As stated by Basu et al., institutions *"are characterized by a combination of multiple and interacting social determinants of infectious disease spread (...) including close and prolonged human contact, poor ventilation, containment of highly susceptible or immunocompromised groups, and significant flows of persons into and out of these institutions"* [8]. It can be expected that, as in other institutional settings, like prisons, military barracks, and schools, migrant centres face specific challenges in preventing and controlling disease transmission. Dimensions such as human resources, medicines/vaccines, sanitation/disinfection, and physical infrastructure are all critical for the prevention, early detection, and outbreak management in institutional settings. It is, however, uncertain what could be priorities for action in migrant reception/detention centres.

In 2016, the European Centre for Disease Prevention and Control (ECDC) developed a "Preparedness checklist tool to strengthen preparedness against communicable disease outbreaks at migrant reception/detention centres" [9]. This tool guides the assessment of gaps in critical dimensions within these centres, and could be useful for decision makers in EU/EEA member states to prioritise investments to enhance routine capacity, as well as preparedness for large sudden influxes of migrants.

The development of this tool was evidence-based, according to a scoping review of the scientific and grey literature. There were two key objectives to this review. The first was to identify challenges for the prevention and control of communicable diseases in migrant centres and similar institutional settings (hereafter objective 1). The second was to identify suitable approaches for assessing strengths and weaknesses in controlling/preventing communicable diseases in migrant centres (hereafter objective 2). This paper presents the results of this scoping study and how those findings impacted the ECDC tool development.

2. Materials and Methods

Studies in peer-reviewed journals and grey literature were included if:

(i) they were published between January 2000 and October 2015 in English, French, or Italian;
(ii) they referred to institutional settings (i.e., institutions hosting "closed" or "semi-open" communities);
(iii) they described types of disease transmission in these settings, and which dimensions were more frequently critical for transmission prevention/outbreak control (so as to address objective 1);
(iv) they described existing assessment tools or prior assessments (so as to address objective 2).

Articles/reports were excluded if they did not address human health and when abstracts/full texts were not retrievable from open source and journal subscriptions available to the Italian Institute of Public Health (ISS) and ECDC. The selection process followed four phases: identification, screening, eligibility, and inclusion, as described in the PRISMA statement [10].

We defined four axes: Exposure, Population, Outcome, Methods, to develop a set of common search roots for the scientific literature search. We identified Medical Subject Headings (MeSH) terms for each search axis, unless term definitions were unrelated to the search context.

The exposure axis included search terms to identify articles on disease transmission; population included terms on institutional settings and methods included terms on assessment tools or prior assessments. The outcome axis included search terms on prevention and control, and on emergency preparedness.

Four search strings were developed by combining the search terms in each axis (Figure 1), systematically giving preference to terms and combinations that provided a greater article yield. Articles were extracted from PubMed on 18 October 2015.

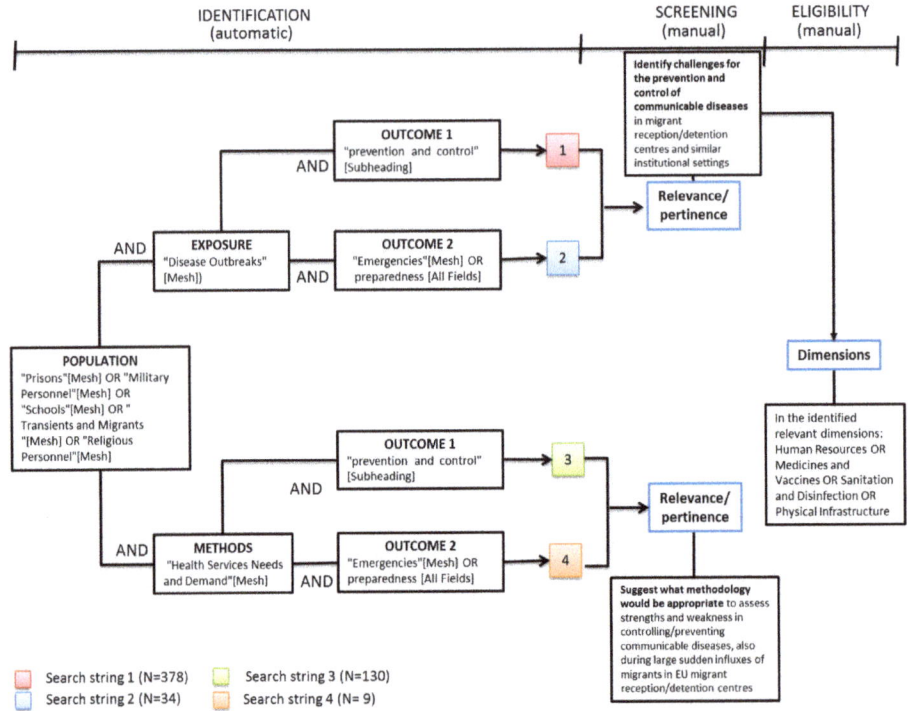

Figure 1. Scientific literature search strategy diagram. EU: European Union.

The same four search axes guided the grey literature search. Articles were "hand-searched" for potentially relevant grey literature from October to December 2015 on the following targeted websites: ECDC, World Health Organization (WHO), the International Organization for Migration (IOM), United Nations High Commissioner for Refugees (UNHCR), Doctors Without Borders (MSF), the Red Cross, the UN Office for the Coordination of Humanitarian Affairs (OCHA).

One reviewer screened each article/report for relevance, to identify which ones would then be analysed in full text, on the basis of the abstracts (scientific literature) and the executive summaries (grey literature). Thereafter, in the eligibility phase, selected articles/reports were analysed in full text to identify if they addressed objective 1 or 2 (or both). For articles addressing objective 1, we also documented which dimensions for communicable disease prevention/control were identified to be critical (dimension analysis).

A dimension was classified as critical when its inadequacy was recognised by authors as one of the causes of outbreak development, or when its reinforcement through response actions was recognised as pivotal for successful outbreak containment. There were four pre-identified dimensions (human resources, medicines/vaccines, sanitation/disinfection, and physical infrastructure). Additional dimensions were documented when identified as critical in the literature (hereby additional dimensions).

3. Results

3.1. Selection Process

We identified 551 scientific articles, of which 522 were screened, and 46 assessed in full text. Three articles were excluded in the eligibility phase because they did not report on actual disease transmission but on mathematical models, and on options to design health policies and strategies (Figure 2). Among the 43 included scientific articles, 72% focused on European/North American countries, and 49% were published after 2010. Most articles (86%) focused on educational institutions (schools, universities, college etc., including both day and boarding institutions) and correctional settings (jails and prisons). Two papers targeted migrant centres [11,12]. Most articles (35) addressed the first objective, the remaining addressed the second.

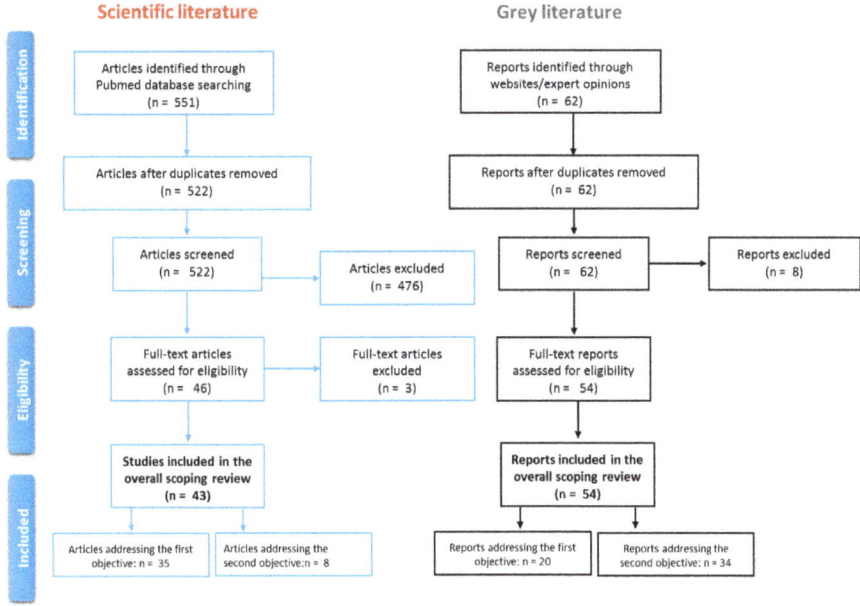

Figure 2. Results of the scientific and grey literature scoping review.

We retrieved 62 grey literature reports and included 54 in the review (Figure 2). Twenty addressed the first objective. All were situation analysis studies focusing on European migrant centres and most (80%) were produced by the WHO PHAME [13] and the IOM EquiHealth Projects [14] between 2013 and 2015. The remaining 34 reports addressed the second objective.

3.2. Challenges for the Prevention and Control of Communicable Diseases in Migrant Centres and Similar Institutional Settings

Fifty-five articles/reports addressed the first objective of this review (35 peer reviewed articles and 20 reports—see Supplementary File 1 for further details). Of those, 27% were published in the Unites States, 20% by WHO, and 11% by IOM. The 35 articles focused on what favoured outbreak development or its control in a wide range of institutional settings from an operational standpoint. Conversely, the 20 reports addressing the same objective focused exclusively on national migrant reception systems and facilities in Europe, generally from a wider public health perspective [15–34].

We found evidence of both direct and indirect transmission of gastrointestinal infections [35,36] in both educational and correctional institutions (Figure 3). In a literature review of reports of gastrointestinal outbreaks in correctional settings, authors found that "*Bacterial agents were associated with 76% of outbreaks, and viral agents were associated with 21%. One outbreak was associated with the protozoan parasite Cryptosporidium, while 'multiple organisms' were associated with an additional outbreak (...) Routes of transmission (...) were foodborne in 67% of cases and person-to-person in 11% of cases*" [36]. Outbreaks of human-to-human transmitted infections were described in different institutions where close physical congregation of individuals occurs [11,37–45]. Conversely, outbreaks of skin infections [46], sexually transmitted diseases (STD), and blood borne viruses (BBV) [47–49] were described more frequently in correctional settings: "*High syphilis prevalence and multiple sexual partnerships result in the potential for extensive syphilis transmission. Condoms are not likely used*" [47]. Some studies have identified factors pointing to an increased risk of transmission among inmates: " *... disproportionate incarceration of people at higher risk for HIV infection, (...) persons with mental illness, substance users, those who trade in sex (...) inmate behaviours that risk HIV transmission—including sex (forced and consensual), injection drug use and tattooing—and the limited availability of condoms and clean needles*" [49]; " *... many prison entrants have histories of injecting drug use (IDU), and thus already have high prevalences of blood borne viruses (BBVs). (...) ... the lack or under-supply of preventive measures (...) combined with extreme social conditions, and consequent prisoner behaviour, creates extra opportunities for BBV transmission. Viruses such as HIV can be transmitted sexually, through sharing injecting drug equipment, by non-sterile tattooing, and transmission of blood or bodily substances during assaults (...) sharing of equipment for shaving and haircutting ...* " [48].

The articles/reports focusing specifically on migrant centres described mainly generic/multiple possible disease exposures and, when specified, the types of transmissions more frequently described were human-to-human and/or via contaminated water/food [11,12,20].

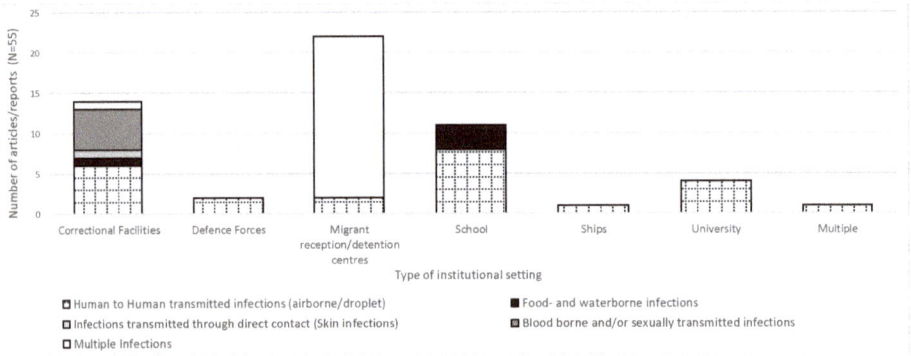

Figure 3. Number of articles or reports addressing the first review objective (*n* = 55), by type of infectious disease transmission and setting.

Specific challenges in preventing and controlling infectious disease spread have been described in correctional settings. In addition to more general challenges in managing health issues within secure environments [50,51], we found evidence that dispersed correctional systems that combine rapid turnover (jails) and longer term (prisons) detention facilities, with frequent interfacility transfers, influence disease transmission dynamics. Rapid turnover creates an inflow of people in rapidly consecutive cohorts (a "revolving doors" effect [52]). An inflow of susceptible people within a closed or semi-open community experiencing an outbreak, has been shown to slow the creation of herd immunity and can act as a transmission amplifier [53,54], while interfacility transfers can facilitate disease spread: "*Contacts occurred during inmate transports between prisons, at a courthouse, and within the prisons (...) Prisons and prison transport vehicles are crowded environments that create potential for the spread of respiratory and other infections including measles, rubella, chickenpox, tuberculosis and meningococcal* disease. The transport system that supports a devolved correctional system, sets this environment apart from other crowded environments such as boarding schools, and aligns it with aspects of military camps" [55]. All this, combined with factors associated with living conditions, can favour infectious disease transmission: *"Detainees are more likely to become infected as a result of significant overcrowding in prisons, poor living conditions, poor nutrition, and physical and emotional stress"* [52]. Finally, it should be noted that *"If an individual is in a correctional institution, the primary purpose of the setting are custody and confinement. Although healthcare is mandated, it is not the priority of custody institutions"* [51].

Overall, sanitation/disinfection was described as critical in 32 articles/reports (58%), followed by medicines/vaccines, physical infrastructure (25 studies/reports; 45% each), and human resources (20; 36%). According to the type of institutional setting, different dimensions were more frequently described as critical. Sanitation/disinfection and medicines/vaccines were more frequently described as critical in articles/reports focusing on educational institutions, while physical infrastructure was the only dimension more frequently described as critical in articles/reports on correctional facilities. Among the 22 articles/reports that specifically focused on migrant reception/detention centres, three dimensions were more frequently described as critical: human resources (15 articles/reports, 68%), physical infrastructure (14 articles/reports, 64%), and sanitation/disinfection (13 articles/reports, 59%). For example, site visits documented that: *" ... suboptimal living conditions, staff numbers and skill mix in detention centres and in open centres are major concerns. Unhygienic surroundings, and in particular toilets, pose further health risks for migrants"* [18]; and, further: *"Unfortunately, the facilities identified as migrant centres were in very poor condition, lacking electricity, heating or proper sanitation systems. Essential services such as food and health care were not systematically delivered"* [28]; *"The infrastructure and the living conditions in reception, refugee, and detention centres vary from one facility to another. The most frequent problem is budget deficit, which affects living conditions (i.e., poor diet, overcrowding, excessive cold or heat, inadequate sanitation, lack of social activities)"* [34]". Shortages in availability of medicines/vaccines were described less frequently (9 studies/reports, 41 %) (Figure 4).

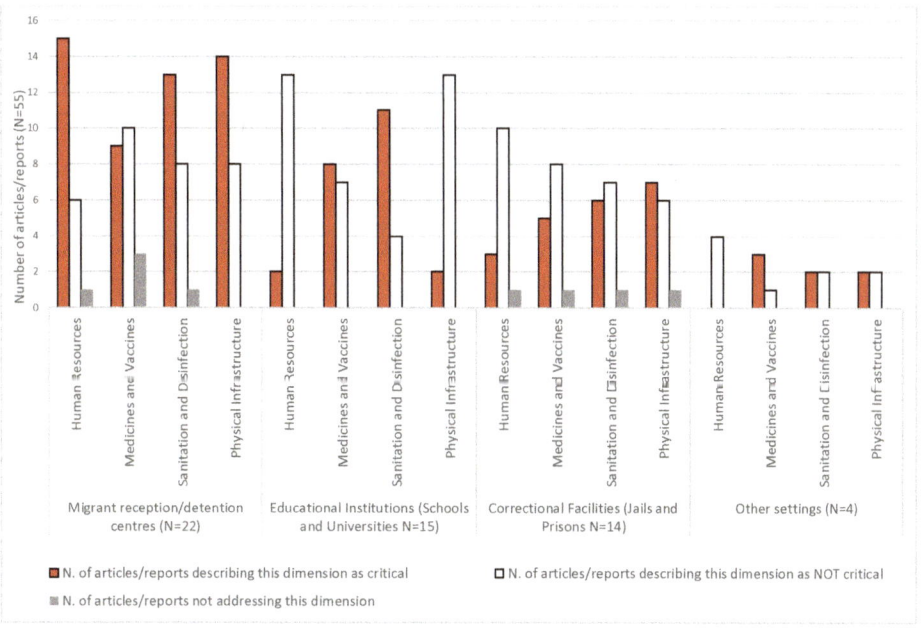

Figure 4. Number of articles or reports addressing the first review objective (*n* = 55), by dimension and institutional setting.

The most frequently identified additional dimension in both articles and reports was overcrowding (24 articles and reports, 55%). The majority (15, 68%) of all articles and reports on migrant facilities reported overcrowding to be an issue.

Among the 35 peer-reviewed articles, five other aspects were also described recurrently as critical. Foremost were early detection and reporting (21 studies, 60%) followed by communication with, and education of, the public (17 studies, 49%), coordination between authorities (14 studies, 40%), staff training (9 studies, 26%), and management of legal/ethical issues (2 studies, 6%). Among those, as shown in Figure 5, early detection and reporting was more frequently described as critical, rather than not critical, in articles/reports focusing on migrant, educational, and correctional settings. Coordination, communication, and staff training emerged as more frequently critical only in articles/reports on correctional facilities.

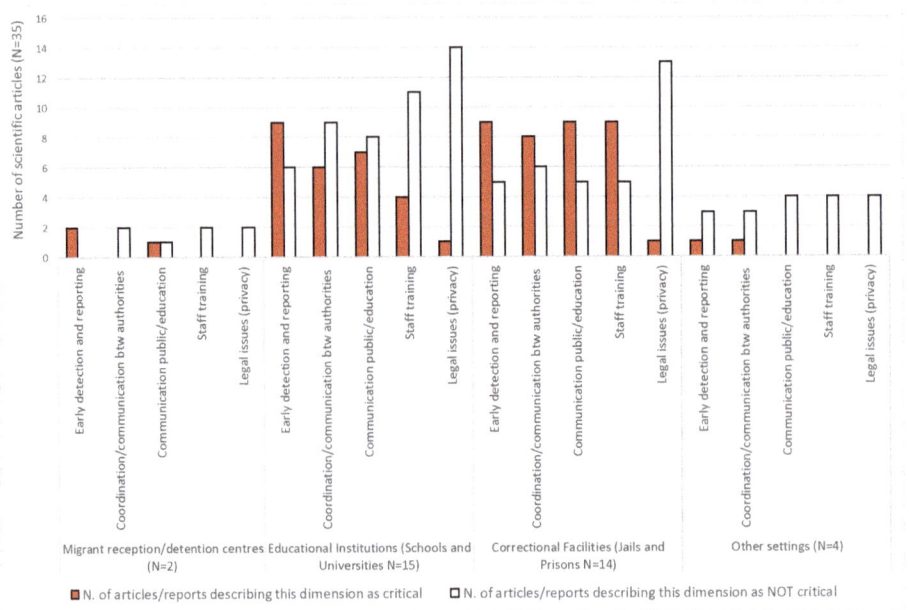

Figure 5. Number of scientific articles addressing the first review objective ($n = 35$), by additional dimension and institutional setting.

The pillars and functions considered by IOM and WHO in the 20 situation analysis studies included in this review only partly matched the dimensions that we had identified (Figure 6). Among those, *health information* (in particular, focusing on surveillance and communication systems) and *health financing* were found by WHO and IOM as recurrently critical within migrant centres. Both did not clearly overlap, neither with the dimensions we had defined before the review, nor with the additional dimensions we identified by analysing the included articles/reports.

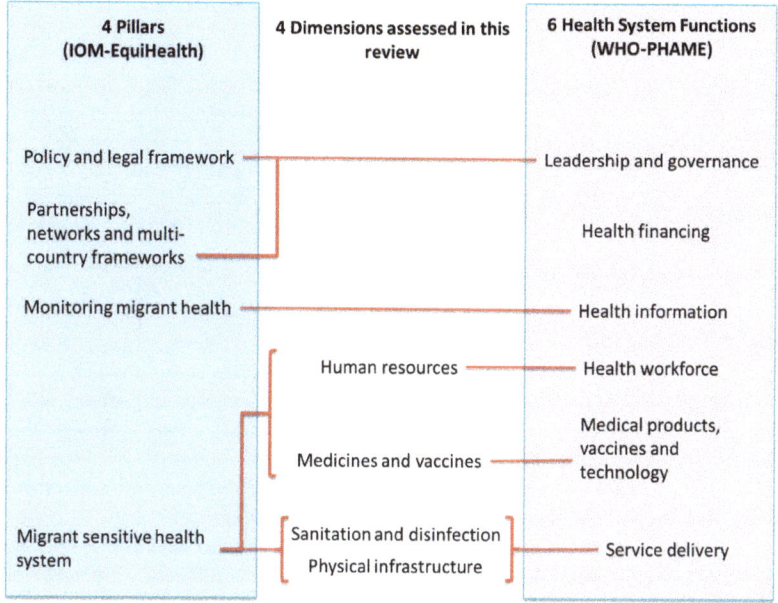

Figure 6. Assessment frameworks used in the International Organization for Migration (IOM) and World Health Organization (WHO) situation assessments in relation to the scoping review dimensions.

3.3. Suitable Approaches for Assessing Strengths and Weaknesses in Controlling/Preventing Communicable Diseases

Forty-two articles/reports addressed the second objective of this review. These included 34 grey literature reports (9 tools and 25 risk/needs assessments and guidance documents) and 8 scientific articles.

The nine tools [56–64] we analysed were principally checklist-based (See Supplementary File 1 for further details). Only one was a self-assessment tool [58]. WHO tools were mainly aimed at assessing health systems [56,59], but also included instruments targeting hospital administrators and emergency managers [60]. Other tools included instruments to assess refugee/displaced population emergencies [61], conduct health needs assessments in prison settings [63,64], or support European parliamentarians visiting immigration detention centres [62]. In addition, while some were clearly oriented to emergency preparedness [56,59,60], another adopted a capacity assessment approach [57] in the framework of the International Health Regulations (IHR) [65].

The methods proposed in the eight scientific articles were more diverse, including mathematical models, the development of a risk assessment tool, a table top exercise, training, the review of preparedness plans, surveys, and a stakeholder analysis.

The 25 risk/needs assessments and guidance documents used different reference standards to measure adequacy within migration holding centres with respect to the dimensions we explored. For example, documents from MSF [61,66], WHO [57,60,67], and UNHCR [68] were cited as standard references in different ECDC documents [15,31,69] included in this review. UNHCR [70] quoted a tool designed to identify strategic humanitarian priorities [71] and the Humanitarian Charter and Minimum Standards in Humanitarian Response (Sphere Project) [72]. Among three documents on migrant holding facilities in Italy: the first document, a WHO situation analysis [21], quoted UNHCR [73] and the Sphere Project; the second document, of the Italian Red Cross [74], quoted a European Red Cross guideline [75]; and the third document, issued by the Veneto Region [76], referred to a WHO guidance [67].

4. Discussion

Disease transmission has been repeatedly documented in institutional settings, including migrant facilities. Human-to-human transmitted and food and waterborne infections have been described in a variety of institutions, while skin infections have been described in correctional and migration settings. These findings are consistent with the results of syndromic surveillance in migration centres in Italy [77,78] and Greece [79,80], that have identified signs/symptoms of scabies, respiratory tract infections, and gastrointestinal infections as the most frequently reported syndromes.

Human resources, medicines/vaccines, sanitation/disinfection, and physical infrastructure were all identified as dimensions to consider for the prevention/control of communicable diseases in migration centres. Among those, we found human resources, physical infrastructure, and sanitation to be most frequently identified as critical. Although cultural mediators are considered essential to provide culturally competent services [81], they were recurrently described as insufficient or unavailable within migrant centres. Poor physical infrastructures, poor environmental hygiene conditions, and a lack of clean clothing, bedding, and personal hygiene equipment were also recurrent challenges [18,28], particularly during large sudden influxes of migrants. However, this was not always the case [34]. The quality of infrastructure/sanitation levels among different migrant holding centres can vary, also within the same country [19]. Challenges in the physical infrastructure of migration facilities might be more evident than in other institutional settings, because surges in migration can rapidly make infrastructures inadequate to host larger numbers of people than initially intended. Conversely, we found medicines/vaccines more often mentioned as critical in educational and other institutional settings. This finding is partly due to the fact that several studies focused on the 2009 pandemic influenza, and largely discussed the use and timing of vaccination and/or antiviral treatments in educational institutions.

This review was conducted embracing a wide range of institutional settings, due to the lack of comprehensive studies with a specific focus on migrant centres and communicable disease transmission and control. The general assumption behind this choice was that a broad spectrum of possible mechanisms drives communicable disease transmission and challenge outbreak control in institutional settings hosting closed or semi-open communities, like migrant centres, and that lessons learned could be translated across settings with similar challenges. We found documents related mainly to three types of institutions: migrant centres, educational institutions, and correctional facilities.

The documents we reviewed with a focus on educational institutional settings described different organisation systems and challenges compared with what could be expected in migrant reception (semi-open) centres. Coherently, the pattern of the most frequently described critical dimensions was different, with human resources and physical infrastructure (the most frequently critical dimensions in migrant centres) identified more frequently as not critical in educational settings.

Conversely, this review highlighted that specific communicable disease transmission dynamics challenge dispersed correctional systems. This is an interesting finding because migration reception in many EU countries is organised in a similar way, with high turnover short-term facilities and reception/detention institutions designed to host migrants for longer periods. We concluded that evidence and experience on communicable disease prevention and control in dispersed correctional settings might be something to consider/assess also in relation to similarly dispersed migrant reception systems. These considerations guided the selection of which key dimensions identified in this review to include in the ECDC preparedness checklist tool to strengthen preparedness in migrant centres [9].

In particular, overcrowding, coordination, health information, and health financing were all dimensions that had not been defined prior to conducting this review. *Overcrowding* emerged as frequently critical, in particular, in migrant centres, and was therefore naturally included in the tool as an element that could increase the risk of outbreaks. The need to develop functional *coordination* among the different actors was instead highlighted, in particular, in dispersed correctional settings. Nonetheless, we included also this aspect in the tool because, like those institutions, migrant detention/reception centres are hubs of many different actors working within and outside the centre itself. *Early detection and reporting* was mentioned as critical in articles on almost all the settings explored and *health information* was a recurring critical element in the WHO/IOM situation analysis reports. This finding is in line with the outcome of an ECDC expert opinion [15] that recommended the implementation of syndromic surveillance systems in migrant centres. ECDC has subsequently developed a "Handbook on implementing syndromic surveillance in migrant centres and other refugee settings" [82], so this aspect was included also in the checklist tool.

Finally, we found that the literature stresses the importance of *health financing* as a relevant dimension in institutional settings. Lack of sustained funding can explain the lack of human resources, stock ruptures in all types of commodities, including pharmaceuticals, inadequate infrastructure, maintenance, and hygiene/sanitation levels. In relation to migration, several EU governments are highly dependent on EU project and emergency funds in facing sudden influxes of migrants [25,31], while in some member state NGOs and international organisations have been supporting national governments by providing services within migrant centres. Thus, health financing sustainability has been proposed as an indicator of the fragility of migration emergency response systems in terms of their viability and surge capacity. For this reason, this aspect was also included in the ECDC checklist tool.

Through this review, it was concluded that common standards and reference tools for the assessment of needs and requirements in EU migrant centres are currently lacking and that the number of studies particularly addressing this topic is still limited. Consequently, the possibility of designing a tool against a pre-established set of standards was precluded.

In conclusion, based upon this review, ECDC developed a checklist tool intended for EU/EEA public health authorities who need to self-assess the capacity for communicable disease prevention and control at reception/detention centres hosting migrants for weeks/months (medium-term) in order to identify gaps and set priorities for development. Its aim is to monitor and support capacity development to prevent the onset, and improve the management of, communicable disease outbreaks at medium-term migrant reception/detention centres, both on a day-to-day basis and in the event of a sudden influx of migrants. The tool aims to assess capacity based on three general objectives:

- Outbreak prevention (covering communicable disease prevention, rapid case detection, and case management)
- Outbreak control (covering outbreak detection and control in the reception/detention centre being assessed)
- Outbreak management during a large sudden influx of migrants (communicable disease prevention, detection, and control during a large sudden influx of refugee migrants at the reception/detention centre being assessed.

One of the first elements adopted from this scoping review was the identification of the appropriate scope for the tool. The tool assesses preparedness capacity in relation to the medium-term accommodation of migrants within centres, thereby complementing an existing tool developed by the WHO PHAME project analysed in this study.

The second general element adopted from the scoping review was to choose a methodological approach that would not assess against a common recognised set of standards, that we found to be missing, but that would be based on capacity, using a health system strengthening approach. Therefore, the tool refers to the International Health Regulations (IHR) as a framework, focusing on capacity development. In terms of methodology, the WHO Assessment Tool for Core Capacity Requirements at Designated Airports, Ports, and Ground Crossings was taken as a model and adapted to the context of medium-term migrant reception/detention facilities.

Finally, the scoping review defined the dimensions to include in the tool, both confirming the relevance of pre-defined ones and incorporating novel ones. In its final version, the tool addressed the following: human resources; medicines and vaccines; physical infrastructure; sanitation; health financing; coordination; health information; overcrowding. A total of 94 statements for self-assessment were designed to cover the objectives of the tool and address all the identified dimensions [9].

Given the broad spectrum of possible mechanisms driving challenges in communicable disease transmission in institutional settings hosting closed or semi-open communities, and the dearth of literature specifically focusing on outbreak prevention and control in migrant centres, we chose to adopt a very broad approach for this review. This approach has intrinsic limitations, due to the diversity of "institutional settings" considered and, within the migration hosting system, the diversity of reception and detention centres in terms of conditions and public health implications. For this reason, the scoping review approach was chosen, as this kind of review allows for the identification of possible issues, even if it will not give a systematic quantification of effects. A scoping review, as described by Arksey and O'Malley [83], while systematic in its collection of data, as opposed to traditional systematic reviews, tends to address broader topics where many different study designs might be applicable, and is less likely to seek to address very specific research questions nor, consequently, to assess the quality of included studies. This type of rapid review might not describe research findings in any detail, but is a useful way of mapping fields of study where it is difficult to visualise the range of material that might be available. The choice of not quantifying effects is also justified because the contribution of each driver to obstacles in communicable disease prevention/control is setting-specific, while the underlying mechanisms can be common across settings with common characteristics. Further, results were stratified by the type of institution, and discussed separately to highlight when data was retrieved directly on migration hosting facilities and when it was evidence originated from other settings that might be relevant also to the migration hosting system. As a result of this methodological choice, limiting the search to PubMed was considered adequate.

While this scoping review study used wide search terms and a long-time frame, we chose to limit our scientific search to articles in English, Italian, and French language. The language choice was guided by the language abilities of the reviewer and led to the inclusion of two globally spoken languages (English, French) and of Italian, the language spoken by one of the EU countries mostly affected by the recent migration crises in the region.

Further, not including other MeSH terms (such as "refugees") limited to our ability to identify articles. The impact of this specific aspect was assessed, and found to be contained (including the term refugee would have led to a non-deduplicated increase of 12% in the number of abstracts. The reason lies in the fact that articles were also captured by the use of the term "migrants and transients", that was included.

A single reviewer was engaged in reading and analysing abstracts and full-text articles/reports, and this could have led to a subjective collection of data. However, the information collected, e.g. if an aspect was mentioned as critical or not, was selected to be as simple and less prone to subjective assessment as possible, and standardised as much as possible in the study protocol to limit any negative impact this choice could have had.

We were limited in our grey literature search to our knowledge of relevant institutions and websites. We considered this not to hinder the general aim of the review that was not to comprehensively assess literature in relation to an intervention, but rather, to gather a general understanding of disease transmission drivers in institutional settings, identify more frequent critical dimensions for outbreak prevention/control, and types of tools that could be adapted to a migrant setting.

5. Conclusions

As discussed, this literature review has looked across different institutional settings to identify the foundations for the development of the ECDC preparedness checklist tool for strengthening preparedness at migrant reception/detention centres [9]. This study enabled us to confirm the need and shape the structure of the tool, identifying human resources, medicines/vaccines, sanitation/disinfection, physical infrastructure, overcrowding, coordination, health information, and health financing as important dimensions for prevention/control of communicable diseases in migration centres. Furthermore, this study highlighted how evidence and experience on communicable disease prevention and control in dispersed correctional settings might be something to consider/assess, also in relation to similarly dispersed migrant reception systems. Moving forward, it will be important to pilot test this tool in field settings, and to generate a broad dialogue aimed at identifying common standards that migrant holding centres could aim to achieve in European settings.

Supplementary Materials: The following are available online at http://www.mdpi.com/1660-4601/15/6/1120/s1, Supplementary File 1: Database supplementary file.

Author Contributions: J.E.S., L.E., S.D. and M.G.D. were in charge of defining the objectives and purpose of the study. S.D. coordinated the study. F.R., J.E.S. and L.E. guided the methodological approach. F.R. reviewed the scientific and grey literature and with A.B. and M.D.M. analysed the data. All authors were actively involved in the interpretation of findings, contributed to drafting and revision of the manuscript and approved the final version.

Acknowledgments: This study was funded through the ECDC specific service contract (No. 4 ECD.5697) implementing the PERPHECT framework contract (No. ECDC/2014/006).

Conflicts of Interest: The authors declare no conflict of interest.

References

1. Riccardo, F.; Dente, M.G.; Kärki, T.; Fabiani, M.; Napoli, C.; Chiarenza, A.; Giorgi Rossi, P.; Munoz, C.V.; Noori, T.; Declich, S. Towards a European Framework to Monitor Infectious Diseases among Migrant Populations: Design and Applicability. *Int. J. Environ. Res. Public Health* **2015**, *12*, 11640–11661. [CrossRef] [PubMed]
2. Migration Policy Debates © OECD May 2014. Available online: https://www.oecd.org/migration/OECD%20Migration%20Policy%20Debates%20Numero%202.pdf (accessed on 11 May 2017).
3. Horton, R. Offline: Migration and health—From aspiration to desperation. *Lancet* **2016**, *388*, 2071. [CrossRef]
4. Riccardo, F.; Giorgi Rossi, P.; Chiarenza, A.; Noori, T.; Declich, S. Letter to the editor: Responding to a call for action—Where are we now? *Eurosurveillance* **2015**, *20*, 30096. [CrossRef] [PubMed]
5. Eurostat. Asylum in the EU Member States: Record Number of over 1.2 Million First Time Asylum Seekers Registered in 2015. Available online: http://ec.europa.eu/eurostat/web/products-press-releases/-/3-04032016-AP (accessed on 11 May 2017).
6. Van Loenen, T.; van den Muijsenbergh, M.; Hofmeester, M.; Dowrick, C.; van Ginneken, N.; Mechili, E.A.; Angelaki, A.; Ajdukovic, D.; Bakic, H.; Pavlic, D.R.; et al. Primary care for refugees and newly arrived migrants in Europe: A qualitative study on health needs, barriers and wishes. *Eur. J. Public Health* **2018**, *28*, 82–87. [CrossRef] [PubMed]
7. Kärki, T.; Napoli, C.; Riccardo, F.; Fabiani, M.; Dente, M.G.; Carballo, M.; Noori, T.; Declich, S. Screening for infectious diseases among newly arrived migrants in EU/EEA countries—Varying practices but consensus on the utility of screening. *Int. J. Environ. Res. Public Health* **2014**, *11*, 11004–11014. [CrossRef] [PubMed]
8. Basu, S.; Stuckler, D.; McKee, M. Addressing institutional amplifiers in the dynamics and control of tuberculosis epidemics. *Am. J. Trop. Med. Hyg.* **2011**, *84*, 30–37. [CrossRef] [PubMed]
9. European Centre for Disease Prevention and Control. *Handbook on Using the ECDC Preparedness Checklist Tool to Strengthen Preparedness against Communicable Disease Outbreaks at Migrant Reception/Detention Centres*; ECDC: Stockholm, Sweden, 2016.
10. Moher, D.; Liberati, A.; Tetzlaff, J.; Altman, D.G.; The PRISMA Group. Preferred Reporting Items for Systematic Reviews and Meta-Analyses: The PRISMA statement. *PLoS Med.* **2009**, *6*, e1000097. [CrossRef] [PubMed]
11. Haas, E.J.; Dukhan, L.; Goldstein, L.; Lyandres, M.; Gdalevich, M. Use of vaccination in a large outbreak of primary varicella in a detention setting for African immigrants. *Int. Health* **2014**, *6*, 203–207. [CrossRef] [PubMed]
12. Valin, N.; Antoun, F.; Chouaïd, C.; Renard, M.; Dautzenberg, B.; Lalande, V.; Ayache, B.; Morin, P.; Sougakoff, W.; Thiolet, J.M.; et al. Outbreak of tuberculosis in a migrants' shelter, Paris, France. *Int. J. Tuberc. Lung Dis.* **2002**, *9*, 528–533.
13. World Health Organization Office for Europe. Migrant Health in the European Region. Available online: http://www.euro.who.int/en/health-topics/health-determinants/migration-and-health/migrant-health-in-the-european-region (accessed on 26 May 2016).

14. International Organization for Migration. EquiHealth Project. Available online: http://equi-health.eea.iom.int/ (accessed on 26 May 2016).
15. European Centre for Disease Prevention and Control. *Expert Opinion on the Public Health Needs of Irregular Migrants, Refugees or Asylum Seekers Across the EU's Southern and Southeastern Borders*; ECDC: Stockholm, Sweden, 2015.
16. United Nations Interagency Health-Needs-Assessment Mission. Southern Turkey, 4–5 December 2012. Available online: http://www.euro.who.int/__data/assets/pdf_file/0006/189213/United-Nations-interagency-health-needs-assessment-mission-final.pdf?ua=1 (accessed on 11 May 2017).
17. WHO Regional Office for Europe. Health Needs Assessment, Malta. 2012. Available online: http://www.euro.who.int/__data/assets/pdf_file/0011/144011/Malta_report.pdf?ua=1 (accessed on 11 May 2017).
18. IOM EquiHealth Assessment Report: The Health Situation at EU Southern Borders Migrant Health, Occupational Health and Public Health Malta. 2013. Available online: http://equi-health.eea.iom.int/images/SAR_Malta_Final.pdf (accessed on 11 May 2017).
19. Medicins Sans Frontieres, Italy. Al di la del muro Viaggio nei Centri per Migrant in Italia. 2010. Available online: http://www.asgi.it/wp-content/uploads/public/al.di.la.del.muro.viaggio.nei.centri.per.migranti.in.italia.pdf (accessed on 11 May 2017).
20. Medici Senza Frontiere. Rapporto sulle Condizioni di Accoglienza nel CPSA Pozzallo. November 2015. Available online: http://archivio.medicisenzafrontiere.it/pdf/Rapporto_CPI_CPSA_Pozzallo_final.pdf (accessed on 11 May 2017).
21. WHO Regional Office for Europe. Increased Influx of Migrants in Lampedusa, Italy. Joint Report from the Ministry of Health, Italy and the WHO Regional Office for Europe Mission of 28–29 March 2011. Available online: http://www.euro.who.int/__data/assets/pdf_file/0004/182137/e96761.pdf?ua=1 (accessed on 11 May 2017).
22. WHO Regional Office for Europe. Second Assessment of Migrant Health Needs Lampedusa and Linosa, Italy. Joint Report on a Mission of the Ministry of Health of Italy, the Regional Health Authority of Sicily and the WHO Regional Office for Europe, 16–19 May 2012. Available online: http://www.euro.who.int/__data/assets/pdf_file/0010/184465/e96796.pdf?ua=1 (accessed on 11 May 2017).
23. WHO Regional Office for Europe. Sicily, Italy: Assessing Health-System Capacity to Manage Sudden Large Influxes of Migrants Joint Report on a Mission of the Ministry of Health of Italy, the Regional Health Authority of Sicily and the WHO Regional Office for Europe. 2014. Available online: http://www.euro.who.int/__data/assets/pdf_file/0007/262519/Sicily-Italy-Assessing-health-system-capacity-manage-sudden-large-influxes-migrantsEng.pdf?ua=1 (accessed on 11 May 2017).
24. IOM EquiHealth Assessment Report: The Health Situation at EU Southern Borders Migrant Health, Occupational Health and Public Health Italy. 2013. Available online: http://equi-health.eea.iom.int/images/SAR_Italy_Final.pdf (accessed on 11 May 2017).
25. WHO Regional Office for Europe. Cyprus: Assessing Health-System Capacity to Manage Sudden Large Influxes of Migrants. Joint Report on a Mission of the Ministry of Health of Cyprus, the International Centre for Migration, Health and Development and the WHO Regional Office for Europe. 2015. Available online: http://www.euro.who.int/__data/assets/pdf_file/0020/293330/Cyprus-Assessment-Report-en.pdf?ua=1 (accessed on 11 May 2017).
26. IOM EquiHealth Assessment Report: The Health Situation at EU Southern Borders Migrant Health, Occupational Health and Public Health Croatia. 2014. Available online: http://equi-health.eea.iom.int/images/SAR_Croatia_Final.pdf (accessed on 11 May 2017).
27. WHO Regional Office for Europe. Serbia: Assessing Health-System Capacity to Manage Sudden Large Influxes of Migrants. Joint Report on a Mission of the Ministry of Health of Serbia and the WHO Regional Office for Europe with the Collaboration of the International Organization for Migration. 2015. Available online: http://www.euro.who.int/__data/assets/pdf_file/0010/293329/Serbia-Assessment-Report-en.pdf?ua=1 (accessed on 11 May 2017).
28. WHO Regional Office for Europe. Assessing Health-System Capacity to Manage Sudden Large Influxes of Migrants Bulgaria. Joint Report on a Mission of the Ministry of Health of Bulgaria and the WHO Regional Office for Europe. 2015. Available online: http://www.euro.who.int/__data/assets/pdf_file/0009/300402/Bulgaria-Assessment-Report-en.pdf (accessed on 11 May 2017).

29. IOM EquiHealth Assessment Report: The Health Situation at EU Southern Borders Migrant Health, Occupational Health and Public Health Bulgaria. 2014–2015. Available online: http://equi-health.eea.iom.int/images/SAR_Bulgaria_Final.pdf (accessed on 11 May 2017).
30. WHO Regional Office for Europe. Portugal: Assessing Health-System Capacity to Manage Sudden Large Influxes of Migrants Joint Report on a Mission of the Ministry of Health of Portugal, the International Centre for Migration, Health and Development and the WHO Regional Office for Europe. 2014. Available online: http://www.euro.who.int/__data/assets/pdf_file/0016/265012/Portugal-assessing-health-system-capacity-to-manage-sudden-large-influxes-of-migrants.pdf?ua=1 (accessed on 11 May 2017).
31. European Centre for Disease Prevention and Control and WHO Regional Office for Europe. Joint ECDC/WHO Regional Office for Europe Mission Report: Increased Influx of Migrants at the Greek–Turkish Border. Greece, 4–8 April 2011. Stockholm: ECDC. 2011. Available online: http://www.euro.who.int/__data/assets/pdf_file/0012/144012/Greece_mission_rep_2011.pdf?ua=1 (accessed on 11 May 2017).
32. WHO Regional Office for Europe. Greece: Assessing Health-System Capacity to Manage Sudden Large Influxes of Migrants. Joint Report on a Mission of the Ministry of Health of Greece, Hellenic Centre for Disease Control and Prevention and WHO Regional Office for Europe. 2015. Available online: http://www.euro.who.int/__data/assets/pdf_file/0007/300400/Greece-Assessment-Report-en.pdf?ua=1 (accessed on 11 May 2017).
33. IOM EquiHealth Assessment Report: The Health Situation at EU Southern Borders Migrant Health, Occupational Health and Public Health Greece. 2013. Available online: http://equi-health.eea.iom.int/images/SAR_Greece_Final.pdf (accessed on 11 May 2017).
34. IOM EquiHealth Assessment Report: The Health Situation at EU Southern Borders Migrant Health, Occupational Health and Public Health Spain. 2013. Available online: http://equi-health.eea.iom.int/images/SAR_Spain_Final.pdf (accessed on 11 May 2017).
35. Lee, M.B.; Greig, J.D. A review of gastrointestinal outbreaks in schools: Effective infection control interventions. *J. Sch. Health* **2010**, *80*, 588–598. [CrossRef] [PubMed]
36. Greig, J.D.; Lee, M.B.; Harris, J.E. Review of enteric outbreaks in prisons: Effective infection control interventions. *Public Health* **2011**, *125*, 222–228. [CrossRef] [PubMed]
37. Tsalik, E.L.; Cunningham, C.K.; Cunningham, H.M.; Lopez-Marti, M.G.; Sangvai, D.G.; Purdy, W.K.; Anderson, D.J.; Thompson, J.R.; Brown, M.; Woods, C.W.; et al. An Infection Control Program for a 2009 influenza A H1N1 outbreak in a university-based summer camp. *J. Am Coll. Health* **2011**, *59*, 419–426. [CrossRef] [PubMed]
38. Leung, J.; Lopez, A.S.; Tootell, E.; Baumrind, N.; Mohle-Boetani, J.; Leistikow, B.; Harriman, K.H.; Preas, C.P.; Cosentino, G.; Bialek, S.R.; et al. Challenges with controlling varicella in prison settings: Experience of California, 2010 to 2011. *J. Correct. Health Care* **2014**, *20*, 292–301. [CrossRef] [PubMed]
39. Jongcherdchootrakul, K.; Henderson, A.K.; Iamsirithaworn, S.; Modchang, C.; Siriarayapon, P. First pandemic A (H1N1) pdm09 outbreak in a private school, Bangkok, Thailand, June 2009. *J. Med. Assoc. Thai* **2014**, *97* (Suppl. 2), S145–S152. [PubMed]
40. Guthrie, J.A.; Lokuge, K.M.; Levy, M.H. Influenza control can be achieved in a custodial setting: Pandemic (H1N1) 2009 and 2011 in an Australian prison. *Public Health* **2012**, *126*, 1032–1037. [CrossRef] [PubMed]
41. Kadlubowski, M.; Wasko, I.; Klarowicz, A.; Hryniewicz, W. Invasive meningococcal disease at a military base in Warsaw, January 2007. *Wkly. Releases* **2007**, *12*, 3147. [CrossRef]
42. Matthews, E.; Armstrong, G.; Spencer, T. Pertussis infection in a baccalaureate nursing program: Clinical implications, emerging issues, and recommendations. *J. Contin. Educ. Nurs.* **2008**, *39*, 419–426. [CrossRef] [PubMed]
43. Bonačić Marinović, A.A.; Swaan, C.; Wichmann, O.; van Steenbergen, J.; Kretzschmar, M. Effectiveness and timing of vaccination during school measles outbreak. *Emerg. Infect. Dis.* **2012**, *18*, 1405–1413. [CrossRef] [PubMed]
44. Kay, D.; Roche, M.; Atkinson, J.; Lamden, K.; Vivancos, R. Mumps outbreaks in four universities in the North West of England: Prevention, detection and response. *Vaccine* **2011**, *29*, 3883–3887. [CrossRef] [PubMed]
45. Crum, N.F.; Wallace, M.R.; Lamb, C.R.; Conlin, A.M.; Amundson, D.E.; Olson, P.E.; Ryan, M.A.; Robinson, T.J.; Gray, G.C.; Earhart, K.C. Halting a pneumococcal pneumonia outbreak among United States Marine Corps trainees. *Am. J. Prev. Med.* **2003**, *25*, 107–111. [CrossRef]

46. Elias, A.F.; Chaussee, M.S.; McDowell, E.J.; Huntington, M.K. Community-based intervention to manage an outbreak of MRSA skin infections in a county jail. *J. Correct. Health Care* **2010**, *16*, 205–215. [CrossRef] [PubMed]
47. Wolfe, M.I.; Xu, F.; Patel, P.; O'Cain, M.; Schillinger, J.A.; St Louis, M.E.; Finelli, L. An outbreak of syphilis in Alabama prisons: Correctional health policy and communicable disease control. *Am. J. Public Health* **2001**, *91*, 1220–1225. [CrossRef] [PubMed]
48. Hellard, M.E.; Aitken, C.K. HIV in prison: What are the risks and what can be done? *Sex Health* **2004**, *1*, 107–113. [CrossRef] [PubMed]
49. Wohl, D.A.; Rosen, D.; Kaplan, A.H. HIV and incarceration: Dual epidemics. *AIDS Read.* **2006**, *16*, 247–250, 257–260. [PubMed]
50. Ehrmann, T. Community-based organizations and HIV prevention for incarcerated populations: Three HIV prevention program models. *AIDS Educ. Prev.* **2002**, *14* (Suppl. 5), 75–84. [CrossRef] [PubMed]
51. Zalumas, J.C.; Rose, C.D. Hepatitis C and HIV in incarcerated populations: Fights, bites, searches, and syringes! *J. Assoc. Nurses AIDS Care* **2003**, *14* (Suppl. 5), 108S–115S. [CrossRef] [PubMed]
52. Van't Hoff, G.; Fedosejeva, R.; Mihailescu, L. Prisons' preparedness for pandemic flu and the ethical issues. *Public Health* **2009**, *123*, 422–425. [CrossRef] [PubMed]
53. Arinaminpathy, N.; Raphaely, N.; Saldana, L.; Hodgekiss, C.; Dandridge, J.; Knox, K.; McCarthy, N.D. Transmission and control in an institutional pandemic influenza A(H1N1) 2009 outbreak. *Epidemiol. Infect.* **2012**, *140*, 1102–1110. [CrossRef] [PubMed]
54. Schwartz, R.D. The impact of correctional institutions on public health during a pandemic or emerging infection disaster. *Am. J. Disaster Med.* **2008**, *3*, 165–170. [PubMed]
55. Levy, M.H.; Quilty, S.; Young, L.C.; Hunt, W.; Matthews, R.; Robertson, P.W. Pox in the docks: Varicella outbreak in an Australian prison system. *Public Health* **2003**, *117*, 446–451. [CrossRef]
56. WHO Regional Office for Europe. Large Influxes of Refugees and Migrants. Toolkit for Assessing Health System Capacity to Manage Large Influxes of Refugees and Migrants in the Acute Phase. 2015. Available online: https://www.escap.eu/bestanden/Care%20(38)/Refugees/toolkit_assessing_hs_capacity_manage_large_influxes_refugees_asylum_seekers_migrants.pdf (accessed on 11 May 2017).
57. World Health Organization. *International Health Regulations (2005): Assessment Tool for Core Capacity Requirements at Designated Airports, Ports and Ground Crossings*; WHO: Geneva, Switzerland, 2009.
58. OSCE. *Self-Assessment Tool for Nations to Increase Preparedness for Cross-Border Implications of Crises*; OSCE Secretariat Transnational Threats Department Borders Unit: Vienna, Austria, 2013.
59. WHO Regional Office for Europe. *Strengthening Health-System Emergency Preparedness. Toolkit for Assessing Health-System Capacity for Crisis Management. Part 1. User Manual*; World Health Organization: Copenhagen, Denmark, 2012.
60. WHO Regional Office for Europe. *Hospital Emergency Response Checklist. An All-Hazards Tool for Hospital Administrators and Emergency Managers*; World Health Organization: Copenhagen, Denmark, 2011.
61. Brown, V.W.; Moren, A.; Paquet, C. *Rapid Health Assessment of Refugee and Displaced Populations*, 3rd ed.; Médecins Sans Frontières: Paris, France, 2006.
62. Council of Europe Visiting Immigration Detention Centres. A Guide for Parliamentarians. 2013. Available online: http://www.apt.ch/content/files_res/guide-for-parliamentarians-visiting-detention-centres-en.pdf (accessed on 11 May 2017).
63. Public Health England. Health and Justice Health Needs Assessment Template: Adult Prisons. 2014. Available online: https://www.gov.uk/government/uploads/system/uploads/attachment_data/file/331628/Health_Needs_Assessment_Toolkit_for_Prescribed_Places_of_Detention_Part_2.pdf (accessed on 11 May 2017).
64. United Nations Office on Drugs and Crime. HIV in Prisons: Situation and Needs Assessment Toolkit. 2010. Available online: http://www.unodc.org/documents/hiv-aids/publications/HIV_in_prisons_situation_and_needs_assessment_document.pdf (accessed on 11 May 2017).
65. International Health Regulations 2005 (second edition) World Health Organization 2008. Available online: http://apps.who.int/iris/bitstream/10665/43883/1/9789241580410_eng.pdf (accessed on 11 May 2017).
66. Medecins Sans Frontiers. Refugee Health. An Approach to Emergency Situations. Available online: http://refbooks.msf.org/msf_docs/en/refugee_health/rh.pdf (accessed on 11 May 2017).

67. World Health Organization. *Communicable Disease Control in Emergencies*; World Health Organization: Copenhagen, Denmark, 2005.
68. United Nations High Commissioner for Refugees. *UNHCR Handbook for Emergencies*, 3rd ed.; UNHCR: Geneva, Switzerland, 2007.
69. European Centre for Disease Prevention and Control. *Outline for Initial Migrant Health Assessment at Point of Entry to the European Union*; European Centre for Disease Prevention and Control: Solna, Sweden, 2011.
70. United Nations High Commissioner for Refugees. Shelter Needs Assessment. Available online: https://emergency.unhcr.org/entry/60439/shelter-needs-assessment (accessed on 11 May 2017).
71. Inter-Agency Standing Committee (IASC) (2012) Multi-Cluster/Sector Initial Rapid Assessment (MIRA). Available online: https://docs.unocha.org/sites/dms/Documents/mira_final_version2012.pdf (accessed on 11 May 2017).
72. The Sphere Project (2011) Humanitarian Charter and Minimum Standards in Humanitarian Response. Available online: http://www.spherehandbook.org/en/how-to-use-this-chapter-2/ (accessed on 11 May 2017).
73. United Nations Refugee Agency. *A Guidance for UNHCR Field Operations on Water and Sanitation Services*; United Nations Refugee Agency: Geneva, Switzerland, 2008.
74. Pacifici, L.E.; Riccardo, F. Manuale di Buone Pratiche. Esperienze da un Centro di Accoglienza per Richiedenti Asilo. Italian Red Cross. 2010. Available online: https://www.cri.it/flex/cm/pages/ServeAttachment.php/L/IT/D/D.5385afb5b4bd69f22d63/P/BLOB%3AID%3D4983/E/pdf (accessed on 11 May 2017).
75. Platform for European Red Cross Cooperation on Refugees, Asylum Seekers and Migrants (PERCO). Guidelines on the Reception of Asylum Seekers for National Red Cross and Red Crescent Societies. Available online: http://www.justice.ie/en/JELR/Irish%20Red%20Cross.pdf/Files/Irish%20Red%20Cross.pdf (accessed on 11 May 2017).
76. Regione del Veneto. Direzione Attuazione Programmazione Sanitaria. Settore Promozione e Sviluppo Igiene e Sanità Pubblica. Protocollo Operativo per il Controllo delle Malattie Infettive e la Profilassi Immunitaria in Relazione All'afflusso di Immigrati. 2 Ottobre 2014. Available online: http://repository.regione.veneto.it/public/2ab9a9def3c4c2ce6140dd9404517dd6.php?dl=true (accessed on 26 July 2017).
77. Napoli, C.; Riccardo, F.; Declich, S.; Dente, M.G.; Pompa, M.G.; Rizzo, C.; Rota, M.C.; Bella, A.; National Working Group. An early warning system based on syndromic surveillance to detect potential health emergencies among migrants: Results of a two-year experience in Italy. *Int. J. Environ. Res. Public Health* **2014**, *11*, 8529–8541. [CrossRef] [PubMed]
78. Riccardo, F.; Napoli, C.; Bella, A.; Rizzo, C.; Rota, M.C.; Dente, M.G.; De Santis, S.; Declich, S. Syndromic surveillance of epidemic-prone diseases in response to an influx of migrants from North Africa to Italy, May to October 2011. *Eurosurveillance* **2011**, *16*, 20016. [CrossRef]
79. Rojek, A.M.; Gkolfinopoulou, K.; Veizis, A.; Lambrou, A.; Castle, L.; Georgakopoulou, T.; Blanchet, K.; Panagiotopoulos, T.; Horby, P.W.; The Epidemic Diseases Research Group field team. Clinical assessment is a neglected component of outbreak preparedness: Evidence from refugee camps in Greece. *BMC Med.* **2018**, *16*, 43. [CrossRef] [PubMed]
80. Veneti, L.; Theocharopoulos, G.; Gkolfinopoulou, K.; Baka, A.; Lytras, T.; Triantafillou, E.; Lambrou, A.; Tsiodras, S.; Georgakopoulou, T.; Mellou, K.; et al. Implementation of infectious disease syndromic surveillance in points of care for refugees/migrants, Greece, April–July 2016. In *ESCAIDE Conference Paper*; European Centre for Disease Prevention and Control (ECDC): Stockholm, Sweden, 2016.
81. Bradby, H.; Humphris, R.; Newall, D.; Phillimore, J. *Public Health Aspects of Migrant Health: A Review of the Evidence on Health Status for Refugees and Asylum Seekers in the European Region*; WHO Regional Office for Europe: Copenhagen, Denmark, 2015.
82. European Centre for Disease Prevention and Control. *Handbook on Implementing Syndromic Surveillance in Migrant Reception/Detention Centres and other Refugee Settings*; ECDC: Stockholm, Sweden, 2016.
83. Arksey, H.; O'Malley, L. Scoping studies: Towards a methodological framework. *Int. J. Soc. Res. Methodol. Theory Pract.* **2005**, *8*, 19–32. [CrossRef]

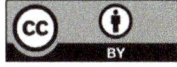

© 2018 by the authors. Licensee MDPI, Basel, Switzerland. This article is an open access article distributed under the terms and conditions of the Creative Commons Attribution (CC BY) license (http://creativecommons.org/licenses/by/4.0/).

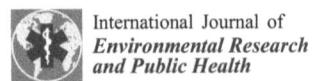

Article

Tuberculosis Specific Interferon-Gamma Production in a Current Refugee Cohort in Western Europe

Alexandra Jablonka [1,2,*,†], Christian Dopfer [3,†], Christine Happle [3,4], Georgios Sogkas [1], Diana Ernst [1], Faranaz Atschekzei [1], Stefanie Hirsch [1], Annabelle Schäll [5], Adan Jirmo [3,4], Philipp Solbach [2,6], Reinhold Ernst Schmidt [1,2], Georg M. N. Behrens [1,2] and Martin Wetzke [2,3]

1. Department of Clinical Immunology and Rheumatology, Hannover Medical School, 30625 Hannover, Germany; sogkas.georgios@mh-hannover.de (G.S.); ernst.diana@mh-hannover.de (D.E.); atschekzei.faranaz@mh-hannover.de (F.A.); hirsch.stefanie@mh-hannover.de (S.H.); schmidt.reinhold.ernst@mh-hannover.de (R.E.S.); behrens.georg@mh-hannover.de (G.M.N.B.)
2. German Center for Infection Research (DZIF), Partner Site Hannover-Braunschweig, 30625 Hannover, Germany; solbach.philipp@mh-hannover.de (P.S.); wetzke.martin@mh-hannover.de (M.W.)
3. Department of Pediatrics, Neonatology and Allergology, Hannover Medical School, 30625 Hannover, Germany; dopfer.christian@mh-hannover.de (C.D.); happle.christine@mh-hannover.de (C.H.); jirmo.adan@mh-hannover.de (A.J.)
4. German Center for Lung Research, Partner Site Hannover BREATH, 30625 Hannover, Germany
5. Hannover Medical School, 30625 Hannover, Germany; annabelle.schaell@stud.mh-hannover.de
6. Department of Gastroenterology, Hepatology and Endocrinology, Hannover Medical School, 30625 Hannover, Germany
* Correspondence: jablonka.alexandra@mh-hannover.de; Tel.: +49-511-532-5337
† These authors contributed equally to this work.

Received: 21 April 2018; Accepted: 11 June 2018; Published: 14 June 2018

Abstract: Background: In 2015, a high number of refugees with largely unknown health statuses immigrated to Western Europe. To improve caretaking strategies, we assessed the prevalence of latent tuberculosis infection (LTBI) in a refugee cohort. Methods: Interferon-Gamma release assays (IGRA, Quantiferon) were performed in n = 232 inhabitants of four German refugee centers in the summer of 2015. Results: Most refugees were young, male adults. Overall, IGRA testing was positive in 17.9% (95% CI = 13.2–23.5%) of subjects. Positivity rates increased with age (0% <18 years versus 46.2% >50 years). Age was the only factor significantly associated with a positive IGRA in multiple regression analysis including gender, C reactive protein, hemoglobin, leukocyte, and thrombocyte count and lymphocyte, monocyte, neutrophil, basophil, and eosinophil fraction. For one year change in age, the odds are expected to be 1.06 times larger, holding all other variables constant (p = 0.015). Conclusion: Observed LTBI frequencies are lower than previously reported in similar refugee cohorts. However, as elderly people are at higher risk for developing active tuberculosis, the observed high rate of LTBI in senior refugees emphasizes the need for new policies on the detection and treatment regimens in this group.

Keywords: tuberculosis; LTBI; refugee; asylum; infection; IGRA; infectious diseases; migrant

1. Introduction

Currently, Western Europe experiences immigration of a large number of immigrants from economically less developed or war-stricken countries such as Syria, Afghanistan, and Iraq [1,2]. In their countries of origin and during their escape or emigration, many migrants lacked access to regular health care and routine vaccination services [3]. During migration, malnutrition, overcrowding, physical and psychological stress, poor water supply, and poor sanitation predispose refugees to infectious diseases [4]. Especially tuberculosis (TB), an infectious disease occurring extremely rarely in immunocompetent persons in Western countries, represents an increasing problem in refugee health care [5]. Based on the recent increase in refugee TB cases, the awareness for this disease grows in Western Europe. In this regard, the identification of migrants at particular risk for TB and their further diagnostic, evaluation, and treatment is a matter of interest [6,7]. Data on the frequency of the TB status of migrants entering Europe is scarce and consequently, diagnostic regimens in migrants have not been harmonized.

In our current work, we performed tuberculosis specific interferon-gamma release assays (IGRA, Quantiferon) to assess the latent or active TB infection in a large, unselective subset of refugees representative of the current refugee crisis in Western Europe. The presentation of this data may help to assess the general risk of TB infections in migrants currently entering Western Europe and, more importantly, may on the long run support evidence-based harmonization of migrant screening for TB.

2. Material and Methods

2.1. Participants

2.1.1. Study Population and Sample Collection

A total of $n = 232$ refugees underwent routine interferon-gamma release assay (IGRA) testing in four Northern German reception centers in August 2015. All subjects presented with acute complaints, mainly common colds or skin diseases such as scabies and were offered a routine blood checkup including the complete blood cell count, C reactive protein, and an IGRA. Further routine testing included the serological analysis of antibodies against vaccine-preventable diseases and parameters indicative for hepatitis. After $n = 232$ subjects, the local health authorities recommended stopping the analysis due to the limited consequence of LTBI in this setting and recommended X-ray examination only.

2.1.2. Data Collection

The interferon-gamma Release Assay QuantiFERON-TB Gold Elisa was used (Quiagen, Hilden, Germany) and a whole blood interferon-gamma test measuring responses to ESAT-6, CFP-10, and TB7.7 (p4) peptide antigens. The laboratory had been certified for routine testing according to DIN EN ISO 15189:2014. For test interpretation, the QFT Analysis Software was used as recommended by the manufacturer, and the age and gender dependent normal values were classified according to the manufacturer suggestions. Specificity was estimated by the manufacturer to be >98%, the sensitivity for active TB was >80%, and the Quantiferon positivity can aid in diagnosing latent or active TB. Complete blood cell counts were obtained by automated analysis and confirmed by microscopic differential blood counts, if necessary. High sensitive CRP was determined by latex-enhanced immunoturbidimetry. All data were extracted from electronic routine patient records. For personal data protection, all data were anonymized before analysis. The date of birth and gender were kept available for analysis. In $n = 5$ patients, information on gender and in $n = 18$ patients, the data on age were unavailable or inconsistent in the records.

2.2. Analysis

Statistical analyses were processed using SPSS version 23.0 or GraphPad Prism version 5.02, the graphs were created using Microsoft Excel version 2003 and/or GraphPad Prism version 5.02. Calculation of LTBI prevalence was conducted by descriptive statistics. Ninety-five percent confidence intervals and standard errors were estimated by bootstrapping (simple, 1000 computations). Fisher exact testing was used for nominal variables for comparison between groups. Multiple regression (backwards, Wald, exclusion <0.10) was used for comparison between groups. Metric values were compared by Student's T-testing. P values < 0.05 were considered significant.

2.3. Study Approval

The Institutional Review Board (Ethics Committee) of Hannover Medical School approved this analysis (#2972-2015). All patient information was anonymized prior to analysis.

3. Results

IGRA testing was performed in n = 232 refugees. Subjects had a median age of 26 years (range 6–74 years, IQR 20–34.75). A total of 74.9% of the tested migrants were male. Figure 1 depicts the age and gender distribution within the cohort.

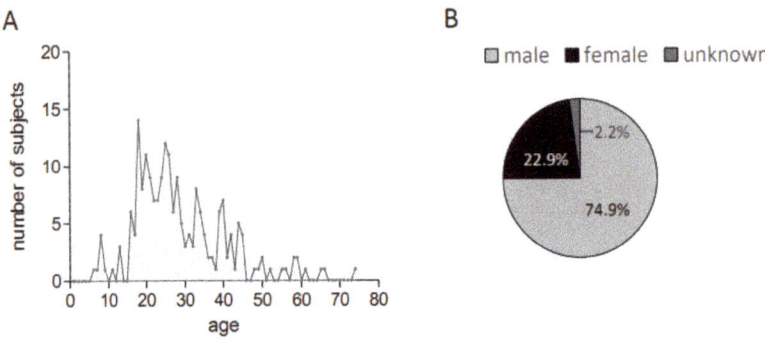

Figure 1. (**A**) The age and (**B**) gender distribution within the analyzed cohort.

In n = 223 (96.1%) subjects, valid IGRA results were obtained. All patients showed in vitro cellular reactivity (reaction to positive control "Mitogen" >0.5 IU/mL), and all negative controls showed no significant reaction. No active, smear-positive tuberculosis was detected in the group. Two refugees were HIV positive, but had a negative IGRA result. Overall, IGRA testing was positive in 17.9% (95% CI = 13.2–23.5%) of subjects. There were no significant differences of the prevalence in male and female refugees [16.8% (95% CI = 11.2–22.8) versus 19.6 (95% CI = 9.8–30.8)]. As shown in Figure 2A, the proportion of positive IGRA testing increased with age (Fisher exact, p = 0.001) (Table 1). While no refugees <18 years displayed positive IGRA testing, 46.2% of refugees >50 years had a positive result. This clear effect was also observed in the male subset of tested refugees that displayed an age-related increase of IGRA positivity with 0% and 9.1% in minor aged and young adults aged 18–24 years as compared to 62.5% in the oldest age group (Figure 2B). In women, however, this effect was not clear, most probably due to the low number of the total subjects (n = 10, Figure 2C).

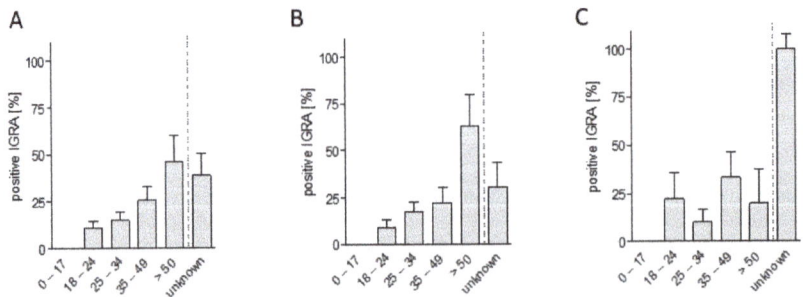

Figure 2. (**A**) Rate of positive IGRA test results in age- specific subgroups of the analyzed refugee cohort; (**B**) Age-related IGRA positivity in male and (**C**) female migrants (bars display the mean plus standard error).

Table 1. Rate of positive IGRA test results in age-specific subgroups of the analyzed refugee cohort.

Age	Total n	% Positive IGRA
0–17 years	21	0
18–24 years	65	10.8
25–34 years	67	14.9
35–49 years	39	25.6
≥50 years	13	46.2
unknown	18	38.9

When comparing the subject-specific parameters in IGRA positive versus IGRA negative subjects, only age yielded a highly significant difference in statistical testing. (Figure 3).

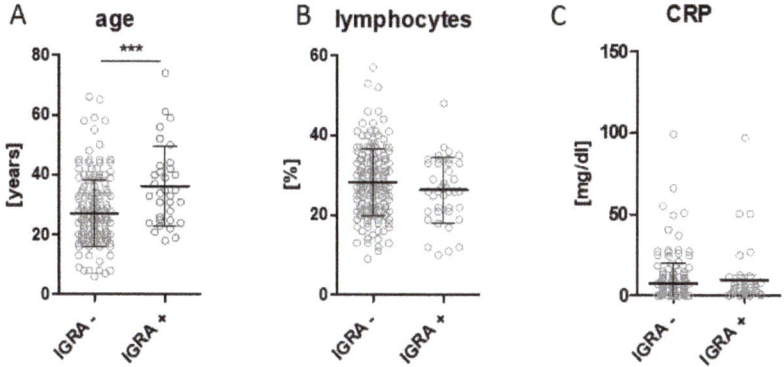

Figure 3. The analysis of subject-specific parameters in refugees with negative (IGRA −) or positive (IGRA +) testing results. (**A**) age; (**B**) CRP; (**C**) hemoglobin (bars display the mean plus standard deviation, Hb: hemoglobin, *** $P < 0.001$).

Age remained the only factor significantly associated with a positive IGRA in multiple regression analysis including gender, C reactive protein, hemoglobin, leukocyte, and thrombocyte count and lymphocyte, monocyte, neutrophil, basophil, and eosinophil fraction. For one year change in age, the odds are expected to be 1.06 times larger, holding all other variables constant (p = 0.015).

4. Discussion

We present data on the age and gender dependent prevalence of TB specific IGRA positivity in migrants entering Europe during the current refugee crisis. The majority of refugees in our cohort were young adults and in all age groups, most migrants were male. As such, the analyzed subset is representative of the current population of refugees seeking asylum in Western Europe which, to the vast majority, consists of young men [8–10]. Overall, we observed 17.9% of positive IGRA tests in the analyzed cohort with an age-dependent increase of positive test results in elder refugees. This is similar to previous publications that report on IGRA positivity rates of 20% in migrants entering the Netherlands in 2012 [11].

In refugees, communicable diseases are a particular threat [3,12–15] as they often times have limited access to health care services or appropriate nutrition or sanitation [16]. While TB is rare in Western countries, the global burden of latent tuberculosis infection has been estimated to be as high as 25% [17]. In 2016, 6.3 million new TB cases were reported [18]. To tackle this worldwide problem, the World Health Organization's (WHO) has formulated updated guidelines and an "End TB Strategy" [19,20]. To reach the WHO target of pre-elimination by 2035, the identification and treatment of active or latent TB infection in immigrants is central [21]. In Western countries, the vast majority of TB cases occur in migrants, for example nearly 65% of active TB cases in the US in 2013 and 73% of all TB infections in the Netherlands in 2009 were in foreign-born persons [22,23].

A central mechanism of migrant health, as well as the TB prevention in the receiving population, is the screening of immigrants for latent and active TB [22,24]. During the current extent of migration to Western Europe, receiving countries have set up different regimens to assess the health status of newly arriving refugees with or without implementation of routine testing for TB infection. Screening regimens are not harmonized. As recently assessed by the WHO and European Respiratory Society (ERS), 86.1% of 38 European national TB screening representatives reported screening for active TB, 50% screened for latent TB, and only 22.2% reported outcomes of latent TB treatment [25]. In 61.1% of European countries taking part in the WHO/ERS survey, screening for active or latent TB was performed in refugee centers. While 75% of countries answered that screening for TB was performed according to national and international guidelines, only 52.7% gave the same answer with regard to latent TB diagnostics [25]. In Germany, asylum law and national infection prevention plans state that all immigrants (except pregnant women) aged 16 years or older living in shared accommodation facilities such as reception centers or shelters for asylum seekers must undergo mandatory chest radiographs, primarily to identify active pulmonary tuberculosis (German Asylum law, § 62 Abs. 1 AsylG). Further measures of upon-entry screening for TB, especially in children or pregnant women, are governed by different policies at the level of the 16 federal states.

The usefulness of screening newly arriving immigrants for latent TB by IGRA is a matter of debate. Mulder et al. estimated the number needed to be treated to prevent one case of TB within 2 years in migrants in the Netherlands, given a positive IGRA and an efficacy of 60% of prophylactic treatment, to be around 350 [11]. Follow up evaluations may include chest radiographs and induced sputum analysis. The assay used in our current work has been described to have a specificity for active TB of around 99% with a sensitivity of about 80% [26,27]. A positive IGRA at entry was associated with an up to 26-fold increased risk for active TB for refugees in the Netherlands in 2012 [11]. In contrast to skin testing (Mantoux tuberculin sensitivity testing), the IGRA assay is not affected by TB vaccination. However, IGRA testing cannot discriminate between TB positive individuals that were recently infected and those with long-standing TB. This is a clinically important distinction as recently infected patients carry a higher risk of reactivation disease progression [28]. As such, appropriate follow up diagnostics and treatment regimens need to be implemented to further evaluate the TB status of IGRA positive refugees.

Unfortunately, we were unable to follow up the refugees with positive IGRA screening in our cohort and cannot report on the chest radiograph or microbiological results or clinical data of these subjects. The observation of zero positive IGRA results in children and adolescents in our cohort is pleasant, previous publications reported latent TB rates of 2.7–6.8% and 0.5% of TB in refugee children entering Europe during the current crisis [29,30]. However, the high IGRA positivity rates in elder refugees of our cohort are critical. Overall, we observed an age-related increase in IGRA positivity with 46.2% of senior refugees above the age of 50 years (62.5% of males >50 years). This finding is of particular concern, as older persons are at increased risk for TB reactivation [31,32]. TB reactivation in elder refugees does not only pose a risk for immigrant health but also for the receiving population, and our data support the notion that health caregivers, during the current refugee crisis, should be particularly aware of the risk for TB in older refugees. However, our analyses are limited by the fact that we only present data on a comparably small number of subjects, only $n = 10$ female refugees ($n = 10$) were IGRA positive, and only $n = 21$ underaged refugees were tested. Another limitation of our work is the fact that we were unable to link the IGRA results to subject-specific countries of origin. It has been reported that migrant TB rates reflect those of their countries of origin [11,21,33–35]. For example, refugees from Sub-Saharan Africa have been reported to be at particular risk for latent TB infections [30,36]. Future studies should include information on the home countries of immigrants to facilitate IGRA based TB risk estimation in specific refugee subgroups.

5. Conclusions

Taken together, we here present the current data on the rates of TB specific IGRA positivity in a representative refugee cohort in Western Europe. The growing population of refugees currently entering Europe challenges receiving healthcare systems and requires effective medical programs based on reliable epidemiological data [16]. Only by stringent screening with appropriate follow-up evaluation and effective therapy, TB associated morbidity can be reduced in the immigrating and receiving population [24]. We hope that our dataset supports the adaptation of appropriate screening and caretaking regimens.

Author Contributions: Research design: A.J., C.D., C.H., G.M.N.B., P.S., R.E.S. Sample collection and analyses: Routine clinical care. Data analysis: M.W., C.H., C.D., A.J., D.E., S.H., G.S., F.A., A.S., A.J. Writing and contributing to the writing of the manuscript: All authors.

Grants and Funding: Martin Wetzke received funding from the Young Academy Clinician/Scientist foundation Hannover Medical School, Germany and the Clinical Leave Clinician/Scientist program of the German Center for Infection Research (DZIF). Christine Happle received funding from the Young Academy Clinician/Scientist foundation and HiLF funding of Hannover Medical School, Germany. Alexandra Jablonka was funded by the Young Academy Clinician Scientist program of Hannover Medical School, Germany. This project was supported by the Geman Center for Infection Research by funding of infrastructure.

Acknowledgments: The authors would like to thank all doctors and personnel involved in the medical care of the migrants for their exceptional work. We would furthermore like to thank Christian Berger, Don-Philipp Dratschke, Matthias Joachim, Jean-Luc Kruppa, Henrick Langner, Bianca Schnake, Arne Steinbrück and Kai Zaengel for the organization of medical care, Annika Hampel for data processing and Torsten Bergemann of Nexave for the extraction from the electronic database.

Conflicts of Interest: The authors have no conflicts of interests to specify.

References

1. Kotsiou, O.S.; Srivastava, D.S.; Kotsios, P.; Exadaktylos, A.K.; Gourgoulianis, K.I. The emergency medical system in Greece: Opening Aeolus' bag of winds. *Int. J. Environ. Res. Public Health* **2018**, *15*, 745. [CrossRef] [PubMed]
2. Bozorgmehr, K.; Wahedi, K. Reframing solidarity in Europe: Frontex, frontiers, and the fallacy of refugee quota. *Lancet Public Health* **2017**, *2*, e10–e11. [CrossRef]
3. Lam, E.; McCarthy, A.; Brennan, M. Vaccine-preventable diseases in humanitarian emergencies among refugee and internally-displaced populations. *Hum. Vaccines Immunother.* **2015**, *11*, 2627–2636. [CrossRef] [PubMed]
4. Kouadio, I.K.; Koffi, A.K.; Attoh-Toure, H.; Kamigaki, T.; Oshitani, H. Outbreak of measles and rubella in refugee transit camps. *Epidemiol. Infect.* **2009**, *137*, 1593–1601. [CrossRef] [PubMed]
5. D'Ambrosio, L.; Centis, R.; Dara, M.; Solovic, I.; Sulis, G.; Zumla, A.; Migliori, G.B. European policies in the management of tuberculosis among migrants. *Int. J. Infect. Dis.* **2017**, *56*, 85–89. [CrossRef] [PubMed]
6. Kuehne, A.; Hauer, B.; Brodhun, B.; Haas, W.; Fiebig, L. Find and treat or find and lose? Tuberculosis treatment outcomes among screened newly arrived asylum seekers in Germany 2002 to 2014. *Euro Surveill.* **2018**, *23*, 17-00042. [CrossRef] [PubMed]
7. Ronald, L.A.; Campbell, J.R.; Balshaw, R.F.; Romanowski, K.; Roth, D.Z.; Marra, F.; Cook, V.J.; Johnston, J.C. Demographic predictors of active tuberculosis in people migrating to British Columbia, Canada: A retrospective cohort study. *CMAJ* **2018**, *190*, E209–E216. [CrossRef] [PubMed]
8. Buber-Ennser, I.; Kohlenberger, J.; Rengs, B.; Al Zalak, Z.; Goujon, A.; Striessnig, E.; Potancokova, M.; Gisser, R.; Testa, M.R.; Lutz, W. Human capital, values, and attitudes of persons seeking refuge in Austria in 2015. *PLoS ONE* **2016**, *11*, e0163481. [CrossRef] [PubMed]
9. Jablonka, A.; Happle, C.; Grote, U.; Schleenvoigt, B.T.; Hampel, A.; Dopfer, C.; Hansen, G.; Schmidt, R.E.; Behrens, G.M. Measles, mumps, rubella, and varicella seroprevalence in refugees in Germany in 2015. *Infection* **2016**, *44*, 781–787. [CrossRef] [PubMed]
10. Jablonka, A.; Behrens, G.M.; Stange, M.; Dopfer, C.; Grote, U.; Hansen, G.; Schmidt, R.E.; Happle, C. Tetanus and diphtheria immunity in refugees in Europe in 2015. *Infection* **2017**, *45*, 157–164. [CrossRef] [PubMed]

11. Mulder, C.; van Deutekom, H.; Huisman, E.M.; Toumanian, S.; Koster, B.F.; Meijer-Veldman, W.; van Loenhout-Rooyackers, J.H.; Appel, M.; Arend, S.M.; Borgdorff, M.W.; et al. Role of the QuantiFERON®-TB gold in-tube assay in screening new immigrants for tuberculosis infection. *Eur. Respir. J.* **2012**, *40*, 1443–1449. [CrossRef] [PubMed]
12. Castelli, F.; Tomasoni, L.R.; El Hamad, I. Migration and chronic noncommunicable diseases: Is the paradigm shifting? *J. Cardiovasc. Med.* **2014**, *15*, 693–695. [CrossRef] [PubMed]
13. Castelli, F.; Sulis, G. Migration and infectious diseases. *Clin. Microbiol. Infect.* **2017**, *23*, 283–289. [CrossRef] [PubMed]
14. Henjum, S.; Barikmo, I.; Strand, T.A.; Oshaug, A.; Torheim, L.E. Iodine-induced goitre and high prevalence of anaemia among Saharawi refugee women. *Public Health Nutr.* **2012**, *15*, 1512–1518. [CrossRef] [PubMed]
15. Blanck, H.M.; Bowman, B.A.; Serdula, M.K.; Khan, L.K.; Kohn, W.; Woodruff, B.A. Angular stomatitis and riboflavin status among adolescent Bhutanese refugees living in southeastern Nepal. *Am. J. Clin. Nutr.* **2002**, *76*, 430–435. [CrossRef] [PubMed]
16. Jakab, Z. Population Movement Is a Challenge for Refugees and Migrants as well as for the Receiving Population. 2015. Available online: http://www.euro.who.int/en/health-topics/health-determinants/migration-and-health/news/news/2015/09/population-movement-is-a-challenge-for-refugees-and-migrants-as-well-as-for-the-receiving-population (accessed on 21 April 2018).
17. Houben, R.M.; Dodd, P.J. The global burden of latent tuberculosis infection: A re-estimation using mathematical modelling. *PLoS Med.* **2016**, *13*, e1002152. [CrossRef] [PubMed]
18. World Health Organisation. *Global Tuberculosis Control 2015*; Document WHO/HTM/BT/2015.22; WHO: Geneva, Switzerland, 2015.
19. Getahun, H.; Matteelli, A.; Abubakar, I.; Aziz, M.A.; Baddeley, A.; Barreira, D.; Den Boon, S.; Borroto Gutierrez, S.M.; Bruchfeld, J.; Burhan, E.; et al. Management of latent mycobacterium tuberculosis infection: WHO guidelines for low tuberculosis burden countries. *Eur. Respir. J.* **2015**, *46*, 1563–1576. [CrossRef] [PubMed]
20. Lonnroth, K.; Migliori, G.B.; Abubakar, I.; D'Ambrosio, L.; de Vries, G.; Diel, R.; Douglas, P.; Falzon, D.; Gaudreau, M.A.; Goletti, D.; et al. Towards tuberculosis elimination: An action framework for low-incidence countries. *Eur. Respir. J.* **2015**, *45*, 928–952. [CrossRef] [PubMed]
21. Korthals Altes, H.; Kloet, S.; Cobelens, F.; Bootsma, M. Latent tuberculosis infection in foreign-born communities: Import versus Transmission in The Netherlands derived through mathematical modelling. *PLoS ONE* **2018**, *13*, e0192282.
22. Alami, N.N.; Yuen, C.M.; Miramontes, R.; Pratt, R.; Price, S.F.; Navin, T.R. Trends in tuberculosis—United States, 2013. *MMWR Morb. Mortal. Wkly. Rep.* **2014**, *63*, 229–233. [PubMed]
23. Van Leth, F.; Kalisvaart, N.A.; Erkens, C.G.; Borgdoff, M.W. Projection of the number of patients with tuberculosis in The Netherlands in 2030. *Eur. J. Public Health* **2009**, *19*, 424–427. [CrossRef] [PubMed]
24. Taylor, E.M.; Painter, J.; Posey, D.L.; Zhou, W.; Shetty, S. Latent tuberculosis infection among immigrant and refugee children arriving in the United States: 2010. *J. Immigr. Minor. Health* **2016**, *18*, 966–970. [CrossRef] [PubMed]
25. Dara, M.; Solovic, I.; Sotgiu, G.; D'Ambrosio, L.; Centis, R.; Tran, R.; Goletti, D.; Duarte, R.; Aliberti, S.; de Benedictis, F.M.; et al. Tuberculosis care among refugees arriving in Europe: A ERS/WHO Europe region survey of current practices. *Eur. Respir. J.* **2016**, *48*, 808–817. [CrossRef] [PubMed]
26. Takasaki, J.; Manabe, T.; Morino, E.; Muto, Y.; Hashimoto, M.; Iikura, M.; Izumi, S.; Sugiyama, H.; Kudo, K. Sensitivity and specificity of QuantiFERON-TB Gold Plus compared with QuantiFERON-TB gold In-Tube and T-SPOT.TB on active tuberculosis in Japan. *J. Infect. Chemother.* **2018**, *24*, 188–192. [CrossRef] [PubMed]
27. Bae, W.; Park, K.U.; Song, E.Y.; Kim, S.J.; Lee, Y.J.; Park, J.S.; Cho, Y.J.; Yoon, H.I.; Yim, J.J.; Lee, C.T.; et al. Comparison of the sensitivity of Quantiferon-TB gold In-Tube and T-SPOT.TB according to patient age. *PLoS ONE* **2016**, *11*, e0156917. [CrossRef] [PubMed]
28. Borgdorff, M.W.; Sebek, M.; Geskus, R.B.; Kremer, K.; Kalisvaart, N.; van Soolingen, D. The incubation period distribution of tuberculosis estimated with a molecular epidemiological approach. *Int. J. Epidemiol.* **2011**, *40*, 964–970. [CrossRef] [PubMed]
29. Pavlopoulou, I.D.; Tanaka, M.; Dikalioti, S.; Samoli, E.; Nisianakis, P.; Boleti, O.D.; Tsoumakas, K. Clinical and laboratory evaluation of new immigrant and refugee children arriving in Greece. *BMC Pediatr.* **2017**, *17*, 132. [CrossRef] [PubMed]

30. Bennet, R.; Eriksson, M. Tuberculosis infection and disease in the 2015 cohort of unaccompanied minors seeking asylum in Northern Stockholm, Sweden. *Infect. Dis.* **2017**, *49*, 501–506. [CrossRef] [PubMed]
31. Piergallini, T.J.; Turner, J. Tuberculosis in the elderly: Why inflammation matters. *Exp. Gerontol.* **2018**, *105*, 32–39. [CrossRef] [PubMed]
32. Mirsaeidi, M.; Sadikot, R.T. Patients at high risk of tuberculosis recurrence. *Int. J. Mycobacteriol.* **2018**, *7*, 1–6. [PubMed]
33. Cohn, D.L.; O'Brien, R.J.; Geiter, L.J.; Rockville, M.D.; Gordin, F.M.; Hershfield, E.; Horsburgh, C.R., Jr.; Jereb, J.A.; Jordan, T.J.; Kaplan, J.E.; et al. Targeted tuberculin testing and treatment of latent tuberculosis infection. *Am. J. Respir. Crit. Care Med.* **2000**, *161*, S221–S247, (Joint statement of the American Thoracic Society (ATS) and the Centers for Disease Control and Prevention (CDC) 1999).
34. Bennett, R.J.; Brodine, S.; Waalen, J.; Moser, K.; Rodwell, T.C. Prevalence and treatment of latent tuberculosis infection among newly arrived refugees in San Diego County, January 2010–October 2012. *Am. J. Public Health* **2014**, *104*, e95–e102. [CrossRef] [PubMed]
35. Cain, K.P.; Haley, C.A.; Armstrong, L.R.; Garman, K.N.; Wells, C.D.; Iademarco, M.F.; Castro, K.G.; Laserson, K.F. Tuberculosis among foreign-born persons in the United States: Achieving tuberculosis elimination. *Am. J. Respir. Crit. Care Med.* **2007**, *175*, 75–79. [CrossRef] [PubMed]
36. Rennert-May, E.; Hansen, E.; Zadeh, T.; Krinke, V.; Houston, S.; Cooper, R. A step toward tuberculosis elimination in a low-incidence country: Successful diagnosis and treatment of latent tuberculosis infection in a refugee clinic. *Can. Respir. J.* **2016**, *2016*, 7980869. [CrossRef] [PubMed]

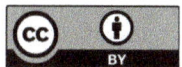

© 2018 by the authors. Licensee MDPI, Basel, Switzerland. This article is an open access article distributed under the terms and conditions of the Creative Commons Attribution (CC BY) license (http://creativecommons.org/licenses/by/4.0/).

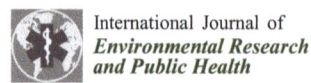

Article

Psychiatric Emergencies of Asylum Seekers; Descriptive Analysis and Comparison with Immigrants of Warranted Residence

Georgios Schoretsanitis [1,2,*], Sarah Eisenhardt [1], Meret E. Ricklin [3], David S. Srivastava [3], Sebastian Walther [1] and Aristomenis Exadaktylos [3]

1. University Hospital of Psychiatry, 3008 Bern, Switzerland; saraheisenhardt11@googlemail.com (S.E.); sebastian.walther@puk.unibe.ch (S.W.)
2. Department of Psychiatry, Psychotherapy and Psychosomatics, and JARA–Translational Brain Medicine, RWTH Aachen University, 52074 Aachen, Germany
3. Department of Emergency Medicine, Inselspital, University Hospital Bern, Freiburgstrasse, 3010 Bern, Switzerland; meret.ricklin@gmail.com (M.E.R.); DavidShiva.Srivastava@insel.ch (D.S.S.); Aristomenis.Exadaktylos@insel.ch (A.E.)
* Correspondence: george.schor@gmail.com; Tel.: +41-31-930-9111

Received: 12 May 2018; Accepted: 19 June 2018; Published: 21 June 2018

Abstract: *Background:* The aim of our study was to assess utilization patterns of psychiatric services by asylum seekers. *Methods:* We included 119 adults who presented themselves at the University Emergency Department between 1 March 2012 and 1 January 2017 for psychiatric consultation. Descriptive data were compared with a control group of non-Swiss individuals with warranted residence permits using Mann-Whitney-U and chi square (χ^2) tests. *Results:* Patients were mainly single, male, residing in reception centers, and presented themselves most frequently due to suicidal ideation. Almost 60% of the patients were assigned to inpatient treatments, with 28 involuntary cases. Compared to the control group, asylum seekers were younger and more often men ($p < 0.001$ for both). Further, they less often had family in Switzerland ($\chi^2 = 9.91$, $p = 0.007$). The proportion of patients coming in as walk-ins was significantly higher in the control group than in asylum seekers ($\chi^2 = 37.0$, $p < 0.001$). Asylum seekers were more frequently referred due to suicidal ideation and aggressive behavior than participants in the control group ($\chi^2 = 80.07$, $p < 0.001$). Diagnoses for asylum seekers infrequently included mood, as they often reported stress-related disorders ($\chi^2 = 19.6$, $p = 0.021$) and they were infrequently released home ($\chi^2 = 9.19$, $p = 0.027$). *Conclusion:* Asylum seekers more frequently demonstrated severe symptoms such as suicidal ideation and aggressive behavior and they were mainly treated as inpatients, potentially due to minimal social resources.

Keywords: asylum seekers; psychiatric emergency services; involuntary treatment; psychiatric hospitalization

1. Introduction

The movement of people currently observed worldwide is comparable in size to the migration during/after the Second World War [1]. In Switzerland, the annual number of asylum seekers from 2008–2013 has remained stable between 40,000 and 43,000 per year, but has substantially increased during the following two years to over 65,000 new applications per year [2].

The vulnerability of asylum seekers and generally displaced persons in terms of mental health issues has been consistently described [3,4]. Despite the methodological inconsistency, there are several studies that suggest an enhanced prevalence of post-traumatic stress disorder and depression among refugees [5]. The factors that account for the deleterious effects of the refugee experience include pre-, peri- and post-migration adversities [6–8].

Epidemiological data of psychiatric emergency services' usage by refugees are now increasingly available and provide a valuable indication of the problems refugees experience [9–12]. This evidence may be instrumental in evolving strategies for improvement of psychiatric services. At the same time, major challenges such as cultural and language barriers need to be addressed [7,13]. Utilization patterns among immigrants in general have already been assessed in the Swiss context [14–16]. Nevertheless, data for asylum seekers are particularly scarce. But information is strongly needed, since refugees and asylum seekers, often considered as a homogenous sample, present prominent differences regarding the psychopathology patterns and prevalence of mental disorders [10,17–19]. Differences also refer to the living arrangements, since asylum seekers in Switzerland mainly, but not exclusively, live in asylum centers. Detention in reception centers has been also connected with a considerable mental health burden [20]. Nevertheless, the majority of claimants face particular problems in accessing mental health services, and frequently, the only available option is a psychiatric consultation in the emergency department. Moreover, it is absolutely worthwhile to study psychiatric emergencies among asylum seekers following the rise in annual numbers of asylum seekers during the past few years (2015–2016). This increase enables a larger-scale epidemiological research, which can focus on particular dimensions of the mental healthcare for asylum seekers, such as the order of compulsory treatment. Such epidemiological data exist mainly for heterogeneous samples of patients, poorly defined as of non-Western or black origin or/and lacking further information of residency status [21–24].

The main aim of this study was to provide first descriptive data on usage of psychiatric emergency services by asylum seekers. We also compared categorical outcomes between asylum seekers and immigrants with residence permits to identify factors that may distinguish these two groups of non-Swiss people.

2. Materials and Methods

This descriptive study included retrospective data from adult asylum seekers (age ≥ 18 years). These individuals were admitted to the University Emergency Department (UNZ) for a psychiatric consultation between the 1 May 2012 and 28 February 2017. The UNZ consists of an organization, which provides 24 h/day psychiatric emergency services and it is responsible for the emergency mental healthcare for the Canton Bern (roughly 1 million citizens) including asylum centers in this catchment area. Consultations were conducted by resident doctors (medical doctors during the psychiatry training program) under supervision of senior doctors. Electronic medical records of patients with migratory background (i.e., non-Swiss nationality) were initially identified. These medical records have fastidiously been scrutinized for asylum seekers leading to 1697 records of patients with migratory background, i.e., non-Swiss nationality. Across asylum seekers there were individuals with pending cases (permit N), persons with rejected asylum application and provisionally admitted refugees (permit F). The last category consisted of foreign nationals, ordered to return to their native countries, but, in those cases, such returners were not admissible, reasonable or possible [25]. These last two subgroups experience different stressors, and were, therefore, also excluded, yielding a final sample of 119 patients (See Figure 1). During the screening process, we identified 1460 medical records of patients with migratory background and warranted residence permits. After removing duplicates and rudimentary records, we identified 1104 patients, who were included in the analysis as the control group.

We were able to extract the following demographic and clinical data from the included medical records: gender, age, nationality, marital status, children, type of residence (reception center or not), the pathway to care (health professionals involved in the referral), the reason for presentation/referral, diagnosis at the time of consultation (according to ICD-10), referral outcome, presence of interpreter during the consultation and contact with psychiatric services prior to the recorded (current) consultation. While classifying patients according to their pathway to care, the following categories were formed: walk-in, general practitioner or other medical doctor (MD), ambulance, police, or reception centers. Note that during the asylum process, the Swiss government provides healthcare coverage on a mandatory basis; everyone is entitled access to a general practitioner. The reasons for presentation/referral were grouped as follows: suicidal thoughts, suicide attempt, auto-aggressive behavior, aggression, mood (depression) symptoms, sleep disorders, acute stress, somatic complaints, psychotic symptoms, psychosocial problems and medication acquisition. If a patient has been registered for more than one reason, the major concern at the time of presentation/referral was used as the main criterion for the outcome. In particular, when suicidal and depressive symptoms co-existed, patients were classified as referred due to suicidal ideation since they were more likely to be referred mainly due to the suicidal than depressive symptoms. Therefore, all patients classified as having depressive symptoms were unlikely to have reported suicidal ideation. Following up on the referral process the possible outcomes were admittance to a psychiatric clinic (voluntary or compulsory) or discharge home. Individuals with rudimentary case files or incomplete medical records were excluded from the analysis. Moreover, for patients who visited the UNZ more than once, only the most recent registration was considered. Based on a rough geographical classification, the origin countries have been formed into six groups; Middle East (Iran, Iraq, Jordan, Lebanon, Syria, Turkey, United Arab Emirates), Eastern Europe (Albania, Belarus, Bosnia-Herzegovina, Chechnya, Macedonia, Kosovo, Russia), sub-Saharan Africa (Angola, Benin, Congo, Eritrea, Ethiopia, Guinea, Nigeria, Somalia, Sudan, Togo), northwestern Africa (Algeria, Libya, Morocco, Tunisia), Central-South Asia (Afghanistan, Bangladesh, China, Sri Lanka).

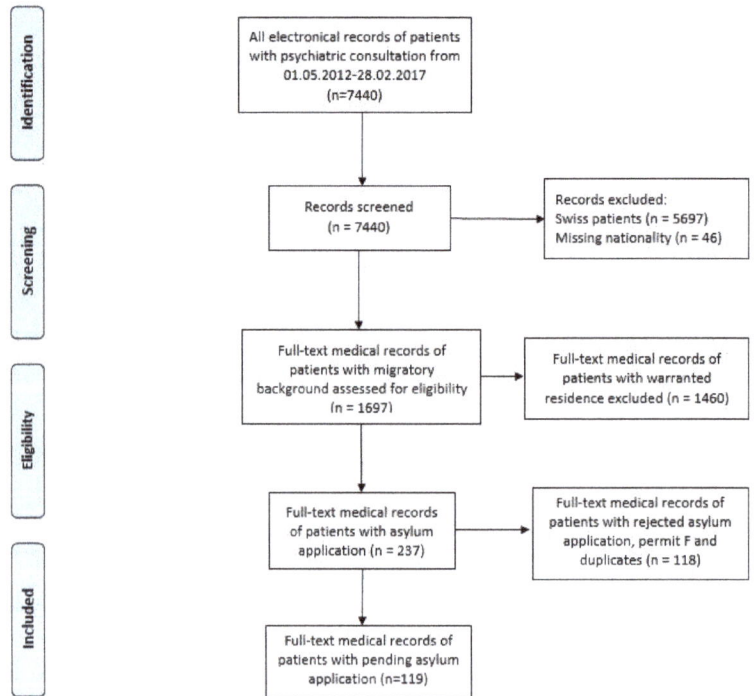

Figure 1. Medical records included in the analysis.

The study was performed retrospectively with health-related patient data that were exported anonymously for analysis. One of the authors (MER) had access to identification patient information and none of the authors was potentially a treating physician of the patients involved. Retrospective analysis of data for this study was in accordance with the local regulatory authority with the Declaration of Helsinki. No informed consent was necessary for this type of study.

3. Statistical Analysis

The data were summarized using descriptive statistics (means and standard deviation). We assessed gender, age, type of residence, referral conditions (reason and referring person), presence of an interpreter and prior contact to psychiatric services. Diagnoses (ICD-10) were classified into diagnostic categories (F10-19, 20-29, 30-39, 40-49, F60-69, F90-99). Demographic characteristics and parameters related to the registered consultation were compared between the group of asylum seekers and a control group of non-Swiss patients with warranted permits: our primary hypothesis was that involuntary treatment orders would be increased in the group of asylum seekers due to issues of integration; we studied referral outcomes as a categorical variable, but we also transformed referral outcomes to a dichotomous variable with '0' for cases of non-compulsory treatment consisting of discharge home and voluntary admissions in the clinic. We used the variable '1' for compulsory treatment consisting of involuntary admissions. The comparison between study groups was based on non-parametrical tests Mann-Whitney-U (M-W-U) test and the chi square test (χ^2) with a significance level of $p < 0.05$. For the computation of possible correlations, cases without data were excluded. All statistical analyses were carried out using IBM SPSS Statistics, version 22.0 (IBM GmbH, Ehningen, Germany).

4. Results

The medical records were scanned for asylum seekers leading to a sample of 119 persons (30 women, 89 men). The mean age was 29.88 ± 9.13 (range 18–57) years (Table 1). In terms of origin, individuals came from a wide range of countries; the most common origin countries were Eritrea ($n = 17$), Afghanistan ($n = 14$) and Morocco ($n = 12$) (Table 2). The majority of the patients were single ($n = 67$, 56.3%) and 72 of the patients did not have children (60.5%). Almost 6 out of 10 patients ($n = 66$, 55.5%) had no relatives in Switzerland. Asylum seekers lived mainly in reception centers ($n = 85$, 71.4%).

Table 1. Sociodemographic characteristics of asylum seekers ($n = 119$) and control group ($n = 1104$).

	Asylum Seekers	Control Group
Females (%)	30 (25.2) *	500 (45.3)
Age (SD)	29.88 (9.13) **	36.98 (12.81)
Marital status (%)		
Never been married	67 (56.3) ***	458 (41.5)
Widowed & Divorced	9 (7.5)	210 (19.0)
Married (Spouse in CH)	13 (10.9)	227 (20.6)
Married (Spouse abroad)	11 (9.2)	101 (9.1)
Unknown	19 (16.0)	108 (9.8)
Children (%)		
No	72 (60.5)	609 (55.2)
Yes (Children in CH)	18 (15.1) ****	348 (31.5)
Yes (Children abroad)	10 (8.4) ****	33 (3.0)
Unknown	19 (16.0)	114 (10.3)
At least one relative in CH, not partner (%)		
No	66 (55.5)	521 (47.2)
Yes	34 (28.6) *****	470 (42.6)
Unknown	19 (16.0)	113 (10.2)

* $\chi^2 = 17.64$, df = 1, $p < 0.001$, ** $p < 0.001$ for M-W-U, *** $\chi^2 = 22.57$, df = 5, $p < 0.001$, **** $\chi^2 = 22.3$, df = 3, $p < 0.001$, ***** $\chi^2 = 9.91$, df = 2, $p = 0.007$.

Table 2. Regions of origin for asylum seekers (n = 119).

Regions of Origin (%)	
Middle East	27 (22.9)
Eastern Europe	11 (9.3)
Sub-Saharan Africa	33 (28.0)
Northwestern Africa	26 (22.0)
Central-South Asia	21 (17.8)

Predominantly, patients came as walk-ins patients (n = 52, 43.7%), whereas 35 patients (29.4%) were referred to the UNZ by the police (Table 3). The most frequent reason of referral was suicidal ideation, reported by 30 patients (25.2%), followed by aggressive behavior, which was the referral reason for 25 patients (21.0%). Seventy patients reported prior contact to psychiatric services (58.8%). The consultation was aided by interpreting service in 29 cases (24.4%) or by the presence of a person who was a speaker of the patient's native language (family member or colleague of the patient) in 9 cases (7.6%), which was not possible in two thirds of the patients (n = 80, 67.2%).

Table 3. Clinical characteristics of asylum seekers (n = 119) and control group (n = 1104).

Variable	Asylum Seekers	Control Group
Pathway to UNZ (%)		
Walk-in	52 (43.7) *	653 (59.1)
General practitioner (or other MDs)	16 (13.4)	101 (9.1)
Ambulance	13 (10.9)	105 (9.5)
Police	35 (29.4)	245 (22.2)
Reception center	3 (2.5)	NA
Referral reason		
Suicidal ideation	30 (25.2) **	122 (11.1)
Suicide attempt	3 (2.5)	43 (3.9)
Auto-aggressive behavior	7 (5.9)	15 (1.4)
Aggressive behavior	25 (21.0) **	103 (9.3)
Psychotic symptoms	11 (9.2) **	186 (16.8)
Depressive symptoms	10 (8.4) **	172 (15.6)
Sleep disorders	8 (6.7)	60 (5.4)
Acute stress	9 (7.6)	91 (8.2)
Somatic complaints	10 (8.4)	73 (6.6)
Psychosocial problems	2 (1.7)	186 (16.8)
Medication acquisition	2 (1.7)	7 (0.6)
Manic symptoms	0 (0)	9 (0.8)
Addiction	0 (0)	23 (2.1)
Other	2 (1.7)	14 (1.3)
ICD diagnoses		
Disorders due to substance use (F10-19)	14 (11.8)	153 (13.9)
Disorders of schizophrenia spectrum (F20-29)	22 (18.5)	243 (22.0)
Affective disorders (F30-F39)	17 (14.3) ***	256 (23.2)
Stress-related disorders (F40-F49)	58 (49.6) ***	398 (36.1)
Personality disorders (F60-69)	6 (5.0)	26 (2.4)
Others	1 (0.8)	23 (2.1)
Referral outcome (%)		
Discharged home	32 (26.9) ****	453 (41.0)
Discharged home with outpatient treatment	16 (13.4)	110 (10.0)
Voluntary admission	42 (35.3)	312 (28.3)
Compulsory admission	29 (24.4)	229 (20.7)

NA: not applicable, * $\chi^2 = 37.0$, df = 4, $p < 0.001$, ** $\chi^2 = 80.07$, df = 15, $p < 0.001$, *** $\chi^2 = 19.6$, df = 9, $p = 0.021$, **** $\chi^2 = 9.19$, df = 3, $p = 0.027$.

The diagnostic picture is dominated by adjustment disorders (F43.2), which comprised one fourth of the diagnoses ($n = 30$, 25.21%). Twenty-two patients (18.5%) received a diagnosis of schizophrenia spectrum disorders, whereas patients were diagnosed with affective and substance use disorders in 14.3% ($n = 17$) and 11.8% ($n = 14$) of the cases, respectively. Regarding the referral outcomes, 59.7% ($n = 71$) of patients were treated as inpatients: 42 voluntary treatment cases and 29 compulsory treatment cases (Table 3).

The group of asylum seekers was compared with a control group of non-Swiss citizens with warranted residence permits in terms of demographic/clinical characteristics and consultation aspects (Table 1). The two groups showed significant differences for age and sex distribution; asylum seekers were younger ($p < 0.001$ for M-W-U), more often men ($\chi^2 = 17.64$, df = 1, $p < 0.001$) and less likely to have been married than participants in the control group ($\chi^2 = 22.57$, df = 5, $p < 0.001$). No differences between groups were reported in the proportion of patients having children; nevertheless, the proportion of asylum seekers with children abroad was higher than in the control group and asylum seekers less frequently reported children living in Switzerland than patients in the control group ($\chi^2 = 22.3$, df = 3, $p < 0.001$). Patients in the control group more frequently had relatives residing in Switzerland compared to asylum seekers ($\chi^2 = 9.91$, df = 2, $p = 0.007$).

Moreover, the two groups differed regarding referral conditions; the proportion of patients presenting as walk-ins was significantly higher for patients of the control group than asylum seekers ($\chi^2 = 37.0$, df = 4, $p < 0.001$). The rest of the referral conditions did not differ between groups ($p > 0.05$ for χ^2 except from referral by the reception center, where no counts were available in the control group and, therefore, no valid analysis was possible. When exploring potential differences in referral reasons between groups, we detected higher rates of suicidal ideation and aggressive behavior but lower rates of depressive and psychotic symptoms in asylum seekers ($\chi^2 = 80.07$, df = 15, $p < 0.001$ for all comparisons). No differences were reported for somatic complaints ($p > 0.05$), whereas analyses were not conducted for the rest of reasons due to small number of counts per reason and group. The ICD diagnoses set by consulting psychiatrists differed for mood disorders (F30-39) and stress-related disorders (F40-49), with the mood disorders occurring proportionally less often and the stress-related disorders occurred proportionally more often in asylum seekers compared to control group ($\chi^2 = 19.6$, df = 9, $p = 0.021$). Regarding referral outcome, the proportion of asylum seekers released home was lower than in the control group ($\chi^2 = 9.19$, df = 3, $p = 0.027$). For assignment to compulsory treatment (using referral outcome as a binary variable), study groups did not demonstrate differences ($\chi^2 = 0.85$, df = 1, $p > 0.05$).

5. Discussion

Our study provides a descriptive and comparative analysis of utilization of psychiatric services for asylum seekers with pending application. To our knowledge, our retrospective assessment adds to previous research because access to mental healthcare for immigrants remains scarce. Nevertheless, this particular subgroup has distinct mental health needs as these patients are exposed to additional mental health risks [26]. Our study, contrasting previous studies, uses the migration status rather than the country of birth or race as a determinant for mental health problems. To our knowledge, specific parameters, such as the order of a compulsory treatment for these individuals, were examined, whereas the main point widely evaded the focus of research. In this context, we chose to include all psychiatric diagnoses, while most of earlier studies focused on refugees with schizophrenic disorders, and particularly first-episode patients. Moreover, the criteria for compulsory admissions largely vary between and even within countries since they strongly depend on the current mental health legislation [27].

The profile of asylum seekers in our sample indicated younger and more often male individuals compared to the control group. They were mainly residing in reception centers and they had no family in Switzerland. Less than the half of patients presented themselves as walk-ins to the UNZ and the most common referral reason was suicidal ideation. Consultants most frequently set a stress-related diagnosis and arranged an inpatient treatment in 40% of the cases. Asylum seekers reported less family support with fewer relatives in Switzerland than controls.

Moreover, the two groups differed regarding referral conditions; the proportion of patients coming in as walk-ins was significantly higher in the control group than asylum seekers. Asylum seekers were consulted more often due to suicidal ideation or aggressive behavior, but less often for psychotic or depressive symptoms compared to controls. Mood disorders were diagnosed in a higher proportion of patients in the control group than in asylum seekers, whereas the rates of stress-related disorders were higher for asylum seekers. Finally, the proportion of individuals released home was smaller in the asylum seekers than in the control group and no differences were reported for assignment to compulsory treatment.

When interpreting these differences, the age difference between study groups seems to be a plausible finding. Regarding the difference pertaining to gender, previous evidence indicated female underrepresentation [11,16,28,29]. In our sample, this finding may be due to the two-fold higher percentages of men in asylum seekers during the years 2011–2015 [2]. Moreover, the high percentage of aggressive behavior as referral reason (almost one out of fourth) for asylum seekers may be accounted for by gender, as aggression is more common in men than in women [30]. The proportion of individuals consulted for suicidal ideation was higher for asylum seekers than for controls; a Danish psychiatric emergency service study also reported suicidal ideas as the most common referral reason for asylum seekers [11]. Likewise, hospital data reported high incidence of suicidal behavior in asylum seekers residing in reception centers in the Netherlands [31]. On the other hand, the low rates of asylum seekers referred for depressive symptoms may be due to the overrepresentation of stress-related disorders in our sample as well as in previous samples [7,17,32], as stress-related disorders may imitate depression in terms of psychopathology [33]. Moreover, an essential amount of asylum seekers with depressive symptoms was classified in the subgroup referred for suicidal ideation. Thus, it would be more precise to say that rates of depressive symptoms without co-existing suicidal ideation were higher in the control group. Further, asylum seekers were less often visiting the UNZ as walk-ins; a previous Irish study reported that asylum seekers tended to visit general practitioners, who may act as primary mental healthcare providers, more frequently than did controls [17]. Alternatively, we speculated that asylum seekers are less familiar with the structure of the health care system in Switzerland, so that they might hesitate to directly visit the UNZ. For both options, the stigmatizing impact of psychiatry may account for the barriers of these individuals to access to mental healthcare [34]. Nevertheless, no differences were reported regarding alternative pathways to mental health care between groups. The finding of high prevalence of stress-related disorders in terms of set diagnoses is no surprise but is in alignment with previous evidence [11,17]. Further, it is also rather expected that a higher proportion of asylum seekers were assigned to inpatient treatment, which may be understood in light of the fact that they showed more severe symptoms such as suicidal ideation and aggressive behavior than the control group. Moreover, controls may have more social resources due to relatives also residing in the country. Thus, the limited social support may account for the higher rates of asylum seekers treated as inpatients. The assignment to inpatient treatment may also relate to the access problems to specific treatments for asylum seekers, which was reported previously in cohort studies, also in the Swiss context [14,35].

Asylum status failed to correlate with assignment to compulsory treatment in our sample. This major counter-intuitive finding introduces a riddle that may demand quantitative data to unravel mediating mechanisms. In a sample of unaccompanied refugee minors with insecure asylum status, researchers reported high rates of involuntary treatment for these individuals referred due to self-harm and suicidal behavior [32]. Nevertheless, in our sample, differences for involuntary treatment between study groups did not reach statistical significance despite the high prevalence of suicidal ideation for asylum seekers.

Anxiety levels for asylum seekers may be strongly related to language issues [29]. The usage of interpreting services in our sample was very low compared to a Danish study [11], which may introduce an important challenge for the improvement of the mental healthcare system. The ethnic distribution of the asylum seekers presented in the emergency department reflects the mosaic of ethnicities of people applying for asylum in the Canton of Bern during the past year (2016). The countries with the most applications included Afghanistan, Eritrea, Syria and Iraq [2].

Due to the retrospective analysis of this database, results must be interpreted with some caution. No standardized general and systemic medical history was taken. Parameters such as socio-economic status, length of stay in Switzerland before presentation, symptom severity and illness onset and duration, were barely provided and therefore could not be included in the analyses. Moreover, asylum seekers in Switzerland invariably are not allowed to work. As a result, we were not able to control for the effects of this variable, although the role of unemployment for compulsory admissions as well as for the psychopathology already has been demonstrated [29,36]. In addition, no data regarding the length of asylum procedure were provided; nevertheless, this parameter has been associated with an increased risk of mental disorders [37–39]. Lastly, the control group was not matched for demographic or clinical characteristics with the group of asylum seekers.

6. Conclusions

Concluding, our data imply that persons presented for psychiatric consultation had severe symptoms and were more likely than persons with permanent permit to be treated as inpatients. The treatment of this distinct patient subgroup introduces a public mental health challenge that needs to be addressed urgently. We strongly hope that this study may inspire the conduction of prospective studies providing a better overview of the mental health of asylum seekers and enabling the minimization of the application of compulsory admissions.

Author Contributions: G.S., S.E., M.E.R., D.S.S., S.W. and A.E. participated in the research design of the study. G.S. performed the initial statistical analyses and wrote the first article draft. S.W. suggested additional analyses and modifications to adjust to the style of this journal. All the authors contributed to the interpretation of data and approved the final manuscript.

Funding: No sources of funding were used for this manuscript.

Acknowledgments: Authors are particularly grateful to C. Ringer, S. Suker, A. Jungnickel, University Hospital of Psychiatry, Bern, Switzerland for their valuable feedback.

Conflicts of Interest: In the last 10 years, Sebastian Walther has received honoraria for serving as a speaker in educational programs from Eli Lilly, Janssen, Lundbeck, and Otsuka. He was an advisory board member for Lundbeck and Otsuka from 2015 to 2016. All other authors declare no conflicts of interest.

References

1. The UN Refugee Agency. *U. Global Trends 2015*; United Nations High Commissioner for Refugees: Geneva, Switzerland, 2016.
2. State Secretariat for Migration, Switzerland. Available online: https://www.sem.admin.ch/sem/de/home/publiservice/statistik/asylstatistik/archiv/2016/11.html (accessed on 12 May 2018).
3. Fazel, M.; Wheeler, J.; Danesh, J. Prevalence of serious mental disorder in 7000 refugees resettled in western countries: A systematic review. *Lancet* **2005**, *365*, 1309–1314. [CrossRef]
4. Bhugra, D.; Gupta, S.; Bhui, K.; Craig, T.; Dogra, N.; Ingleby, J.D.; Kirkbride, J.; Moussaoui, D.; Nazroo, J.; Qureshi, A.; et al. Wpa guidance on mental health and mental health care in migrants. *World Psychiatry Off. J. World Psychiatr. Assoc.* **2011**, *10*, 2–10. [CrossRef]
5. World Health Organisation Regional Office for Europe. *Policy Brief on Migration and Health: Mental Health Care for Refugees*; World Health Organisation: Copenhagen, Denmark, 2015.
6. Carswell, K.; Blackburn, P.; Barker, C. The relationship between trauma, post-migration problems and the psychological well-being of refugees and asylum seekers. *Int. J. Soc. Psychiatry* **2011**, *57*, 107–119. [CrossRef] [PubMed]
7. Silove, D.; Sinnerbrink, I.; Field, A.; Manicavasagar, V.; Steel, Z. Anxiety, depression and PTSD in asylum-seekers: Assocations with pre-migration trauma and post-migration stressors. *Br. J. Psychiatry J. Ment. Sci.* **1997**, *170*, 351–357. [CrossRef]

8. Hassan, G.; Ventevogel, P.; Jefee-Bahloul, H.; Barkil-Oteo, A.; Kirmayer, L.J. Mental health and psychosocial wellbeing of Syrians affected by armed conflict. *Epidemiol. Psychiatr. Sci.* **2016**, *25*, 129–141. [CrossRef] [PubMed]
9. Deans, A.K.; Boerma, C.J.; Fordyce, J.; De Souza, M.; Palmer, D.J.; Davis, J.S. Use of royal darwin hospital emergency department by immigration detainees in 2011. *Med. J. Aust.* **2013**, *199*, 776–778. [CrossRef] [PubMed]
10. Iversen, V.C.; Morken, G. Differences in acute psychiatric admissions between asylum seekers and refugees. *Nord. J. Psychiatry* **2004**, *58*, 465–470. [CrossRef] [PubMed]
11. Reko, A.; Bech, P.; Wohlert, C.; Noerregaard, C.; Csillag, C. Usage of psychiatric emergency services by asylum seekers: Clinical implications based on a descriptive study in Denmark. *Nord. J. Psychiatry* **2015**, *69*, 587–593. [CrossRef] [PubMed]
12. McColl, H.; Johnson, S. Characteristics and needs of asylum seekers and refugees in contact with London community mental health teams: A descriptive investigation. *Soc. Psychiatry Psychiatr. Epidemiol.* **2006**, *41*, 789–795. [CrossRef] [PubMed]
13. Sandhu, S.; Bjerre, N.V.; Dauvrin, M.; Dias, S.; Gaddini, A.; Greacen, T.; Ioannidis, E.; Kluge, U.; Jensen, N.K.; Lamkaddem, M.; et al. Experiences with treating immigrants: A qualitative study in mental health services across 16 European countries. *Soc. Psychiatry Psychiatr. Epidemiol.* **2013**, *48*, 105–116. [CrossRef] [PubMed]
14. Maier, T.; Schmidt, M.; Mueller, J. Mental health and healthcare utilization in adult asylum seekers. *Swiss Med. Wkly.* **2010**, *140*, w13110. [CrossRef] [PubMed]
15. Chatzidiakou, K.; Schoretsanitis, G.; Schruers, K.R.; Müller, T.J.; Ricklin, M.E.; Exadaktylos, A.K. Acute psychiatric problems among migrants living in switzerland- a retrospective study from a Swiss University emergency department. *Emerg. Med. (Los Angel.)* **2016**, *6*. [CrossRef]
16. Pfortmueller, C.A.; Schwetlick, M.; Mueller, T.; Lehmann, B.; Exadaktylos, A.K. Adult asylum seekers from the Middle East including Syria in Central Europe: What are their health care problems? *PLoS ONE* **2016**, *11*, e0148196. [CrossRef] [PubMed]
17. Toar, M.; O'Brien, K.K.; Fahey, T. Comparison of self-reported health & healthcare utilisation between asylum seekers and refugees: An observational study. *BMC Public Health* **2009**, *9*, 214.
18. Ryan, D.A.; Benson, C.A.; Dooley, B.A. Psychological distress and the asylum process: A longitudinal study of forced migrants in Ireland. *J. Nerv. Ment. Dis.* **2008**, *196*, 37–45. [CrossRef] [PubMed]
19. Silove, D.; Steel, Z.; Susljik, I.; Frommer, N.; Loneragan, C.; Chey, T.; Brooks, R.; le Touze, D.; Ceollo, M.; Smith, M.; et al. The impact of the refugee decision on the trajectory of ptsd, anxiety, and depressive symptoms among asylum seekers: A longitudinal study. *Am. J. Disaster Med.* **2007**, *2*, 321–329. [PubMed]
20. Steel, Z.; Momartin, S.; Bateman, C.; Hafshejani, A.; Silove, D.M.; Everson, N.; Roy, K.; Dudley, M.; Newman, L.; Blick, B.; et al. Psychiatric status of asylum seeker families held for a protracted period in a remote detention centre in Australia. *Aust. N. Z. J. Public Health* **2004**, *28*, 527–536. [CrossRef] [PubMed]
21. Mulder, C.L.; Koopmans, G.T.; Selten, J.P. Emergency psychiatry, compulsory admissions and clinical presentation among immigrants to The Netherlands. *Br. J. Psychiatry J. Ment. Sci.* **2006**, *188*, 386–391. [CrossRef] [PubMed]
22. Norredam, M.; Garcia-Lopez, A.; Keiding, N.; Krasnik, A. Excess use of coercive measures in psychiatry among migrants compared with native Danes. *Acta Psychiat. Scand.* **2010**, *121*, 143–151. [CrossRef] [PubMed]
23. Davies, S.; Thornicroft, G.; Leese, M.; Higgingbotham, A.; Phelan, M. Ethnic differences in risk of compulsory psychiatric admission among representative cases of psychosis in London. *BMJ* **1996**, *312*, 533–537. [CrossRef] [PubMed]
24. Mann, F.; Fisher, H.L.; Major, B.; Lawrence, J.; Tapfumaneyi, A.; Joyce, J.; Hinton, M.F.; Johnson, S. Ethnic variations in compulsory detention and hospital admission for psychosis across four UK early intervention services. *BMC Psychiatry* **2014**, *14*, 256. [CrossRef] [PubMed]
25. State Secretariat for Migration, Switzerland. Available online: https://www.sem.admin.ch/sem/en/home/themen/aufenthalt/nicht_eu_efta/ausweis_f__vorlaeufig.html (accessed on 12 May 2018).
26. Momartin, S.; Steel, Z.; Coello, M.; Aroche, J.; Silove, D.M.; Brooks, R. A comparison of the mental health of refugees with temporary versus permanent protection visas. *Med. J. Aust.* **2006**, *185*, 357–361. [PubMed]
27. Riecher-Rossler, A.; Rossler, W. Compulsory admission of psychiatric patients—An international comparison. *Acta Psychiat. Scand.* **1993**, *87*, 231–236. [CrossRef] [PubMed]

28. Crepet, A.; Rita, F.; Reid, A.; Van den Boogaard, W.; Deiana, P.; Quaranta, G.; Barbieri, A.; Bongiorno, F.; Di Carlo, S. Mental health and trauma in asylum seekers landing in sicily in 2015: A descriptive study of neglected invisible wounds. *Confl. Health* **2017**, *11*, 1. [CrossRef] [PubMed]
29. Hocking, D.C.; Kennedy, G.A.; Sundram, S. Mental disorders in asylum seekers: The role of the refugee determination process and employment. *J. Nerv. Ment. Dis.* **2015**, *203*, 28–32. [CrossRef] [PubMed]
30. Witt, K.; van Dorn, R.; Fazel, S. Risk factors for violence in psychosis: Systematic review and meta-regression analysis of 110 studies. *PLoS ONE* **2013**, *8*, e55942. [CrossRef]
31. Goosen, S.; Kunst, A.E.; Stronks, K.; van Oostrum, I.E.; Uitenbroek, D.G.; Kerkhof, A.J. Suicide death and hospital-treated suicidal behaviour in asylum seekers in The Netherlands: A national registry-based study. *BMC Public Health* **2011**, *11*, 484. [CrossRef] [PubMed]
32. Ramel, B.; Taljemark, J.; Lindgren, A.; Johansson, B.A. Overrepresentation of unaccompanied refugee minors in inpatient psychiatric care. *SpringerPlus* **2015**, *4*, 131. [CrossRef] [PubMed]
33. McColl, H.; McKenzie, K.; Bhui, K. Mental healthcare of asylum-seekers and refugees. *Adv. Psychiatr. Treat.* **2008**, *14*, 452–459. [CrossRef]
34. Bartolomei, J.; Baeriswyl-Cottin, R.; Framorando, D.; Kasina, F.; Premand, N.; Eytan, A.; Khazaal, Y. What are the barriers to access to mental healthcare and the primary needs of asylum seekers? A survey of mental health caregivers and primary care workers. *BMC Psychiatry* **2016**, *16*, 336. [CrossRef] [PubMed]
35. Sundvall, M.; Tidemalm, D.H.; Titelman, D.E.; Runeson, B.; Baarnhielm, S. Assessment and treatment of asylum seekers after a suicide attempt: A comparative study of people registered at mental health services in a Swedish location. *BMC Psychiatry* **2015**, *15*, 235. [CrossRef] [PubMed]
36. Braam, A.W.; van Ommeren, O.W.; van Buuren, M.L.; Laan, W.; Smeets, H.M.; Engelhard, I.M. Local geographical distribution of acute involuntary psychiatric admissions in subdistricts in and around Utrecht, The Netherlands. *J. Emerg. Med.* **2016**, *50*, 449–457. [CrossRef] [PubMed]
37. Hollifield, M.; Warner, T.D.; Lian, N.; Krakow, B.; Jenkins, J.H.; Kesler, J.; Stevenson, J.; Westermeyer, J. Measuring trauma and health status in refugees: A critical review. *JAMA* **2002**, *288*, 611–621. [CrossRef] [PubMed]
38. Hallas, P.; Hansen, A.R.; Staehr, M.A.; Munk-Andersen, E.; Jorgensen, H.L. Length of stay in asylum centres and mental health in asylum seekers: A retrospective study from Denmark. *BMC Public Health* **2007**, *7*, 288. [CrossRef] [PubMed]
39. Sultan, A.; O'Sullivan, K. Psychological disturbances in asylum seekers held in long term detention: A participant-observer account. *Med. J. Aust.* **2001**, *175*, 593–596. [PubMed]

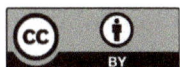

© 2018 by the authors. Licensee MDPI, Basel, Switzerland. This article is an open access article distributed under the terms and conditions of the Creative Commons Attribution (CC BY) license (http://creativecommons.org/licenses/by/4.0/).

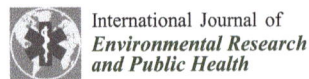

Review

Sexual Health Help-Seeking Behavior among Migrants from Sub-Saharan Africa and South East Asia living in High Income Countries: A Systematic Review

Donna Angelina Rade [1], Gemma Crawford [2], Roanna Lobo [2], Corie Gray [2,*] and Graham Brown [2,3]

1. School of Public Health, Curtin University, Kent Street, Bentley, WA 6102, Australia; d.rade@postgrad.curtin.edu.au
2. Collaboration for Evidence, Research and Impact in Public Health, School of Public Health, Curtin University, Kent Street, Bentley, WA 6102, Australia; g.crawford@curtin.edu.au (G.C.); roanna.lobo@curtin.edu.au (R.L.); Graham.Brown@latrobe.edu.au (G.B.)
3. Australian Research Centre in Sex, Health and Society School of Psychology and Public Health, La Trobe University, Bundoora, VIC 3086, Australia
* Correspondence: corie.gray@curtin.edu.au

Received: 16 May 2018; Accepted: 18 June 2018; Published: 22 June 2018

Abstract: The number of migrants has increased globally. This phenomenon has contributed to increasing health problems amongst migrants in high-income countries, including vulnerability for HIV acquisition and other sexual health issues. Adaptation processes in destination countries can present difficulties for migrants to seek help from and gain access to health services. This study examined migrants' from sub-Saharan Africa (SSA) and South East Asia (SEA) sexual health help-seeking behavior in high-income countries with universal health coverage. The systematic review followed PRISMA guidelines and was registered with PROSPERO. Several databases were searched from 2000 to 2017. Of 2824 studies, 15 met the inclusion criteria. These consisted of 12 qualitative and three quantitative studies conducted in Australia, Spain, the United Kingdom, Belgium, Scotland, Ireland, and Sweden. Migrants experienced a range of difficulties accessing health services, specifically those related to sexual health, in high-income countries. Few studies described sources of sexual health help-seeking or facilitators to help-seeking. Barriers to access were numerous, including: stigma, direct and indirect costs, difficulty navigating health systems in destination countries and lack of cultural competency within health services. More culturally secure health services, increased health service literacy and policy support to mitigate costs, will improve health service access for migrants from SSA and SEA. Addressing the structural drivers for stigma and discrimination remains an ongoing and critical challenge.

Keywords: migrants; sexual health; help-seeking behavior; systematic review

1. Introduction

The number of migrants has been increasing globally, with an estimate of 258 million international migrants in 2017 [1]. Between 1990 and 2017, the number of international migrants increased from 152.5 million to 257.7 million—a rise of over 69% [1]. Half (51%) of these migrants were situated in only 10 countries—nine of which are classified as high-income countries (HIC) by the World Bank, including United States of America (USA), France, Canada and Australia [2]. A documented migrant is defined as someone "who entered a country lawfully and remains in the country in accordance with his or her admission criteria" [3]. Australia, as an example, has a substantial proportion of documented international migrants [4] with the Australian Bureau of Statistics [4] recently reporting that the number of overseas migrants has reached its highest point in 20 years.

There are multiple and complex reasons for migration to HIC, including: safety and security, health, labour, economic inequalities between high and low-income countries, and family reunification [5–7]. There are a range of health issues associated with migration; with increased vulnerability during the migration process [8]. Research from HIC indicates migrants from low and middle-income countries (LMIC) may have different health and health care needs than the destination population [8]. This vulnerability may lead to specific problems regarding sexual and reproductive health (SRH) and service provision [9]. The complexity of migrants' diverse religions, cultural backgrounds, educational levels, migration histories, present living conditions and legal statuses may all influence their sexual health (SH), including their vulnerability for HIV acquisition [9].

Research with migrants in Australia, Canada, the United Kingdom (UK), France, Switzerland and the Netherlands highlight vulnerability for HIV acquisition, with some overseas born populations overrepresented in HIV notifications [10]. In the case of Australia, people born in sub-Saharan Africa and North and Southeast Asia have some of the highest rates of HIV diagnoses by region of birth and are overrepresented in late or advanced presentation of HIV infection [11]. It has been suggested that a range of risk factors have contributed to the higher number of HIV cases from these two regions, such as: low levels of HIV literacy; high rates of undiagnosed and therefore untreated HIV infections; significant levels of stigma attached to HIV which prevents people from being tested, treated, or from seeking information; and misconceptions that Australia is free from HIV [12].

Personal, interpersonal, social life, environmental, and cultural factors play important roles in influencing migrants' sexual health help-seeking behavior. Previous Australian research shows SEA and SSA face a range of challenges, such as the adaptation process, cultural and gender differences and norms, level of control over decision-making, lack of familiarity with the Australian health system, lack of English language proficiency and inequities in health service access, including to HIV testing [12]. Whilst not explored in this review, it is acknowledged that there are further barriers to accessing health services for undocumented migrants.

A better understanding of the facilitators and barriers faced by documented migrants from SSA and SEA in utilizing SRH services may inform the development of tailored and innovative health promotion strategies [13] and more comprehensive, appropriate, and accessible health services for migrants in high income countries. The aim of this systematic review is to explore, from the perspective of migrants, types of help-seeking behavior and the barriers and enabling factors that influence documented migrants in gaining access to SRH services and HIV testing in high income countries (such as Australia) with universal health coverage (UHC).

2. Methods

This systematic review was conducted according to the Preferred Reporting Items for Systematic Reviews and Meta-Analyses (PRISMA) guidelines [14]. It followed procedures previously used by other systematic reviews conducted by the research team [15–17]. The review was registered in the International Prospective Register of Systematic Reviews (PROSPERO) to ensure quality adherence, reporting and dissemination (registration number: CRD42015023330).

2.1. Search Strategy and Information Sources

A total of seven databases were searched: PsycINFO, MEDLINE, ProQuest, PubMed, Scopus, Global Health and Web of Science. Google Scholar was also used to verify the results of the database searches. Lastly, an examination of reference lists from the relevant studies was undertaken to assess whether database results were exhaustive.

Search terms included: (migrant*, immigra*, "sexual health", "reproductive health", "help-seeking behavio?r, "health seeking behavio?r"). All relevant variations, including Medical Subject Headings

(MeSH) [18] terms were used depending on database requirements and specifications (see Table 1). Searched fields were keywords, title, and abstract.

Table 1. Search terms and databases used in the systematic review.

Databases	PsycINFO, MEDLINE, ProQuest, PubMed, Scopus, Global Health and Web of Science.
Concept 1: Migrants	"Ethnic group*" OR "Culturally and Linguistically Diverse" OR "Non-English speaking" OR "Ethnic minority*" OR "Transient*" OR "migra*" OR "Immigra*" OR "International student*" OR "Migrant worker*" OR "Labour migra*" OR "Minority group*" OR "Asylum seeker" OR "Displaced people"
Concept 2: Sexual health	"Sexual behavio*" OR "Sexual risk behavio*" OR "Sexual practice*" OR "HIV infection*" OR "Sexually transmitted disease*" OR "Genital disease*" OR "Sexually transmitted infection*" OR "Unsafe sex" OR "Sex education" OR "sexual literacy" OR "sexual health" OR "reproductive health" OR STI OR STD OR HIV
Concept 4: Help-seeking	"Health seeking behavio?r" OR "Help-seeking behavio?r" OR "Health system" OR "Health care" OR "Health service accessibility" OR "Health service" OR "Health information" OR "Health education" OR "Social support" OR "Primary health care" OR "HIV testing"

This review considered qualitative or quantitative evidence from primary studies related to adult migrant sexual health help-seeking behavior in HIC. For the purposes of this study, HIC were those nominated by the World Bank as Organization for Economic Co-operation and Development (OECD) countries with Gross National Income (GNI) per capita above $12,236 [2]. Only articles with a focus on sexual health were included. Help-seeking behaviour was described as "the behaviour of actively seeking help" and included formal (e.g., from health professionals), informal (e.g., from friends and family) and self-help sources [19].This review was interested in studies of documented migrants, and studies that focused solely on undocumented migrants were not included. This was due to the fact that undocumented migrants experience unique barriers to accessing health services compared to documented migrants. Studies were incorporated if they included migrants from sub-Saharan African and Southeast Asian countries, aged above 18 years old, and residing in high income countries for more than 1 year. This review was interested in the migrant experience, and as such, articles on the perspectives of healthcare providers were not included.

The review included only studies conducted in countries that had Universal Health Coverage (UHC), such as Australia, Spain, the United Kingdom, Belgium, Scotland, the Republic of Ireland, and Sweden. Description of what UHC entails, who is entitled to UHC, and a definition of UHC, has been debated [20] and as such, there are discrepancies in its applications between countries for migrants. This review used as the definition of UHC a "health care system that provides healthcare and financial protection to more than 90% of the citizens of a particular country" [21]. Data from the Global Residence Index was used to determine countries with UHC [21]. From this list, only two HIC were without UHC—the United States of America and Saint Kitts and Nevis. It is acknowledged that UHC is often not extended to all migrants. For example, those on temporary visas (including international students and workers) in Australia are not eligible to Medicare (Australia's UHC system) [22]. Likewise, for those seeking asylum in Australia, health care is reported to have been below Australian standards, with long delays in accessing medical professionals [23]. Broader articles on help-seeking or reproductive health only were not included.

Only full text, peer-reviewed journal articles, published in English, between the years 2000–2017 were included in the review. Every study identified through the database searches was examined based on information in the abstract and title. The full text from relevant studies that met the inclusion criteria was then retrieved.

Title and abstract were screened by two reviewers for potential eligible articles. The results were then checked by another member of the team based on the inclusion and exclusion criteria. Forty-two articles were eligible. Quality appraisal was conducted by two reviewers using a checklist adapted from the Joanna Briggs series of assessment and review instruments [24] and the National Institute for Health and Care Excellence (NICE) Quality Appraisal Checklist [25]. Criteria considered in the quality appraisal checklist included: study population, methodology, outcomes and analysis. Meetings to discuss quality appraisal with the broader research team identified additional articles for exclusion based on the income of the host country, UHC status and migrant country of birth. Final judgment regarding the quality of selected studies was based on the overall assessment of the article, methods, and study objectives and their relevance. Studies that were excluded at this point ($n = 27$) included those without ethical approval or insufficient content on sexual health and HIV. A final 15 studies were included. Figure 1 shows the process of study selection.

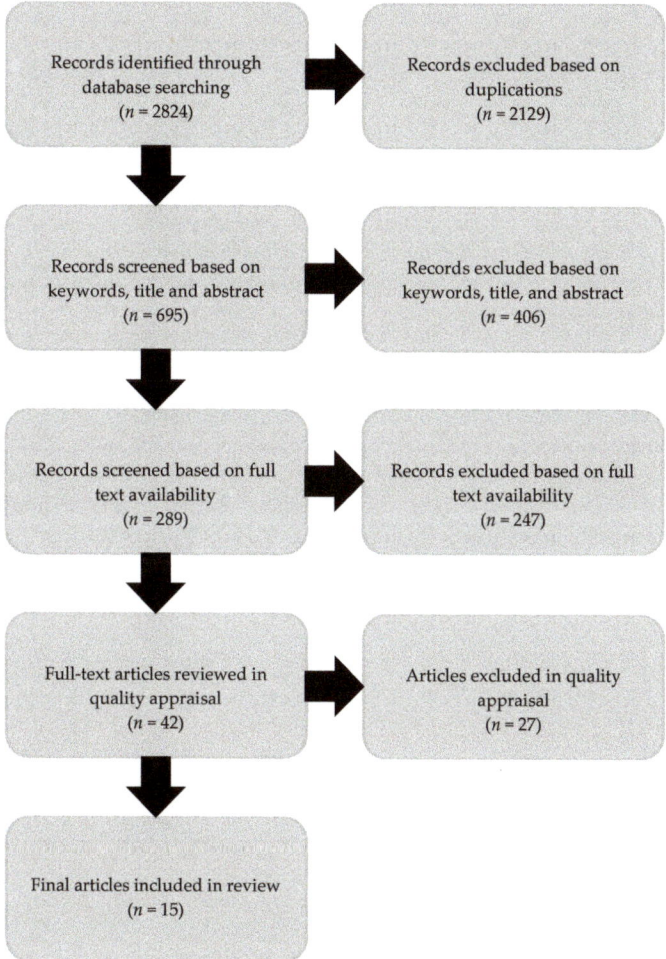

Figure 1. Flow diagram of review process.

2.2. Data Extraction

Two researchers independently performed data extraction on the selected articles using a standardized data extraction form [24]. The data extracted included author and title, research objective, study design, and key conclusions and recommendations. The final studies were classified into three broad areas: (1) Sources of sexual health help-seeking of migrants, (2) enabling factors for sexual health help-seeking behavior of migrants, and (3) barriers to sexual health help-seeking behavior of migrants.

3. Results

Fifteen studies met the inclusion criteria for the review (see Table 2). All selected studies included migrants from Southeast Asia and sub-Saharan African countries living in high income countries, specifically those with UHC. Of these 15 studies, seven were conducted in Australia [26–32]; two in the UK [33,34] and one study in Sweden [35], Ireland [36], Spain [37], Belgium [38], and Scotland respectively [39]. Of the 15 studies, eight studies examined migrants from sub-Saharan African countries [29,31,33,34,36,38–40]; two studies examined migrants from Southeast Asia countries [26,35]; and five studies explored migrants from mixed regions [27,28,30,32,37].

Twelve of the studies were qualitative [26,27,30–38,40]; and three were quantitative studies [28,29,39]. Of the 12 qualitative studies, six used focus group discussions [26,27,31,33,34,38], three used in-depth interviews [32,35–37], and three used a mix of focus group discussions and interviews [30,36,40]. Nine of the studies included both male and female participants [27,28,30,32–34,36,38,40], with the remaining six studies completed with female participants [26,29,31,35,37,39]. Three of the studies focused only on refugees [26,29,30], and four of the studies had a mean arrival to destination country of less than five years [27,29,35,36]. The studies varied in participant age with the majority including participants between 18 and 60 years. Two studies included participants aged 16 and over [30,39]. Two of the studies were conducted with people living with HIV [32,37]. All studies received ethics approval from a human research ethics committee [26–40].

Results have been reported on in the following domains:

- Sources of help-seeking—sources of information for sexual health and sources for treatment.
- Facilitating factors—social support and patient-healthcare provider relationship.
- Barriers—personal factors; interpersonal and cultural factors; cultural competency of healthcare provider; healthcare cost and location; confidentiality and relationship with healthcare provider.
- Study recommendations—policy, practice (clinical and health promotion) and research.

Table 2. General study characteristics, quality appraisal, and findings of fourteen studies addressing migrant sexual health help-seeking behavior in high income countries.

Title	Research Objective	Study Design	Conclusions/Recommendations
Adedimeji et al. (2015) [36] Increasing HIV testing among African immigrants in Ireland: Challenges and opportunities	To identify barriers for African migrants to access voluntary HIV testing, and to assess possible solutions to increase rates of HIV testing among this population.	• Setting: Ireland • Inclusion criteria/eligibility: Migrants from Africa, lived in Ireland more than 2 years and not previously diagnosed with HIV. • Sample: 60 participants—focus groups (n = 56), interviews (n = 4). Mean of 4.7 years since migrating to Ireland. • Age range: 18–64 years old • Gender: Male and female • Type of study: Qualitative; semi-structured interviews and focus groups • Recruitment: Convenience and snowball sampling • Ethical approval: Yes	**Conclusions:** • Barriers to HIV testing in African migrants in Ireland were found, including fear of consequences of an HIV diagnosis (residency status and social relations) and test affordability. **Recommendations:** • Involve stakeholders (immigrant group leaders, policy makers, health providers and religious leaders) in interventions to increase HIV testing to ensure cultural acceptability.
Agu et al. (2016) [27] Migrant sexual health help-seeking and experiences of stigmatization and discrimination in Perth, Western Australia: Exploring barriers and enablers	To explore barriers and enablers to sexual health help-seeking behaviors, and experiences of stigma and discrimination among migrants from sub-Saharan Africa and Southeast Asia living in Perth, Western Australia.	• Setting: Australia • Inclusion criteria/eligibility: Born in SEA or SSA, lived in Australia more than one year. • Sample: 45 participants—21 from SSA, 19 SEA, 5 from other regions. 35 (76%) of participants had arrived in Australia less than 5 years. • Age range: 18–50 years old • Gender: Male and female • Type of study: Qualitative; focus groups • Recruitment: Purposive and snowball sampling techniques. • Ethical approval: Yes	**Conclusions:** • Barriers and enablers to sexual help-seeking behaviors included sociocultural and religious influence, financial constraints and knowledge dissemination to reduce stigma. • Common experiences of stigma and discrimination (including in health care settings) and the social and self-isolation of people living with HIV. **Recommendations:** • Address stigma and discrimination in health care settings. • Provide culturally-appropriate sexual health knowledge that is group specific rather than targeted at migrants universally.
Akerman et al. (2017) [35] Healthcare-seeking behaviour in relation to sexual and reproductive health among Thai-born women in Sweden: a qualitative study	To explore sexual health help-seeking behaviors and views of HIV among Thai women living in Sweden.	• Setting: Sweden • Inclusion criteria/eligibility: Born in Thailand and living in Sweden less than five years • Sample: 19 participants • Age range: 24–50 years old • Gender: Female • Type of study: Qualitative; in-depth, semi-structured interviews • Recruitment: Purposive sampling • Ethical approval: Yes	**Conclusions:** • Low sexual and reproductive health care use and low uptake of HIV testing. Women expressed low perception of risk to HIV. • Barriers to healthcare included: language difficulties and low knowledge about the healthcare system. This resulted in a dependence on partners to access health services, or a preference to seek medical help in Thailand. **Recommendations:** • Offer HIV testing as part of cervical cancer screening. • Offer free health examinations to Thai migrants.

Table 2. *Cont.*

Title	Research Objective	Study Design	Conclusions/Recommendations
Drummond et al. (2011) [29] Barriers to accessing health care services for West African refugee women living in Western Australia	To examine barriers in accessing and utilizing health services of West African women refugees compared to Australian women.	• **Setting:** Australia • **Inclusion criteria/eligibility:** Refugee women from Liberia or Sierra Leone • **Sample:** 51 women from Liberia or Sierra Leone and 100 Australian women (comparison). Women were newly arrived (less than 5 years) and had lived in refugee camps up to 10 years before resettlement. • **Age range:** 20–67 years (West African), 18–90 years (Australian) • **Gender:** Female • **Type of study:** Quantitative; comparison study • **Recruitment:** Snowball sampling • **Ethical approval:** Yes	**Conclusions:** • Barriers to accessing health care were negatively correlated with longer residence and higher education • Emotional factors and service provider perceptions were major barriers to access healthcare services. **Recommendation:** • Implement intensive health promotion campaigns through social networks and ethnic media.
Dune et al. (2017) [28] Culture Clash? Investigating constructions of sexual and reproductive health from the perspective of 1.5 generation migrants in Australia using Q methodology	To investigate the role of culture in constructions of sexual and reproductive health and health care seeking behavior from the perspective of 1.5 generation migrants	• **Setting:** Australia • **Inclusion criteria/eligibility:** Not described • **Sample:** 42 participants with majority from SSA (43%) and SEA/EA (29%). Other regions included: Europe, Middle East and the Americans. 43% had arrived in the last 10 years. • **Age range:** 18–39 years • **Gender:** Male and female • **Type of study:** Quantitative; Q methodology • **Recruitment:** Purposive; flyers posted at relevant venues • **Ethical approval:** Yes	**Conclusions:** • Some migrants' constructs of sexual and reproductive health changed when in a new culture; others had difficulty integrating new cultural values. • Culture may be more easily adapted as many aspects of home (e.g., political, economically, etc.) do not exist in new country. Religion is portable, and may be the reason for an experience of 'culture clash' for some migrants.
Guionnet et al. (2014) [37] Immigrant women living with HIV in Spain: A qualitative approach to encourage medical follow-up	To examine the facilitators and barriers to medical follow-up among immigrant women living in Spain	• **Setting:** Spain • **Inclusion criteria/eligibility:** Women living with HIV; born in Spain, SSA or Latin America • **Sample:** 26 participants—10 from SSA, 8 from Latin America, and 8 from Spain. • **Age range:** 25–55 years old • **Gender:** Female • **Type of study:** Qualitative; semi-structured interviews • **Recruitment:** Purposive sampling • **Ethical approval:** Yes	**Conclusions:** • Barriers for immigrant women living with HIV in continuing treatment included cultural, social, and gender roles, relationship with the healthcare system, and self-perception. **Recommendations:** • Health professionals to work to identify and overcome barriers faced by patients in adhering to treatment

Table 2. Cont.

Title	Research Objective	Study Design	Conclusions/Recommendations
Korner (2007) [32] 'If I Had My Residency I Wouldn't Worry': Negotiating Migration and HIV in Sydney, Australia	To describe the interrelationships between migration and resettlement, the Australian immigration system and living with HIV.	• **Setting:** Australia • **Inclusion criteria/eligibility:** People living with HIV, born in a non-English country, or speaking a language other than English at home • **Sample:** 29 participants—16 (55%) in Asia, remainder from South America and Southern Europe; 11 (38%) were permanent residents, 12 (43%) had been in Australia longer than 10 years. • **Age range:** 29 to 58 years • **Gender:** Male and female • **Type of study:** Qualitative; interviews • **Recruitment:** Purposive sampling via a non-government organisation and a sexual health clinic • **Ethical approval:** Yes	**Conclusions:** • Main issue faced by migrants living with HIV was migration • Uncertain immigration status can be a barrier to treatment, health care and support. **Recommendations:** • Reduce barriers to accessing health services, including reviewing the practice of rejecting permanent residency applications of people living with HIV • Address HIV-related stigma in migrant communities
Lindkvist et al. (2015) [40] Fogging the issue of HIV—Barriers for HIV testing in a migrated population from Ethiopia and Eritrea	To identify barriers faced by Eritrean and Ethiopian migrants in Stockholm, Sweden for HIV testing.	• **Setting:** Sweden • **Inclusion criteria/eligibility:** Born in Ethiopia or Eritrea • **Sample:** 28 participants; focus groups (n = 21), interviews (n = 7). Arrival in Sweden ranged from 2 to 25 years. • **Age range:** Age not reported • **Gender:** Male and female • **Type of study:** Qualitative; focus groups and interviews • **Recruitment:** Purposive sampling • **Ethical approval:** Yes	**Conclusions:** • Main barrier was 'fogging the issue of HIV'—categorised as hiding the truth, living in denial and seeking help outside the healthcare system. This was due to distrust of the healthcare system and fearing the consequences of living with HIV. **Recommendation:** • Provide culturally appropriate information on HIV-related issues, in combination with offers of HIV testing early on arrival to Sweden.
Manirankunda et al. (2009) [38] "It's better not to know": Perceived barriers to HIV voluntary counselling and testing among sub-Saharan African migrants in Belgium	To examine the barriers, needs, and perceptions of HIV voluntary counselling and testing (VCT) among sub-Saharan African migrants in Belgium	• **Setting:** Belgium • **Inclusion criteria/eligibility:** Identified as SSA; English or French speaking. • **Sample:** 70 participants. Mean duration of stay 8.5 years. • **Age range:** 18–49 years • **Gender:** Male and female • **Type of study:** Qualitative; focus groups • **Recruitment:** Purposive sampling • **Ethical approval:** Yes	**Conclusions:** • Multiple barriers to VCT identified including: fear of dying of AIDS, fear of stigma or discrimination and low perceived risk of acquisition. **Recommendation:** • Implement VCT with pre- and post-test counselling, including via health services and via community outreach testing.

Table 2. *Cont.*

Title	Research Objective	Study Design	Conclusions/Recommendations
McMichael and Gifford (2009) [30] "It is Good to Know Now... Before it's Too Late": Promoting Sexual Health Literacy Amongst Resettled Young People With Refugee Backgrounds	To explore young refugees' accessibility to health information	• **Setting:** Australia • **Inclusion criteria/eligibility:** From refugee background. • **Sample:** 142 participants—interviews (n = 14), focus groups (n=128). Most participants were from Iraq, Afghanistan, Burma, Sudan, Liberia and the Horn of Africa. • **Age range:** 16–25 years • **Gender:** Male and female • **Type of study:** Qualitative; focus group discussions and interviews • **Recruitment:** Purposive sampling • **Ethical approval:** Yes	**Conclusions:** • Similar barriers were found to health service access as other young people • Experiences of forced migration, displacement, and resettlement brings additional challenges. **Recommendation:** • Improve accessibility of sexual health services to reduce poor sexual health outcomes and increase sexual health literacy.
Rogers and Earnest (2014) [31] A cross-generational study of contraception and reproductive health among Sudanese and Eritrean women in Brisbane, Australia	To assess knowledge and access to contraception and reproductive health of mothers and daughters from Sudanese and Eritrean backgrounds living in Brisbane	• **Setting:** Australia • **Inclusion criteria/eligibility:** Sudan or Eritrean women from refugee or migrant background • **Sample:** 13 participants—8 aged between 35–55 years, 5 aged 18–30. • **Age range:** 18–30 years, or 35–55 years • **Gender:** Female • **Type of study:** Qualitative; focus group discussions • **Recruitment:** Purposive and snowball sampling • **Ethical approval:** Yes	**Conclusions:** • A range of barriers found to health service access and contraceptive use included: lack of cultural competency and ineffective communication by health care workers; poor knowledge of health care system and intergenerational culture clash in relation to sexual health education in the home. **Recommendations:** • Provide sexual health information for new migrants during process of resetting • Develop partnerships between health care professionals and CaLD communities • Provide translated health information and access to interpreters • Design culturally sensitive strategies for parents to communicate with their children about sexual health and enable parent-daughter transfer of health information.
Shangase and Egbe (2014) [33] Barriers to accessing HIV services for Black African communities in Cambridgeshire, the United Kingdom	To examine barriers faced by Black African communities to accessing HIV healthcare services.	• **Setting:** United Kingdom • **Inclusion criteria/eligibility:** From African communities. • **Sample:** 30 participants; most aged in their twenties and thirties • **Age range:** 21–65 years • **Gender:** Male and female • **Type of study:** Qualitative; focus group discussions • **Recruitment:** Purposive sampling • **Ethical approval:** Yes	**Conclusions:** • A range of barriers found including language, limited knowledge of HIV, preference for traditional medicines and lack of cultural diversity among health service workers. **Recommendations:** • Plan health services considering cultural diversity, including use of traditional medicine • Ensure HIV workforce undertakes cultural competency training, and is culturally diverse.

Table 2. Cont.

Title	Research Objective	Study Design	Conclusions/Recommendations
Thomas et al. (2010) [34] "If I cannot access services, then there is no reason for me to test": the impacts of health service charges on HIV testing and treatment amongst migrants in England	To examine the influence of England's government health policy on migrants' health seeking and HIV testing.	• **Setting:** United Kingdom • **Inclusion criteria/eligibility:** Living in the UK as a migrant • **Sample:** 70 participants from South Africa, Zimbabwe, and Zambia • **Age range:** Above 18 years • **Gender:** Male and female • **Type of study:** Qualitative; focus group discussions • **Recruitment:** Purposive sampling • **Ethical approval:** Yes	**Conclusions:** • Changes in policy resulted in difficulties in accessing healthcare services due to cost and difficultly registering. **Recommendations:** • Reverse the policy changes made • Provide clear information and guidelines to both migrants and health workers in regards to accessing free health services.
Yakubu et al. (2010) [39] Sexual health information and uptake of sexual health services by African women in Scotland: A pilot study	To identify sources of sexual health information sought by African women in Scotland.	• **Setting:** Scotland • **Inclusion criteria/eligibility:** Women from Africa • **Sample:** 96 survey respondents; 47% had lived in the UK less than 5 years. • **Age range:** 16–55 years old • **Gender:** Female • **Type of study:** Quantitative; cross-sectional survey • **Recruitment:** Purposive sampling • **Ethical approval:** Yes	**Conclusions:** • Poor knowledge of STIs and HIV and low uptake of sexual health services and regular screening. **Recommendation:** • Develop collaboration between African communities in Scotland with the sexual health services to develop better HIV prevention program.
Ussher et al. (2012) [26] Purity, privacy and procreation: Constructions and experiences of sexual and reproductive health in Assyrian and Karen women living in Australia	To assess experiences of Karen and Assyrian woman refugees in utilizing SRH services in Australia	• **Inclusion criteria/eligibility:** Women from Karen and Assyrian communities who arrived as refugees • **Setting:** Australia • **Sample:** 42 participants—28 (67%) from Karen communities. Karen participants had arrived on average 3.5 years ago. • **Age range:** 25–45 years • **Gender:** Female • **Type of study:** Qualitative; focus group discussions • **Recruitment:** Purposive sampling • **Ethical approval:** Yes	**Conclusions:** • Constructions and experiences of sexual health were closely tied to cultural, religious and gendered family views. **Recommendations:** • Further research to explore interaction of gender, culture and migration process in the construction of sexual health.

3.1. Sources of Sexual Health Help-Seeking

Of the 15 included studies, four studies reported findings on the sources of sexual health information sought by migrants from sub-Saharan African and Southeast Asian countries living in high-income countries [27,30,33,35,39].

Migrants used a range informational sources including health professionals, TV and radio, books and magazines, and friends and family. Generally, there was a preference for information to come from a professional source; however, this was not easily accessed [30,39]. For example, in a survey with African women in Scotland (n = 92), Yakubu et al., found that the majority of women received SH information from books and magazines (79%); TV/radio (76%); and friends and family (70%); and only around a third from a family doctor (35%) [39]. However, preferences on where to receive information were firstly from a doctor (57%), a sexual health clinic (46.6%) and TV/radio (39.7%), with only a small proportion wishing to receive information from family and friends (27%).

A study by McMichael and Gifford used focus groups and interviews to explore access to sources of sexual health information and services among young (16–25 years old) refugees in Australia (n = 142). They found a preference for participants to seek sexual health information from doctors, who were seen as having expertise and the ability to provide accurate information [30]. However, it was highlighted that the participants only sought help from a doctor in relation to symptoms of an STI, for contraception or for an unplanned pregnancy [30]. In addition, participants tended to discuss sexual health with their peers, however, they reflected that they could not rely on their friends' information because it was sometimes unreliable and incomplete. Participants found it difficult to seek SH information from their parents due to religious and cultural factors; fear of judgement; and dislike for responses that focused on warnings or personal responsibility [30].

In this study, media (including radio and TV) and written material (books and magazines) were common sources of information; however, young refugees suggested that some of these materials presented were uninteresting, or provided exaggerated or inconsistent information [30]. Instead, the study found preference for using the internet as a source of sexual health information, as users can remain anonymous [30].

In semi-structured interviews with Thai women in Sweden (n = 19), Akerman et al. found that most women would discuss sexual health information with their partner in the first instance [35]. In the case of contraceptives or other women's health issues (i.e., pregnancy), women would seek information from other women, including Thai friends, family, or their partner's family [35]. Women also used the internet before visiting their GP (accessed via their partners) [35].

A survey by Drummond et al. with newly arrived (less than 5 years) West African women in Australia (n = 51) found that most women would access a medical clinic (94%) or a hospital clinic (67%) if they thought they had a STI [29]. They were least likely to seek treatment from a religious leader (8%), self-help groups, family or friends or traditional healers (all 10%) [29].

3.2. Facilitators for Sexual Health Help-Seeking Behavior

Of the 15 studies, five studies described factors that facilitated migrants to access and utilize sexual health services [27,28,30,35,37]; however, these were often not the main research objective.

In some studies, participants described attending healthcare services if there was a physical symptom that they could not fix [30,35]. Social support was not only a source of information on SRH, but also supported help-seeking behavior [27,28,35,37]. In semi-structured interviews by Guionnet et al. with women living with HIV in Spain (n = 26), participants reflected that having the support of loved ones assisted them to adhere to treatment, process the information from their doctor and encouraged them to continue their treatment [37]. Likewise, positive relationships with their healthcare provider encouraged participants to attend appointments and adhere to treatment. Positive interaction included: the doctor being an expert on the issue, providing emotional support and translation of scientific terms to lay language [37]. A trustworthy relationship with healthcare providers was also found to facilitate access to sexual health services [30,37].

3.3. Barriers to Sexual Health Help-Seeking Behavior

Fourteen of the 15 studies highlighted factors that inhibited migrants from accessing health services in high income countries [27–36,38,40]. From these studies, the following barriers to accessing health care services were described.

3.3.1. Personal Factors

Studies indicated that many migrants from sub-Saharan African and Southeast Asian countries had inadequate information about the health system in destination countries and experienced difficulty navigating access, such as how to make appointments or knowing the necessary documents required [27,32,34,35,40]. Poor knowledge and understanding of primary healthcare also limited migrants' access [30,38]. In addition, many studies reported a lack of knowledge of available SRH services and their location [27,33,35,38].

3.3.2. Interpersonal and Cultural Factors

Eight of the 15 studies examined interpersonal factors preventing migrants from seeking help from health services [26,27,29,30,33,34,36,38]. Barriers cited by study participants were: feeling afraid of being judged by the health provider; feeling afraid and ashamed about what other people would think; and feeling embarrassed to discuss sexual health [26,27,29,30,36,40]. In a study by Drummond et al., participants who were asked about accessing services for an STI expressed concern about losing their job, being afraid of treatment and medication used, and were of the belief they could cope with the problem themselves [29].

In focus groups (n = 70 participants) by Manirankunda et al., sub-Saharan African migrants living in Belgium expressed HIV-related stigma, guilt and shame, which included a belief that people living with HIV were "*at fault*" for their diagnosis [38]. This type of stigma resulted in participants feeling that they were not at risk (as they had not engaged in 'bad' behavior) or avoiding testing due to fear of being diagnosed [38]. Additionally, in focus groups and interviews (n = 60 participants) by Adedimeji et al., sub-Saharan African participants living in Ireland expressed concern about the perception that HIV is only for "*people from Africa*", which created feelings of mistrust and suspicion among their own migrant communities [36]. Participants also reflected that HIV stigma was an issue, particularly among religious and community leaders. This resulted in gossip surrounding the HIV diagnosis of an individual, and in the individual feeling isolated and unsupported by their community. These experiences had a negative impact on people's willingness to test for HIV [36].

Likewise, there was a perception among participants in a number of studies that a sexual health issue (such as a pregnancy outside of marriage or a HIV diagnosis) would result in social isolation [26,38,40]. Guionnet et al. found that women living with HIV did not wish to disclose their status due to fear of being socially rejected, fear of being labelled as 'positive' or associated with negative stereotypes, and fear of hurting loved ones [37]. All women who did not disclose their status to a loved one stopped treatment [37]. In focus groups and interviews by Lindkvist with migrants from Ethiopia and Eritrea living in Sweden (n = 28), fear of being known to be living with HIV resulted in people not telling loved ones about their diagnosis and travelling to other cities for testing and treatment [40].

In a quantitative study using Q methodology (n = 42), Dune et al. found that for migrants living in Australia, perception by others influenced help-seeking behavior [28]. Lack of support for issues such as STIs and having sex outside of marriage made people reluctant to seek professional care or seek appropriate resources (i.e., condoms) [28,30,37,40]. Focus groups by Roger et al. with Sudanese and Eritrean mothers and daughters in Australia highlighted a lack of discussion around SRH topics in their communities, with sexual health considered taboo [31]. As a result, many women were hesitant to discuss sexual health with a healthcare provider and had difficultly using the correct terms for SRH [31]. This finding was similar across a number of other studies [26,27,30].

In focus groups with refugee women from Karen (*n* = 42) living in Australia, Ussher et al. found conflict between refugees' culture and beliefs and Australia's approach to sexual education [26]. While older women expressed concern that teaching young girls about sexual health would encourage sex outside marriage, they found it difficult to control access to movies featuring representations of sex, sexual health education at school and interaction with sexually active friends. For young women, the taboo nature of sexual health made them reluctant to seek information or access services regarding their sexual health.

For women from Thailand in the Åkerman et al. study, access to health services was delayed or avoided due to perceived dependence on their male partner [35]. The male partner was first consulted, before he would then arrange for his female partner to attend a health service. Likewise, in interviews with migrants living with HIV in Australia (*n* = 29) in a study by Korner et al., women also indicated dependence on their husband to arrange healthcare appointments [32].

In some studies, participants preferred the use of traditional medicines—either entirely, or in conjunction with prescribed medication [33,34,38]. Participants also reported self-medicating until they were "really" sick, before seeking professional treatment [34].

3.3.3. Cultural Competency of Healthcare Provider

Cultural competency issues were reported as barriers in eight studies [27,31–33,35–37]. As an example, in a study by Adedimeji et al., sub-Saharan African migrants living in Ireland expressed reluctance to seek healthcare due to perceived poor service from providers; with the perception that health providers were insensitive and arrogant [36]. This was instigated by a lack of appropriate interpreter services and a perception that providers believed *"everyone from Africa is living with HIV"*, resulting in perceived discrimination [36]. This was also a concern expressed in focus groups by Agu et al., with migrants from SSA and SEA in Australia (*n* = 45), with some participants believing they had been tested without giving consent [27]. Testing without consent was also the experience for some migrants diagnosed with HIV in Australia in the Korner et al. study, who indicated that they were not aware they had been tested when they found out their HIV diagnosis [32]. Experiences of discrimination in the destination country outside of healthcare services also limited willingness to seek professional services [27,33].

The cultural background of a service provider was an important factor in accessing health services [31,33]. In a study by Shangase and Egbe, focus group discussions with Africans living in the UK (*n* = 30) found that participants perceived a *"negative attitude"* from healthcare providers based on their ethnicity [33]. Migrants in some studies suggested that people outside their own culture would be unable to understand their specific needs and would not be in a position to help navigate them through the differences in culture [31,33]. Dune et al. found that participants reported a difference in the culture of their country of origin to Australia in relation to SRH. The study highlighted a belief among participants that healthcare providers were not equipped to deal with their unique needs [28]. Several studies also described the importance of the gender of the healthcare provider, with many women unwilling to discuss sexual health with a male [31,33].

Additionally, a number of studies identified that language was a barrier [30–33,35,37,40], in that either a provider would not use simple descriptions, or an appropriate interpreter was not available or offered. This resulted in confusion around diagnosis and treatment, including correct dosage [33]. In the Åkerman et al. study with Thai women living in Sweden, male partners were often their interpreter, although they also struggled with the language used in consultations [35]. Participants in this study also expressed a preference to seek healthcare in their country of origin, due to the barriers experienced in accessing their destination country's health system [35].

In a study by Lindkvist with migrants from Ethiopia and Eritrea living in Sweden, some participants described the misuse of interpreters [40]. Participants described being provided an interpreter without being consulted on whether they needed one which was experienced as an insult. Issues arose when interpreters had conflicting translations, or provided incomplete translation, which created further confusion [40].

3.3.4. Healthcare Cost and Location

Five of the 15 studies found that the cost of healthcare and location were factors that inhibited migrants from accessing health services [27,29,34,36,38].

Adedimeji et al. reported that the cost for GP-provided HIV testing, approximately 40–50 Euros, was the largest barrier to testing for participants [36]. Many participants self-identified as having a low-income, but were not eligible for a medical card (for low-cost health services) [36]. For those able to access government funded health services, there were long waiting times, which resulted in missed opportunities for early diagnosis and linkages to care [36]. Focus groups with sub-Saharan African migrants (n = 70) in England by Thomas et al., identified instances of individuals using false identities in order to access free health services [34].

Several studies also found that beyond the cost of consultation, there were other costs experienced by migrants in accessing healthcare [34,36]. These included contraception, pharmaceuticals, time off work, childcare and transport [36–38]. In the study by Thomas et al., participants reported importing medication from their country of origin due to the cheaper price [34]. Likewise, in a study by Korner et al., temporary residents living with HIV in Australia indicated they were unable to afford HIV treatment and instead imported treatment from their country of origin [32].

Location of health services was also highlighted as a factor inhibiting access to testing [36,37,40]. Adedimeji et al. reported that most participants were accustomed to seeking treatment from main hospitals, and were unaware there were several private HIV testing services in the capital city of Ireland (Dublin) [36]. The respondents of the study were opposed to accessing treatment in the hospitals due to perceived lack of privacy [36].

3.3.5. Confidentiality and Relationship with Healthcare Provider

Seven of 15 studies addressed the healthcare provider and patient relationship [27,28,30,32–34,36].

In a number of studies, participants expressed concern about the confidentiality of their consultation [27,30,31,36,37,40], with some preferring a person outside the community to conduct testing. Additionally, participants in some studies expressed concern about an HIV diagnosis reported to the government or immigration authorities, which they perceived would result in them being deported [27,32,34,36,38].

Negative relationships and previous negative experiences with healthcare providers also limited uptake of health services and testing [37].

3.4. Study Recommendations

Fourteen of the 15 studies made recommendations relating to policy, health promotion and clinical practice and research. Recommendations generally related to improvements in clinical practice or for interventions to increase education and access to services [27,29,33,36,37,39,41], such as outreach HIV testing, increased sexual health education, addressing HIV-related stigma, or cultural competency training of clinical staff. Recommendations for policy are generally related to cost of health services and promoting free services [34,35,40], or development of migration policies for people living with HIV [32]. Recommendations for research centered on the need for better understanding of the construction of health and sexual health among migrants and additional barriers to accessing sexual health services [26,28].

4. Discussion

There is an upward trend in the number of migrants moving to high income countries [42]. As a result, the number of health issues experienced by SSA and SEA migrants living in those countries has increased, including increases in STIs, HIV and other SRH problems. In many countries, there is concern about delayed access for SRH issues, particularly in relation to late diagnosis of HIV [43–45]. Despite these concerns, there are limited peer-reviewed studies assessing SSA and SEA migrant sexual health help seeking behavior in high income countries. This review explored sources of information on sexual health and the barriers and facilitators influencing SSA and SEA migrants to gain access to SH services and testing in high income countries. The review identified 15 peer-reviewed articles that met the inclusion criteria published between 2000 and 2017. The articles selected identified a range of barriers, and to a lesser extent, facilitators and sources of help-seeking across a number of levels.

4.1. Overview of Findings

Few articles described sources of help-seeking in this review. For most migrants, healthcare providers were often considered to be the preference for information on SRH [27,30,39]. However, issues relating to access to health services, or a reluctance to discuss sexual health topics, resulted in limited knowledge transfer from these 'trusted' sources [30,39]. Combined with low levels of access to trusted sources, several studies identified topics of sexual health as being taboo—particularly for young people who were unmarried [26,27,31]. This contributed to low levels of knowledge on sexual health (mainly on safe sex practices) [46]. Indeed, previous research in Australia has identified lower knowledge on a broad range of sexual health topics among SSA and SEA migrants [47–51]. Knowledge regarding transmission and the process of testing for HIV has been shown to increase rates of testing [52,53].

This review identified very few enabling factors to accessing SRH services for SSA and SEA migrants. For most studies, symptoms relating to an SRH issue were most often the motivator for seeking professional help, which is problematic in regards to STIs and BBVs that can be asymptomatic for a period of time, such as HIV. This is consistent with previous research which has identified a reluctance to seek professional help unless physical symptoms are present, for both sexual health issues and other physical and mental health issues [29,44,52,54].

Barriers to sexual health help seeking were commonly reported and were mostly consistent within this review. The main barriers identified included: low knowledge of healthcare system in the destination country and where to access SRH services; the taboo nature of SRH within communities and lack of perceived social support; lack of cultural competency within the healthcare system; the cost and location of healthcare and concerns of confidentiality [27–36,38].

In some studies, perceived shame and stigma relating to HIV and STIs limited uptake of health services, even when symptoms were apparent. Expectations of community isolation for issues such as HIV, STIs and unplanned pregnancy contributed to low levels of testing and interactions with healthcare providers [29,31]. In the case of HIV, there was a perception that HIV only happened to 'bad' people, which lowered individual perception of risk [55]. Previous studies have identified the important role that addressing stigma and increasing social support has in improving knowledge, safe sex behavior and improving sexual health service uptake [44,52,56–58].

For the most part, studies in this review identified a lack of responsiveness within health systems to address the needs of migrants as well as low levels of cultural competency among healthcare providers. Difficulties navigating the healthcare system, booking appointments and knowing how to link into health services were described in this review. Pathways to care are often quite different between origin and destination countries and migrants may bring expectations of health services to their new country [59,60]. The perceived culture regarding SRH between origin and destination country are often conflicted for migrants, with 'Western' countries suggested to be generally more liberal in their approach [28,59]. In some cases, a perceived invisibility of community within healthcare services limited uptake. Non-community members were perceived as being unable to help navigate cultural differences, creating difficulty in accessing services [33]. For some sub-Saharan African migrants, this was evidenced by preferences for traditional medication and expressed mistrust of 'Western' medicine [33]. In previous studies, general practitioners have identified gaps in their own knowledge and understanding of culture, which have negatively impacted on their delivery of care [61]. There is a need for health systems and providers to be able to understand and engage with cultural beliefs and practices, to better address the SH of migrants in their destination country [59,62].

In some studies, migrants perceived healthcare providers to be discriminatory or unable to address language barriers [30–33,35,37,40]. Sub-Saharan African migrants reported feeling 'targeted' by healthcare providers in relation to HIV, who were perceived as assuming *"everyone from Africa is living with HIV"* [36] and incidences of lack of consent to test for HIV were reported [27,32]. Additionally, where language was a barrier, studies identified the lack of interpreter services, and partners or other family members being used instead. In many cases, healthcare providers were criticized for using overly complicated or scientific terms, rather than lay language [30–33,35,37,40]. Previous research has identified healthcare providers as being integral to facilitating access to health services, and encouraging BBV and STI testing [62]. It is therefore critical that healthcare providers have the cultural competency to build positive, trusting relationships with migrant patients and have adequate resources (such as interpreters or bicultural workers) to support engagement and perceived cultural security [60,61,63].

4.2. Implications for Health Promotion, Clinical Practice, Policy and Research

This review highlighted a number of considerations for practice, policy and research. These implications are based on the results and recommendations made in the included studies, unless otherwise stated. These implications are broad, acknowledging that sub-Saharan Africa and Southeast Asian migrants are not homogenous and have a range of experiences that influence barriers and facilitators to help seeking. As recommended by a number of articles from this review, community involvement is critical in the uptake of strategies to improve access to sexual health services to address unique barriers [64,65].

4.2.1. Implications for Research

Studies discussed the differences in cultural beliefs and practices regarding health, preventative health and sexual health. A better working knowledge of communities' understanding of health and health behaviors is needed to tailor health services and health promotion interventions [44,66]. Future research should consider segmentation of migrant groups by country of birth, gender, age and other relevant factors to better identify and address specific issues for priority groups.

Many of the studies described barriers to health services, with very little discussion on the sources of or facilitators to help-seeking. Better understanding of what works and why is needed, with a focus on successful interventions in health promotion, service delivery and policy changes [36]. Research that focuses on the pathways of care for migrants in seeking help for sexual health issues will provide better working knowledge of experiences of testing and treatment [67].

4.2.2. Implications for Health Promotion Practice

A number of studies made recommendations regarding sexual education, including safe sex practices. All these studies stressed the importance of culturally appropriate material and delivery of information [27,36]. Indeed, there is need for health promotion interventions to consider the role of culture, sexuality, resettlement process, understanding of preventative health and gender norms in sexual health help-seeking [35,44,60,66]. Previous research with healthcare providers have also acknowledged the need for resources to extend beyond language, and to also consider cultural factors [68]. Points of education recommended included: school-based education [30], during the settlement process [31,35], and social and ethnic media and community events [58].

The role of community and social support was acknowledged in some studies [36]. Studies also highlighted a need for direct involvement of affected communities in the development of targeted prevention and testing programs [39]. Recommendations included involving community and religious leaders in delivery of sexual education and in addressing stigma and judgment associated with unplanned pregnancy, STIs and HIV within communities. Additionally, developing partnerships between communities, healthcare services and health promotion organisations may help develop trust and facilitate access to relevant services by migrants [31]. Diversifying opportunities to access sexual health services may also increase help-seeking behavior [69]. Community-based testing for HIV, STI and hepatitis B have been successful [70], particularly in conjunction with information sessions from healthcare providers [38].

4.2.3. Implications for Clinical Practice

Access to health services and cultural competency of services were the most cited barriers to help-seeking. As global migration continues to increase, there is a need for countries and health services to be more responsive to the needs of their culturally diverse populations. This should be considered in planning health services to ensure that pathways of care are clear and accessible, there is a diversity of staff (both ethnic group and gender), appropriate interpreters and bilingual workers are accessible when required, and staff have cultural competency training [27,33,60,63,66]. Sufficient time must also be available to explain confidentiality and privacy, health concepts, procedures and treatment options fully, and to listen to and discuss concerns regarding cultural practices and beliefs [33,36].

While not a focus of this review, other studies have cited low knowledge of priority populations for specific sexual health issues, such as HIV and hepatitis B, among healthcare providers [61,67]. Additional training, or systems to prompt sexual health discussions, may be a consideration [41]. However, identifying high risk populations may result in communities feeling 'targeted', or reify existing differences [36]. Accordingly, strategies to minimize this need to be considered with relevant communities.

4.2.4. Implications for Policy

Cost and location were frequent barriers to accessing health services. Consequently, direct and indirect (i.e., transport, time off work, childcare etc.) costs of access need to be considered by governments in planning the delivery of health services [36]. Experiences of migrants not being eligible for low-cost health service within countries with universal health coverage, particularly in the case of the UK [34], questions whether UHC is accessible for all people within a country [20]. In other cases, where migrants are able to access UHC, issues may pertain to the location of free health services, difficultly in applying for low-cost health care, differences in gender norms in relation to sexual behavior and help-seeking decision making, experiences of stigma and discrimination or lack of clear pathways of care [44,60,66]. Relevant issues need to be identified for specific populations of migrants to encourage uptake of services.

In many of these studies, documented migrants expressed concern regarding deportation, particularly in relation to HIV. Implications of an HIV diagnosis need to be made clearer in cases of mandatory testing (such as in Australia) [27], to avoid creating additional barriers to healthcare access [32].

4.3. Study Design and Reporting Strengths and Limitations

Most studies indicated methodological limitations of the research. Limitations that were frequently reported in included studies were: lack of interpreter or translated material and subsequent exclusion of those who did not speak the destination country language/s; convenience sampling (participants were often those connected to a non-government organisation working in sexual health) and social desirability bias. In some instances, studies provided little detail about country of birth, age range and other sociodemographic details, as well as legal status in host country. Most studies recruited participants from multiple countries of birth, had large age ranges and included both male and female participants, with subsequent reporting of very broad, common issues and experiences. Very few studies provided more specific detail for particular groups. Poor understanding of variations between cultures can result in incorrect assumptions about migrant health needs and subsequent low health service utilisation. Positively, all included studies sought ethical approval.

The majority of studies ($n = 12$) reported were qualitative. As such, the association between barriers and facilitators and help-seeking outcomes were not able to be assessed. However, the qualitative nature of these studies does provide further insight into the facilitators and barriers and provided greater detail and context regarding migrants' experiences. Most studies provided detail about the methodological and theoretical framework and analysis process; however, some were limited in their reporting against best-practice reporting criteria.

Quantitative studies acknowledged the limitation of small sample sizes, with all studies recruiting less than 100 participants, and two studies less than 50. These studies focused on constructs and attitudes towards sexual health help-seeking but did not report on behavior or other help-seeking outcomes.

4.4. Strengths and Limitations of the Systematic Review

This systematic review is the first known study to assess sub-Saharan African and Southeast Asian migrants' sexual health help seeking in high-income countries in relation to sources of help-seeking, facilitators and barriers. The use of seven databases and multiple search terms across 17 years of peer-review literature provided a broad scope of studies. Inclusion of both quantitative and qualitative studies provided both descriptive data alongside participants' lived experiences and the context of these experiences. Multiple researchers reviewed database search results and assessed the quality of the studies for inclusion to reduce error. The review was registered with the PROSPERO International Prospective Register of Systematic Reviews. While the studies had different research questions, many of the barriers described in this review were consistent.

The limitations of this systematic review were that it included only peer-reviewed studies and those published in English. The exclusion of grey literature in this review may have limited the results, which has implications for external validity. Additionally, only articles published in English were included due to limited resources, which may have narrowed the scope of this review. It is likely that studies in other languages may have provided valuable contributions. No meta-analysis was conducted due to the heterogeneity of the included studies.

The SR only focused on high-income countries that have a universal health care system, therefore the results may not be transferable to countries such as the USA. The selected studies focused only on migrants with legal status in their destination country and there may be additional barriers for undocumented migrants. Future reviews could look at the barriers specific to undocumented migrants, as these are unique factors not relevant to documented migrants. The results of this review were context specific and are unlikely to be transferable to all sub-Saharan African and Southeast Asian migrant populations residing in high-income countries, though the findings may be valuable for a number of countries and provide broad insights and recommendations for research, policy and practice. Many of the studies included focused on barriers to health service access, making it difficult to comment on sources of help-seeking and facilitators.

This review was only interested in migrants' perspectives. It is acknowledged that studies on healthcare provider perspectives contain a rich range of information, which is not described here. Further work is planned to review this.

5. Conclusions

Growth in global migration has seen increases in the acquisition of STIs and BBVs amongst migrants. For migrants travelling to high-income countries from countries in regions of higher HIV prevalence, a range of factors may increase vulnerability for HIV acquisition. This study found barriers to access included: stigma relating to STIs and BBVs, direct and indirect cost associated with access, difficulty navigating health systems in destination country and lack of cultural competency within health services. Very few studies described sources of sexual health help-seeking or facilitators to help-seeking.

Early diagnosis of STIs and BBVs is crucial to prevent onwards transmission and reduce the burden of associated healthcare. Accordingly, a better understanding is required of the structural drivers of inequality including culture and gender along with targeted, resourced and evidence-informed strategies to address these barriers.

Author Contributions: D.A.R. served as the primary author performing initial database searches and drafting the initial manuscript. G.C. and R.L. were the research supervisors conceptualizing research questions, assisting with database searching and quality appraisal, and providing critical feedback and editing of the manuscript. C.G. undertook updated searches and final article selection for inclusion in the study, drafted components of the manuscript and is the corresponding author. G.B. provided guidance on the research process and critical feedback and editing on the manuscript. All authors read and approved the final manuscript for submission.

Acknowledgments: The author would like to express appreciation to Diana Blackwood (Curtin Health Sciences Librarian) for her valuable feedback during consultation about search terms and databases. We would like to thank Yoshua Tanto for his support with database searching.

Conflicts of Interest: The authors declare no conflict of interest.

References

1. United Nations. *International Migration Report 2017 (ST/ESA/SER.A/403)*; United Nations: New York, NY, USA, 2017.
2. The World Bank. World Bank Country and Lending Groups. Available online: https://datahelpdesk.worldbank.org/knowledgebase/articles/906519#East_Asia_and_Pacific (accessed on 21 June 2018).
3. International Organization for Migration: Country Office for Belgium and Luxembourg. Key Migration Terms. Available online: http://belgium.iom.int/key-migration-terms%E2%80%8B (accessed on 15 June 2018).
4. Australian Bureau of Statistics. Overseas Born Aussies Hit a 120 Year Peak. Available online: http://abs.gov.au/ausstats/abs@.nsf/latestProducts/3412.0Media%20Release12013-14 (accessed on 5 May 2015).
5. Abraído-Lanza, A.F.; Armbrister, A.N.; Flórez, K.R.; Aguirre, A.N. Toward a theory-driven model of acculturation in Public Health Research. *Am. J. Public Health* **2006**, *96*, 1342–1346. [CrossRef] [PubMed]
6. Du, H.; Li, X. Acculturation and HIV-related sexual behaviours among international migrants: A systematic review and meta-analysis. *Health Psychol. Rev.* **2015**, *9*, 103–122. [CrossRef] [PubMed]
7. Magaña, C.G.; Hovey, J.D. Psychosocial stressors associated with Mexican migrant farmworkers in the midwest United States. *J. Immigr. Health* **2003**, *5*, 75–86. [CrossRef] [PubMed]
8. Norredam, M.; Nielsen, S.S.; Krasnik, A. Migrants' utilization of somatic healthcare services in Europe: A systematic review. *Eur. J. Public Health* **2010**, *20*, 555–563. [CrossRef] [PubMed]
9. Rademakers, J.; Mouthaan, I.; De Neef, M. Diversity in sexual health: Problems and dilemmas. *Eur. J. Contracept. Reprod. Healthc.* **2005**, *10*, 207–211. [CrossRef] [PubMed]
10. Fakoya, I.; Alvarez-del Arco, D.; Woode-Owusu, M.; Monge, S.; Rivero-Montesdeoca, Y.; Delpech, V.; Rice, B.; Noori, T.; Pharris, A.; Amato-Gauci, A.; et al. A systematic review of post-migration acquisition of HIV among migrants from countries with generalised HIV epidemics living in Europe: Implications for effectively managing HIV prevention programmes and policy. *BMC Public Health* **2015**, *15*, 561. [CrossRef] [PubMed]
11. The Kirby Institute. *HIV, Viral Hepatitis and Sexually Transmissible Infections in Australia: Annual Surveillance Report 2015*; The Kirby Institute, UNSW: Sydney, Australia, 2015.
12. Guy, R.J.; McDonald, A.M.; Bartlett, M.J.; Murray, J.C.; Giele, C.M.; Davey, T.M.; Appuhamy, R.D.; Knibbs, P.; Coleman, D.; Hellard, M.E. HIV diagnoses in Australia: Diverging epidemics within a low-prevalence country. *Med. J. Aust.* **2007**, *187*, 437. [PubMed]
13. Gama, A.; Fraga, S.; Dias, S. Impact of socio-demographic factors on HIV testing among African immigrants in Portugal. *J. Immigr. Minor. Health* **2010**, *12*, 841–846. [CrossRef] [PubMed]
14. Moher, D.; Liberati, A.; Tetzlaff, J.; Altman, D.G.; Group, P. Preferred reporting items for systematic reviews and meta-analyses: The PRISMA statement. *PLoS Med.* **2009**, *6*, e1000097. [CrossRef] [PubMed]
15. Leavy, J.E.; Crawford, G.; Leaversuch, F.; Nimmo, L.; McCausland, K.; Jancey, J. A Review of Drowning Prevention Interventions for Children and Young People in High, Low and Middle Income Countries. *J. Commun. Health* **2016**, *41*, 424–441. [CrossRef] [PubMed]

16. Leavy, J.E.; Crawford, G.; Portsmouth, L.; Jancey, J.; Leaversuch, F.; Nimmo, L.; Hunt, K. Recreational drowning prevention interventions for adults, 1990–2012: A review. *J. Commun. Health* **2015**, *40*, 725–735. [CrossRef] [PubMed]
17. Crawford, G.; Lobo, R.; Brown, G.; Macri, C.; Smith, H.; Maycock, B. HIV, Other Blood-Borne Viruses and Sexually Transmitted Infections amongst Expatriates and Travellers to Low-and Middle-Income Countries: A Systematic Review. *Int. J. Environ. Res. Public Health* **2016**, *13*, 1249. [CrossRef] [PubMed]
18. Segen's Medical Dictionary. Medical Subject Headings. In *The Free Dictionary*; Farlex: Huntingdon Valley, PA, USA, 2012.
19. Rickwood, D.; Deane, F.P.; Wilson, C.J.; Ciarrochi, J. Young people's help-seeking for mental health problems. *Aust. e-J. Adv. Ment. Health* **2005**, *4*, 218–251. [CrossRef]
20. O'Connell, T.; Rasanathan, K.; Chopra, M. What does universal health coverage mean? *Lancet* **2014**, *383*, 277–279. [CrossRef]
21. Global Residence Index. The 2018 STC Health Index. Available online: http://globalresidenceindex.com/hnwi-index/health-index/ (accessed on 11 June 2018).
22. Australian Government Department of Home Affairs. Health Insurance. Available online: https://www.homeaffairs.gov.au/trav/stud/more/health-insurance (accessed on 18 June 2018).
23. Sanggaran, J.-P.; Haire, B.; Zion, D. The health care consequences of Australian immigration policies. *PLoS Med.* **2016**, *13*, e1001960. [CrossRef] [PubMed]
24. Joanna Briggs Institute. *Joanna Briggs Institute Reviewers' Manual*; The Joanna Briggs Institute: Adelaide, Australia, 2014.
25. National Institute for Clinical Excellence. *Methods for the Development of NICE Public Health Guidance*; NICE: London, UK, 2006.
26. Ussher, J.M.; Rhyder-Obid, M.; Perz, J.; Rae, M.; Wong, T.W.; Newman, P. Purity, privacy and procreation: Constructions and experiences of sexual and reproductive health in Assyrian and Karen women living in Australia. *Sex. Cult. Interdiscip. Q.* **2012**, *16*, 467–485. [CrossRef]
27. Agu, J.; Lobo, R.; Crawford, G.; Chigwada, B. Migrant Sexual Health Help-Seeking and Experiences of Stigmatization and Discrimination in Perth, Western Australia: Exploring Barriers and Enablers. *Int. J. Environ. Res. Public Health* **2016**, *13*, 485. [CrossRef] [PubMed]
28. Dune, T.; Perz, J.; Mengesha, Z.; Ayika, D. Culture Clash? Investigating constructions of sexual and reproductive health from the perspective of 1.5 generation migrants in Australia using Q methodology. *Reprod. Health* **2017**, *14*, 50. [CrossRef] [PubMed]
29. Drummond, P.D.; Mizan, A.; Brocx, K.; Wright, B. Barriers to accessing health care services for West African refugee women living in Western Australia. *Health Care Women Int.* **2011**, *32*, 206–224. [CrossRef] [PubMed]
30. McMichael, C.; Gifford, S. "It is good to know now...before it's too late": Promoting sexual health literacy amongst resettled young people with refugee backgrounds. *Sex. Cult. Interdiscip. Q.* **2009**, *13*, 218–236. [CrossRef]
31. Rogers, C.; Earnest, J. A cross-generational study of contraception and reproductive health among Sudanese and Eritrean women in Brisbane, Australia. *Health Care Women Int.* **2014**, *35*, 334–356. [CrossRef] [PubMed]
32. Korner, H. 'If I had my residency I wouldn't worry': Negotiating migration and HIV in Sydney, Australia. *Ethn. Health* **2007**, *12*, 205–225. [CrossRef] [PubMed]
33. Shangase, P.; Egbe, C.O. Barriers to Accessing HIV Services for Black African Communities in Cambridgeshire, the United Kingdom. *J. Commun. Health* **2014**, *40*, 20–26. [CrossRef] [PubMed]
34. Thomas, F.; Aggleton, P.; Anderson, J. "If I cannot access services, then there is no reason for me to test": The impacts of health service charges on HIV testing and treatment amongst migrants in England. *AIDS Care* **2010**, *22*, 526–531. [CrossRef] [PubMed]
35. Åkerman, E.; Essén, B.; Westerling, R.; Larsson, E. Healthcare-seeking behaviour in relation to sexual and reproductive health among Thai-born women in Sweden: A qualitative study. *Cult. Health Sex.* **2017**, *19*, 194–207. [CrossRef] [PubMed]
36. Adedimeji, A.A.; Asibon, A.; O'Connor, G.; Carson, R.; Cowan, E.; McKinley, P.; Leider, J.; Mallon, P.; Calderon, Y. Increasing HIV testing among African immigrants in ireland: Challenges and opportunities. *J. Immigr. Minor. Health* **2015**, *17*, 89–95. [CrossRef] [PubMed]

37. Guionnet, A.; Navaza, B.; Pizarro de la Fuente, B.; Perez-Elias, M.J.; Dronda, F.; Lopez-Velez, R.; Perez-Molina, J.A. Immigrant women living with HIV in Spain: A qualitative approach to encourage medical follow-up. *BMC Public Health* **2014**, *14*, 1115. [CrossRef] [PubMed]
38. Manirankunda, L.; Loos, J.; Alou, T.A.; Colebunders, R.; Nöstlinger, C. "It's better not to know": Perceived barriers to HIV voluntary counseling and testing among sub-Saharan African migrants in Belgium. *AIDS Educ. Prev.* **2009**, *21*, 582–593. [CrossRef] [PubMed]
39. Yakubu, B.D.; Simkhada, P.; Teijlingen, E.v.; Eboh, W. Sexual health information and uptake of sexual health services by African women in Scotland: A pilot study. *Int. J. Health Promot. Educ.* **2010**, *48*, 79–84. [CrossRef]
40. Lindkvist, P.; Johansson, E.; Hylander, I. Fogging the issue of HIV—Barriers for HIV testing in a migrated population from Ethiopia and Eritrea. *BMC Public Health* **2015**, *15*, 82. [CrossRef] [PubMed]
41. Manirankunda, L.; Loos, J.; Debackaere, P.; Nostlinger, C. "It is not easy": Challenges for provider-initiated HIV testing and counseling in Flanders, Belgium. *AIDS Educ. Prev.* **2012**, *24*, 456–468. [CrossRef] [PubMed]
42. United Nations. *Trends in International Migrant Stock: The 2008 Revision*; New York, NY, USA, 2009.
43. Kall, M.M.; Smith, R.D.; Delpech, V.C. Late HIV diagnosis in Europe: A call for increased testing and awareness among general practitioners. *Eur. J. Gen. Pract.* **2012**, *18*, 181–186. [CrossRef] [PubMed]
44. Korner, H. Late HIV diagnosis of people from culturally and linguistically diverse backgrounds in Sydney: The role of culture and community. *AIDS Care* **2007**, *19*, 168–178. [CrossRef] [PubMed]
45. The Kirby Institute. *HIV, Viral Hepatitis and Sexually Transmissible Infections in Australia, Annual Surveillance Report 2016*; The Kirby Institute, UNSW Sydney: Sydney, Australia, 2016.
46. Dean, J.; Mitchell, M.; Stewart, D.; Debattista, J. Intergenerational variation in sexual health attitudes and beliefs among Sudanese refugee communities in Australia. *Cult. Health Sex.* **2017**, *19*, 17–31. [CrossRef] [PubMed]
47. Dean, J.; Mitchell, M.; Stewart, D.; Debattista, J. Sexual health knowledge and behaviour of young Sudanese Queenslanders: A cross-sectional study. *Sex. Health* **2017**, *14*, 254–260. [CrossRef] [PubMed]
48. McGregor, S.; Mlambo, E.; Gunaratnam, P.; Wilson, D.; Guy, R. *HIV Knowledge, Risk Behaviour and Testing: A Community Survey in People From Culturally and Linguistically Diverse (CALD) Backgrounds in NSW, Australia*; The Kirby Institute UNSW Sydney: Sydney, Australia, 2017.
49. Song, A.; Richters, J.; Crawford, J.; Kippax, S. HIV and sexual health knowledge and sexual experience among Australian-born and overseas-born students in Sydney. *J. Adolesc. Health* **2005**, *37*, 243. [CrossRef] [PubMed]
50. Drummond, P.D.; Mizan, A.; Wright, B. HIV/AIDS knowledge and attitudes among West African immigrant women in Western Australia. *Sex. Health* **2008**, *5*, 251–259. [CrossRef] [PubMed]
51. Gray, C.; Crawford, G.; Reid, A.; Lobo, R. HIV knowledge and use of health services among people from South East Asia and sub-Saharan Africa living in Western Australia. *Health Promot. J. Aust.* **2018**. [CrossRef] [PubMed]
52. Blondell, S.J.; Kitter, B.; Griffin, M.P.; Durham, J. Barriers and Facilitators to HIV Testing in Migrants in High-Income Countries: A Systematic Review. *AIDS Behav.* **2015**, *19*, 2012–2024. [CrossRef] [PubMed]
53. Alvarez-del Arco, D.; Monge, S.; Azcoaga, A.; Rio, I.; Hernando, V.; Gonzalez, C.; Alejos, B.; Caro, A.M.; Perez-Cachafeiro, S.; Ramirez-Rubio, O. HIV testing and counselling for migrant populations living in high-income countries: A systematic review. *Eur. Public Health* **2013**, *26*, 1039–1045. [CrossRef] [PubMed]
54. Collaboration for Evidence Research and Impact in Public Health. *"I Want to Test but I'm Afraid": Barriers to HIV Testing among People Born in South East Asia and sub-Saharan Africa: Final Report*; Curtin University: Perth, Australia, 2018.
55. Bova, C.; Nnaji, C.; Woyah, A.; Duah, A. HIV Stigma, Testing Attitudes and Health Care Access Among African-Born Men Living in the United States. *J. Immigr. Minor. Health* **2016**, *18*, 187–193. [CrossRef] [PubMed]
56. Sutton, M.Y.; Parks, C.P. HIV/AIDS Prevention, Faith, and Spirituality among Black/African American and Latino Communities in the United States: Strengthening Scientific Faith-Based Efforts to Shift the Course of the Epidemic and Reduce HIV-Related Health Disparities. *J. Relig. Health* **2013**, *52*, 514–530. [CrossRef] [PubMed]
57. Hood, J.E.; Friedman, A.L. Unveiling the hidden epidemic: A review of stigma associated with sexually transmissible infections. *Sex. Health* **2011**, *8*, 159–170. [CrossRef] [PubMed]

58. Drummond, P.D.; Mizan, A.; Brocx, K.; Wright, B. Using peer education to increase sexual health knowledge among West African refugees in Western Australia. *Health Care Women Int.* **2011**, *32*, 190–205. [CrossRef] [PubMed]
59. Mengesha, Z.B.; Dune, T.; Perz, J. Culturally and linguistically diverse women's views and experiences of accessing sexual and reproductive health care in Australia: A systematic review. *Sex. Health* **2016**, *13*, 299–310. [CrossRef] [PubMed]
60. Mengesha, Z.B.; Perz, J.; Dune, T.; Ussher, J. Refugee and migrant women's engagement with sexual and reproductive health care in Australia: A socio-ecological analysis of health care professional perspectives. *PLoS ONE* **2017**, *12*, e0181421. [CrossRef] [PubMed]
61. Johnson, D.R.; Ziersch, A.M.; Burgess, T. I don't think general practice should be the front line: Experiences of general practitioners working with refugees in South Australia. *Aust. N. Z. Health Policy* **2008**, *5*, 20. [CrossRef] [PubMed]
62. Boateng, L.; Nicolaou, M.; Dijkshoorn, H.; Stronks, K.; Agyemang, C. An exploration of the enablers and barriers in access to the Dutch healthcare system among Ghanaians in Amsterdam. *BMC Health Serv. Res.* **2012**, *12*, 75. [CrossRef] [PubMed]
63. Sheikh-Mohammed, M.; MacIntyre, C.R.; Wood, N.J.; Leask, J.; Isaacs, D. Barriers to access to health care for newly resettled sub-Saharan refugees in Australia. *Med. J. Aust.* **2006**, *185*, 594–597. [PubMed]
64. Ogilvie, L.D.; Burgess-Pinto, E.; Caufield, C. Challenges and approaches to newcomer health research. *J. Transcult. Nurs.* **2008**, *19*, 64–73. [CrossRef] [PubMed]
65. Wilson, D.; Neville, S. Culturally safe research with vulnerable populations. *Contemp. Nurse* **2009**, *33*, 69–79. [CrossRef] [PubMed]
66. Henderson, S.; Kendall, E. Culturally and linguistically diverse peoples' knowledge of accessibility and utilisation of health services: Exploring the need for improvement in health service delivery. *Aust. J. Prim. Health* **2011**, *17*, 195–201. [CrossRef] [PubMed]
67. Burns, F.M.; Imrie, J.Y.; Nazroo, J.; Johnson, A.M.; Fenton, K.A. Why the(y) wait? Key informant understandings of factors contributing to late presentation and poor utilization of HIV health and social care services by African migrants in Britain. *AIDS Care* **2007**, *19*, 102–108. [CrossRef] [PubMed]
68. Botfield, J.R.; Newman, C.E.; Zwi, A.B. Drawing them in: Professional perspectives on the complexities of engaging 'culturally diverse' young people with sexual and reproductive health promotion and care in Sydney, Australia. *Cult. Health Sex.* **2017**, *19*, 438–452. [CrossRef] [PubMed]
69. Deblonde, J.; De Koker, P.; Hamers, F.F.; Fontaine, J.; Luchters, S.; Temmerman, M. Barriers to HIV testing in Europe: A systematic review. *Eur. J. Public Health* **2010**, *20*, 422–432. [CrossRef] [PubMed]
70. Driver, G.; Debattista, J.; Gu, Z.; Lemoire, J.; Hooper, J. HIV testing within the African community using home-based self collection of oral samples. *Aust. N. Z. J. Public Health* **2017**, *44*, 446. [CrossRef] [PubMed]

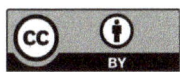

© 2018 by the authors. Licensee MDPI, Basel, Switzerland. This article is an open access article distributed under the terms and conditions of the Creative Commons Attribution (CC BY) license (http://creativecommons.org/licenses/by/4.0/).

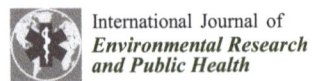

Article

Verbal and Non-Verbal Aggression in a Swiss University Emergency Room: A Descriptive Study

Dominic Kaeser [1], Rebekka Guerra [1], Osnat Keidar [1], Urs Lanz [2], Michael Moses [1], Christian Kobel [3], Aristomenis K. Exadaktylos [1] and Meret E. Ricklin [1,*]

1. Department of Emergency Medicine, Inselspital, University Hospital Bern, Freiburgstrasse, 3010 Bern, Switzerland; dominic.kaeser@gmail.com (D.K.); rebekkav@hotmail.com (R.G.); osnat.keidar@insel.ch (O.K.); drmikemoses@gmail.com (M.M.); aristomenis.exadaktylos@insel.ch (A.K.E.)
2. Security Service, Inselspital, University Hospital Bern, Freiburgstrasse, 3010 Bern, Switzerland; urs.lanz@insel.ch
3. Legal service, Inselspital, University Hospital Bern, Freiburgstrasse, 3010 Bern, Switzerland; christian.kobel@insel.ch
* Correspondence: meret.ricklin@gmail.com; Tel.: +41-31-632-2402

Received: 1 June 2018; Accepted: 4 July 2018; Published: 6 July 2018

Abstract: Workplace violence (WPV) by patients and visitors is a hazard in many emergency departments (ED), with serious consequences for both staff and patients. Patients with a migratory background seem to be prone to being involved in WPV. We therefore reviewed all reports of ED staff who experienced WPV over a 4-year period (2013–2016). We analyzed data on the reasons for the incident, the time of day, the manner of violence, the consequences, and the migratory background of the aggressor. In total, 83 cases of WPV were reported over a four-year period. The average age of the violent person was 33.1 years; in 35 cases (42.0%), aggressors were younger than 30 years old, 53 (63.8%) were male, 49 (59%) were of Swiss nationality, and 35–40% had a migratory background. The odds ratio of people originating from a low- to middle-income country versus those originating from a high-income country was 1.8. Furthermore, 45.8% of the patients arrived by ambulance ($n = 38$) and 19 patients (22.9%) were self-presenting. Most cases (92.8%) involved verbal aggression, but in more than half of the cases, physical assault (56.6%) was also reported. In addition, 43 (51.8%) of the events occurred during the night. Results also showed that 42 (50.6%) of patients who were involved in WPV were under the influence of alcohol and 29 (34.9%) suffered from psychiatric disorders. Security personnel and police were involved in 53 (63.9%) and 47 (56.6%) cases, respectively. Twenty patients (24.1%) were sedated and 16 (19.3%) were restrained. In 18 cases (21.7%), the psychiatrist ordered compulsory hospitalization in a psychiatric institution. Taken together, WPV is a relatively common event in our ED and persons with a migratory background are involved more often relative to their frequency of ED visits.

Keywords: aggression; emergency department; workplace violence; migrants

1. Introduction

Workplace violence (WPV) by patients and visitors is a reality in many emergency departments (ED) all over the world [1–9]. Previous studies have shown that in North America and Great Britain, 74% of doctors were victims of verbal abuse (VA) and 28% were victims of physical abuse (PA) over a one year period. Furthermore, 81% of nurses experienced VA and 26% experienced PA over a one month period [10–12]. Depending on the setting, rates of VA may be up to 100% within the last twelve months. However, published data about WPV in the ED setting reports very different crime rates depending on the setting and location [13–19].

WPV is not only a hazard to the ED staff, but also to other patients as it can disturb the departmental workflow and impact patient safety [20]. In addition, WPV can lead to personal consequences, such as stress, increased rates of missed workdays, burnout, job dissatisfaction, high consumption of alcohol or drugs, relationship breakdown, and post-traumatic stress disorder [11,13,21].

Various risk factors have been reported to contribute to WPV. These include patient-related risk factors, such as social, economic and cultural factors, male gender, alcohol intoxication, substance abuse, mental disorder, and language barrier that leads to frustration [20,22–24]. These factors are often found in migrants, especially those who originate from low- and middle-income countries [25]. With these reasons and the recent increase of patients with migratory backgrounds seeking ED assistance, as well as previous reports indicating that migrants are prone to be at higher risk for aggressive behavior [26], the aim of this study was to define the incidence of and characterize cases of WPV that were reported at the ED of a Swiss university hospital. Our data indicates that the investigated ED had a relatively low level of WPV with an increased odds-ratio of people originating from low- to middle-income countries to be involved in aggressive behavior.

2. Materials and Methods

This single centre retrospective study that was done in a Level one university hospital emergency department in Bern, the capital of Switzerland, used the report folder for "threat and aggression" where all reports were filed by ED staff who experienced and reported WPV. The study included all cases of WPV where the patient was 16 years or older.

After identifying the cases from January 2013 to December 2016 and cross-referencing the information with our clinical information system, we generated an anonymised data spreadsheet. The cases were analysed by patient criteria, such as age, gender, nationality, migratory background, main diagnosis, and reason for hospital admission. Furthermore, we analysed the incidence, the categorisation of PA, VA, threat, sexual harassment, stalking, damage to property, or theft, and the time of the aggression according to shift time (07:00–15:00; 15:00–23:00; 23:00–07:00). Necessary interventions were grouped by the involvement of police and/or security personnel, psychiatrist consultation, use of sedative medication, or restraint of the patient. Possible consequences included letters of complaint, expulsion from the hospital, refusal of future admissions to the hospital area, pressing charges against the patient, or compulsory hospitalisation in a psychiatric institution ordered by the psychiatrist. The cases were analysed by year in order to identify trends and developments.

According to the international organization for migration (IOM), a migrant is any person who is moving or has moved across an international border or within a State away from his/her habitual place of residence [27]. However, we used a different categorization. We calculated the odds and odds ratio for people of low- to middle-income countries versus high-income countries with a gross national income per capita of above $12,236 for 2018 using Microsoft Excel [28].

The study was performed according to Swiss law and consent of the cantonal ethic commission was given (KEK No. 390/15).

3. Results

The study center was an emergency department of a Swiss Level one university hospital with a catchment area of about 2 million people, which treats about 45,000 patients per year [29]. In the time period of the study, 159,388 patients were seen in total, with 13.7% of patients originating from low- to middle-income countries. A total of 84 cases of WPV were reported from January 2013 to December 2016. No cases were excluded. From January to December 2013, there were 4.5 cases of WPV per 10,000 patients who were treated in the ED, in 2014 there were 6.3 cases, in 2015 there were 4.9 cases, and in 2016 there were 4.3 cases per 10,000 patients.

The mean age of the aggressors was 33.1 years. In 53 cases (63.9%), the aggressor was male. Thirty-five (42.0%)—23 males and 12 females—were between 16 and 30 years of age (Table 1).

The gender of the perpetrator was not recorded in seven cases, nor was it possible to determine it properly. The same was true for the age of the perpetrator in six cases.

Table 1. Characteristics of the aggressor.

Characteristic	Total	16–20 AIY	21–30 AIY	31–40 AIY	41–50 AIY	51–60 AIY	>60 AIY
Male	50 (59.5)	6 (7.2)	18 (20.5)	11 (13.3)	5 (6.0)	3 (3.6)	7 (8.4)
Female	27 (32.1)	5 (6.0)	8 (8.4)	8 (9.6)	1 (1.2)	4 (4.8)	1 (1.2)
Unknown	7 (8.4)						
Nationality	Swiss	Western E	East E	African	Asian	Other/Unknown	
	50 (59.2)	9 (10.8)	8 (9.6)	3 (3.6)	4 (4.8)	10 (12)	
Country of Origin	L&M-IC	H-IC	Unknown				
	17	56	12				
Year	2013	2014	2015	2016	Total		
Total of WPV cases	17	25	22	20	84		
RR M	0.4	0.4	0.29	0.35	0.31		
Admission Self-admission Ambulance	Self-admission	Ambulance	Police	Psychiatrist	Physician	Other/Unknown	
	19 (22.9)	38 (45.9)	9 (10.8)	3 (3.6)	5 (6.0)	9 (10.8)	
Diagnosis	Psychiatric	Alcohol	Intox	Injury	Other	Unknown	
	29 (34.9)	42 (50.6)	11 (17.5)	12 (19.0)	18 (21.7)	6 (7.2)	

AIY: Age in years, N (%). Multiple diagnoses may be given. E. = Europe; L&M-IC: low- and middle-income country; H-IC: high-income country. Intoxications were not included under psychiatric diseases; alcohol intoxication was not included under intoxication. 7 were of unknown gender. RR of M = relative risk of persons with a migratory background to be involved in WPV.

Over the study period, WPV incidences were between 17 and 25 per year. And of these perpetrators, we observed a twofold increase between 2013 and 2016—from 7 to 14 cases. Most patients possessed a Swiss passport (49; 59.2%) or passports from other high-income countries (23; 31.9%). The percentage of patients with a migratory background with origins in a low- to middle-income country who were involved in WPV was 22%. In comparison to this, 22% of foreigners in total live in the Bern area [30]. Compared to high-income countries, patients from low- and middle-income countries had an elevated incidence of aggression with an odds ratio of 1.81.

Most patients were admitted to the hospital by ambulance (45.9%) or were self-presenting (22.9%), and nine (10.8%) were brought to the department by the police.

The most common main diagnosis on admission was intoxication with alcohol ($n = 42$) or other substances ($n = 11$). Next were mental disorders (34.9%) without additional intoxication. Most cases of mental disorders were suicidal ideation (26.1% of psychiatric patients), followed by schizophrenia (17.4% of psychiatric patients). Twelve (19.0%) aggressors were admitted to the ED due to injuries. Eighteen (21.7%) patients were treated for internal medical problems other than intoxication.

Most cases of WPV involved VA (92.8%); in half of the cases, PA (56.6%) was involved. In 24.1% of cases, there were threats against the ED staff, and five cases (6.0%) of property damage and two cases (2.4% of patients) of sexual harassment were also reported. In five cases, relatives were involved in WPV and in four cases, a weapon was present.

In total, 15 (18.1%) cases of WPV occurred between 07:00 and 15:00, 24 (28.9%) between 15:00 and 23:00, and 43 (51.8%) between 23:00 and 07:00 (Table 2).

Assistance by internal security personnel was necessary in 63.9% of cases and in 56.6% of cases, the police were involved. Psychiatrist consultation was requested in 34.9% of patients who were involved in WPV, in 24.1% sedative medication was requested, and in 19.3% of cases, fixation was deemed necessary.

More than half of the patients (53%) who were involved in WPV received a letter of complaint from the hospital. Six patients (7.2%) were told to leave the hospital area and 3 patients (3.6%) were banned from returning to the hospital area. In 21.7% of cases, a psychiatrist ordered compulsory hospitalisation in a psychiatric institution. This figure increased from zero in 2013 to ten in 2015 and dropped to five in 2016. In 9.6% of cases, charges were pressed against the patient, however it is unknown how often this led to a conviction. The charges included four PA and four with PA in combination with sexual harassment, damage of property, and threat. Nineteen (29%) patients who were involved in PA (55.8%) received a letter of complaint, charges were pressed against seven (20.6%), and in seven cases (9.5%), the aggression had no consequences.

Table 2. Case characteristics of WPV.

Characteristic	N (%)	N (%)	N (%)	N (%)	N (%)	N (%)
Time of incidents	07:00–15:00 15 (18.1)	15:00–23:00 24 (28.9)	23:00–07:00 43 (51.8)			
Type of aggression	Verbal 77 (92.8)	Physical 47 (56.6)	Sexual 2 (2.4)	Threat 20 (24.1)	Damage 5 (6)	
Intervention	Security 53 (63.9)	Police 47 (56.6)	Psychiatrist 29 (34.9)	Sedatives 20 (24.1)	Fixation 16 (19.3)	
Consequences	None 8 (9.6)	Expulsion 6 (7.2)	Refusal of admission 3 (3.6)	Letter of complaint 44 (53.0)	äFU 18 (21.7)	Charges pressed 8 (9.6)

äFU = compulsory hospitalization in a psychiatric institution; RR = relative risk of migrants to be involved in WPV.

4. Discussion

The aim of this study was to characterize the reported WPV over a 4-year period from January 2013 to December 2016 in the ED of a Swiss Level one university hospital and to describe the associated factors, necessary interventions, and the consequences of these incidents.

Even though the personnel anecdotally reported an increase in cases of WPV, actual reported cases did not increase over the last few years. However, numbers of reported cases were very low. It is not certain if the number of reported cases is a true image of the situation. It may be that awareness of WPV is increasing, but that the staff remain reluctant to accept the importance of reporting it. Most studies estimate that 50% to 75% of cases are unreported [31]. The principle barriers to reporting are fear of retaliation, absence of physical injury, fear of inconvenience from reporting WPV, or the potential effect on customer satisfaction; ED staff often think that it is an inherent part of the job [32].

It is easy to imagine the impact on staff and patients—especially if the large numbers of unreported cases are considered—to be similar to that in previous studies [13,19]. In the present study, we believe that there may be a high degree of underreporting, since only the most serious cases were reported—those with a major consequence to or significant impact on the affected person. This is shown by the fact that in 2014, only 4 of 25 cases were reported where there was no PA or threat involved and in nearly 60% of all cases, intervention by the police was necessary. Those cases are very severe. On one hand, the fact that these make up 60% of the reported cases indicates that only the top of the iceberg is being reported. On the other hand, it indicates that in the ED of this study, we have a selection bias of cases as small institutions do not need to accept to treat the agitated, intoxicated, and partially persons with a migratory background as this University ED does.

In other studies, stalking or theft were mentioned as further categories of WPV, but in our cases, no such incidences were identified [13].

Comparable to other studies, most patients were young and male [13]. The number of patients with a migratory background from low- to middle-income countries in WPV was stable, with 35 to 40%—what is about double of the foreign population living in the Bern region, which was 22% in 2016 [33]. In the same period, the frequency of asylum seekers attending the ED increased by 45% from 465 to 653 per year [29]. Unfortunately, in most of the studies that were published about WPV, no information about the migratory background of the aggressors can be found. However, a study by Knutzen et al. showed that the rate of the use of restraint in the emergency department was significantly higher in patients with an immigrant background, especially in younger age groups, and a Swedish study reported violence as one of the problems that nurses experienced by working with migrants in emergency care [30,34]. In our study, the data did not allow us to draw conclusions about the motive or reason of the patients for the violence. However, other studies show that factors like the potential language barrier, cultural differences, or differences in the health care system might lead to frustration and therefore to aggression [34–36]. To meet the need of this increasing population who are visiting the ED, our ED regularly trains the health care professionals on intercultural competence in health care by the Red Cross. Other methods for de-escalation are to address the psychological and emotional distress and the unmet needs of the people involved. Furthermore, skilled communication with no confrontation, trust-building, and negotiation are suggested to be good ways to manage critical situations and to avoid harm [37].

The risk factors for WPV that have been found in this study were the same as in prior studies [13]. These were mainly male gender, alcohol intoxication, substance abuse, and mental disorders. Apart from male gender, these are all factors that lead to scenarios where the patient may not be able to rationally interpret the situation and might feel threatened or fear for loss of dignity. The severity of the cases shown in this study and the fact that many cases involved more than one category of aggression show that patients who might not be capable of coping with these unusual circumstances use every possible action to defend themselves from what they see as a threat [20,22,23]. An additional risk factor in our population was admission to hospital by ambulance or police.

Because of the lack of available information, it was not possible to identify other risk factors, such as waiting time, pain, and surroundings, or to show the impact of WPV for ED staff, as for data protection reasons, we were not able to obtain the interviews of either the patients who were involved in the WPV or the staff. Another limitation of this single center study is the low caseload of WPV, despite the high amount of people who were seen. To shed more light on the situation, a better reporting system might be needed, and to describe the situation in Switzerland, a multicenter study might be helpful that includes all large EDs.

As reported before, nearly all cases of WPV included VA [13]. VA might be the starting point for the escalation of the situation and therefore, could be a point for the prevention of PA. A study from Fernandes et al. from 2002 showed that there was an initial decrease in violent events 3 months after violence reduction workshops. However, there was a slight increase by 6 months after the workshop—what was assumed to be a positive effect of the training that was extinguished over time—but this could possibly be regained with refresher courses [38]. For threat and sexual harassment, nearly half of the cases involved PA, and security personal and police were almost always involved. Most cases happened between 23:00–07:00, when fewer staff were present and the number of patients with alcohol intoxication was highest. Only 8 of 47 cases of PA happened between 07:00–15:00. Most cases where restraint was necessary occurred between 15:00–23:00 or 23:00–07:00. Hyland et al. analysed the cases of aggressive behaviour of the patients over a 12-month period in an Australian ED and found a similar trend, with 76.5% of cases of WPV from 17:00–08:00 [39]. These findings show that security personnel ought to be rapidly available at all times and especially during night shifts.

5. Conclusions

In this single center study, we described the 4-year incidence of WPV in a Swiss university hospital. Patients with a migratory background originating from low- or middle-income countries, compared to high-income countries, had an elevated prevalence of aggression with an odds ratio of 1.8 to show aggressive behavior. Other factors that could be related to aggression were male gender, alcohol intoxication, substance abuse, and mental disorders.

As only one tool of WPV reporting was available and the nurses mainly reported the events, we have to assume that substantial numbers of the cases were not reported. We recommend the introduction of a reporting platform where all ED staff, including security personnel, can rapidly and simply report WPV. Furthermore, it will be necessary to improve staff awareness of the importance of reporting cases of WPV. The number of cases and the time period in this study were relatively small. Future studies should include more cases in order to confirm and extend the findings and to assess the effect of preventive measures taken, such as staff training and access to intercultural translators.

Furthermore, we suggest qualitative studies in parallel to understand in detail the motivation of aggression and sequelae for the staff.

Author Contributions: Conceptualization, U.L., A.K.E. and M.E.R.; Formal Analysis, D.K. and R.G.; Investigation, C.K.; Methodology, U.L., C.K. and A.K.E.; Project Administration, M.E.R.; Validation, O.K.; Writing-Original Draft, D.K.; Writing-Review & Editing, R.G., O.K., M.M., A.K.E. and M.E.R.

Funding: This research received no external funding.

Conflicts of Interest: The authors declare no conflict of interest.

References

1. Tadros, A.; Kiefer, C. Violence in the emergency department: A global problem. *Psychiatr. Clin. N. Am.* **2017**, *40*, 575–584. [CrossRef] [PubMed]
2. Abdellah, R.F.; Salama, K.M. Prevalence and risk factors of workplace violence against health care workers in emergency department in Ismailia, Egypt. *Pan Afr. Med. J.* **2017**, *26*, 21. [CrossRef] [PubMed]
3. Han, C.Y.; Lin, C.C.; Barnard, A.; Hsiao, Y.C.; Goopy, S.; Chen, L.C. Workplace violence against emergency nurses in Taiwan: A phenomenographic study. *Nurs. Outlook* **2017**, *65*, 428–435. [CrossRef] [PubMed]
4. Bayram, B.; Cetin, M.; Colak Oray, N.; Can, I.O. Workplace violence against physicians in Turkey's emergency departments: A cross-sectional survey. *BMJ Open* **2017**, *7*, e013568. [CrossRef] [PubMed]
5. Shafran-Tikva, S.; Zelker, R.; Stern, Z.; Chinitz, D. Workplace violence in a tertiary care Israeli hospital—A systematic analysis of the types of violence, the perpetrators and hospital departments. *Isr. J. Health Policy Res.* **2017**, *6*, 43. [CrossRef] [PubMed]
6. Ramacciati, N.; Ceccagnoli, A.; Addey, B.; Rasero, L. Violence towards emergency nurses. The Italian national survey 2016: A qualitative study. *Int. J. Nurs. Stud.* **2018**, *81*, 21–29. [CrossRef] [PubMed]
7. Partridge, B.; Affleck, J. Verbal abuse and physical assault in the emergency department: Rates of violence, perceptions of safety, and attitudes towards security. *Australas. Emerg. Nurs. J.* **2017**, *20*, 139–145. [CrossRef] [PubMed]
8. Shi, L.; Zhang, D.; Zhou, C.; Yang, L.; Sun, T.; Hao, T.; Peng, X.; Gao, L.; Liu, W.; Mu, Y.; et al. A cross-sectional study on the prevalence and associated risk factors for workplace violence against Chinese nurses. *BMJ Open* **2017**, *7*, e013105. [CrossRef] [PubMed]
9. Rosenthal, L.J.; Byerly, A.; Taylor, A.D.; Martinovich, Z. Impact and prevalence of physical and verbal violence toward healthcare workers. *Psychosomatics* **2018**, in press. [CrossRef] [PubMed]
10. Hassankhani, H.; Parizad, N.; Gacki-Smith, J.; Rahmani, A.; Mohammadi, E. The consequences of violence against nurses working in the emergency department: A qualitative study. *Int. Emerg. Nurs.* **2018**, *39*, 20–25. [CrossRef] [PubMed]
11. Kowalenko, T.; Walters, B.L.; Khare, R.K.; Compton, S. Michigan College of Emergency Physicians Workplace Violence Task Force. Workplace violence: A survey of emergency physicians in the state of Michigan. *Ann. Emerg. Med.* **2005**, *46*, 142–147. [CrossRef] [PubMed]
12. Ryan, D.; Maguire, J. Aggression and violence—A problem in Irish accident and emergency departments? *J. Nurs. Manag.* **2006**, *14*, 106–115. [CrossRef] [PubMed]
13. Phillips, J.P. Workplace violence against health care workers in the United States. *N. Engl. J. Med.* **2016**, *374*, 1661–1669. [CrossRef] [PubMed]
14. Magnavita, N.; Heponiemi, T. Workplace violence against nursing students and nurses: An Italian experience. *J. Nurs. Scholarsh.* **2011**, *43*, 203–210. [CrossRef] [PubMed]
15. Lin, Y.H.; Liu, H.E. The impact of workplace violence on nurses in south taiwan. *Int. J. Nurs. Stud.* **2005**, *42*, 773–778. [CrossRef] [PubMed]
16. Kamchuchat, C.; Chongsuvivatwong, V.; Oncheunjit, S.; Yip, T.W.; Sangthong, R. Workplace violence directed at nursing staff at a general hospital in southern thailand. *J. Occup. Health* **2008**, *50*, 201–207. [CrossRef] [PubMed]
17. Hegney, D.; Eley, R.; Plank, A.; Buikstra, E.; Parker, V. Workplace violence in Queensland, Australia: The results of a comparative study. *Int. J. Nurs. Pract.* **2006**, *12*, 220–231. [CrossRef] [PubMed]
18. AbuAlRub, R.F.; Khalifa, M.F.; Habbib, M.B. Workplace violence among Iraqi hospital nurses. *J. Nurs. Scholarsh.* **2007**, *39*, 281–288. [CrossRef] [PubMed]

19. Chapman, R.; Perry, L.; Styles, I.; Combs, S. Consequences of workplace violence directed at nurses. *Br. J. Nurs.* **2009**, *18*, 1256–1261. [CrossRef] [PubMed]
20. Ray, M.M. The dark side of the job: Violence in the emergency department. *J. Emerg. Nurs.* **2007**, *33*, 257–261. [CrossRef] [PubMed]
21. Jackson, D.; Clare, J.; Mannix, J. Who would want to be a nurse? Violence in the workplace—A factor in recruitment and retention. *J. Nurs. Manag.* **2002**, *10*, 13–20. [CrossRef] [PubMed]
22. James, A.; Madeley, R.; Dove, A. Violence and aggression in the emergency department. *Emerg. Med. J.* **2006**, *23*, 431–434. [CrossRef] [PubMed]
23. Kerrison, S.A.; Chapman, R. What general emergency nurses want to know about mental health patients presenting to their emergency department. *Accid. Emerg. Nurs.* **2007**, *15*, 48–55. [CrossRef] [PubMed]
24. Holmes, D.; Rudge, T.; Perron, A. *(Re)thinking Violenc in Health Care Settings. A Critical Approach*; Routledge. Taylor and Francis Group: London, UK; New York, NY, USA, 2012.
25. McMahon, E.M.; Corcoran, P.; Keeley, H.; Cannon, M.; Carli, V.; Wasserman, C.; Sarchiapone, M.; Apter, A.; Balazs, J.; Banzer, R.; et al. Mental health difficulties and suicidal behaviours among young migrants: Multicentre study of European adolescents. *BJPsych Open* **2017**, *3*, 291–299. [CrossRef] [PubMed]
26. Graetz, V.; Rechel, B.; Groot, W.; Norredam, M.; Pavlova, M. Utilization of health care services by migrants in Europe—A systematic literature review. *Br. Med. Bull.* **2017**, *121*, 5–18. [CrossRef] [PubMed]
27. IOM. Iom Glossary on Migration. International Migration Law Series no. 25. Available online: Https://www.iom.int/key-migration-terms (accessed on 25 June 2018).
28. The Wolrd Bank. World Bank Country and Lending Groups. Available online: https://datahelpdesk.worldbank.org/knowledgebase/articles/906519-world-bank-country-and-lending-groups (accessed on 25 June 2018).
29. Muller, M.; Klingberg, K.; Srivastava, D.; Exadaktylos, A.K. Consultations by asylum seekers: Recent trends in the emergency department of a Swiss university hospital. *PLoS ONE* **2016**, *11*, e0155423. [CrossRef] [PubMed]
30. Knutzen, M.; Sandvik, L.; Hauff, E.; Opjordsmoen, S.; Friis, S. Association between patients' gender, age and immigrant background and use of restraint—A 2-year retrospective study at a department of emergency psychiatry. *Nord. J. Psychiatry* **2007**, *61*, 201–206. [CrossRef] [PubMed]
31. Emergency Nurses Association. *Emergency Department Violence Surveillance Study*; Institute for Emergency Nursing Research: Des Plaines, IL, USA, 2011.
32. Emergency Nurses Association. *Position Statement: Violence in the Emergency Care Setting*; Emergency Nurses Association: Des Plaines, IL, USA, 2014.
33. Swiss Federal Statistical Office. *Police Crime Statistics*; Swiss Federal Statistical Office: Neuchatel, Switzerland, 2016.
34. Ozolins, L.-L.; Hjelm, K. Nurses' experiences of problematic situations with migrants in emergency care in Sweden. *Clin. Eff. Nurs.* **2003**, *7*, 84–93. [CrossRef]
35. Priebe, S.; Sandhu, S.; Dias, S.; Gaddini, A.; Greacen, T.; Ioannidis, E.; Kluge, U.; Krasnik, A.; Lamkaddem, M.; Lorant, V.; et al. Good practice in health care for migrants: Views and experiences of care professionals in 16 European countries. *BMC Public Health* **2011**, *11*, 187. [CrossRef] [PubMed]
36. Segalowitz, N.; Ehayia, E. Exploring the determinants of language barriers in health care (LBHC): Toward a research agenda for the language sciences. *Can. Mod. Lang. Rev.* **2011**, *67*, 480–507. [CrossRef]
37. Harwood, R.H. How to deal with violent and aggressive patients in acute medical settings. *J. R. Coll. Physicians Edinb.* **2017**, *47*, 94–101. [CrossRef] [PubMed]
38. Fernandes, C.M.; Raboud, J.M.; Christenson, J.M.; Bouthillette, F.; Bullock, L.; Ouellet, L.; Moore, C.; Violoence in the Emergency Department Study, G. The effect of an education program on violence in the emergency department. *Ann. Emerg. Med.* **2002**, *39*, 47–55. [CrossRef] [PubMed]
39. Hyland, S.; Watts, J.; Fry, M. Rates of workplace aggression in the emergency department and nurses' perceptions of this challenging behaviour: A multimethod study. *Australas. Emerg. Nurs. J.* **2016**, *19*, 143–148. [CrossRef] [PubMed]

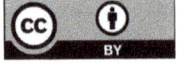

© 2018 by the authors. Licensee MDPI, Basel, Switzerland. This article is an open access article distributed under the terms and conditions of the Creative Commons Attribution (CC BY) license (http://creativecommons.org/licenses/by/4.0/).

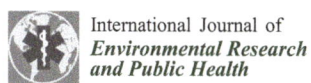

Article

Upon Rejection: Psychiatric Emergencies of Failed Asylum Seekers

Georgios Schoretsanitis [1,2,*], Dinesh Bhugra [3], Sarah Eisenhardt [1], Meret E. Ricklin [4], David S. Srivastava [4], Aristomenis Exadaktylos [4] and Sebastian Walther [1]

1. University Hospital of Psychiatry, 3008 Bern, Switzerland; saraheisenhardt11@googlemail.com (S.E.); sebastian.walther@upd.unibe.ch (S.W.)
2. Department of Psychiatry, Psychotherapy and Psychosomatics, and JARA-Translational Brain Medicine, RWTH Aachen University, 52074 Aachen, Germany
3. Institute of Psychiatry, King's College London, De Crespigny Park, London SE5 8AF, UK; dinesh.bhugra@kcl.ac.uk
4. Department of Emergency Medicine, Inselspital, University Hospital Bern, Freiburgstrasse, 3010 Bern, Switzerland; meret.ricklin@gmail.com (M.E.R.); DavidShiva.Srivastava@insel.ch (D.S.S.); Aristomenis.Exadaktylos@insel.ch (A.E.)
* Correspondence: george.schor@gmail.com; Tel.: +41-31-930-9111; Fax: +41-31-930-9404

Received: 18 June 2018; Accepted: 14 July 2018; Published: 16 July 2018

Abstract: *Background:* The status of a refugee or asylum seeker is only recognised after legal processes. The uncertainty of these procedures or the rejection itself may severely impact mental well-being. *Methods:* We surveyed the patterns of psychiatric services used by patients whose applications for asylum had been rejected. In a retrospective investigation of admissions to the University Emergency Department in Bern, Switzerland between 1 March 2012 and 28 February 2017, we studied patients receiving a psychiatric consultation after their applications had been rejected. The primary endpoint was based on the comparison of these individuals with controls who were asylum seekers with pending asylum applications using the Mann-Whitney U test and the chi-square test (χ^2) with a significance level of 0.05. *Results:* Thirty-eight cases were identified. There were more men than women and the mean age was 30.08 ± 9.62 years. Patients predominantly presented as walk-in patients ($n = 16$, 42.1%), most frequently due to suicidal ideation ($n = 16$, 42.1%). Stress-related disorders were the most common diagnosis ($n = 29$, 76.3%) and patients were mainly referred to inpatient treatment ($n = 28$, 73.7%). Patients with rejected applications were less likely to be living in reception centres than patients with a pending application ($\chi^2 = 17.98$, $p < 0.001$). *Conclusion:* The profile of asylum seekers whose applications had been rejected reflects individuals with high-stress levels, potentially aggravated by the negative asylum decision.

Keywords: failed asylum seekers; psychiatric emergency services; psychiatric hospitalisation; acute stress

1. Introduction

Immigrants and asylum seekers comprise a highly vulnerable group exposed to factors that may increase their risk of developing mental health problems [1,2]. Over the past few years, there has been an extensive study of factors mediating the negative effects of migration on mental health. These factors are often classified as pre-, peri- or post-migration adversities [3–5]. Those individuals seeking refuge and/or asylum are defined by law. It has been shown that asylum seekers comprise a subgroup of immigrants requiring increasing attention [6–8]. The asylum process invariably includes the reception, registration, and examination of the application. Depending on the legislation of the host country, persons are allocated in reception centres during this procedure. In fact, asylum seekers are exposed to specific risk factors that relate directly to the asylum process—including insecurity, stress and the fear of involuntary repatriation [7,9,10], which may explain why the whole process of asylum determination may aggravate the severity of claimants' symptoms [11]. Furthermore, it is not surprising that the length of the procedure itself may correlate with the prevalence of psychiatric symptoms [6,12], whereas detention in reception centres poses an additional challenge due to the limitations placed on the claimants' freedoms. Moreover, the application outcome may amplify precedent psychopathology or trigger new psychiatric symptoms [7,8,13–15]. The claimants may suffer additional stress if they are due to be expelled [8,16,17]. Data are available on the use of mental health care services by asylum seekers and these results reflect valuable aspects of claimants' needs [18–21]. As an increasing number of these patients require mental health services, this evidence may be instrumental in developing strategies to improve psychiatric services. Claimants may often have difficulties in accessing treatment [22]. The situation might be further aggravated by cultural and language barriers [4,23]. A previous study has investigated the mental health of rejected asylum seekers compared to groups of claimants with a pending or approved residence permit in Switzerland based on interviews and standardized questionnaires [14]. Nevertheless, there are no specific data on the use of mental health care services by rejected asylum seekers because the available evidence does not separate these individuals from persons with applications in various stages of the asylum process [24,25]. This methodological issue is of crucial importance as the asylum process may last for years and asylum seekers are a widely heterogeneous group with respect to psychopathology and the prevalence of mental disorders [7,10,19,26]. Likewise, the only available specified service for immigrants in Canton Bern is aimed at mental health care for all types of immigrants regardless of the asylum process phase; further, all persons during the asylum process are entitled to health insurance coverage with some restrictions.

The debate on the needs of rejected asylum seekers is not restricted to psychiatry as it involves other health care fields [27]. Therefore, it is helpful to assess psychiatric emergencies in failed asylum seekers separately from other emergencies. The increase in the numbers of asylum applications, in turn, makes it easier to collect large-scale data and, thus, to investigate the specific needs of failed asylum seekers. The main aim of the current study was to provide descriptive data on the use of psychiatric emergency services by failed asylum seekers. We also compared categorical outcomes between patients with failed and pending applications, in order to identify factors that may distinguish these two groups of patients. This control group (asylum seekers with pending application) was considered a better option than a group of immigrants with warranted residence or the population because it should yield smaller social and cultural differences from the rejected asylum-seeking group. We hypothesised that deleterious effects would be associated with the negative decision, therefore leading to more severe symptoms in the rejected patients.

2. Methods

This descriptive study included retrospective data from adult patients (age ≥ 18 years) admitted to the University Emergency Department (Universitäres Notfallzentrum, UNZ, Bern, Switzerland) for a psychiatric consultation (during an interdisciplinary medical examination or a specific psychiatric evaluation) between 1 March 2012 and 28 February 2017. The UNZ provides 24 h/day psychiatric emergency services and it is responsible for emergency mental health care in Canton Bern, Switzerland (with a population of over 1,000,000 inhabitants) including asylum centres in this catchment area. Consulting clinicians are mainly resident doctors under the supervision of senior doctors. The screening process of the medical records is described in detail in a previous paper [28].

First, we reviewed electronic medical records to detect patients with a migration background (i.e., non-Swiss nationality), which led to 1697 records. Second, we reviewed records in order to identify patients with an asylum application, which yielded 237 records. Lastly, we separated the records of patients subject to deportation (failed applications). Apart from the sociodemographic characteristics (age, gender, nationality, marital status, children, relatives in Switzerland), we were able to extract the following clinical data: the pathway to care (health professionals involved in the referral), the reason for presentation/referral, the ICD-10 diagnosis set by the consulting person, the referral outcome, the presence of an interpreter during the consultation and contact with psychiatric services prior to the recorded (current) consultation.

The pathway to care was classified as follows: walk-in, general practitioner or another medical doctor, ambulance, police, or reception centres. The reasons for presentation/referral were grouped as follows: suicidal thoughts, attempted suicide, auto-aggressive behaviour, aggression, depressive symptoms, sleep disorders, acute stress, somatic complaints, psychotic symptoms, psychosocial problems and use of medication. Diagnoses (ICD-10) were classified in accordance with diagnostic categories (F10–19, 20–29, 30–39, 40–49, F60–69, F90–99). The possible referral outcomes were admittance to a psychiatric clinic (voluntary or compulsory) or discharge home. For patients who visited the UNZ more than once, only the most recent registration was considered; six patients had two registrations, while there were three registrations for two other persons. The asylum decision predated all registrations for the persons being consulted more than once. Rudimentary case files or incomplete medical records were excluded from the analysis ($n = 46$).

The health-related patient data were exported anonymously for analysis. Only one author (MER) had access to the information that could identify the patient. None of the authors were potentially an attending physician of the patients involved. Retrospective analysis of data for this study was in accordance with the local regulatory authority and with the Declaration of Helsinki. No informed consent was necessary for this case note type of study. The protocol was approved by the Ethics Committee of Canton Bern (Project-ID Number 2018-00198).

Statistical Analysis

The data were summarised using descriptive statistics. Comparisons were conducted between persons with pending and failed asylum application. The Mann-Whitney U test (M-W-U) was used for age and gender distributions, and the chi-square test (χ^2) for categorical variables. When the latter test was not possible due to the small number of cases, Fisher's exact test was conducted. A significance level of 0.05 was used for all comparisons. Referral outcome was transformed to a dichotomous variable; '0' was used for cases of non-compulsory treatment consisting of discharge home and voluntary admissions in the clinic, whereas '1' encoded compulsory (inpatient) treatment. This analysis was repeated using the type of treatment, as well as with out-vs-inpatient as a dummy variable. All statistical analyses were carried out using IBM SPSS Statistics, version 22.0 (IBM GmbH, Ehningen, Germany).

3. Results

We were able to identify 38 records of patients (15 women and 23 men) with a rejected asylum application (Table 1). In 31 cases, the patients were informed of the application outcome within 2 weeks prior to the psychiatric consultation (81.6%); 3 patients had previously presented at least once at UNZ shortly after the outcome of the application (7.89%); 3 patients had presented due to other triggers (7.89%); 1 patient presented shortly before the deportation day (2.6%). The mean age was 30.08 ± 9.62 years. In terms of origin, the individuals came from a range of countries; the most common countries of origin were Russia ($n = 5$), Eritrea ($n = 3$), Sri Lanka ($n = 3$), Syria ($n = 3$) and Vietnam ($n = 3$) (Table 2). One-third of the patients were single ($n = 13$, 34.2%), whereas 10 were married (26.3%). Seventeen patients (44.7%) did not have children, while 10 patients (26.3%) did (in 7 cases, the children lived in Switzerland). For 11 patients (28.9%), no information regarding children was available. Almost half of the patients ($n = 18$, 47%) had no relatives in Switzerland (see Table 1).

Table 1. The sociodemographic characteristics of patients with rejected (n = 38) and pending application (n = 119).

Variable	Rejected Application	Pending Application	
Females (%)	15 (39.5)	30 (25.2)	p = 0.092
Age (SD)	30.08 (9.62)	29.88 (9.13)	p = 0.964
Marital status (%)	n (%)	n (%)	
Never been married	13 (34.2)	67 (56.3)	
Widowed and Divorced	5 (13.2)	9 (7.5)	χ^2 = 7.518, df = 5,
Married (Spouse in CH)	7 (18.4)	13 (10.9)	p = 0.185
Married (Spouse abroad)	3 (7.9)	11 (9.2)	
Unknown	10 (26.3)	19 (16.0)	
Children (%)	n (%)	n (%)	
No	17 (44.7)	72 (60.5)	
Yes (Children in CH)	7 (18.4)	18 (15.1)	χ^2 = 4.008, df = 5,
Yes (Children abroad)	3 (7.9)	10 (8.4)	p = 0.261
Unknown	11 (28.9)	19 (16.0)	
At least one relative in CH, not partner (%)	n (%)	n (%)	
No	18 (47.4)	66 (55.5)	
Yes	10 (26.3)	34 (28.6)	χ^2 = 2.075, df = 2,
Unknown	10 (26.3)	19 (16.0)	p = 0.354
Residing in reception center (%)	n (%)	n (%)	
Yes	14 (36.8) *	85 (71.4)	
No	23 (60.5) *	28 (23.5)	* χ^2 = 17.98,
Unknown	1 (2.6)	6 (5)	df = 2, p < 0.001

*: Statistically significant. Age provided in years, CH: Switzerland.

Table 2. The regions of the origin of persons with a rejected application (n = 38).

Regions of Origin (%)	
Middle East	7 (18.4)
Eastern Europe	8 (21.1)
Sub-Saharan Africa	11 (28.9)
Northwestern Africa	4 (10.5)
Central-South Asia	8 (21.1)

Patients predominantly came as walk-in patients (n = 16, 42.1%), whereas 10 (26.3%) were referred to the UNZ by the ambulance service (Table 3). Patients were most frequently referred due to suicidal thoughts (n = 16, 42.1%). Stress-related disorders (F40–49) comprised the most common diagnoses (n = 29, 76.3%). Consultants diagnosed an adjustment disorder (F43.2) in 14 cases (36.8%) and an acute stress reaction (F43.0) in 8 cases (21.1%).

Table 3. The clinical characteristics of rejected ($n = 38$) and pending applications ($n = 119$).

Variable	Rejected Application	Pending Application	
Pathway to UNZ Emergency Department	n (%)	n (%)	
Walk-in	16 (42.1)	52 (43.7)	
General practitioner (or other MDs)	2 (5.3)	16 (13.4)	$\chi^2 = 7.771$, df = 4,
Ambulance	10 (26.3)	13 (10.9)	$p = 0.1$
Police	8 (21.1)	35 (29.4)	
Reception center	2 (5.3)	3 (2.5)	
Referral reasons	n (%)	n (%)	
Suicidal ideation	16 (42.1)	30 (25.2)	
Suicide attempt	5 (13.2)	3 (2.5)	
Auto-aggressive behavior	3 (7.9)	7 (5.9)	
Aggressive behavior	3 (7.9)	25 (21.0)	
Psychotic symptoms	2 (5.3)	11 (9.2)	
Depressive symptoms	2 (5.3)	10 (8.4)	$\chi^2 = 15.968$, df = 11,
Sleep disorders	2 (5.3)	8 (6.7)	$p = 0.142$
Acute stress	3 (7.9)	9 (7.6)	
Somatic complaints	1 (2.6)	10 (8.4)	
Psychosocial problems	1 (2.6)	2 (1.7)	
Medication acquisition	0 (0)	2 (1.7)	
Other	0 (0)	2 (1.7)	
ICD diagnoses	n (%)	n (%)	
Disorders due to substance use (F10–19)	2 (5.3)	14 (11.8)	
Schizophrenia spectrum disorders (F20–29)	2 (5.3)	22 (18.5)	
Affective disorders (F30–F39)	3 (7.9)	17 (14.3)	* $\chi^2 = 17.59$, df = 7,
Stress-related disorders (F40–F49)	29 (76.3) *	58 (49.6)	$p = 0.014$
Personality disorders (F60–69)	0 (0)	6 (5.0)	
Others	2 (5.3)	1 (0.8)	
Referral outcome	n (%)	n (%)	
Discharged home	4 (10.5)	32 (26.9)	
Discharged home with outpatient treatment	6 (15.8)	16 (13.4)	$\chi^2 = 4.412$, df = 3,
Voluntary admission	16 (42.1)	42 (35.3)	$p = 0.22$
Compulsory admission	12 (31.6)	29 (24.4)	

*: Statistically significant. ICD: International Classification of Diseases; MD: medical doctor; UNZ: University Emergency Department.

The researchers found that 7 of the 8 patients with a diagnosis of acute stress reaction were informed about the negative asylum decision shortly before referral. Twenty-four patients had prior contact with psychiatric services (63.2%). The consultation was aided by an interpreting service in 9 cases (23.7%) or by the presence of a person who could speak the patient's native language (family member or friend of the patient) in 5 cases (13.2%), which was not required or possible for the majority of the patients ($n = 23$, 60.5%).

Regarding the referral outcomes, patients were mainly treated as inpatients ($n = 28$, 73.7%); in 12 of these cases (31.6%), treatment was voluntary. A detailed description of sociodemographic and clinical characteristics of the patients with a pending application (control group) is provided elsewhere [28]. No association was detected between interpretation (by interpreting service or person from the patient's environment) and compulsory treatment ($p = 0.58$ for Fisher exact test).

No differences for age and gender distribution were reported between asylum seekers with failed and pending applications ($p > 0.05$ for M-W-U for both comparisons). Nevertheless, there was a non-significant trend for gender, with proportionally more women in the group of patients with a rejected application than in the group of patients with a pending application ($p = 0.092$). Groups did not differ in the basic demographics, e.g., being single, having children or relatives in Switzerland ($p > 0.05$ in both cases). Nor did the groups differ in terms of prior contact with mental health care or in the presence of an interpreter during the consultation ($p > 0.05$ in both cases). A lower proportion of failed asylum seekers resided in reception centres than claimants with pending applications ($\chi^2 = 17.98$, df = 2, $p < 0.001$). Regarding referral reasons, the rates of suicidal ideation and attempted suicide were higher in patients with a rejected application rather than with a pending application, whereas aggressive behavior was more frequent in patients with a pending application; nevertheless, these differences did not reach statistical significance ($\chi^2 = 15.97$, df = 11, $p = 0.14$). Although the ambulance was more frequently involved in the referral process for failed claimants, this trend was not significant ($\chi^2 = 7.77$, df = 4, $p = 0.1$). In the same comparison, the police were more frequently involved for patients with pending than with rejected application. Regarding diagnoses, the proportion of individuals receiving a stress-related diagnosis (F40–49) was higher for rejected asylum seekers than for the control group ($\chi^2 = 17.59$, df = 7, $p = 0.014$). No differences were reported for referral outcomes, assignment to compulsory treatment or to inpatient setting ($p > 0.05$ for all three comparisons), although the inpatient admission rates were numerically higher in patients with a rejected application than a pending application (73.7% vs. 59.7%).

4. Discussion

Our retrospective study assessed psychiatric emergencies as reflected in patterns of use of mental health care services by persons with a failed asylum application. This subgroup of asylum seekers has not been widely studied, as they are commonly considered together with other individuals with asylum applications in various phases of the determination process [20].

Asylum seekers with rejected applications were predominantly young, male and single. In almost 90% of the cases, the negative refugee decision triggered severe psychic symptoms that led to psychiatric consultations at UNZ. The major pathway to the mental health care system was self-referrals (for 40.5% of patients); patients presented themselves to the facility most frequently for reported suicidal thoughts (40% of cases) followed by an evaluation after a suicide attempt (in 13.2%). In a Danish study with 61% of rejected asylum seekers, researchers reported suicidal ideation as the most common reason for consultation [20]. One out of three failed asylum seekers was given a diagnosis of adjustment disorders, which is in alignment with previous data reporting high-stress levels and depressive symptoms for patients with rejected applications [7,10,22].

Another finding deserving particular attention is the high percentage of patients treated as inpatients, which may relate to the lack of outpatient or social resources for these patients [29]. Alternatively, this finding might be related to the alarmingly high levels of stress and psychological symptoms suffered by rejected asylum seekers [22,24]. On the other hand, for involuntary inpatient treatment, there were no differences between persons with rejected and pending applications.

Moreover, the proportion of individuals diagnosed with a stress-related disorder was higher for the failed asylum seekers than for the control group of asylum seekers with pending decisions. In fact, the rates of acute stress reactions were 3 times higher for the failed asylum seekers than for the control group of asylum seekers with pending decisions (21% vs. 7.6%). Note that 7 out of 8 rejected asylum seekers receiving the diagnosis of acute stress reaction were referred shortly (within 24 h) after the negative asylum decision. Because severe symptoms have been reported in many claimants even during the determination process [28], we posit that the decision may have aggravated pre-existing symptoms, rather than triggering them. Here, we have to consider the possible adverse effects of the pending status as well. Ambulances were used for one-fourth of these patients–indicating that the symptoms were severe in the acute phase, but the differences were not statistically significant. Although suicide attempts were more frequent in failed claimants than in claimants with pending decisions, this difference also did not reach significance.

There were significant differences in the type of residence between rejected asylum seekers and persons with a pending application: the proportion of failed asylum seekers residing in reception centres was lower than for claimants with a pending application. This result may have occurred because claimants with a pending application are forced to stay in reception centres for long periods.

Nevertheless, data for the duration of stay in Switzerland were not consistently available in the medical records, so we cannot control for this confounding variable.

The number of consultations supported by the presence of an interpreting service (n = 9, 24.3%) was low compared to previous hospital data [20], but this may be due to bilingualism in Canton Bern, where German and French are the official languages. A group of immigrants came from French-speaking North African and Arabic countries and, therefore, French may offer a common language for them when contacting health care services. The association between interpretation (by interpreting service or person from the patient's environment) and compulsory treatment for patients with a rejected application was not significant; this may also result from the small size of the group.

Our study has some major limitations that need to be remembered when interpreting the findings. This retrospective study was based on case notes. These case notes are of variable quality and may be unreliable. Thus, some patients were excluded due to incomplete information. The selection of the time period was rather arbitrary and relates to the availability of the electronic records. Parameters, such as the previous socio-economic status in the home country, the duration of stay in Switzerland before presentation or decision, symptom duration and severity assessed with established questionnaires, housing type (for the persons not residing in reception centres), and the reasoning for the organization of interpreting services were not available and therefore could not be considered. Moreover, no data were provided on the length of the asylum procedure before the decision. Nevertheless, these data seem to be crucial and their inclusion in the analysis could have provided valuable insight [30]. When multiple registrations per patient were available, we included the most recent. This highlights the need for follow-up data, which are widely lacking. Further, information regarding the duration or outcome of the inpatient treatment (for the patients referred to inpatient setting) was not available. Lastly, given the naturalistic design of this study, the control group was not matched for demographic or clinical characteristics with the group of asylum seekers.

5. Conclusions

Our observations indicate that persons with rejected applications entering mental health care facilities are relatively likely to suffer from severe psychiatric symptoms such as suicidal ideation as well as high levels of stress; under these circumstances, the asylum rejection decision may trigger additional acute stress, leading to psychiatric emergencies and consultations. These individuals are invariably treated as inpatients, which may reflect high levels of psychological symptoms and/or the scarce social resources of these patients. Although findings indicate that failed claimants exhibit more acute symptoms, such as suicidal ideation or suicide attempts, than patients with pending status, these differences were not statistically significant. One possibility is that there is a continuum of severe symptoms during the determination process, which may be aggravated by the rejection decision. Providers should be aware of the particular psychopathology patterns in these highly vulnerable individuals. Given the limited social resources of these patients, inpatient treatment may be more appropriate for these patients than for other patient groups. Finally, an intensive support might prevent symptom aggravation during the final phase of the asylum procedure, i.e., shortly before and after the application outcome is announced.

Author Contributions: G.S., D.B., S.E., M.E.R., D.S.S., S.W. and A.E. participated in the research design of the study. G.S. performed the initial statistical analyses and wrote the first draft. S.W. suggested additional analyses and modifications to adjust to the style of this journal. All the authors contributed to the interpretation of data and approved the final manuscript.

Funding: This research received no external funding.

Acknowledgments: Authors are particularly grateful to Christoph Ringer, Samir Suker, Arne Jungnickel from the University Hospital of Psychiatry, Bern, for their valuable feedback.

Conflicts of Interest: The authors declare no conflict of interest.

References

1. Fazel, M.; Wheeler, J.; Danesh, J. Prevalence of serious mental disorder in 7000 refugees resettled in western countries: A systematic review. *Lancet* **2005**, *365*, 1309–1314. [CrossRef]
2. Bhugra, D.; Gupta, S.; Bhui, K.; Craig, T.; Dogra, N.; Ingleby, J.D.; Kirkbride, J.; Moussaoui, D.; Nazroo, J.; Qureshi, A.; et al. WPA guidance on mental health and mental health care in migrants. *World Psychiatry* **2011**, *10*, 2–10. [CrossRef] [PubMed]
3. Carswell, K.; Blackburn, P.; Barker, C. The relationship between trauma, post-migration problems and the psychological well-being of refugees and asylum seekers. *Int. J. Soc. Psychiatry* **2011**, *57*, 107–119. [CrossRef] [PubMed]
4. Silove, D.; Sinnerbrink, I.; Field, A.; Manicavasagar, V.; Steel, Z. Anxiety, depression and ptsd in asylum-seekers: Assocations with pre-migration trauma and post-migration stressors. *Br. J. Psychiatry* **1997**, *170*, 351–357. [CrossRef] [PubMed]
5. Hassan, G.; Ventevogel, P.; Jefee-Bahloul, H.; Barkil-Oteo, A.; Kirmayer, L.J. Mental health and psychosocial wellbeing of syrians affected by armed conflict. *Epidemiol. Psychiatr. Sci.* **2016**, *25*, 129–141. [CrossRef] [PubMed]
6. Laban, C.J.; Gernaat, H.B.; Komproe, I.H.; Schreuders, B.A.; De Jong, J.T. Impact of a long asylum procedure on the prevalence of psychiatric disorders in iraqi asylum seekers in The Netherlands. *J. Nerv. Ment. Dis.* **2004**, *192*, 843–851. [CrossRef] [PubMed]
7. Silove, D.; Steel, Z.; Susljik, I.; Frommer, N.; Loneragan, C.; Chey, T.; Brooks, R.; le Touze, D.; Ceollo, M.; Smith, M.; et al. The impact of the refugee decision on the trajectory of ptsd, anxiety, and depressive symptoms among asylum seekers: A longitudinal study. *Am. J. Dis. Med.* **2007**, *2*, 321–329.
8. Sundvall, M.; Tidemalm, D.H.; Titelman, D.E.; Runeson, B.; Baarnhielm, S. Assessment and treatment of asylum seekers after a suicide attempt: A comparative study of people registered at mental health services in a swedish location. *BMC Psychiatry* **2015**, *15*, 235. [CrossRef] [PubMed]
9. Momartin, S.; Steel, Z.; Coello, M.; Aroche, J.; Silove, D.M.; Brooks, R. A comparison of the mental health of refugees with temporary versus permanent protection visas. *Med. J. Aust.* **2006**, *185*, 357–361. [PubMed]
10. Ryan, D.A.; Benson, C.A.; Dooley, B.A. Psychological distress and the asylum process: A longitudinal study of forced migrants in Ireland. *J. Nerv. Ment. Dis.* **2008**, *196*, 37–45. [CrossRef] [PubMed]
11. Hocking, D.C.; Kennedy, G.A.; Sundram, S. Mental disorders in asylum seekers: The role of the refugee determination process and employment. *J. Nerv. Ment. Dis.* **2015**, *203*, 28–32. [CrossRef] [PubMed]
12. Hallas, P.; Hansen, A.R.; Staehr, M.A.; Munk-Andersen, E.; Jorgensen, H.L. Length of stay in asylum centres and mental health in asylum seekers: A retrospective study from denmark. *BMC Public Health* **2007**, *7*, 288. [CrossRef] [PubMed]
13. Davis, R.M.; Davis, H.T. PTSD symptom changes in refugees. *Torture Q. J. Rehabil. Torture Vict. Prev. Torture* **2006**, *16*, 10–19.
14. Mueller, J.; Schmidt, M.; Staeheli, A.; Maier, T. Mental health of failed asylum seekers as compared with pending and temporarily accepted asylum seekers. *Eur. J. Public Health* **2011**, *21*, 184–189. [CrossRef] [PubMed]
15. Jakobsen, M.; Meyer DeMott, M.A.; Wentzel-Larsen, T.; Heir, T. The impact of the asylum process on mental health: A longitudinal study of unaccompanied refugee minors in norway. *BMJ Open* **2017**, *7*, e015157. [CrossRef] [PubMed]
16. Noll, G. Rejected asylum seekers: The problem of return. *Int. Migr.* **1999**, *37*, 267–288. [CrossRef] [PubMed]
17. Sanchez-Mazas, M. The construction of "official outlaws". Social-psychological and educational implications of a deterrent asylum policy. *Front. Psychol.* **2015**, *6*, 382. [CrossRef] [PubMed]
18. Deans, A.K.; Boerma, C.J.; Fordyce, J.; De Souza, M.; Palmer, D.J.; Davis, J.S. Use of royal darwin hospital emergency department by immigration detainees in 2011. *Med. J. Aust.* **2013**, *199*, 776–778. [CrossRef] [PubMed]
19. Iversen, V.C.; Morken, G. Differences in acute psychiatric admissions between asylum seekers and refugees. *Nord. J. Psychiatry* **2004**, *58*, 465–470. [CrossRef] [PubMed]
20. Reko, A.; Bech, P.; Wohlert, C.; Noerregaard, C.; Csillag, C. Usage of psychiatric emergency services by asylum seekers: Clinical implications based on a descriptive study in Denmark. *Nord. J. Psychiatry* **2015**, *69*, 587–593. [CrossRef] [PubMed]

21. McColl, H.; Johnson, S. Characteristics and needs of asylum seekers and refugees in contact with london community mental health teams: A descriptive investigation. *Soc. Psychiatry Psychiatr. Epidemiol.* **2006**, *41*, 789–795. [CrossRef] [PubMed]
22. Schwarz-Nielsen, K.H.; Elklitt, A. An evaluation of the mental status of rejected asylum seekers in two danish asylum centers. *Torture Q. J. Rehabil. Torture Vict. Prev. Torture* **2009**, *19*, 51–59.
23. Sandhu, S.; Bjerre, N.V.; Dauvrin, M.; Dias, S.; Gaddini, A.; Greacen, T.; Ioannidis, E.; Kluge, U.; Jensen, N.K.; Lamkaddem, M.; et al. Experiences with treating immigrants: A qualitative study in mental health services across 16 european countries. *Soc. Psychiatry Psychiatr. Epidemiol.* **2013**, *48*, 105–116. [CrossRef] [PubMed]
24. Maier, T.; Schmidt, M.; Mueller, J. Mental health and healthcare utilization in adult asylum seekers. *Swiss Med. Wkly.* **2010**, *140*, w13110. [CrossRef] [PubMed]
25. Pfortmueller, C.A.; Schwetlick, M.; Mueller, T.; Lehmann, B.; Exadaktylos, A.K. Adult asylum seekers from the middle east including syria in central europe: What are their health care problems? *PLoS ONE* **2016**, *11*, e0148196. [CrossRef] [PubMed]
26. Toar, M.; O'Brien, K.K.; Fahey, T. Comparison of self-reported health & healthcare utilisation between asylum seekers and refugees: An observational study. *BMC Public Health* **2009**, *9*, 214.
27. Romero-Ortuno, R. Eligibility of non-residents for nhs treatment: Failed asylum seekers should not be denied access to free nhs care. *BMJ* **2004**, *329*, 683. [CrossRef] [PubMed]
28. Schoretsanitis, G.; Eisenhardt, S.; Ricklin, M.E.; Srivastava, D.S.; Walther, S.; Exadaktylos, A. Psychiatric emergencies of asylum seekers; descriptive analysis and comparison with immigrants of warranted residence. *Int. J. Environ. Res. Public Health* **2018**, *15*, 1300. [CrossRef] [PubMed]
29. Procter, N.G. Providing emergency mental health care to asylum seekers at a time when claims for permanent protection have been rejected. *Int. J. Ment. Health Nurs.* **2005**, *14*, 2–6. [CrossRef] [PubMed]
30. Sultan, A.; O'Sullivan, K. Psychological disturbances in asylum seekers held in long term detention: A participant-observer account. *Med. J. Aust.* **2001**, *175*, 593–596. [PubMed]

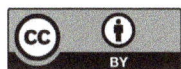

© 2018 by the authors. Licensee MDPI, Basel, Switzerland. This article is an open access article distributed under the terms and conditions of the Creative Commons Attribution (CC BY) license (http://creativecommons.org/licenses/by/4.0/).

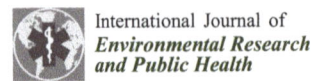

Concept Paper

A Brief Introduction to the Multidimensional Intercultural Training Acculturation Model (MITA) for Middle Eastern Adolescent Refugees

Atefeh Fathi *, Usama El-Awad, Tilman Reinelt and Franz Petermann

Zentrum für Klinische Psychologie und Rehabilitation, Universität Bremen, Grazer Str. 6, 28359 Bremen, Germany; elawad@uni-bremen.de (U.E.-A.); reinelt@uni-bremen.de (T.R.); fpeterm@uni-bremen.de (F.P.)
* Correspondence: fathi@uni-bremen.de; Tel.: +49-0421-218-68634

Received: 11 June 2018; Accepted: 13 July 2018; Published: 18 July 2018

Abstract: The large number of adolescent refugees around the world constitutes a great challenge for societies. However, current models of acculturation have been developed for migrants, but not specifically for adolescent refugees. Crucial factors to describe adolescent refugee acculturation, such as intentions to return to their homeland, especially with respect to adolescent refugees with temporary residency and experiences of potentially traumatic events, are missing. Hence, the Multidimensional Intercultural Training Acculturation (MITA) model is introduced. The model proposes that two major concerns for adolescent refugees, which are socio-cultural adjustment and mental health, are predicted by intercultural and social–emotional competence, intentions to return to their homeland, and experiences of traumatic events. Moreover, the effects of three modes of acculturation are also proposed in the model. It is expected that these variables mediate the effects of intercultural competence, social–emotional competence, intentions to return to the homeland, and experiences of traumatic events on socio-cultural adjustment as well as mental health. Finally, it is also expected that in-group social support and out-group social support moderate the direct connection between the experiences of traumatic events and mental health.

Keywords: multidimensional intercultural training acculturation model (MITA); intercultural competence; traumatic events; mental health; Middle Eastern refugee adolescents

1. Introduction

According to the United Nations Refugee Agency' reports, the number of people around the world forced from home because of war, human rights violations, persecution, or generalized violence and who need resettlement increased from 33.9 million in 1997 to 65.6 million in 2017 [1]. Altogether, more than half (55 percent) of all refugees worldwide come from Middle Eastern countries. Syrians are considered to be the largest resettled population, with 12 million refugees at the end of 2016. Afghans are the second largest group, followed by Iraqis [1]. Among European countries, Germany has received the largest number of refugees, at about 746,649 in 2017. Nearly one-third of these refugees were under the age of 18 [2]. The most common Middle Eastern country of origin for refugee adolescents and children was Afghanistan, followed by Syria and Iraq [1]. Some of these adolescent refugees may be psychologically vulnerable due to the experience of potentially traumatic events such as experiencing separation from their parents or close family members, or even their deaths. In addition, they may be confronted with cultural identity confusion during the process of resettlement. This complicated mixture of experiences may make their process of acculturation especially stressful [3].

Acculturation is defined as a cultural modification of individuals by adapting to another culture. In other words, acculturation is the process of cultural and psychological changes that occur because of the interaction between immigrants and members of the host culture [4]. At the cultural level, both the host and origin cultures usually have some priorities or targets for immigrants to attain (e.g., form of communication, eating habits, and dressing style) which lead them to choose different types of acculturation strategies [4]. At the psychological level that comprises cultural shedding, culture learning, and cultural conflict, behavioral rules change, which is usually non-problematic. Although cultural shedding and cultural learning may be selective, accidental, or deliberate, they productively allow the individual to adapt to the society of settlement [4]. However, cultural conflicts are expected to be problematic and affect refugees' social behaviors and jeopardize their mental health [5]. This is especially relevant for adolescent refugees, as their identity development is positively related with some crucial factors such as belonging to a peer group and good social relationships based on mutual respect and acceptance [6,7]. Therefore, adolescent refugees need long-term and comprehensive solutions to rebuild their fractured identities [8]. For example, psychological and social supports and offers from youth welfare services are able to reduce many difficulties and prepare valuable comprehensive care services [9,10]. Moreover, some multimodal psychosocial supports and school-based programs [11] as well as some specific training programs for adolescent refugees that concentrate both on changing the environment and changing the adolescent refugees' skill sets (e.g., emotional skills such as emotional regulation, social skills such as conversational skills, and behavioral skills such as assertiveness and empathy) might be especially promising [12,13].

However, despite the overwhelming numbers of adolescent refugees, all current acculturation models are specific to immigrants or adult refugees (e.g., the Multidimensional Individual Differences Acculturation model: MIDA [14], the Relative Acculturation Extended Model: RAEM [15], and Rudmin's model of acculturation as second-culture acquisition [16]). Therefore, a new acculturation model specific to adolescent refugees is needed to improve the knowledge on this population, especially on those from the Middle East living in European countries, and more importantly to evaluate their social behaviors and mental health. The model we propose, builds on and combines elements from three different models of acculturation: (1) Berry's bi-dimensional model of acculturation [17], (2) the Multidimensional Individual Differences Acculturation model [14], and (3) Rudmin's [16] acculturative learning model.

1.1. Bi-Dimensional Model of Acculturation

According to Berry's bi-dimensional model of acculturation [17], there are two principal factors in estimating acculturation: (1) retention of the heritage culture, and (2) attainment of the new culture. These two principal factors result in four acculturation strategies which are as follows: integration (i.e., retention of the heritage culture as well as attainment of the new culture), separation (i.e., retention of the heritage culture but no attainment of the new one), assimilation (i.e., abandonment of the heritage culture and adoption of the new culture), and marginalization (i.e., abandonment of the heritage culture as well as failure to adapt to the new culture) [18]. Inconsistencies and conflicts between these different acculturation strategies can lead to psychological difficulties [18]. Hence, acculturative stress may be observed when acculturation experiences result in psychological problems for refugees. Berry discussed that although bi-cultural (integrated) individuals must be more under pressure from both the heritage and host culture communities, they generally have a better psychological adaptation [4] and if their acculturation strategy does not lead to success, they are sufficiently flexible to modify it [18]. Separated individuals have more contact with people of their heritage culture and receive more support from them. However, they report more pressure from the host society to adapt to the receiving culture and are most likely to face discrimination from members of the host society [19]. Assimilated people are characterized by low ethnic identity as well as a high national identity of the host country. Although they may have more contact with people of the host country and report fewer experiences of discrimination, they suffer from low support from their family and the members of their ethnic groups. Marginalized individuals demonstrate "cultural identity confusion" [18,20]. They show a higher degree of lack of interpersonal trust, self-assurance, and neuroticism [21]. Berry [4] noted that the idea of marginality was synonymous with the concept of deculturation, which is broadly used as the process where aspects of one culture are lost after contact with another one. Individuals with a marginalization strategy are highly averted from their original culture as well as the culture of the dominant group. Marginalized people profoundly suffer from acculturative stress, which is the psychological effect of adaptation to a new culture [22,23]. Acculturative stress is defined as a reduction in the psychological health of immigrants and refugees [24].

1.2. The Acculturative Learning Model

Rudmin discussed that the concentration on acculturative stress neglects the motivation to acculturate [25]. For example, sojourners, skilled workers, missionaries, business agents, and students show that it is achievable to acculturate purely because of some motivational reasons, even if the attitudes to the host culture are not entirely positive or are even negative. Moreover, acculturation as a process that requires resources such as mental energy, money, time, and social capital, and in some cases the risks of negative consequences, may necessitate some cost–benefit estimations [16]. Rudmin's model contains three steps, including acculturative motivation, acculturative learning, and alterations in the individuals. Rudmin's model [16] of acculturation as second-culture acquisition explains that the motivation to acculturate leads to acculturative learning, which may bring about some changes in individuals (e.g., such as communication style, lifestyle, values, moral codes, clothing, the way of thinking, social activities). The alterations that arise from acculturative learning may be outcomes of the family situation, successes, failures, political activities, and creativity as well as discrimination. Motivation to acculturate can involve: (1) cultural attitudes, (2) ethnic identity, (3) reacting to stress, and (4) utility, involving the risks and costs of second-culture acquisition [16]. This model claims that the four main methods of acculturative learning are: (1) information about the new culture, (2) instructions, (3) imitation of new culture behaviors, and (4) mentoring by persons competent in the host culture and caring enough about the acculturating person to be individually supportive. Finally, in Rudmin's model, perceptions about the socioeconomic status as well as discrimination are considered as control variables. They can influence how an individual is learning a second culture. However, these factors alone do not result in acculturation. Therefore, these variables are not considered as learning a second culture [26].

1.3. The Multidimensional Individual Differences Acculturation Model

The Multidimensional Individual Difference Acculturation (MIDA) model was initially developed by Safdar et al. [14] using first-generation Iranian immigrants living in Canada. This model was empirically examined with immigrants of diverse ethnic origins living in urban and rural areas in Canada [14], Iranian immigrants living in the Netherlands, the United Kingdom, and the United States [27], and Indian and Russian immigrants living in Canada [28]. Primarily, the MIDA model suggested that acculturation attitudes and coping resources are more essential predictors of psycho-physical health outcomes than demographic variables [14]. In the MIDA model, three factors are predictors of acculturation attitudes and adaptation outcomes. These predictor variables are: (1) psychosocial resources, (2) co-national connectedness, and (3) hassles. Psycho-social resources contain three components: resilience, cultural competence, and out-group social support (social support from the host society). Resilience focuses on the existence of positive psychological functioning. Cultural competence refers to immigrants' communication abilities in the host society and their cultural efficacy. Out-group social support refers to the social support from members of the host society [14]. Co-national connectedness is the second predictive factor that consists of three components: ethnic identity, family allocentrism, and perceived family and in-group social support. Ethnic identity focuses on the identification with the heritage group. Family allocentrism refers to the quality of family ties and relationships [14]. In-group social support refers to the perceived support from family and in-group members. In the MIDA model, distinguishing between in-group social support and out-group social support is very important to predict the immigrants' psychological well-being. Hassles allude to chronic irritants that individuals frequently face, such as time pressure, financial difficulties, arguing with friends/family members, and being overburdened with responsibilities [14]. The outcome variables in this model are in-group behavior from Co-national connectedness, out-group behavior from psycho-social resources, and psycho-physical distress from hassles [27,28]. Types of acculturation strategies [17] are also evaluated in MIDA model, which are attitudes toward old culture maintenance (separation) and new culture acquisition (assimilation). These types of acculturation strategies are considered as mediating variables in connecting the MIDA model's psychological constructs to the output [14]. In this mediating situation, co-national connectedness predicts separation or old culture maintenance and separation predicts in-group contact [27,28]. Hassles predict separation as well as psychophysical distress. Psycho-social resources predict assimilation or new culture acquisition and assimilation predicts out-group contact [14,27].

1.4. Limitation of the Acculturation Models Regarding Adolescent Refugees

Traditionally, Berry's model of acculturation has been the dominant paradigm in acculturation studies. However, a common criticism of Berry's acculturation model is that it has primarily concentrated on the acculturation of permanent adult migrants and has been mainly employed with voluntary adult refugee and immigrant samples. Therefore, some critical factors such as intercultural competence as well as acculturative learning [25], which can play essential roles in acculturation orientation (especially for adolescent refugees with temporary residency), have been ignored.

Although some essential factors related to acculturative learning are included in Rudmin's model [16], there are still some deficiencies that should be taken into consideration. First of all, information has rarely been scrutinized for its effectiveness as a procedure of second-culture learning, including informal information found in movies, novels, and music [29,30]. Furthermore, instructions, as intercultural training, have commonly concentrated on preparing students, skilled workers, and sojourners [31]. Thus, proper information about the host culture and the concept of culture itself, as well as intercultural training, are needed to be applied more broadly (e.g., most important for adolescent refugees who come from completely different cultures and ethnicities). Finally, considering the utility decision that works by the decision between the costs and the benefits [16], intentions to return to the homeland should be taken into consideration. Intentions to return to the homeland can affect the motivation of adolescent refugees to establish and to maintain their intercultural relationships. Therefore, a new model for adolescent refugees needs to fill the gap by applying intentions to return to the homeland as well as intercultural competence as factors, which mainly contain motivation to acculturate, cultural knowledge, and intercultural training as their latent components.

In addition, some critical factors, including social–emotional competencies and experiences of traumatic events, which can affect adolescent refugees' mental health and socio-cultural adjustment as well as acculturation orientations, are mainly neglected in the MIDA model. Because of the nature of its variables, the MIDA model is essentially culture non-specific. Moreover, its outcome variables, including out-group/in-group contacts as well as psychological/physical health, are fundamental issues in multicultural societies as well as common goals of all immigrants. However, this model has been applied mostly to educated immigrants or adult individuals with immigration backgrounds [14,27,28]. Adolescent refugees with temporary residency, lower education, and insufficient social experiences are not considered.

In general, some crucial factors, such as intentions to return to the homeland (especially for adolescent refugees with temporary residency and experiences of potentially traumatic events which make the adolescent refugees psychologically fragile and vulnerable), can differentiate the acculturation models specific to refugee populations from the models of acculturation specific to immigrants. To overcome all these limitations, we propose the Multidimensional Intercultural Training Acculturation Model (MITA).

2. The Multidimensional Intercultural Training Acculturation Model (MITA)

The MITA model has derived some elements from three different models of acculturation, including three modes of acculturation (assimilation, separation, and integration) from Berry's bi-dimensional model of acculturation [17], out-group social support, in-group social support, and mental health from Multidimensional Individual Differences Acculturation model (MIDA) [14], and intercultural competence as acculturative learning from Rudmin's model [16] as second-culture acquisition. The MITA model has also derived some elements from different approaches to acculturation research, including Berry's [4,17,18] two dimensions of adoption of the host culture and maintenance of the heritage culture and the difference between socio-cultural adjustment and psychological adjustment [32]. The MITA model has added some new elements, including intentions to return to the homeland, the experience of traumatic events, and socio-cultural adjustment. Furthermore, The MITA model is supported by a number of theoretical approaches within clinical, social, and cross-cultural psychology, including acculturation attitudes [17] and Hammer et al.'s [33] theoretical framework of Intercultural Communicating Competence (ICC) for conceptualizing intercultural competence. To conceptualize social–emotional competence, empathy from prosocial behaviors [34], and among appraisal theories, the emotion regulation strategies of Gross [35], including: (1) situation selection, (2) situation modification, (3) attentional deployment, (4) cognitive change, and (5) response-focused strategies, are selected. In the MITA model, four factors are predictors of mental health and socio-cultural adjustment. These predictor variables are (1) intercultural competence, (2) social–emotional competence, (3) intentions to return to the homeland, and (4) experiences of traumatic events.

The outcome variables in this model are socio-cultural adjustment from intercultural competence, social–emotional competence, and intentions to return to the homeland and mental health from social–emotional competence, as well as the experience of traumatic events.

Modes of acculturation [17] including integration, separation, and assimilation, are also proposed in the MITA model. These modes of acculturation are considered as mediating variables in connecting the MITA model's psychological constructs to the output variables. In this mediating situation, intentions to return to the homeland predict separation and separation predicts socio-cultural adjustment as well as mental health. Intercultural competence predicts integration and integration predicts socio-cultural adjustment as well as mental health. Social–emotional competence predicts assimilation and assimilation predicts socio-cultural adjustment. Experience of traumatic events predicts separation and separation predicts socio-cultural adjustment.

Moreover, the direct connection between intercultural and social–emotional competence/experiences of traumatic events, and the three modes of acculturation is influenced by two variables, including out-group social support and in-group social support. It is expected that these two variables would play some moderated mediating roles in linking intercultural competence, social–emotional competence, and experiences of traumatic events to modes of acculturation. In this moderated mediating situation, out-group social support affects the connection between intercultural and social–emotional competence and integration as well as assimilation. In-group social support affects the connection between the experience of traumatic events and assimilation. Finally, in-group social support and out-group social support are considered as moderating variables in connecting the experience of traumatic events to mental health. The connections among predictor variables, output variables, mediating variables, moderating variables, and moderated mediating variables are shown in Figure 1.

In sections to follow, each of these variables mentioned above in the MITA model is discussed further.

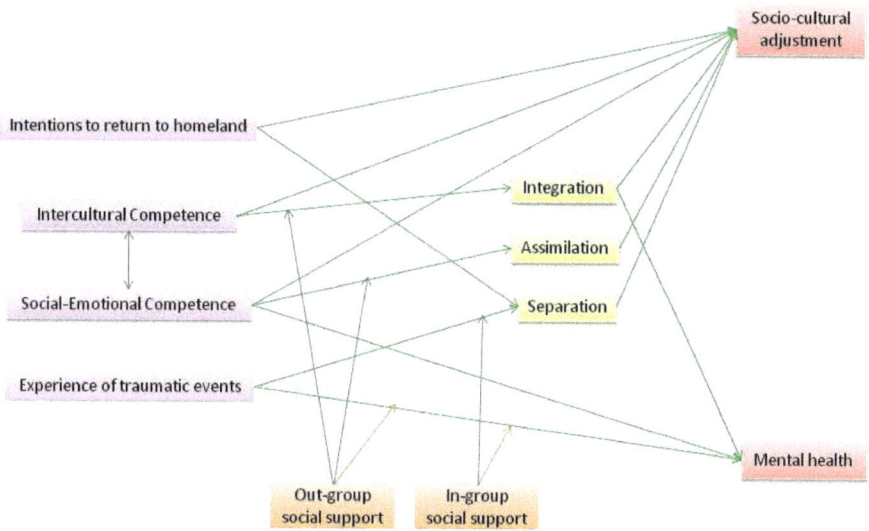

Figure 1. Multidimensional Intercultural Training Acculturation Model (MITA).

2.1. Intercultural Competence

The term intercultural competence describes the capability to appropriately and effectively carry out social interactions and communicate with people from various cultures [32]. The refugees' ability to communicate can facilitate all other aspects of adaptation and adjustment in the host culture. Therefore, intercultural competence may be considered as the fundamental process as well as the main outcome of the acculturation process [32]. According to Berry [17], there are three phases of acculturation processes, including contact, conflict, and adaptation. In these phases contact is a core concept for acculturation. In the contact phase, communication is remarkably important and needs to be constructive and without failures and misunderstandings as much as it is possible [17]. According to Hammer et al., [33] communication in the contact phase to acculturation is viewed as one of the common processes of intercultural competence. Based on this, there is an increase in intercultural sensitivity to cultural differences during acculturation [33]. Intercultural sensitivity comprises the ability to experience and distinguish pertinent cultural differences and is considered a focal competence for intercultural communication [36]. Hence, to understand acculturation successfully, the interactional context in which this process takes place needs to be clarified [37]. As most of the current adolescent refugees in the Western countries are from non-European backgrounds [38], the term culture has become an important element to understand the process of acculturation. As acculturation refers to cultural change, it is a requisite to determine how the term culture is described [39]. According to Shore [40], culture refers to shared understandings, meanings, or referents kept by a specific group of people. As noted by Rudmin [25], the similarity between the host culture and the heritage culture can clarify how much acculturation is needed to adapt to the host culture. Therefore, research on the concept of cultural awareness, cultural similarities, and differences can play a constructive role in socio-cultural adjustment. However, different cultural groups can bring up racial [41] as well as ethnic stereotypes [42], which might result in stereotype threat. Stereotype threat emerges when a person is in a situation having a fear of behaving in a way that would accidentally confirm a negative stereotype [43]. It should be mentioned that stereotype threat can lead to spotlight anxiety which may bring about vigilant worry and this experience of emotional distress can undermine social and emotional performance [43]. Therefore, it is expected that increasing knowledge about different types of stereotypes can be helpful to reduce its threat to social and emotional and consequently, to improve the socio-cultural adjustment. Hence, based on these explanations, in the MITA model, intercultural competence contains three components as follows: (1) cultural awareness, (2) knowledge about cultural similarities and differences, and (3) knowledge about stereotypes. In the MITA model, intercultural competence predicts socio-cultural adjustment. Moreover, the connection between intercultural competence and mental health is mediated by integration.

2.2. Social–Emotional Competence

Social–emotional competence is defined as the ability to interact with people, regulate emotions and behaviors properly, solve problems reasonably, and communicate impressively. In the MITA model, social–emotional competence contains two components as follows: (1) emotion regulation and (2) empathy.

Emotion regulation is the ability to react to different experiences with the range of emotions in a way that is socially acceptable as well as the ability to postpone impulsive reactions when needed [44]. According to Gross [45], improving one's ability for emotion regulation will lead to a greater ability to respond to emotional experiences appropriately. Several studies have confirmed the link between emotion dysregulation and impaired anger management ability [46–48]. Moreover, there is some experimental evidence that the execution of adaptive emotion regulation strategies can significantly diminish rage and aggression [49,50]. Although studies so far mostly have failed to confirm the link between post-migration living difficulties and emotion dysregulation, it might be the case that these daily living difficulties also affect refugees' capability to regulate their emotions appropriately. Consequently, impaired emotion regulation might act as a mechanism for empowering the connection between refugees' experiences and mental health outcomes [9,51]. This means that the experience of extreme emotional distress in connection with trauma and post-migration living difficulties might force the refugees to use dysfunctional emotion regulation strategies and the lack of access to functional strategies may thus empower the association between post-migration living difficulties and psychological difficulties [9]. Therefore, in the proposed MITA model, emotion regulation is added as one of the components of the social–emotional competence. Another component of social–emotional competence that is strongly linked to an appropriate emotion regulation is empathy [52]. According to Hammer et al. [33], empathy enables a person's adaptation to differences in the course of intercultural sensitivity. According to Bar-Tal [34], empathy is a fundamental motivating factor for prosocial behavior, which is defined as a social behavior that benefits society or other individuals as a whole and emotion regulation can moderate the degree to which empathy is associated with prosocial behavior [53]. Several studies revealed that people with better abilities to regulate their emotions properly show a greater increase in prosocial behavior and empathy [54,55]. Hence, because of this significant positive association between empathy and emotion regulation, empathy is also added as one of the components of social–emotional competence. Therefore, in MITA model, social–emotional competence predicts mental health as well as socio-cultural adjustment. Moreover, it is also expected that assimilation mediates the connection between social–emotional competence and socio-cultural adjustment.

2.3. Intentions to Return to the Homeland

According to Lu [55], because of different reasons (including economic, social and political restrictions), not all refugees who intend to return to their homeland necessarily go back. Refugees' intentions to "return" can give us a great understanding of their future plans as well as their opinions about their experiences in the host countries. This information may help researchers and mental health practitioners in the domain to develop training programs which can enhance refugees' skills and experiences in areas that they need the most [56,57]. Intentions to return to the homeland can affect the desire to acquire knowledge of the host culture, to develop connections with members of the host society, and to learn about the host country's social and cultural environments which all considered as motivation to acculturate [58]. If acculturation is considered to be the process of acquiring knowledge of a host culture [17], intentions to return to the homeland can affect the willingness to take part in this process [59]. Its impact on the adolescent refugees, however, is still poorly investigated. Therefore, in the MITA model, intention to return to homeland is added as a predictor of socio-cultural adjustment. In the mediating situation, intentions to return to homeland predict separation and separation predicts socio-cultural adjustment as well as mental health.

2.4. Experience of Traumatic Events

Exposure to violence (both pre- and post-migration) as well as parents or close family members' exposure to violence is the most studied risk factor for mental health difficulties for adolescent refugees [60]. In a study of adolescent Iraqi refugees, the experience of traumatic events predicted mental health difficulties [61]. In addition, the adolescents of non-tortured refugee families from different Middle Eastern countries appeared to have healthier mental states than the adolescent refugees from Iraq [62]. Despite the important effects of the experience of potentially traumatic events on adolescent refugees' mental health [51,63], none of the models of acculturation have considered it as an important factor. Therefore, in the MITA model, the experience of traumatic events is added to predict the mental health of adolescent refugees. In-group/out-group social support also moderates the connection between experiences of traumatic events and mental health. Moreover, in the MITA model, the connection between experiences of traumatic events and socio-cultural adjustment is mediating by separation.

2.5. Modes of Acculturation

The modes of acculturation, which have been identified by Berry [17] as separation, assimilation, integration, and marginalization, refer to ways of adapting to the new culture. However, as the acculturation mode of marginalization can be considered as a psychopathological process rather than an acculturation mode [14], only separation, assimilation, and integration are included in the model. These three modes of acculturation are considered as mediating variables in connecting the MITA model's psychological constructs to the output variables. In this mediating situation, intentions to return to homeland predict separation and separation predicts socio-cultural adjustment as well as mental health. Intercultural competence predicts integration and integration predicts socio-cultural adjustment as well as mental health. Social–emotional competence predicts assimilation and assimilation predicts socio-cultural adjustment. Experience of traumatic events predicts separation and separation predicts socio-cultural adjustment.

2.6. Mental Health

Psychological health during the acculturation process is a common goal of refugees and host countries [64]. Refugees, especially adolescent refugees, are of particular interest, as they are arguably the most at-risk group for mental disorders among all immigrants [65]. Adolescent refugees might experience acculturative stress when being confronted with different languages, dressing styles, or eating habits [66]. Hence, adolescent refugees often suffer from mental disorders such as depression, anxiety, and in some cases psychosis [52,67]. There are numerous studies examining the mental health issues experienced by refugee children and adolescents, and all of them have come to an agreement that the process of the resettlement can make them extremely vulnerable and fragile because of their underdevelopment of psycho-social and coping skills [68], inability to handle and manage certain life events, dependency, and incomplete biological development [62]. As almost half the world's refugee population includes children and adolescents [2], to clarify the process of acculturation, any model of acculturation specific to adolescent refugees should ultimately be involved with the state of psychological health. Therefore, mental health as an outcome variable is added to the MITA model.

2.7. Socio-Cultural Adjustment

In general, adjustment refers to the changes which occur in oneself (such as thoughts, emotions, actions, strategies) and the interaction that facilitates the process of adaptation [17,18]. Socio-cultural adjustment is a behavioral as well as a practical feature of adapting to a host culture. Socio-cultural adjustment can be defined as an ability to fit in properly or interact with members of the host culture, effectively [32].

During the process of acculturation, socio-cultural adjustment can be challenging. Some factors, such as cultural distance, quantity and quality of social interactions with both host and heritage cultures, acculturation attitudes toward the host society, intercultural training, emotional skills (e.g., emotional regulation), social skills (conversational skills), behavioral skills (e.g., assertiveness, empathy), previous cross-cultural experiences [69], interest in the host culture's national events, and sharing interest and friendships with members of the host culture [32,69] were found to be combined with socio-cultural adjustment. Therefore, in the MITA model, the socio-cultural adjustment is added as an outcome variable which is predicted from intercultural competence, social–emotional competence and intentions to return to the homeland. In the mediating situation, the connection between intentions to return to the homeland and socio-cultural adjustment is mediated by separation. Integration mediates the connection between intercultural competence and socio-cultural adjustment. Social–emotional competence predicts assimilation and assimilation predicts socio-cultural adjustment. Experience of traumatic events predicts separation and separation predicts socio-cultural adjustment.

2.8. Out-Group Social Support/In-Group Social Support

In general, social support may have a remarkable influence on the mental state. A high amount of available social support in the new culture and the nature of the host society can have a considerable effect on minimizing acculturative stress and empower individuals to handle the difficulties of living in a diverse environment [70,71]. Availability of support systems is an important post-migration factor that can facilitate successful adaptation for adolescent refugees even when they have gone through traumatic experiences [72–74]. Conversely, a lack of social support can be related to a poor psychological adaptation [75,76]. With respect to the positive effect of social support, the connection with the close ethnic groups has been found to have a positive effect on mental health in children and adolescents [77,78]. Furnham and Bochner [79] reported an opposite relationship between the prevalence of mental disorders and the perceived social support from the members of the heritage culture. The protective nature of positive peer relationships, as well as good parental mental health, have been highlighted in various studies [74,80–82]. Adolescent refugees in close contact with their nuclear families and close family members showed less emotional distress and greater adjustment than those who survived the refugee process alone [82].

Therefore, in the proposed model, out-group and in-group social support are added as moderated mediating variables to affect the connection between intercultural and social–emotional competence/experiences of traumatic events and modes of acculturation. In this moderated mediating situation, out-group social support affects the connection between intercultural and social–emotional competence and integration as well as assimilation. In-group social support affects the connection between the experience of traumatic events and assimilation. Moreover, in-group social support and out-group social support are also considered as moderating variables in connecting the experience of traumatic events to mental health.

3. Discussion

Overall, the MITA model proposes that two major concerns of adolescent refugees, including socio-cultural adjustment and mental health, are predicted by intercultural as well as social–emotional competence, intentions to return to the homeland, and experiences of traumatic events. In addition to the direct influence of intercultural competence, social–emotional competence, intentions to return to the homeland, and experiences of traumatic events on mental health and socio-cultural adjustment, the effects of three modes of acculturation (integration, separation, and assimilation) are also proposed in the model. It is expected that these variables mediate the effects of intercultural competence, social–emotional competence, intentions to return to the homeland, and experiences of traumatic events on socio-cultural adjustment as well as mental health.

Moreover, the direct connection between intercultural and social–emotional competence/experiences of traumatic events and the three modes of acculturation is influenced by two variables, including out-group social support and in-group social support. It is expected that these two variables would play some moderated mediating roles in linking intercultural competence, social–emotional competence, and experiences of traumatic events to modes of acculturation. Finally, it is also expected that in-group social support and out-group social support moderate the direct connection between experiences of traumatic events and mental health. This proposed model can help researchers in the domain to understand adolescent refugees' behaviors, lifestyle, and beliefs in different ethnicities by evaluating aspects of intercultural and social–emotional competence, which are not addressed in current acculturation models. For instance, considering intentions to return to the homeland, our proposed model can clarify the reasons why adolescent refugees with different ethnicities and socio-cultural characteristics may select different acculturation strategies, even when they live in the same society. Moreover, using intercultural and social–emotional competence, the model can explain why adolescent refugees from the same countries and socio-cultural backgrounds or even same families may choose different acculturation strategies. At the clinical level, this model highlights socio-cultural reasons behind some mental health problems among adolescent refugees. The relationship between acculturation strategies and the social traditions in the host society can explain why adolescent refugees get involved with psychological problems. Besides, for intervention purposes, it can help clinicians to apply some special training programs involving the socio-cultural characteristics of adolescent refugees (e.g., group intercultural competence training [56]). Despite the theoretical evidence, a great deal of applied and basic research is still required to test the fundamental assumptions of the MITA model.

4. Limitations of the MITA model

Because of the nature of this concept paper, the proposed MITA model has not been tested yet, and therefore, its factors should be taken with caution and viewed as hypotheses. Moreover, time is not explicitly considered in the proposed model: levels of intercultural and social–emotional competence, intentions to return to the homeland, and their relations with the modes of acculturation as well as socio-cultural adjustment and mental health may vary with the length of residency in the host country. Finally, the levels of connections among the variables in the proposed model are mostly defined according to monocultural societies (or societies that promote monoculturalism). Therefore, the relations among the variables might differ in multicultural societies.

5. Implications for Future Research

In the future, the proposed model should be tested and validated empirically. Furthermore, the model should be tested using samples of refugee adolescents from different ethnicities (e.g., such as those of African, Indian, Asian, and Pakistani origin). This would be an important step in assuring the contribution of the present model to acculturation processes and the intercultural and social–emotional competence of various ethnicities. Finally, it is essential to test the MITA model and especially its proposed moderators and mediators over time in various countries with different approaches to culture, for example with Canadian multiculturalism and German monoculturalism.

6. Conclusions

To the best of our knowledge, no research study has been accomplished on establishing an acculturation model specific to adolescent refugees connecting social–emotional and intercultural competence, the experience of traumatic events, and intentions to return to the homeland to mental health as a psychological outcome, and socio-cultural adjustment as a behavioral outcome using acculturation attitudes as mediating variables and in-group/out-group social support as moderating as well as moderated mediating variables. In this sense, the MITA model is best regarded as exploratory, with further investigation required.

Author Contributions: A.F. designed the MITA model and wrote the paper; U.E.-A. commented on the manuscript and the MITA model, T.R. commented on the manuscript as well as the MITA model and lead the project; F.P. commented on the manuscript as well as the MITA model and supervised the project. All authors discussed the components in the MITA model and commented on the manuscript at all stages.

Funding: The research was supported by the Porticus Foundation.

Conflicts of Interest: The authors declare no conflicts of interest.

References

1. United Nations Population Fund-UNFPA. *232 Million International Migrants Living Abroad Worldwide-New UN Global Migration Statistics Reveal*; UN Department of Public Information: New York, NY, USA, 2018.
2. Bundesamt Für Migration und Flüchtlinge. *Aktuelle Zahlen zu Asyl. Den Menschen im Blick. Schützen. Integrieren*; Bundesamt Für Migration und Flüchtlinge: Nuremberg, Germany, 2017.
3. Reinelt, T.; Vasileva, M.; Petermann, F. Refugee children's mental health problems: Beyond posttraumatic stress disorder. *Kindheit und Entwicklung* **2016**, *25*, 231–237. [CrossRef]
4. Berry, J.W.; Phinney, J.S.; Sam, D.L.; Vedder, P. Immigrant youth: Acculturation, identity, and adaptation. *Appl. Psychol. Int. Rev.* **2006**, *55*, 303–332. [CrossRef]
5. Berry, J.W. Acculturation: Living successfully in two cultures. *Int. J. Intercult. Relat.* **2005**, *29*, 697–712. [CrossRef]
6. Reinelt, T.; Schipper, M.; Petermann, F. Different Pathways to Resilience: On the utility of the resilience concept in clinical child psychology and child psychiatry. *Kindheit und Entwicklung* **2016**, *25*, 189–199. [CrossRef]
7. Ragelienė, T. Links of Adolescents Identity Development and Relationship with Peers: A Systematic Literature Review. *J. Can. Acad. Child Adolesc. Psychiatry* **2016**, *25*, 97–105.
8. Schwartz, S.J.; Unger, J.B.; Zamboanga, B.L.; Szapocznik, J. Rethinking the Concept of Acculturation. Implications for Theory and Research. *Am. Psychol.* **2010**, *65*, 237–251. [CrossRef] [PubMed]
9. Nickerson, A.; Bryant, R.A.; Silove, D.; Steel, Z. A critical review of psychological treatments of posttraumatic stress disorder in refugees. *Clin. Psychol. Rev.* **2011**, *31*, 399–417. [CrossRef] [PubMed]
10. Nitkowski, D.; Laakmann, M.; Petersen, R.; Petermann, U.J.; Petermann, F. Emotion Training with Students: An effectiveness study concerning the relation between subjective well-being, emotional awareness, and emotion expression. *Kindheit und Entwicklung* **2017**, *26*, 175–183. [CrossRef]
11. Anders, M.; Christiansen, H. Unaccompanied refugee minors: A systematic review of psychological interventions. *Kindheit und Entwicklung* **2016**, *25*, 216–230. [CrossRef]
12. Petermann, F.; Petermann, U. Refugee Minors. *Kindheit und Entwicklung* **2016**, *25*, 201–203. [CrossRef]
13. Norhayati, Z. The effects of cross-cultural training on the acculturation process of the global workforce. *Int. J. Manpower* **2000**, *21*, 492–510. [CrossRef]
14. Safdar, S.; Lay, C.; Struthers, W. The process of acculturation and basic goals: Testing a multidimensional individual difference acculturation model with Iranian immigrants in Canada. *Appl. Psychol. Int. Rev.* **2003**, *52*, 555–579. [CrossRef]
15. Navas, M.; Rojas, A.J.; García, M.; Pumares, P. Acculturation strategies and attitudes according to the Relative Acculturation Extended Model (RAEM): The perspectives of natives versus immigrants. *Int. J. Intercult. Relat.* **2007**, *31*, 67–86. [CrossRef]
16. Rudmin, F.W. Constructs, measurements and models of acculturation and acculturative stress. *Int. J. Intercult. Relat.* **2009**, *33*, 106–123. [CrossRef]
17. Berry, J.W. Immigration, acculturation, and adaptation. *Appl. Psychol.* **1997**, *46*, 5–68. [CrossRef]
18. Berry, J.W.; Kim, U.; Power, S.; Young, M.; Bujaki, M. Acculturation Attitudes in Plural Societies. *J. Appl. Psychol.* **1989**, *38*, 185–206. [CrossRef]

19. Berry, J.W. Mutual intercultural relations among immigrants and ethnocultural groups in Canada. *Int. J. Intercult. Relat.* **2006**, *30*, 719–734. [CrossRef]
20. Ward, C.; Kennedy, A. Acculturation strategies, psychosocial adjustment, and sociocultural competence during cross-cultural transitions. *Int. J. Intercult. Relat.* **1994**, *18*, 329–343. [CrossRef]
21. Piontkowski, U.; Florack, A.; Hölker, P.; Obdzrálek, P. Predicting acculturation attitudes of dominant and non-dominant groups. *Int. J. Intercult. Relat.* **2000**, *24*, 1–26. [CrossRef]
22. Schwartz, S.J.; Zamboanga, B.L. Testing Berry's Model of Acculturation: A Confirmatory Latent Class Approach. *Cult. Divers. Ethn. Minor. Psychol.* **2008**, *14*, 275–285. [CrossRef] [PubMed]
23. Ward, C.; Leong, C.; Low, M. Personality and sojourner adjustment: An explanation of the Big Five and the cultural fit position. *J. Cross-Cult. Psychol.* **2004**, *35*, 137–151. [CrossRef]
24. Berry, J.W.; Kim, U.; Minde, T.; Mok, D. Comparative studies of acculturative stress. *Int. Migr. Rev.* **1987**, *21*, 491–511. [CrossRef]
25. Rudmin, F.W. Critical History of the Acculturation Psychology of Assimilation, Separation, Integration, and Marginalization. *Rev. Gen. Psychol.* **2003**, *7*, 3–37. [CrossRef]
26. Castro, J.F.P. Acculturation in the Portuguese overseas experience with Japan: A Rudmin Model application. *Daxiyangguo: Revista Portuguesa de Estudos Asiáticos* **2016**, *20*, 89–120.
27. Safdar, S.; Struthers, W.; van Oudenhoven, P.J. Acculturation of Iranians in the United States, the United Kingdom, and the Netherlands: A test of multidimensional individual difference acculturation model. *J. Cross-Cult. Psychol.* **2009**, *40*, 468–491. [CrossRef]
28. Safdar, S.; Calvez, S.; Lewis, J.R. Multi-group analysis of the MIDA model: Acculturation of Indian and Russian immigrants in Canada. *Int. J. Intercult. Relat.* **2017**, *36*, 200–212. [CrossRef]
29. Rudmin, F.W.; Villemo, C.; Olsen, B. Acculturation of the majority population: How Norwegians adopt minority ways. *Psykologisk Tidsskrift* **2007**, *11*, 43–51.
30. Sierles, F.S. Using film as the basis of an American culture course for first-year psychiatry residents. *Acad. Psychiatry* **2005**, *29*, 100–104. [CrossRef] [PubMed]
31. Osman-Gani, A.M.; Rockstuhl, T. Cross-cultural training, expatriate self-efficacy, and adjustments to overseas assignments: An empirical investigation of managers in Asia. *Int. J. Intercult. Relat.* **2009**, *33*, 277–290. [CrossRef]
32. Searle, W.; Ward, C. The prediction of psychological and sociocultural adjustment during cross cultural transitions. *Int. J. Intercult. Relat.* **1990**, *14*, 449–464. [CrossRef]
33. Hammer, M.R.; Bennett, M.J.; Wiseman, R. Measuring intercultural sensitivity: The intercultural development inventory. *Int. J. Intercult. Relat.* **2003**, *27*, 421–443. [CrossRef]
34. Bar-Tal, D. *Prosocial Behavior: Theory and Research*; Hemisphere Publishing Corp: Washington, DC, USA, 1976; pp. 154–196.
35. Gross, J.J. The Emerging Field of Emotion Regulation: An Integrative Review. *Rev. Gen. Psychol.* **1998**, *2*, 271–299. [CrossRef]
36. Arasaratnam, L.A. The development of a new instrument of intercultural communication competence. *J. Intercult. Commun.* **2009**, *20*, 1404–1634.
37. Rohmann, A.; Piontkowski, U.; van Randenborgh, A. When Attitudes Do Not Fit: Discordance of Acculturation Attitudes as an Antecedent of Intergroup Threat. *Personal. Soc. Psychol. Bull.* **2008**, *34*, 337–352. [CrossRef] [PubMed]
38. Steiner, I. Spatial selectivity and demographic impact of recent German immigrants in the Swiss regions. *Eur. Reg.* **2014**, *19*, 56–68.
39. Triandis, H.C.; Gelfland, M.J. Converging measurement of horizontal and vertical individualism and collectivism. *J. Personal. Soc. Psychol.* **1998**, *74*, 118–128. [CrossRef]
40. Shore, C. Audit culture and Illiberal governance. *Anthropol. Theor.* **2008**, *8*, 278–298. [CrossRef]
41. Fiske, S.T. Prejudices in Cultural Contexts: Shared Stereotypes (Gender, Age) Versus Variable Stereotypes (Race, Ethnicity, Religion). *Perspect. Psychol. Sci.* **2017**, *12*, 791–799. [CrossRef] [PubMed]
42. Garg, N.; Schiebinger, L.; Jurafsky, D.; Zou, J. Word embeddings quantify 100 years of gender and ethnic stereotypes. *Proc. Natl. Acad. Sci. USA* **2018**, *115*, E3635–E3644. [CrossRef] [PubMed]
43. Spencer, S.J.; Logel, C.; Davies, P.G. Stereotype Threat. *Annu. Rev. Psychol.* **2016**, *67*, 415–437. [CrossRef] [PubMed]

44. Frank, D.W.; Dewitt, M.; Hudgens-Haney, M.E.; Schaeffer, D.J.; Ball, B.H.; Schwarz, N.F.; Hussein, A.A.; Smart, L.M.; Sabatinelli, D. Emotion regulation: Quantitative meta-analysis of functional activation and deactivation. *Neurosci. Biobehav. Rev.* **2014**, *45*, 202–211. [CrossRef] [PubMed]
45. Gross, J.J. Emotion regulation: Affective, cognitive, and social consequences. *Psychophysiology* **2002**, *39*, 281–291. [CrossRef] [PubMed]
46. Mauss, I.B.; Cook, C.L.; Cheng, J.Y.; Gross, J.J. Individual differences in cognitive reappraisal: Experiential and physiological responses to an anger provocation. *Int. J. Psychophysiol.* **2007**, *66*, 116–124. [CrossRef] [PubMed]
47. Memedovic, S.; Grisham, J.R.; Denson, T.F.; Molds, M.L. The effects of trait reappraisal and suppression on anger and blood pressure in response to provocation. *J. Res. Personal.* **2010**, *44*, 540–543. [CrossRef]
48. Shorey, R.C.; Cornelius, T.L.; Idema, C. Trait anger as a mediator of difficulties with emotion regulation and female-perpetrated psychological aggression. *Violence Vict.* **2011**, *26*, 271–282. [CrossRef] [PubMed]
49. Denson, T.F.; Moulds, M.L.; Grisham, J.R. The effects of analytical rumination, reappraisal, and distraction on anger experience. *Behav. Ther.* **2012**, *43*, 355–364. [CrossRef] [PubMed]
50. Szasz, P.L.; Szentagotai, A.; Hofmann, S.G. The effect of emotion regulation strategies on anger. *Behav. Res. Ther.* **2011**, *49*, 114–119. [CrossRef] [PubMed]
51. Carswell, K.; Blackburn, P.; Barker, C. The relationship between trauma, post-migration problems and the psychological well-being of refugees and asylum seekers. *Int. J. Soc. Psychiatry* **2011**, *57*, 107–119. [CrossRef] [PubMed]
52. Saarni, C. Children's emotional-expressive behaviors as regulators of others' happy and sad states. *New Dir. Child Dev.* **1992**, *55*, 91–106. [CrossRef]
53. Hein, S.; Röder, M.; Fingerle, M. The role of emotion regulation in situational empathy-related responding and prosocial behaviour in the presence of negative effect. *Int. J. Psychol.* **2016**, *10*, 19–28. [CrossRef]
54. Lockwood, P.L.; Seara-Cardoso, A.; Viding, E. Emotion Regulation Moderates the Association between Empathy and Prosocial Behavior. *PLoS ONE* **2014**, *9*, e96555. [CrossRef] [PubMed]
55. Lu, M. Determinants of Residential Satisfaction: Ordered Logit vs. Regression Models. *Growth Chang.* **1999**, *30*, 264–287. [CrossRef]
56. EL-Awad, U.; Fathi, A.; Petermann, F.; Reinelt, T. Promoting Mental Health in Unaccompanied Refugee Minors: Recommendations for Primary Support Programs. *Brain Sci.* **2017**, *7*, 146. [CrossRef] [PubMed]
57. McCormick, B.; Wahba, J. Overseas Work Experience, Savings and Entrepreneurship amongst Return Migrants to LDCs. *Scott. J. Political Econ.* **2001**, *48*, 164–178. [CrossRef]
58. Chirkov, V.I.; Vansteenkiste, M.; Tao, R.; Lynch, M. The role of self-determined motivation and goals for study abroad in the adaptation of international students. *Int. J. Intercult. Relat.* **2007**, *31*, 199–222. [CrossRef]
59. Dentakos, S.; Wintre, M.; Chavoshi, S.; Wright, L. Acculturation Motivation in International Student Adjustment and Permanent Residency Intentions: A Mixed-Methods Approach. *Emerg. Adulthood* **2017**, *5*, 27–41. [CrossRef]
60. Fazel, M.; Reed, R.V.; Panter-Brick, C.; Stein, A. Mental health of displaced and refugee children resettled in high-income countries: Risk and protective factors. *Lancet* **2012**, *379*, 266–282. [CrossRef]
61. Kira, I.A.; Lewandowski, L.; Chiodo, L.; Ibrahim, A. Advances in systemic trauma theory: Traumatogenic dynamics and consequences of backlash as a multi-systemic trauma on Iraqi refugee Muslim adolescents. *Psychology* **2014**, *5*, 389–412. [CrossRef]
62. Kocijan-Hercigonja, D.; Rijavec, M.; Marusic, A.; Hercigonja, V. Coping strategies of refugee, displaced, and non-displaced children in a war area. *Nordic J. Psychiatry* **1998**, *52*, 45–50. [CrossRef]
63. Daud, A.; af Klinteberg, B.; Rydelius, P.A. Resilience and vulnerability among refugee children of traumatized and non-traumatized parents. *Child Adolesc. Psychiatry Ment. Health* **2008**, *2*, 7. [CrossRef] [PubMed]
64. Ellis, B.H.; Miller, A.B.; Baldwin, H.; Abdi, S. New Directions in Refugee Youth Mental Health Services: Overcoming Barriers to Engagement. *J. Child Adolesc. Trauma* **2011**, *4*, 69–85. [CrossRef]
65. Motti-Stefanidi, F.; Asendorpf, J.B.; Masten, A.S. The adaptation and well-being of adolescent immigrants in Greek schools: A multilevel, longitudinal study of risks and resources. *Dev. Psychol.* **2012**, *24*, 451–473. [CrossRef] [PubMed]
66. Sam, D.L.; Berry, J.W. *Cambridge Handbook of Acculturation Psychology*; Cambridge University Press: Cambridge, UK, 2006; pp. 132–170.

67. Hovey, J.D. Acculturative Stress, Depression, and Suicidal Ideation among Central American Immigrants. *Suicide Life-Threat. Behav.* **2000**, *30*, 125–139. [CrossRef]
68. Ajdukovic, M.; Ajdukovic, D. Impact of displacement on the psychological well-being of refugee children. *Int. Rev. Psychiatry* **1998**, *10*, 186–195. [CrossRef]
69. Ward, C.; Kennedy, A. Psychological and Socio-Cultural Adjustment during Cross-Cultural Transitions: A Comparison of Secondary Students Overseas and at Home. *Int. J. Psychol.* **2007**, *28*, 129–147. [CrossRef]
70. Jerusalem, M.; Hahn, A.; Schwarzer, R. Social bonding and loneliness after network disruption: A longitudinal study of East German refugees. *Soc. Indic. Res.* **1996**, *38*, 229–243. [CrossRef]
71. Kok, J.K.; Lee, M.N.; Low, S.K. Coping abilities and social support of Myanmar teenage refugees in Malaysia. *Vulnerable Child. Youth Stud. Int. Interdiscip. J. Res. Policy Care* **2016**, *12*, 71–80. [CrossRef]
72. Fox, P.G.; Cowell, M.J.; Montgomery, A.C. The effects of violence on health and adjustment of Southeast Asian refugee children: An integrative review. *Public Health Nurs.* **1994**, *11*, 195–201. [CrossRef] [PubMed]
73. Renner, W.; Laireiter, A.-R.; Maier, M.J. Social support as a moderator of acculturative stress among refugees and asylum seekers. *Soc. Behav. Personal.* **2012**, *40*, 129–146. [CrossRef]
74. Wong, C.W.S.; Schweitzer, R.D. Individual, premigration and postsettlement factors, and academic achievement in adolescents from refugee backgrounds: A systematic review and model. *Transcult. Psychiatry* **2017**, *54*, 756–782. [CrossRef] [PubMed]
75. Jupp, J.J.; Luckey, J. Educational experiences in Australia of indo-Chinese adolescent refugees. *Int. J. Ment. Health* **1990**, *18*, 78–91. [CrossRef]
76. Kovacev, L.; Shute, R. Acculturation and social support in relation to psychosocial adjustment of adolescent refugees resettled in Australia. *Int. J. Behav. Dev.* **2004**, *28*, 259–267. [CrossRef]
77. Betancourt, T.S.; Salhi, C.; Buka, S.; Leaning, J.; Dunn, G.; Earls, F. Connectedness, social support and internalizing emotional and behavioral problems in adolescents displaced by the Chechen conflict. *Disasters* **2012**, *36*, 635–655. [CrossRef] [PubMed]
78. Rousseau, C.; Said, T.M.; Gagné, M.J.; Bibeau, G. Resilience in unaccompanied minors from the north of Somalia. *Psychoanal. Rev.* **1998**, *85*, 615–637. [PubMed]
79. Furnham, A.; Bochner, S. *Culture Shock, Psychological Reactions to Unfamiliar Environment*; Routledge: London, UK, 1990; pp. 110–156.
80. Almqvist, K.; Broberg, A.G. Mental health and social adjustment in young refugee children 3 1/2 years after their arrival in Sweden. *J. Am. Acad. Child Adolesc. Psychiatry* **1999**, *38*, 723–730. [CrossRef] [PubMed]
81. Simich, L.; Beiser, M.; Mawani, F.N. Social Support and the Significance of Shared Experience in Refugee Migration and Resettlement. *West. J. Nurs. Res.* **2003**, *25*, 872–891. [CrossRef] [PubMed]
82. Weine, S. Family Roles in Refugee Youth Resettlement from a Prevention Perspective. *Child Adolesc. Psychiatr. Clin. N. Am.* **2012**, *17*, 515–518. [CrossRef] [PubMed]

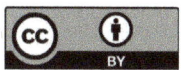

© 2018 by the authors. Licensee MDPI, Basel, Switzerland. This article is an open access article distributed under the terms and conditions of the Creative Commons Attribution (CC BY) license (http://creativecommons.org/licenses/by/4.0/).

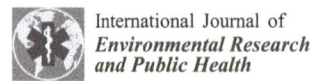

Commentary

Linkage to Care Is Important and Necessary When Identifying Infections in Migrants

Manish Pareek [1,2,*], Teymur Noori [3], Sally Hargreaves [4,5] and Maria van den Muijsenbergh [6,7]

1. Department of Infection, Immunity and Inflammation, University of Leicester, Leicester, LE1 7RH, UK
2. Department of Infection and Tropical Medicine, University Hospitals Leicester NHS Trust, Leicester LE1 5WW, UK
3. European Centre for Disease Prevention and Control, 16973 Solna, Sweden; Teymur.Noori@ecdc.europa.eu
4. Section of Infectious Diseases and Immunity, Department of Medicine, Imperial College London, Hammersmith Hospital, London W12 0HS, UK; s.hargreaves@imperial.ac.uk
5. The Institute for Infection and Immunity, St George's, University of London, London WC1E 7HU, UK
6. Department of Primary and Community Care, Radboud University Medical Center, 6525 GA Nijmegen, The Netherlands; Maria.vandenMuijsenbergh@radboudumc.nl
7. Pharos, Dutch Centre of Expertise on Health Disparities, 3507 LH Utrecht, The Netherlands
* Correspondence: mp426@le.ac.uk

Received: 23 June 2018; Accepted: 17 July 2018; Published: 22 July 2018

Abstract: Migration is an important driver of population dynamics in Europe. Although migrants are generally healthy, subgroups of migrants are at increased risk of a range of infectious diseases. Early identification of infections is important as it prevents morbidity and mortality. However, identifying infections needs to be supported by appropriate systems to link individuals to specialist care where they can receive further diagnostic tests and clinical management. In this commentary we will discuss the importance of linkage to care and how to minimise attrition in clinical pathways.

Keywords: migration; health; infection; linkage; care

Migration is an important driver of population dynamics in Europe with numbers of both internal (European Union) and external, both regular and irregular, migrants increasing over the last few decades [1]. Although the types of migrants arriving to Europe is highly diverse, in general, the majority of migrants are healthy [2]. However, there are subgroups of migrants arriving from low- and middle-income countries who bear a disproportionate burden of a range of infectious diseases—in particular HIV, tuberculosis (TB), multi-drug resistant TB, and hepatitis B and C (both undiagnosed and previously diagnosed but not treated). Whilst our understanding of infectious diseases and migrant health has improved, there is still a gap in the evidence-base relating to migrants in Europe. Nonetheless, the reasons for the higher prevalence of these infections in migrant populations appear to include, amongst many, a higher prevalence of infection in their countries of origin, low levels of screening and vaccination, increased levels of post-migration acquisition of certain infections (for example HIV) [3–5], barriers to healthcare on arrival, and low socioeconomic status [2]; however, further studies in European settings relating to the prevalence of infections and reasons for the higher prevalence (including sexual behaviour with respect to post-migration HIV acquisition) are required. As a matter of equity it is important that clinicians and policy-makers, in partnership with migrant communities, consider the specific and different needs of migrants when developing screening and vaccination programmes to reduce the burden of infection.

Identifying infectious diseases early is important as it mitigates adverse clinical outcomes and in some instances onward transmission; yet considerable heterogeneity exists across Europe as to how to approach migrant screening, and it is as yet unclear what represents a cost-effective approach [6,7]. Implementing migrant screening requires a clear understanding of how to screen migrants, where screening should happen (transit, arrival, or post-arrival) and the costs of having the testing done. In response, the European Centre for Disease Prevention and Control are developing evidence-based guidance on infectious disease screening for migrants [8]. This guidance, the product of intense work with key infectious disease experts across the European Union, will help to inform policy-makers and front-line clinicians on how to approach implementation of screening and vaccination in newly arrived migrants.

Integral to the development of the European Centre for Disease Prevention and Control (ECDC) guidance is an understanding of the importance of, and interventions for, each element of the care pathway from access to appropriate health services, to testing/screening, and then to follow-up treatment through to treatment completion and/or adherence.

We know from previous work relating to a range of infections that post-testing cascades of care occur with drop-out at each point in the clinical pathway including a failure to get results after testing, failure to attend specialist services to commence treatment, and failure to complete treatment [9]; data for migrants is less clear [10] but the principle remains the same—drop-outs in the post-screening/diagnostic testing services need to be minimised.

Drop-outs at each step of the care pathway (both in terms of attendance but also poor adherence to medication) can be caused by the plethora of personal and system-level barriers migrants may face in accessing statutory health/appropriate health services on arrival and subsequently, due to the lack of clarity about the organisation and financing of care compounded by linguistic and cultural barriers [11]. Many vulnerable migrant groups are not entitled to free statutory health care on arrival which will undoubtedly impact on uptake of screening and attendance at specialist services. Additional concerns for new migrants to European countries include competing psycho-social priorities such as housing, employment, concerns about family reunion, relationships, mental health issues, and chronic diseases. These problems not only interfere with testing, but also have the potential to increase the risks or consequences of infectious diseases. This synergistic interaction linked to socially disadvantaged circumstances, known as syndemics, calls for an integrated approach of public health and primary care, addressing biomedical as well as psychosocial problems [12].

Therefore, it is important that ease of access, making health services responsive, and engaging migrant communities is considered at an early stage when developing clinical pathways relating to screening for infection and appropriate vaccination. Engagement includes providing the necessary information and tailoring services to the needs and possibilities of the migrants involved [13]. Whilst this early work may seem less important, it likely sets in motion the basis for future community engagement, co-development of services, rapport and trust—particularly important when dealing with individuals who come from often marginalised and neglected communities.

Pathways of care should be designed with an understanding that the method in which the offer/rationale of testing is framed may well impact on whether individuals accept testing as well as how they view the subsequent result and, if necessary, follow-up with specialist care. Testing on its own achieves relatively little for the migrant with an infection if they do not attend follow-up and complete the necessary treatment. It is critical to always bear in mind that testing for infections is only one element of the migrants' care pathway. A decision to test, by necessity, equates to an intention/decision to refer for assessment and, if required, treat. It is the linkage from testing to referral and attendance for specialist care which requires care and attention when designing care pathways and providing appropriate levels of education and information to migrants and front-line healthcare professionals. One specific area to consider when designing pathways of care is to consider how to make them as simple as possible for the migrant, with many professionals keen to move beyond working in infection silos (for example just screening for TB) but to consider multiple infections and vaccination, alongside other health needs. This will require working more closely with migrant communities to ascertain their view and concerns, but certain elements should be incorporated [14]:

1. Collaboration between primary care, public health, and specialist care in order to ensure continuity of care tailored to all the needs of the person involved.

2. Single point-of-referral to a migrant-friendly clinical service with culturally competent staff that deal with migrants and infectious diseases (as well as other health needs). This clinic could be facilitated by being staffed by specialists with a broad range of skill-sets who can manage all infections alongside interpreters and other support services to support treatment adherence and completion.
3. Robust data collection to facilitate sharing of best practice with respect to linkage to care and treatment completion for migrants with infectious diseases.

Although the patterns of migration across Europe are highly mixed, a lack of good quality data and limited sharing of best practice means that it remains unclear how best to deliver screening, vaccination, and treatment to migrants arriving in Europe. Evidence-based guidance emphasising methods of implementation supported by appropriate resources and migrant communities' views have the potential to aid the design of stream-lined pathways of care for infectious diseases which address, and maximise, linkage to specialist care so that we have migrant services that meet the needs of a rapidly changing Europe.

Author Contributions: Conceptualization M.P., M.v.d.M., T.N., S.H.; Methodology M.P., M.v.d.M., T.N., S.H.; Draft preparation M.P. and M.v.d.M.; Writing-Review & Editing M.P., M.v.d.M., T.N., S.H.

Funding: This work is supported by the European Health Group and European Centre for Disease Prevention and Control (ECDC): FWC No ECDC/2015/016, Specific Contract No 1 ECD.5748. MP is supported by the National Institute for Health Research (NIHR Post-Doctoral Fellowship, Manish Pareek, PDF-2015-08-102). The views expressed in this publication are those of the author(s) and not necessarily those of the NHS, the National Institute for Health Research or the Department of Health. SH is funded by the Imperial NIHR Biomedical Research Centre, the Wellcome Trust (Grant number 209993/Z/17/Z), and the European Society for Clinical Microbiology and Infectious Diseases (ESCMID) through an ESCMID Study Group for Infections in Travellers and Migrants (ESGITM) research grant.

Acknowledgments: We thank the anonymous peer-reviewers for their helpful comments.

Conflicts of Interest: M.P. reports an institutional grant (unrestricted) for project related to blood-borne virus testing from Gilead Sciences outside the submitted work. All other authors report no conflict of interest.

References

1. United Nations Department of Economic and Social Affairs. *International Migration Report 2015*; United Nations Department of Economic and Social Affairs: Geneva, Switzerland, 2015.
2. European Centre for Disease Prevention and Control. *Migrant Health: Background Report to the ECDC Report on Migration and Infectious Diseases in the EU*; European Centre for Disease Prevention and Control: Stockholm, Sweden, 2009.
3. Alvarez-del Arco, D.; Fakoya, I.; Thomadakis, C.; Pantazis, N.; Touloumi, G.; Gennotte, A.-F.; Zuure, F.; Barros, H.; Staehelin, C.; Göpel, S.; et al. High levels of postmigration HIV acquisition within nine European countries. *AIDS* **2017**, *31*, 1979–1988. [CrossRef] [PubMed]
4. Desgrées-du-Loû, A.; Pannetier, J.; Ravalihasy, A.; Gosselin, A.; Supervie, V.; Panjo, H.; Bajos, N.; Lert, F.; Lydié, N.; Dray-Spira, R. Sub-Saharan African migrants living with HIV acquired after migration, France, ANRS PARCOURS study, 2012 to 2013. *Eurosurveillance* **2015**, *20*, 31–38. [CrossRef] [PubMed]
5. Marsicano, E.; Lydié, N.; Bajos, N. 'Migrants from over there' or 'racial minority here'? Sexual networks and prevention practices among sub-Saharan African migrants in France. *Cult. Health Sex.* **2013**, *15*, 819–835. [CrossRef] [PubMed]
6. Greenaway, C.; Pareek, M.; Abou Chakra, C.-N.; Walji, M.; Makarenko, I.; Alabdulkarim, B.; Hogan, C.; McConnell, T.; Scarfo, B.; Christensen, R.; et al. The effectiveness and cost-effectiveness of screening for active tuberculosis among migrants in the EU/EEA: A systematic review. *Eurosurveillance* **2018**, *23*, 170–542. [CrossRef] [PubMed]

7. Kärki, T.; Napoli, C.; Riccardo, F.; Fabiani, M.; Dente, M.G.; Carballo, M.; Noori, T.; Declich, S. Screening for Infectious Diseases among Newly Arrived Migrants in EU/EEA Countries—Varying Practices but Consensus on the Utility of Screening. *Int. J. Environ. Res. Public Health* **2014**, *11*, 11004–11014. [CrossRef] [PubMed]
8. Pottie, K.; Mayhew, A.D.; Morton, R.L.; Greenaway, C.; Akl, E.A.; Rahman, P.; Zenner, D.; Pareek, M.; Tugwell, P.; Welch, V.; et al. Prevention and assessment of infectious diseases among children and adult migrants arriving to the European Union/European Economic Association: A protocol for a suite of systematic reviews for public health and health systems. *BMJ Open* **2017**, *7*, e014608. [CrossRef] [PubMed]
9. Alsdurf, H.; Hill, P.C.; Matteelli, A.; Getahun, H.; Menzies, D. The cascade of care in diagnosis and treatment of latent tuberculosis infection: A systematic review and meta-analysis. *Lancet Infect. Dis.* **2016**, *16*, 1269–1278. [CrossRef]
10. Nellums, L.B.; Rustage, K.; Hargreaves, S.; Friedland, J.S. Multidrug-resistant tuberculosis treatment adherence in migrants: A systematic review and meta-analysis. *BMC Med.* **2018**, *16*, 27. [CrossRef] [PubMed]
11. van Loenen, T.; van den Muijsenbergh, M.; Hofmeester, M.; Dowrick, C.; van Ginneken, N.; Mechili, E.A.; Angelaki, A.; Ajdukovic, D.; Bakic, H.; Pavlic, D.R.; et al. Primary care for refugees and newly arrived migrants in Europe: A qualitative study on health needs, barriers and wishes. *Eur. J. Public Health* **2018**, *28*, 82–87. [CrossRef] [PubMed]
12. Singer, M.; Bulled, N.; Ostrach, B.; Mendenhall, E. Syndemics and the biosocial conception of health. *Lancet* **2017**, *389*, 941–950. [CrossRef]
13. Van den Muijsenbergh, M.; van Weel-Baumgarten, E.; Burns, N.; O'Donnell, C.; Mair, F.; Spiegel, W.; Lionis, C.; Dowrick, C.; O'Reilly-de Brún, M.; de Brun, T.; et al. Communication in cross-cultural consultations in primary care in Europe: The case for improvement. The rationale for the RESTORE FP 7 project. *Prim. Health Care Res. Dev.* **2013**, *15*, 122–133. [CrossRef] [PubMed]
14. Pareek, M.; Greenaway, C.; Noori, T.; Munoz, J.; Zenner, D. NIHR PDF-2015-08-102: Impact, acceptability and cost-effectiveness of identifying infectious diseases amongst migrants in primary care. *BMC Med.* **2016**, *14*, 48.

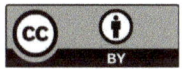

© 2018 by the authors. Licensee MDPI, Basel, Switzerland. This article is an open access article distributed under the terms and conditions of the Creative Commons Attribution (CC BY) license (http://creativecommons.org/licenses/by/4.0/).

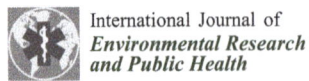

Review

A Systematic Review of Sexual and Reproductive Health Knowledge, Experiences and Access to Services among Refugee, Migrant and Displaced Girls and Young Women in Africa

Olena Ivanova [1,*], Masna Rai [1] and Elizabeth Kemigisha [2]

1. Division of Infectious Diseases and Tropical Medicine, Medical Centre of the University of Munich (LMU), 80802 Munich, Germany; masnarai11@gmail.com
2. Faculty of Interdisciplinary Studies, Mbarara University of Science and Technology, P.O. Box 1410, Mbarara, Uganda; ekemigisha@must.ac.ug
* Correspondence: olena.ivanova@lrz.uni-muenchen.de

Received: 28 June 2018; Accepted: 23 July 2018; Published: 26 July 2018

Abstract: Adolescent girls and young women are an overlooked group within conflict- or disaster-affected populations, and their sexual and reproductive health (SRH) needs are often neglected. Existing evidence shows that forced migration and human mobility make girls and women more vulnerable to poor SRH outcomes such as high risk sexual behaviors, lack of contraception use, STIs and HIV/AIDS. We performed a systematic literature review to explore knowledge, experiences and access to SRH services in this population group across the African continent. Two databases (PubMed and Web of Science) were searched and from 896 identified publications, 15 peer-reviewed articles published in English met the inclusion criteria for this review. These consisted of eight applied qualitative, five quantitative and two mixed-method study designs. The quality of the studies was evaluated by the mixed-methods appraisal tool (MMAT) using scores in percentages (0–100%). Available evidence indicates that knowledge of young women and girls regarding contraceptive methods, STIs and HIV/AIDS are limited. This population group often experiences gender-based and sexual violence and abuse. The access and availability of SRH services are often limited due to distances, costs and stigma. This review demonstrates that there is still a dearth of peer-reviewed literature on SRH related aspects among refugee, migrant and displaced girls and young women in Africa. The data disaggregation by sex and age should be emphasized for future research in this field.

Keywords: sexual and reproductive health; adolescent; refugee; migrant; young women; knowledge; access; experiences; systematic review; Africa

---

1. Introduction

Every year, thousands of people around the world flee their homes to escape conflict, disasters and violence within their own country or by crossing international borders. During these humanitarian emergencies, refugees and internally displaced persons (IDPs) suffer a great pressure which affects their health. Adolescent girls and young women (10–24 years old) are an overlooked group within conflict- or disaster-affected populations, and their sexual and reproductive health (SRH) needs remain largely unmet [1]. As such, the synergy of crisis as well as the neglect of SRH needs, increases vulnerability of adolescent girls to unwanted pregnancies, HIV and sexually transmitted infections (STIs), maternal death and sexual violence [2–4]. Adolescent girls in humanitarian settings experience increased exposure to early and forced marriage, coerced sex and early childbearing, as well as increased risk-taking associated with gender roles in family circles [5]. The girls in refugee camps are also vulnerable to sexual exploitation and trafficking [6].

Use and knowledge of SRH services and commodities, including family planning, are also often low among women and girls in humanitarian settings. One of the very few studies on this subject by McGinn et al. demonstrated that knowledge and use of modern contraceptive methods was low among married or in-union women of reproductive age in six reproductive health program locations (North Darfur, West Darfur, South Darfur, Southern Sudan, Northern Uganda and Eastern Congo) in three conflict-affected countries—Sudan, Uganda and the Democratic Republic of Congo [7].

The access to SRH services is challenging for young women and girls living in refugee settlements or dispersed across host countries. The minimum health care package in humanitarian setting requires inclusion of sexual and reproductive health services [8]. A systematic review by Casey et al. established that implementation of SRH programs is possible in a humanitarian setting, however their utilization depends on their quality [9]. Furthermore, the review highlighted minimal provision of adolescent SRH services [9]. In 2004 a global evaluation of reproductive health services for refugees and IDPs concluded that most people affected by conflict lack adequate SRH care [10]. The evaluation found that contraceptive methods offered were frequently limited to pills and condoms. Long-acting contraceptives or permanent methods were rarely offered, and for all methods, supplies were often not reliable. The evaluation also pointed that adolescents were often underserved [10]. Since then, much progress has been made in the field of SRH in crisis settings in terms of policy, guidance and practice and steps have been taken toward integrating SRH into humanitarian response including increased program funding to implement SRH services [11]. Nevertheless, most conflict-affected girls and women still do not have adequate access to SRH services with family planning services often being particularly neglected. From 2012 to 2014, the Inter-agency Working Group (IAWG) undertook a second global evaluation of reproductive health in humanitarian settings. One of the series of reviews and articles concluded that although services are being provided, the availability of good quality SRH services was inconsistent across different settings. There was still a limited knowledge of available services and socio-cultural barriers to accessing them among communities [12].

Although, the research on the SRH of conflict- and disaster-affected populations is gaining attention globally, there is very scarce information on the needs and experiences of young refugees and IDPs in humanitarian settings, who are likely to be at particularly high risk of adverse SRH outcomes. Enhancing the weak evidence base on needs and experiences of crisis-affected girls and women will provide the tools for the research community and humanitarian actors to identify better ways to serve the SRH needs of these population groups. This systematic review aims at exploring and synthetizing the available evidence on sexual and reproductive health knowledge, experiences and access to services among refugee, migrant and displaced girls and young women in Africa.

2. Materials and Methods

A mixed methods systematic review, exploring qualitative and quantitative data, was conducted to assess our aim. Sandelowski et al. identified three general frameworks through which to conduct mixed methods systematic reviews—segregated, integrated, and contingent [13]. We have applied the integrated methodology for our review. In integrated designs, the methodological differences between qualitative and quantitative studies are minimized and the studies are grouped for synthesis by results addressing the same research questions, or describing the same aspects of a target phenomenon [13].

2.1. Search Strategy

We adhered to the Preferred Reporting Items for Systematic Reviews and Meta-Analyses (PRISMA) guidelines for systematic reviews [14]. Two electronic databases—PubMed and Web of Science were searched. Search terms for sexual and reproductive health covered the topics relevant to conflict-affected situations, e.g., sexual violence, maternal health, as well as the topics of a particular relevance to young girls and women, e.g., sexuality education, teenage pregnancies, etc. Our choice was also guided by the SRH definitions from the International Conference on Population and Development (ICPD) in 1994. Search terms are described in Table 1. Data search was performed between the end of

March and the beginning of April 2018. In addition, we completed a manual search of the reference lists of relevant articles. All records were exported into Mendeley—an online bibliographic management program produced by Elsevier. After we removed the duplicates, titles and abstracts were screened for inclusion.

Table 1. Search terms used in PubMed and Web of Science.

Category	Search Terms Combined with AND
Age Group	youth OR teenager OR teen OR girl OR young female OR adolescent OR woman OR young woman OR women OR young person OR adolescence OR female OR reproductive age
Age	10 to 24
Status	refugee OR migrant OR displaced OR displaced person OR foreigner OR immigrant OR ethnic minority OR indigenous OR internally displaced OR asylum
SRH topics	sexual OR sexual health OR reproductive health OR early marriage OR child marriage OR female genital mutilation OR cutting OR female circumcision OR circumcised OR sexual behavior OR sexual experience OR sexual activity OR early sexual debut OR sexual initiation OR menstruation OR menstrual hygiene OR contraception OR family planning OR pregnancy OR antenatal OR birth OR post-natal OR sexually transmitted infection OR STI OR sexual intercourse OR HIV OR violence OR sexuality education OR reproduction OR sexual well-being OR condom OR human immunodeficiency virus OR AIDS OR sex education OR sex OR relationship OR physical relationship OR sexual coercion OR rape OR sexual violence OR sexual abuse OR abortion OR maternal health OR fistula OR motherhood OR gender OR forced sex OR intimate partner violence OR gender based violence OR transactional sex OR sex work OR HPV OR cervical cancer
Outcome	need OR unmet need OR access OR knowledge OR availability OR experience OR awareness OR perception
Countries/regions	Africa OR Algeria OR Angola OR Benin OR Botswana OR Burkina Faso OR Burundi OR Cameroon OR Cape Verde OR Central African Republic OR Chad OR Comoros OR Congo OR Democratic Republic of the Congo OR Cote d'Ivoire OR Djibouti OR Egypt OR Equatorial Guinea OR Eritrea OR Ethiopia OR Gabon OR Gambia OR Ghana OR Guinea OR Guinea-Bissau OR Kenya OR Lesotho OR Liberia OR Libya OR Madagascar OR Malawi OR Mali OR Mauritania OR Mauritius OR Morocco OR Mozambique OR Namibia OR Niger OR Nigeria OR Rwanda OR Sao Tome OR Senegal OR Seychelles OR Sierra Leone OR Somalia OR South Africa OR Sudan OR South Sudan OR Swaziland OR Tanzania OR Togo OR Tunisia OR Uganda OR Zambia OR Zimbabwe, NOT (Europe OR EU OR European Union OR Australia OR US OR New Zeeland OR United States OR France OR Greece OR Italy OR Austria OR Belgium OR Latvia OR Bulgaria OR Lithuania OR Croatia OR Luxembourg OR Cyprus OR Malta OR Czech Republic OR Netherlands OR Denmark OR Poland OR Estonia OR Portugal OR Finland OR Romania OR France OR Slovakia OR Germany OR Slovenia OR Greece OR Spain OR Hungary OR Sweden OR Ireland OR United Kingdom OR UK OR America OR Asia OR Brazil OR South America OR Latin America)

2.2. Study Selection

This review was limited to peer-reviewed, full-text articles published in English before March 2018. While we initially planned to search the grey literature, our time and financial resources did not permit us to explore this literature. Studies providing insufficient information, for example letters, abstracts or conference papers, were excluded. Study population of interest included refugee, migrant or displaced women and girls. For refugee, migrants and internally displaced populations (IDPs) we applied the official definitions of The United Nations (UN) and International Organization for Migration (IOM). Only studies which included results on adolescent and young women (10–24 years old) were considered. The UN define adolescents as individuals being 10–19 years old and youth as those persons between the ages of 15 and 24 years. We excluded studies which reported results on SRH of migrants and refugees without sex and age disaggregation. Only studies, which were conducted in African countries were included. Studies related to refugees of African origin settled in other region other than Africa were excluded. Details of the study selection are summarized in Figure 1.

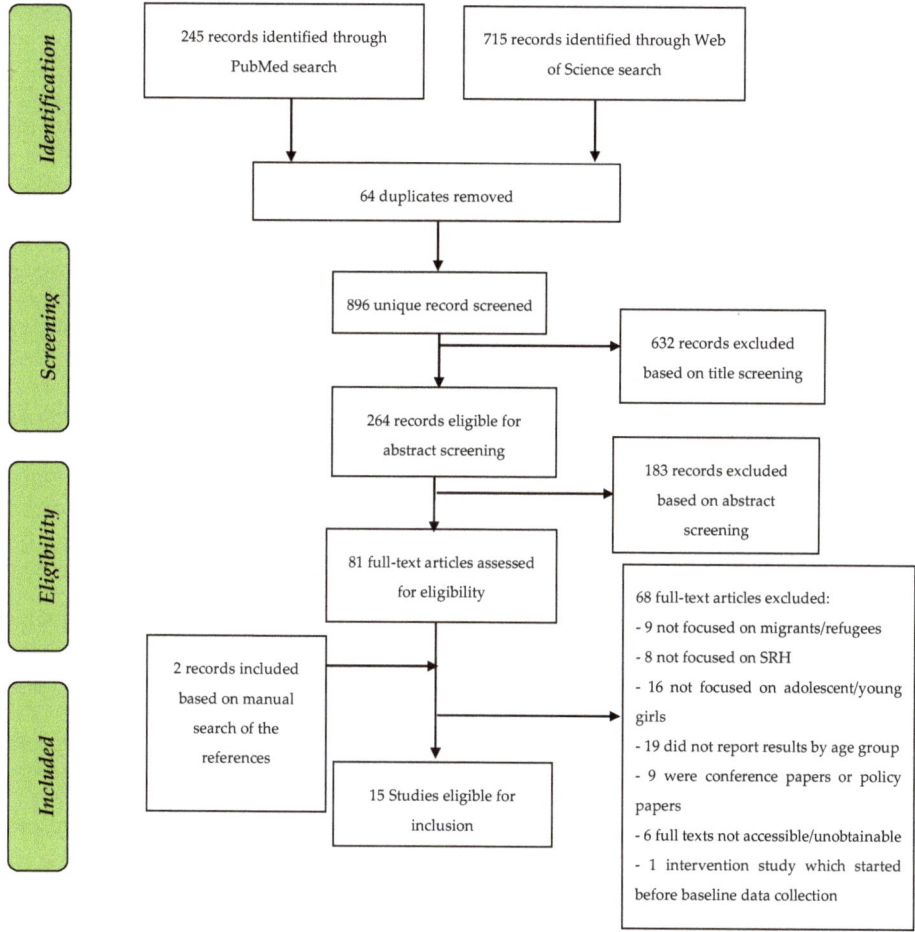

Figure 1. PRISMA Flow Diagram.

2.3. Critical Appraisal

Two researchers independently reviewed the full texts for quality and suitability. Eligible papers then underwent a quality appraisal using the MMAT tool [15]. This tool was designed for systematic mixed studies reviews. The tool helps to examine the appropriateness of the study aim, adequacy and methodology, study design, data collection, study selection, data analysis, presentation of findings, author's discussions and conclusions. For each of the included studies, the relevant four quality questions were asked corresponding to the study type, e.g., qualitative, quantitative descriptive or mixed methods. The studies were scored using percentages (0–100%). Any discrepancies were discussed until a consensus was reached.

2.4. Data Extraction and Analysis

Two authors independently read all included articles and completed a data extraction form created to gather the following: authors, study setting, main study objectives, study population, study design and study findings. Due to the inclusion of studies using qualitative and quantitative design, conducting a meta-analysis of the data was not appropriate. A descriptive narrative synthesis was chosen as the most relevant and suitable method of data synthesis for this review. The results are supported with original quotations and examples.

3. Results

3.1. Study Characteristics

From 960 records, 15 studies met the inclusion criteria. They were conducted in nine African countries which included Uganda, Ethiopia, DR Congo, Somalia, Kenya, Nigeria, Djibouti, Rwanda and Sierra Leone [6,16–29]. These consisted of eight applied qualitative, five quantitative and two mixed-method study designs. Three studies were performed exclusively with young girls and women of age groups 10–24, 12 other studies included them as one of the groups in total population, e.g., among women of reproductive age or adolescents including boys and girls. One study [16] reported the results before and after the intervention. For the purpose of this review we have used the baseline data from the above mentioned study on HIV/STDs knowledge and attitudes among young displaced girls. In the case of the study performed by Stark et al. [26] we only used the qualitative data for this review because the quantitative data were previously reported within a bigger sample in Stark et al. [25]. Tanabe et al. [28] focused on refugee adolescent girls living with disabilities. Four studies also included data collected in Asian or Middle East countries apart of African countries [27–29]. Further details on the methodology and the main objectives of the included studies are presented in Table 2.

3.2. Sexual and Reproductive Health Knowledge

Six articles reported on knowledge and misconceptions regarding contraception, HIV/AIDS and STIs [16,18,19,21,27,28]. Overall, the knowledge of refugee and displaced young women and girls on the full range of contraceptive methods were limited. Also, the adolescents were less aware about modern methods of contraception than the adults in the same setting [27]. Nevertheless, the young participants could name at least one method of contraception [21,28]. Two studies demonstrated that the misinformation about contraceptive methods is widespread preventing young women and girls from using them [18,21]. Knowledge of routes of HIV transmission and HIV prevention were also limited [16,19]. Casey et al. [16] demonstrated that 25% of female youth did not know any correct route of HIV transmission, while 28.7% did not know any effective means of avoiding HIV. Harrison et al. [19] showed that comprehensive correct knowledge of HIV/AIDS among refugee females in Uganda aged 15–24 was 33.5%. Casey et al. [16] also found low knowledge among female youth in Sierra Leone regarding STIs —33.2% of participants did not know any signs of STIs.

Table 2. Characteristics of studies included in the review.

N	Author	Year	Country	Population	Age Group Included in the Review	Design	Main Research Objective/Aim	Quality of Studies (MMAT)
1	Casey et al. [16]	2006	Sierra Leone	Youth displaced by conflict (244 female and 293 male participants)	15–24	Quantitative Cross-sectional Survey (baseline data)	Explore the HIV/AIDS/STD knowledge, attitudes and behaviors of youth	50%
2	Feseha et al. [17]	2012	Ethiopia	Refugee women (422) including 40 girls of 15–19 years old and 156 of 20–24 years old	15–24	Quantitative Cross-sectional Questionnaire	Assess the magnitude of intimate partner physical violence and associated factors among women	100%
3	Gure et al. [18]	2015	Somalia	Unmarried girls in displacement camps (5) among total sample of 21 married and unmarried women	18–20	Qualitative Cross-sectional FGDs	Explore women's knowledge of, experiences with, and need for reproductive health services	50%
4	Harrison et al. [19]	2009	Uganda	Refugees and host communities (1600) with 120 (19.8%) of total female refugees (607) being girls of age 15–19 and 100 (16.6%) of 20–24 years old	15–24	Quantitative Cross-sectional Standardized behavioral surveillance survey (BSS)	Provide data on HIV related knowledge, attitudes and behavior among refugees and surrounding hosts populations to allow for targeted HIV interventions	100%
5	Iyakaremye and Mukagatare [6]	2016	Rwanda	Adolescent girls from DRC(10) in total sample (17) of boys, mothers, fathers and staff	Adolescent girls age not mentioned	Qualitative Cross-sectional Interviews and FGDs	Explore the experience of sexual abuse of adolescent girls in refugee camp	75%
6	Kägesten et al. [20]	2017	Ethiopia and Thailand	Young Somali adolescents (406) in Kobe refugee camp, from which 214 (52.7%) were girls; and young adolescents from Myanmar (399)	10–14	Quantitative Cross-sectional Household survey	Describe transition into puberty and access to SRH information among very young adolescents in humanitarian setting	75%
7	Okanlawon et al. [21]	2010	Nigeria	Youth in Oru refugee camp (116 female of total 208)	10–24	Qualitative and Quantitative Cross-sectional Self-administered questionnaire, in depth interviews and FGDs	Examine the perceptions, beliefs, knowledge and attitudes of refugee youths towards contraceptive use and also the access to and use of contraceptives in this refugee camp	Qualitative—75% Quantitative—50% Mixed—50%
8	Ortiz-Echevarria et al. [22]	2017	Ethiopia	Somali refugees and host community (126–32 adults and 94 adolescents including 46 refugee girls)	10–16	Qualitative Cross-sectional FGD with community mapping and photo	Understand lived realities of very young adolescents in Kobe refugee camp, their health and development needs, expectations and goals	75%
9	Patel et al. [23]	2012	Uganda	Acholi girls (67) and adult women (65) in three displacement camps in Gulu district	14–19	Qualitative Cross-sectional In-depth interviews and FGD	Provide a better understanding of adolescent girl's enhanced risk for HIV infection in conflict settings and to inform the development of appropriate sexual education and HIV prevention initiatives in this population group	100%

Table 2. Cont.

N	Author	Year	Country	Population	Age Group Included in the Review	Design	Main Research Objective/Aim	Quality of Studies (MMAT)
10	Schlecht et al. [24]	2013	Uganda	Displaced and refugee men and women from Uganda and DRC (133)	10–24	Qualitative Cross sectional FGDKey informant interviews	Describe the factors which contribute to early relationships and informal marriages in conflict and post-conflict settings	75%
11	Stark et al. [25]	2017	DRC and Ethiopia	Displaced, conflict-affected adolescent girls (1296)	13–19	Quantitative Cross-sectional Survey questionnaire using computer-assisted personal interview and computer-assisted self-interview	Assess the prevalence and related risk factors of physical, emotional, and sexual violence	100%
12	Stark et al. [26]	2017	DRC and Ethiopia	87 internally displaced adolescent girls from DRC and 78 Sudanese girls in Ethiopian refugee camps	10–19	Qualitative Cross-sectional Qualitative participatory mapping activity	Provide insight into assessing gender based violence from two methodological approaches	75%
13	Tanabe et al. [28]	2015	Kenya, Nepal and Uganda	352 refugee female and male participants from them44 adolescent girls with any type of impairment in Kenya and Uganda	15–19	Qualitative Cross-sectional Individual interviews and FGDs	Explore the specific risks, needs and barriers for persons with disabilities to access SRH services, and the capacities and practical ways through which the challenges could be addressed	75%
14	Tanabe et al. [27]	2017	Djibouti, Kenya, Uganda, Bangladesh, Jordan and Malaysia	Adolescents, women and men in refugee settings	15–19	Qualitative and Quantitative Cross-sectional Household survey, in-depth interviews, FGDs and facilities assessment	Document the knowledge of family planning, belief and practices of refugees, and the state of service provision	Qualitative—50% Quantitative—50% Mixed—50%
15	Whelan [29]	2007	Uganda, Yemen and DRC	Refugees (816) including sample of 78 girls from Uganda and DRC participating in FGDs	Adolescent girls age not mentioned	Qualitative Cross-sectional FGDs and interviews	Identify factors that facilitate or hinder access to, use of, and satisfaction with RH services in refugee settings	50%

3.3. Sexual and Reproductive Health Experiences and Practices

All studies shared findings on the experiences and practices of female youth including contraceptive use, gender-based and sexual violence, child marriages, transactional sex, puberty changes and decision-making. Half of the studies reported on the prevalence of and fears related to gender-based or sexual violence and abuse in humanitarian settings [6,17,22,23,25,26,29]. In the study of Feseha et al. [17] the magnitude of partner's physical violence in the last 12 months in the Schimelba refugee camp in northern Ethiopia among girls aged 15–19 was 10% and 41% among girls 20–24 years old. High prevalence of violence (51.6%) among conflict-affected girls 13–19 years old was also reported in DRC and Ethiopia by Stark et al. [25]. The qualitative study from Iyakaremye and Mukagatare [6] performed with adolescents in Kigeme refugee camp in Rwanda found that rape, unwanted physical touching, sexual exploitation, commercial sex, early marriage and trafficking were the main forms of sexual abuse. Forced sex and rape among young women were also reported in the qualitative study of Whelan et al. [29]. Sexual violence was also mentioned by the majority of girls in Ethiopia and DRC and was considered to be the most serious type of violence affecting the community: *"sometimes there are drunk men who rape girls along the road"* (age 15, Ethiopia) [26]. This sexual abuse leaves girls with consequences such as unwanted pregnancies leading to unsafe abortions, rejection and harassment in their families [6]. The topic of child/early marriages was raised in qualitative studies and it was seen as an important concern among young adolescents [6,22]. It was perceived as a barrier to pursue education and often resulted in early pregnancies: *"(for) the ladies, it's possible that they may not continue with the education and they may end up in early marriage"* (girls, 13–14 years old). [22].

Transactional and commercial sex, so called "survival sex" in exchange for goods, food, menstrual hygiene products and money was highlighted in some studies [6,19,21,23,29]. *"Many girls in this camp sleep with men in order to survive. We are here in Nigeria with nothing and nobody to help us and we have to survive"* (18 year old young women) [21]. Harrison et al. [19] found that 66.7% of sexually active females aged 15-24 had a transactional partner in the past 12 months. At the same time only 16.7% of them used a condom during the last sexual encounter. The low condom use was also documented in three other studies [16,21,27]. This also applies to other contraceptive methods. The main reasons identified for non-use were partner refusal, misinformation, religion, fear of side effects and stigma. One girl from the Oru refugee camp in Nigeria commented: *"I like using condom during sex but I didn't use it the last time I had sex because I didn't want to buy it in the camp. I don't want anyone to think I'm a prostitute. I remember the last time I went to buy condom and pills in a chemist in the camp; I was embarrassed by some women. They asked me what a young girl like me wanted to do with condom and pills. I was so ashamed that I had to lie that someone sent me. So, I prefer buying it outside the camp, a little bit far away, where no one knows me."* [21]. Only one study explored body/puberty changes in refugee adolescent girls which is an important aspect of adolescents' sexual and reproductive health [20].

3.4. Access to Sexual and Reproductive Health Services, Commodities and Information

Several studies addressed the access to SRH services and information [18,20–23,27–29]. Girls and young women stated parents (mostly mothers), siblings and peers as main sources of SRH information on pregnancy, puberty, menstruation, etc. [20,22,23]. Lack of information regarding different areas of SRH was documented in the above studies. For example, the majority of Somali girls (95.2%) indicated having learned about body changes before they occurred, however 66.8% would like to have had more information and very few girls of age 10-14 reported learning about pregnancy (18.2%) [20]. Patel et al. [23] in a qualitative inquiry found that many participants reported access to information on HIV/AIDS and very few (6%) had access to information on contraception, sexuality, abortion and pregnancy. The same study showed that girls younger 18 years old face problems to access information about family planning: *"When they (family planning services) are teaching about condoms, they usually restrict it to people of 18 years and above. They are the ones who are advised to use it. The use of family planning is for married women (those with husbands) not for girls. . . young girls in the ages of 12–14 years don't have any knowledge about condoms."* (adolescent girl) [23].

Adolescent girls also lacked access to SRH commodities including menstrual hygiene products and contraception. Only 61.5% of Somali girls in Kobe refugee camp stated having sufficient access to soap and water, but less than one girl in five (19.2%) had access to cloth/pads to use during menstruation [20]. Three studies documented a limited access to contraceptive methods including condoms [21,23,27]. A high proportion (60 to 91%) of adolescent girls found it difficult to obtain contraceptives in the camps [21,23]. The main barriers were distance to the health care facilities, costs, lack of knowledge about sources of contraception, stigma and judgmental attitudes. For example, adolescent girls in Nakivale camp, Uganda reported that they often find the condom dispensers in the settlement empty [27]. Costs and distance to the health care services were highlighted in the study of Okanlawon et al. [21]: *"Before, contraceptives like pills, IUD, injectables, etc., were free in this camp, but since the camp clinic was closed in 2007, we now go to hospitals in the surrounding community to receive the service. It's no longer free. Some of us like to use it, but we can't get it in the camp. That's the problem."* (24 years old young women).

The last point we would like to highlight is the quality of provided SRH services. Refugee women and girls complained about lack of facilities for STI testing, lack of acceptable and affordable contraceptives, stock outs, long waiting times, language barriers and discrimination [21,27–29].

3.5. Criticial Appraisal of Included Studies

The majority of studies (10 of 15) scored 75% and more, five other studies scored 50% and no study was assigned less than 50% (Table 2). Overall, we could conclude that the quality of included articles was from moderate to high.

4. Discussion

The aim of this review was to combine the existing evidence on SRH knowledge, experiences and access to services of young women and girls aged 10–24 in crisis and humanitarian situations. Such studies were largely absent and thus this review pointed out the lack of available peer-reviewed literature on SRH of girls and young women in the African region, where multiple conflicts are ongoing for decades, putting their health, including SRH at risk. To summarize, the young women and girls are lacking knowledge on SRH issues; access to this information is often hindered because of many different factors including stigma related to young age; access to SRH services and commodities is challenging because of distance, costs and quality.

The studies in this review show us the limited SRH knowledge and awareness among adolescent girls and the misconceptions about the contraceptives which cause the adolescents to refrain from using them. As a result, insufficient uptake of family planning contributes to morbidity and mortality in women and girls of reproductive age via pregnancy-related complications and deaths [30]. The studies have also explored the access to and sources of SRH knowledge and education in humanitarian settings but the sources preferred by the adolescent for obtaining SRH information has not been very well documented. An effective way of educating the adolescents about SRH would be through the sources they prefer.

The studies show high prevalence of sexual violence, coerced sex, transactional sex and other forms of sexual exploitations. In a few studies, this sexual harassment or physical violence may be instigated by own family members or partner [17,25]. Sexual exploitation by family members or close relatives may be quite difficult to assess as the adolescents may not be willing to open up to report such incidences. However, we believe that quite a large number of girls are suffering from sexual exploitations and harassments by their family members and close relatives apart from their partners. This finding has been reported previously in other studies in Africa in non-humanitarian settings [31]. These cases of sexual exploitations also need to be extensively studied.

In addition, we would like to discuss the main points which could help to strengthen future data collection in this field. Firstly, although many identified studies report on SRH of refuges and migrants, few of them disaggregate findings by age and sex of respondents. During the full text review and data extraction process we faced challenges to separate results for youth and for female participants, excluding several studies from this review. Some of the included studies also stressed the necessity to perform target research in this age group [20]. A number of studies have been performed on SRH of women of reproductive age. The results which are not segregated by age, may confuse the current situation and needs of the adolescents with those of the women of higher reproductive age.

Secondly, multi-setting studies provide reach and comparable information across different humanitarian settings. However, here the disaggregation of results by setting plays an important role as the findings of one humanitarian settings cannot be generalized onto the other due to the differences between the settings. The differences may exist due to cultural values and background of the refugees and the infrastructural and economic differences of the hosts.

Limitations

This systematic review has a number of limitations. Only studies written in English were included. The MMAT appraisal tool for mixed-method research was used to assess the quality of reporting in the studies, but more specialized quality assessment tools such as the Cochrane Collaboration's tool for assessing risk of bias would have provided more in-depth reviews of quality. Unfortunately due to time constraints and funding, this review did not include grey literature, such as UNFPA and UNHCR reports and studies conducted by non-governmental organizations working in humanitarian settings. These studies could have provided valuable data on SRH indicators and situation of girls and women affected by conflicts and disasters. Although PubMed and Web of Science are the most often used search databases, we might have missed some relevant studies included to other databases, e.g., Global Health or EMBASE. Some of the peer-reviewed studies which could not be accessed, were also not included.

5. Conclusions

Results of this review demonstrate the gaps in the existed evidence on SRH of migrant, refugee and displaced girls and women living in Africa. The necessity of disaggregation by sex and age should be addressed in future research. Targeting young refugee, displaced and migrant adolescents of 10–14 years old is very important enabling the complexity of body and physiological changes and the paucity of information from this age and population group to be taken into account.

Author Contributions: O.I. designed the review, led the searching, screening, and analysis of records and drafted the article. M.R. performed a literature search, quality assessment of the publications and contributed to the article writing process. E.K. provided conceptual insight and feedback on revisions. All authors critically reviewed and approved the final manuscript.

Funding: This review was funded by the Friedrich-Baur-Stiftung, Medical Faculty of Ludwig Maximilian University of Munich (LMU), Germany.

Acknowledgments: We would like to thank our colleagues—Andrea Rachow, Kathrin Held, Lisa Rogers and Michael Hoelscher for their support and guidance during the funding acquisition stage and review process.

Conflicts of Interest: The authors declare no conflict of interest.

Abbreviations

AIDS	Acquired immune deficiency syndrome
HIV	Human immunodeficiency virus
IAWG	Inter-agency Working Group (IAWG)
IDP	Internally displaced people
FGD	Focus group discussion
MMAT	Mixed Methods Appraisal Tool
PRISMA	Preferred Reporting Items for Systematic Reviews and Meta-Analyses
SRH	Sexual and reproductive health

STI	Sexually transmitted infection
UNFPA	United Nations Population Fund
UNHCR	The United Nations Refugee Agency

References

1. UNFPA; Save the Children USA. *A Companion to the Inter-Agency Field Manual on Reproductive Health in Humanitarian Settings: A Companion to the Inter-Agency Field Manual on Reproductive Health in Humanitarian*, 1st ed.; UNFPA: New York, NY, USA; Save the Children USA: Fairfield, CT, USA, 2009; pp. 1–92.
2. Ward, J.; Marsh, M. Sexual Violence against Women and Girls in War and Its Aftermath: Realities, Responses, and Required Resources. Available online: http://www.svri.org/sites/default/files/attachments/2016-01-15/CCEF504C15AB277E852571AB0071F7CE-UNFPA.pdf (accessed on 15 May 2018).
3. Jamieson, D.J.; Meikle, S.F.; Hillis, S.D.; Mtsuko, D.; Mawji, S.; Duerr, A. An evaluation of poor pregnancy outcomes among Burundian refugees in Tanzania. *JAMA* **2000**, *3*, 397–402. [CrossRef]
4. Bartlett, L.A.; Jamieson, D.J.; Kahn, T.; Sultana, M.; Wilson, H.G.; Duerr, A. Maternal mortality among Afghan refugees in Pakistan, 1999–2000. *Lancet* **2002**, *359*, 643–649. [CrossRef]
5. UNFPA. *Adolescent Girls in Disaster & Conflict: Interventions for Improving Access to Sexual and Reproductive Health Services*, 1st ed.; UNFPA: New York, NY, USA, 2016; pp. 1–88.
6. Yakaremye, I.; Mukagatare, C. Forced migration and sexual abuse: Experience of congolese adolescent girls in Kigeme refugee camp, Rwanda. *Health Psychol. Rep.* **2016**, *4*, 261–271. [CrossRef]
7. McGinn, T.; Austin, J.; Anfinson, K.; Amsalu, R.; Casey, S.E.; Fadulalmula, S.I.; Langston, A.; Lee-Jones, L.; Meyers, J.; Mubiru, F.K.; et al. Family planning in conflict: results of cross-sectional baseline surveys in three African countries. *Confl. Health* **2011**, *5*, 11. [CrossRef] [PubMed]
8. UNFPA. *Inter-Agency Field Manual on Reproductive Health in Humanitarian Settings: 2010 Revision for Field Review*, 1st ed.; Inter-Agency Working Group (IAWG) on Reproductive Health in Crises: New York, NY, USA, 2010; pp. 1–217.
9. Casey, S.E. Evaluations of reproductive health programs in humanitarian settings: A systematic review. *Confl. Health* **2015**, *9*, S1. [CrossRef] [PubMed]
10. UNHCR. Inter-Agency Global Evaluation of Reproductive Health Services for Refugees and Internally Displaced Persons. 2004. Available online: http://www.unhcr.org/41c846f44.pdf (accessed on 15 May 2018).
11. Chynoweth, S.K. Advancing reproductive health on the humanitarian agenda: The 2012–2014 global review. *Confl. Health.* **2015**, *9*, I1. [CrossRef]
12. Casey, S.E.; Chynoweth, S.K.; Cornier, N.; Gallagher, M.C.; Wheeler, E.E. Progress and gaps in reproductive health services in three humanitarian settings: Mixed-methods case studies. *Confl. Health* **2015**, *9*, S3. [CrossRef] [PubMed]
13. Sandelowski, M.; Voils, C.I.; Barroso, J. Defining and designing mixed research synthesis studies. *Res. Sch.* **2006**, *13*, 29. [PubMed]
14. Moher, D.; Liberati, A.; Tetzlaff, J.; Altman, D.G.; PRISMA Group. Preferred reporting items for systematic reviews and meta-analyses: The PRISMA statement. *PLoS Med.* **2009**, *151*, 264–269.
15. Pace, R.; Pluye, P.; Bartlett, G.; Macaulay, A.C.; Salsberg, J.; Jagosh, J.; Seller, R. Testing the reliability and efficiency of the pilot Mixed Methods Appraisal Tool (MMAT) for systematic mixed studies review. *Int. J. Nurs. Stud.* **2012**, *49*, 47–53. [CrossRef] [PubMed]
16. Casey, S.E.; Larsen, M.M.; McGinn, T.; Sartie, M.; Dauda, M.; Lahai, P. Changes in HIV/AIDS/STI knowledge, attitudes, and behaviours among the youth in Port Loko, Sierra Leone. *Glob. Public Health* **2006**, *1*, 249–263. [CrossRef] [PubMed]
17. Feseha, G.; Gerbaba, M. Intimate partner physical violence among women in Shimelba refugee camp, northern Ethiopia. *BMC Public Health* **2012**, *12*, 125. [CrossRef] [PubMed]
18. Gure, F.; Yusuf, M.; Foster, A.M. Exploring Somali women's reproductive health knowledge and experiences: Results from focus group discussions in Mogadishu. *Reprod. Health Matters* **2015**, *23*, 136–144. [CrossRef] [PubMed]
19. Harrison, K.M.; Claass, J.; Spiegel, P.B.; Bamuturaki, J.; Patterson, N.; Muyonga, M.; Tatwebwa, L. HIV behavioural surveillance among refugees and surrounding host communities in Uganda, 2006. *Afr. J. AIDS Res.* **2009**, *8*, 29–41. [CrossRef] [PubMed]

20. Kågesten, A.E.; Zimmerman, L.; Robinson, C.; Lee, C.; Bawoke, T.; Osman, S.; Schlecht, J. Transitions into puberty and access to sexual and reproductive health information in two humanitarian settings: A cross-sectional survey of very young adolescents from Somalia and Myanmar. *Confl. Health* **2017**, *11*, 24. [CrossRef] [PubMed]
21. Okanlawon, K.; Reeves, M.; Agbaje, O.F. Contraceptive use: Knowledge, perceptions and attitudes of refugee youths in Oru Refugee Camp, Nigeria. *Afr. J. Reprod. Health* **2010**, *14*, 16–25. [PubMed]
22. Ortiz-Echevarria, L.; Greeley, M.; Bawoke, T.; Zimmerman, L.; Robinson, C.; Schlecht, J. Understanding the unique experiences, perspectives and sexual and reproductive health needs of very young adolescents: Somali refugees in Ethiopia. *Confl. Health* **2017**, *11*, 26. [CrossRef] [PubMed]
23. Patel, S.H.; Muyinda, H.; Sewankambo, N.K.; Oyat, G.; Atim, S.; Spittal, P.M. In the face of war: Examining sexual vulnerabilities of Acholi adolescent girls living in displacement camps in conflict-affected Northern Uganda. *BMC Int. Health Hum. Rights* **2012**, *12*, 38. [CrossRef] [PubMed]
24. Schlecht, J.; Rowley, E.; Babirye, J.; Schlecht, J.; Rowley, E. Early relationships and marriage in conflict and post-conflict settings: Vulnerability of youth in Uganda. RHM. *Reprod. Health Matters* **2013**, *21*, 234–242. [CrossRef]
25. Stark, L.; Asghar, K.; Yu, G.; Bora, C.; Baysa, A.A.; Falb, K.L. Prevalence and associated risk factors of violence against conflict-affected female adolescents: A multi-country, cross-sectional study. *J. Glob. Health* **2017**, *7*, 10416. [CrossRef] [PubMed]
26. Stark, L.; Sommer, M.; Davis, K.; Asghar, K.; Baysa, A.A.; Abdela, G.; Tanner, S.; Falb, K. Disclosure bias for group versus individual reporting of violence amongst conflict-affected adolescent girls in DRC and Ethiopia. *PLoS ONE* **2017**, *12*, e0174741. [CrossRef] [PubMed]
27. Tanabe, M.; Myers, A.; Bhandari, P.; Cornier, N.; Doraiswamy, S.; Krause, S. Family planning in refugee settings: Findings and actions from a multi-country study. *Confl. Health* **2017**, *11*, 9. [CrossRef]
28. Tanabe, M.; Nagujjah, Y.; Rimal, N.; Bukania, F.; Krause, S. Intersecting sexual and reproductive health and disability in humanitarian settings: Risks, needs, and capacities of refugees with disabilities in Kenya, Nepal, and Uganda. *Sex. Disabil.* **2015**, *33*, 411–427. [CrossRef] [PubMed]
29. Whelan, A.; Blogg, J. 'Halfway people': Refugee views of reproductive health services. *Glob. Public Health* **2007**, *2*, 373–394. [CrossRef] [PubMed]
30. Ackerson, K.; Zielinski, R. Factors influencing use of family planning in women living in crisis affected areas of Sub-Saharan Africa: A review of the literature. *Midwifery* **2017**, *54*, 35–60. [CrossRef] [PubMed]
31. Lalor, K. Child Sexual Abuse in Sub-Saharan Africa: Child Protection Implications for Development Policy Makers and Practitioners. 2005. Available online: https://arrow.dit.ie/aaschsslrep/2/ (accessed on 1 June 2018).

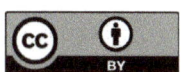

© 2018 by the authors. Licensee MDPI, Basel, Switzerland. This article is an open access article distributed under the terms and conditions of the Creative Commons Attribution (CC BY) license (http://creativecommons.org/licenses/by/4.0/).

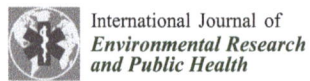

Article

Obesity Inequalities According to Place of Birth: The Role of Education

Elena Rodriguez-Alvarez [1,2,*], Nerea Lanborena [1,2] and Luisa N. Borrell [2,3]

1 Department of Nursing I, University of the Basque Country (UPV/EHU), 48940 Leioa, Spain; nerea.lamborena@ehu.eus
2 OPIK-Research Group for Social Determinants of Health and Demographic Change, University of the Basque Country (UPV/EHU), 48940 Leioa, Spain
3 Department of Epidemiology & Biostatistics, Graduate School of Public Health & Health Policy, City University of New York, New York, NY 10027, USA; Luisa.Borrell@sph.cuny.edu
* Correspondence: elena.rodriguez@ehu.eus; Tel.: +34-94-601-5593; Fax: +34-94-601-3059

Received: 28 June 2018; Accepted: 25 July 2018; Published: 31 July 2018

Abstract: This study examined obesity inequalities according to place of birth and educational attainment in men and in women in Spain. A cross-sectional study was conducted using data from the Spanish National Health Survey 2011–2012 and from the European Health Survey in Spain 2014. We used data for 27,720 adults aged 18–64 years of whom 2431 were immigrants. We used log-binomial regression to quantify the association of place of birth with obesity before and after adjusting for the selected characteristics in women and in men. We found a greater probability of obesity in immigrant women (PR: 1.42; 95% CI: 1.22–1.64) and a lower probability of obesity in immigrant men (PR: 0.73; 95% CI: 0.59–0.89) relative to natives after adjustment. Significant heterogeneity was observed for the association of place of birth and obesity according to education in men (p-interactions = 0.002): Men with lower educational levels (PR: 0.47; 95% CI: 0.26–0.83) have a protective effect against obesity compared with their native counterparts. This study suggests that place of birth may affect obesity in women and in men. However, this effect may be compounded with education differently for women and men.

Keywords: obesity; immigration; education; inequalities; health survey

1. Introduction

Obesity currently represents a world-wide public health problem, given its impact on chronic diseases and premature mortality [1,2]. In addition, obesity is associated with a high financial burden for health care utilization [3]. Over the past four decades, the global prevalence of obesity in adults has tripled in men (3.2% to 10.8%) and doubled in women (6.4% to 14.9%). Projections for 2025 indicate that the overall prevalence of obesity will reach 18% in men and exceeds 21% in women [4]. Currently, more than half of adults are overweight and almost one in six adults in Europe is obese [5]. It is estimated that a 5% reduction in body mass index (BMI) in the European population would entail a 16.7% decrease in the prevalence of obesity related-diseases such cancer, stroke, and type 2 diabetes [6].

In recent years, extant evidence suggests that health status is conditioned by the unequal distribution of social determinants [7,8]. For instance, place of birth and socioeconomic position may explain inequalities in risks associated with health and/or disease, as a result of the different opportunities and resources people may have to achieve good health [9]. In fact, place of birth and the migratory process from the least developed countries to those of greater economic development, such as the countries of the European Union with a very high Human Development Index (HDI), represent a crucial factor for the study of social inequalities in health [10]. Therefore, most studies conclude that the worst socioeconomic and labor conditions, the lowest social support and the highest discrimination of the immigrant population may explain their poor mental and physical health outcomes compared to the native population [11–13]. With regards to obesity in Europe, studies report higher prevalence estimates of obesity among immigrant population compared to their native counterparts [14–17]. However, this difference may be explained by the lower socioeconomic position of the immigrant population. In contrast, European studies on native population only show that educational attainment, as an indicator of socioeconomic position, is the main determinant in obesity inequalities, exhibiting a clear direct social gradient, i.e., higher prevalence of obesity with lower education attainment [18–20]. However, and in contrast to the USA, where the role of education on immigrants' health depends on gender and country of birth [21,22], no studies have examined the effect of place of birth and education together on obesity inequalities in European men and women.

Spain is one of the countries with the highest prevalence of obesity (17% in men and 16% in women) in the European Union and among countries presenting greater obesity inequalities among the native population by educational attainment, especially among women [18,20,23]. Moreover, Spain is the fourth country in the European Union when it comes to the proportion of immigrants (13.6% in 2017) [24]. Specifically, during the last two decades, Spain has experienced an intense growth of the immigrant population from less developed countries for economic reasons. Most immigrants are coming from Latin America (38%; mainly from Ecuador, Colombia, Peru and Bolivia) Maghreb (14%; mainly from Morocco), sub-Saharan Africa (4%; mainly Senegal and Nigeria), Asia (7%; mainly China) and the rest of non-very high developed European Union countries (10%; mainly Romania). However, and despite this trend as well as the importance of place of birth and the migratory process as determinants of inequality [10], few studies have focused on obesity inequalities between immigrant and native populations in Spain [25,26]. Furthermore, the immigrant population usually has a lower level of education than the native population [27]. Therefore, this study aimed to examine (a) obesity inequalities between immigrant and native populations; and (b) the combined effect of place of birth and educational attainment in men and in women in Spain for the years 2011–2014.

2. Materials and Methods

2.1. Data Source and Study Population

The study was based on a cross-sectional analysis of data obtained from the Spanish National Health Survey (SNHS) of 2011–2012 and from the European Health Survey in Spain (EHSS) of 2014 conducted by the Ministry of Health, Social Services and Equality in collaboration with the National Institute of Statistics. The surveys used representative samples of the non-institutionalized population in Spain through a stratified multistage sampling. More detailed information on the methodology of these surveys has been described elsewhere [23]. Analyses were based on information obtained from the individual questionnaires conducted in selected households, with a sample of 21,007 adults for the 2011–2012 SNHS and 22,842 adults for the 2014 EHSS. The response rates were 71% for both surveys. For the 43,849 people who completed the individual questionnaires, we excluded records of individuals under 18 years of age (n = 941) and older than 64 years (n = 12,416), those born in countries with an HDI considered as very high in 2015 (>0.80; n = 738), and those missing info on BMI (n = 1105), occupation (n = 570) and other covariates (n = 359). These exclusions yielded an analytical sample of 27,720 of whom 2431 were immigrants. This study used publicly available data obtained from the Ministry of Health Social Services and Equity in Spain. Thus, ethical approval for the study was not required.

2.2. Variables

The dependent variable was obesity, defined according to the World Health Organization (WHO) as BMI ≥ 30 kg/m^2, and calculated using self-reported weight and height [28]. The independent variable was place of birth categorized as native for those born in Spain, and immigrants for those born in a country with non-very high HDI in 2015 (Europe, Africa, Latin America and Asia). In addition, educational attainment was considered as an effect measure modifier and was categorized as primary education or less, secondary and graduate or higher education [25].

Consistent with previous studies, we included the following covariates as potential confounders: age (18–24, 25–44 and 45–64 years) [26], living arrangement (married/couple and other), employment (employed, unemployed and other) and social class (using the classification of the Spanish Society of Epidemiology as non-manual workers for class I, II and III and manual workers for class IV and V) [29]. Consistent with a previous study [30], self-reported health responses were aggregated as good (very good and good) and poor (fair, bad and very bad). Finally, for health behaviors, we included smoking (current, former and never smoker) consumption of alcohol (frequent, occasional and not last year/never), physical activity at work and at leisure time (active and sedentary) and daily consumption of fruits and vegetables (yes/no) [25].

2.3. Statistical Analysis

Descriptive statistics for selected characteristics were calculated for the total population and according to place of birth in women and in men. In addition, prevalence estimates for obesity were calculated for each covariate according to place of birth in women and in men. Chi-square of independence and Cochran-Mantel-Haenszel statistics were used to assess significance associations between each covariate and (1) place of birth, and (2) place of birth and obesity in women and in men. Similarly, t-tests were used to assess differences for age and BMI according to place of birth in women and in men. We used log-binomial regression to quantify the association of place of birth with obesity in women and men before and after controlling for selected covariates. We tested interactions terms between place of birth and educational attainment in the fully-adjusted model for women and for men.

Data management procedures were carried out using SPSS 24.0. (IBM, Armonk, NY, USA) whereas the statistical analyses were conducted using SUDAAN 11.0.1 (RTI, Research Triangle Park, NC, USA) to take into account the complex sampling design and yield unbiased standard error estimates. Sample sizes presented in Table 1 were a-weighted, but all other estimates (proportions, standard errors, prevalence ratios [PR] and their 95% confidence intervals (95% CI) were weighted.

3. Results

Table 1 shows the distribution of selected sociodemographic, health status and health behavior characteristics for immigrant and native women and men. Around half of the immigrant population came from Latin America (54% men and 45% women). Immigrant women were younger, less educated, more likely to be employed as manual workers, have a partner, and rate their health status as worse than native women (all p-values < 0.001). In relation to health behaviors, immigrant women were less likely to be smokers, consume alcohol, be sedentary at work but more likely to have leisure time than their native counterparts (all p-values < 0.01). There was no association between consumption of fruits and vegetables and place of birth in women. As with women, immigrant men were younger, less educated, more likely to be employed as manual workers and to have a partner than their native counterparts (all p-values < 0.001). Immigrant men were also less likely to smoke, consume alcohol, be sedentary at work but more likely to have leisure time than native men (p-values < 0.01).

Table 1. Distribution of sociodemographic, self-rated health and health behavior characteristics for participants of the Spanish National Health Survey 2011–2012 and European Health Survey in Spain 2014.

Characteristic	Women				Men			
	Immigrants $n = 1338$	Natives $n = 12,624$	Total $n = 13,962$	p-Value *	Immigrants $n = 1093$	Natives $n = 12,665$	Total $n = 13,758$	p-Value *
	% (SE) **	% (SE)	% (SE)		% (SE)	% (SE)	% (SE)	
Survey year				<0.001				<0.001
2011	50.6 (1.7)	49.4 (0.5)	49.6 (0.5)		52.7 (1.9)	49.6 (0.5)	49.9 (0.5)	
2014	49.4 (1.7)	50.6 (0.5)	50.6 (0.5)		47.3 (1.9)	50.4 (0.5)	50.1 (0.5)	
Region of origin								
Europe	24.3 (1.5)				22.7 (1.6)			
Africa	16.2 (1.4)				27.0 (1.7)			
Latin America	54.2 (1.7)				44.8 (1.9)			
Asia	5.3 (0.8)				5.5 (0.9)			
Age (years)	36.8 (0.35)	41.9 (0.14)	41.2 (0.13)	<0.001	36.8 (0.42)	41.7 (0.14)	41.1 (0.13)	<0.001
18–24	11.3 (1.2)	10.6 (0.4)	10.7 (0.4)	<0.001	13.8 (1.4)	10.3 (0.4)	10.7 (0.4)	<0.001
25–44	65.2 (1.6)	45.4 (0.5)	48.3 (0.5)		62.4 (1.9)	46.8 (0.5)	48.7 (0.5)	
45–64	23.4 (1.4)	44.0 (0.5)	41.0 (0.5)		23.8 (1.6)	42.9 (0.5)	40.6 (0.5)	
Educational attainment				<0.001				<0.001
Primary or less	18.3 (1.4)	13.7 (0.4)	14.4 (0.4)		18.6 (1.5)	14.5 (0.4)	15.0 (0.4)	
Secondary	67.8 (1.6)	61.1 (0.5)	62.0 (0.5)		69.0 (1.7)	66.5 (0.5)	66.8 (0.5)	
Graduate or higher	13.9 (1.1)	25.3 (0.5)	23.6 (0.4)		12.3 (1.1)	19.1 (0.4)	18.2 (0.4)	
Social Class				<0.001				<0.001
Manual	83.1 (1.2)	55.9 (0.5)	59.8 (0.5)		84.0 (1.4)	58.4 (0.5)	61.4 (0.5)	
Non-manual	16.9 (1.2)	44.1 (0.5)	40.2 (0.5)		16.0 (1.4)	41.6 (0.5)	38.6 (0.5)	
Employment status				<0.001				<0.001
Employed	52.4 (1.7)	54.4 (0.5)	54.1 (0.5)		56.6 (1.9)	66.4 (0.5)	65.3 (0.5)	
Unemployed	22.8 (1.4)	17.2 (0.4)	18.0 (0.4)		33.5 (1.8)	18.2 (0.4)	20.0 (0.4)	
Others	24.7 (1.5)	28.5 (0.5)	27.9 (0.5)		9.9 (1.2)	15.4 (0.4)	14.7 (0.4)	
Living arrangement				<0.001				<0.001
Married/Couple	43.7 (1.7)	41.0 (0.5)	41.4 (0.5)		61.7 (1.8)	58.0 (0.5)	58.4 (0.5)	
Other	56.3 (1.7)	59.0 (0.5)	58.6 (0.5)		38.3 (1.8)	42.0 (0.5)	41.6 (0.5)	
Self-rated health				<0.001				<0.001
Good	71.1 (1.6)	76.0 (0.4)	75.3 (0.4)		81.1 (1.5)	81.2 (0.4)	81.2 (0.4)	
Poor	28.9 (1.6)	24.0 (0.4)	24.7 (0.4)		18.9 (1.5)	18.8 (0.4)	18.8 (0.4)	
Smoking status				<0.001				<0.001
Current Smoker	17.0 (1.2)	29.4 (0.5)	27.6 (0.5)		32.4 (1.5)	35.9 (0.5)	35.5 (0.5)	
Former Smoker	10.8 (1.0)	21.2 (0.4)	19.7 (0.4)		18.7 (1.5)	26.1 (0.5)	25.2 (0.4)	
Never smoked	72.2 (1.5)	49.5 (0.5)	52.7 (0.5)		48.9 (1.9)	38.0 (0.5)	39.3 (0.5)	
Alcohol consumption				<0.001				<0.001
Frequent	16.9 (1.2)	28.6 (0.5)	26.9 (0.4)		36.5 (1.8)	55.4 (0.5)	53.2 (0.5)	
Occasional	36.8 (1.6)	36.2 (0.5)	36.3 (0.5)		28.8 (1.7)	28.3 (0.5)	28.3 (0.5)	
Not last year/never	46.3 (1.7)	35.2 (0.5)	36.8 (0.5)		34.7 (1.8)	16.3 (0.4)	18.5 (0.4)	
Workplace physical activity				<0.001				<0.001
Sedentary	77.6 (1.4)	85.8 (0.4)	84.6 (0.4)		68.0 (1.7)	76.6 (0.4)	75.6 (0.4)	
Active	22.4 (14)	14.2 (0.4)	15.4 (0.4)		32.0 (1.7)	23.4 (0.4)	24.4 (0.4)	
Leisure-time physical activity				<0.001				<0.001
Sedentary	54.4 (1.7)	41.1 (0.5)	43.0 (0.5)		40.5 (1.9)	33.2 (0.5)	34.0 (0.5)	
Active	45.6 (1.7)	58.9 (0.5)	570 (0.5)		59.5 (1.9)	66.8 (0.5)	66.0 (0.5)	
Daily Consumption of fruit and vegetable				<0.001				<0.001
Yes	37.5 (1.7)	39.6 (0.5)	39.3 (0.5)		29.2 (1.7)	28.8 (0.5)	28.8 (0.5)	
No	62.5 (1.7)	60.4 (0.5)	60.7 (0.5)		70.8 (1.7)	71.2 (0.5)	71.2 (0.5)	
BMI, Kg/M^2	25.7 (0.18)	24.5 (0.05)	24.7 (0.05)	<0.001	25.9 (0.13)	26.4 (0.04)	26.3 (0.04)	<0.001

* p-values from Chi-square statistics and t-tests. ** Means and SEs presented for age and BMI.

Table 2 presents the prevalence estimates for obesity for selected characteristics according to place of birth in men and in women. For women, the prevalence of obesity was higher in immigrants (20%) than in native women (12.5%), with the highest prevalence among those from Africa (30.9%). When compared to native women, older age, low educational attainment, manual social class, married or living couple, and poor perceived health were associated with higher prevalence estimates of obesity among immigrants (all p-values < 0.001). In addition, lower prevalence of obesity was associated with smoking status, alcohol consumption, and physical activity at the work place and leisure in immigrant women relative to their native counterparts (all p-values < 0.05).

Table 2. Prevalence estimates for obesity according to place of birth in women and in men: Spanish National Health Survey 2011–2012 and European Health Survey in Spain 2014.

Characteristic	Women				Men			
	Immigrants n = 1338	Natives n = 12,624	Total n = 13,962	p-Value *	Immigrants n = 1093	Natives n = 12,665	Total n = 13,758	p-Value *
	% (SE)	% (SE)	% (SE)		% (SE)	% (SE)	% (SE)	
Overall	20.0 (1.4)	12.5 (0.3)	13.6 (0.4)	<0.001	12.5 (1.2)	16.9 (0.4)	16.4 (0.4)	<0.001
Survey year				0.257				0.192
2011	16.3 (1.9)	12.7 (0.5)	13.2 (0.5)		12.9 (1.7)	17.4 (0.6)	16.9 (0.5)	
2014	23.8 (2.1)	12.3 (0.5)	14.0 (0.5)		12.0 (2.1)	16.5 (0.5)	16.0 (0.5)	
Region of origin								
Europe	15.4 (2.8)				13.4 (2.6)			
Africa	30.9 (4.3)				10.7 (2.3)			
Latin America	20.5 (1.9)				13.8 (1.9)			
Asia	2.7 (1.7)				6.1 (3.4)			
Age (years)				<0.001				<0.001
18–24	6.4 (2.5)	4.4 (0.8)	4.7 (0.8)		2.8 (1.5)	5.4 (0.9)	5.0 (0.8)	
25–44	18.4 (1.7)	9.7 (0.5)	11.4 (0.5)		12.4 (1.5)	13.7 (0.5)	13.5 (0.5)	
45–64	30.9 (3.4)	17.3 (0.6)	18.4 (0.6)		18.4 (3.0)	23.2 (0.6)	22.9 (0.6)	
Educational attainment				<0.001				<0.001
Primary or less	35.2 (4.4)	25.6 (1.2)	27.4 (1.3)		10.3 (2.8)	24.8 (1.2)	22.7 (1.1)	
Secondary	17.5 (1.6)	12.3 (0.4)	13.2 (0.5)		12.5 (1.5)	17.1 (0.5)	16.5 (0.5)	
Graduate or higher	12.1 (2.7)	5.8 (0.5)	6.3 (0.5)		15.5 (3.4)	10.5 (0.7)	10.9 (0.7)	
Social class				<0.001				<0.001
Manual	21.7 (1.6)	15.7 (0.5)	16.9 (0.5)		11.8 (1.3)	19.5 (0.5)	18.3 (0.5)	
Non-manual	11.4 (2.5)	8.4 (0.4)	8.6 (0.4)		16.0 (3.2)	13.3 (0.5)	13.5 (0.5)	
Employment status				<0.001				0.016
Employed	16.1 (1.8)	9.4 (0.4)	10.3 (0.4)		12.1 (1.5)	16.2 (0.5)	15.7 (0.4)	
Unemployed	22.1 (2.9)	16.0 (1.0)	17.1 (0.9)		15.2 (2.5)	18.9 (1.0)	18.2 (0.9)	
Others	26.2 (3.4)	16.3 (0.7)	17.6 (0.8)		5.3 (2.5)	18.0 (1.0)	17.0 (1.0)	
Living arrangement				<0.001				<0.001
Married/Couple	23.4 (2.1)	14.2 (0.5)	15.5 (0.5)		16.7 (1.8)	20.0 (0.5)	19.5 (0.5)	
Other	15.6 (1.9)	10.0 (0.5)	10.9 (0.5)		5.6 (1.1)	12.8 (0.5)	12.0 (0.5)	
Self-rated health				<0.001				<0.001
Good	14.8 (1.5)	9.6 (0.4)	10.3 (0.4)		11.9 (1.3)	14.9 (0.4)	14.5 (0.4)	
Poor	32.7 (3.2)	21.6 (0.9)	23.5 (0.9)		14.9 (1.3)	26.0 (1.0)	24.6 (1.0)	
Smoking status				0.032				<0.001
Current smoker	21.0 (3.5)	10.9 (0.6)	11.8 (0.6)		9.2 (1.9)	15.5 (0.6)	14.8 (0.6)	
Former smoker	22.0 (3.9)	12.4 (0.8)	13.1 (0.8)		17.3 (3.2)	23.2 (0.8)	22.7 (0.8)	
Never smoked	19.4 (1.7)	13.5 (0.5)	14.7 (0.5)		12.8 (1.8)	14.0 (0.6)	13.8 (0.6)	
Alcohol consumption				<0.001				0.110
Frequent	14.0 (2.7)	8.8 (0.5)	9.2 (0.6)		13.8 (2.1)	16.4 (0.5)	16.2 (0.5)	
Occasional	17.5 (2.2)	11.2 (0.5)	12.2 (0.6)		14.2 (2.5)	16.3 (0.7)	16.1 (0.7)	
Not last year/never	24.1 (2.3)	16.8 (0.7)	18.1 (0.7)		9.7 (1.8)	20.0 (1.1)	17.7 (0.9)	
Workplace physical activity				0.718				0.273
Sedentary	19.7 (1.6)	12.5 (0.4)	13.4 (0.4)		12.8 (1.5)	17.2 (0.4)	16.7 (0.4)	
Active	20.9 (3.1)	12.7 (0.9)	14.4 (1.0)		11.7 (2.2)	16.2 (0.8)	15.5 (0.7)	
Leisure-time physical activity				<0.001				<0.001
Sedentary	22.8 (2.1)	16.0 (0.6)	17.2 (0.6)		12.2 (1.8)	24.0 (0.8)	22.4 (0.7)	
Active	16.7 (1.9)	10.1 (0.4)	10.8 (0.4)		12.7 (1.6)	13.4 (0.4)	13.3 (0.4)	
Daily Consumption of fruit and vegetables				0.409				0.471
Yes	19.8 (2.4)	13.0 (0.5)	13.4 (0.5)		12.5 (1.2)	17.4 (0.7)	16.8 (0.7)	
No	20.1 (1.8)	12.2 (0.4)	13.9 (0.6)		12.4 (1.5)	16.8 (0.5)	16.2 (0.4)	

* p-values from Cochran-Mantel-Haenszel statistics.

In men, the prevalence of obesity was lower among immigrants relative to their native peers (12.5% vs. 16.9%; $p < 0.001$), especially among those coming from Asia (6.1%). Immigrant men exhibited lower prevalence estimates for obesity associated with age, employment status, living arrangement, self-rated health, smoking status and leisure-time physical activity compared with native men (all p-values < 0.05). Moreover, low educational attainment and manual social class were associated with lower prevalence of obesity among immigrant men whereas the opposite was true for native men (p-values < 0.001).

Table 3 shows unadjusted and adjusted prevalence ratios for obesity with their 95% confidence intervals (CI) for immigrant men and women relative to their native counterparts. For women, the probability of obesity was 1.60 (95% CI: 1.38–1.86) times higher in immigrants compared with natives. This probability increased after adjusting for age and self-rated health (PR: 1.73; 95% CI: 1.50–2.00). However, the association while attenuated remained significant in the fully-adjusted model (Model 5: PR: 1.42; 95% CI: 1.22–1.64). For men, the probability of obesity was 26% (PR: 0.74; 95% CI: 0.60–0.89) lower in immigrants relative to natives. This lower probability of obesity remained significant and nearly unchanged in the final model (PR: 0.73; 95% CI: 0.59–0.89).

Table 3. Prevalence ratios and their 95% confidence intervals of obesity for place of birth in women and in men: Spanish National Health Survey 2011–2012 and European Health Survey in Spain 2014.

Place of Birth	Unadjusted	Model 1 *	Model 2	Model 3	Model 4	Model 5
Women						
Natives	1.00	1.00	1.00	1.00	1.00	1.00
Immigrants	1.60 (1.3–1.86)	1.60 (1.3–1.86)	1.73 (1.5–2.00)	1.73 (1.5–2.01)	1.56 (1.3–1.81)	1.42 (1.2–1.64)
Men						
Natives	1.00	1.00	1.00	1.00	1.00	1.00
Immigrants	0.74 (0.60–0.89)	0.73 (0.6–0.89)	0.83 (0.6–1.01)	0.79 (0.6–0.95)	0.75 (0.6–0.92)	0.73 (0.5–0.89)

* Model 1 adjusted for survey year; model 2 additionally adjusted for age and self-rated health; model 3 additionally adjusted for employment status and living arrangement; model 4 additionally adjusted for physical activity at work and at leisure time, smoking, alcohol consumption and daily consumption of fruits and vegetables; and model 5 additionally adjusted for social class and education attainment.

Heterogeneity for the association between place of birth and obesity was observed according to education in men (*p*-interaction = 0.002) but not in women (*p*-interaction = 0.94). Figure 1 shows that immigrant men with at least a primary (PR: 0.47; 95% CI: 0.26–0.83) and secondary (PR: 0.75; 95% CI: 0.59–0.95) education have a protective effect against obesity compared with their native counterparts. Immigrant women have higher probability of obesity than native women regardless of educational attainment. However, the probability of obesity was greater among immigrant women with a graduate or higher education.

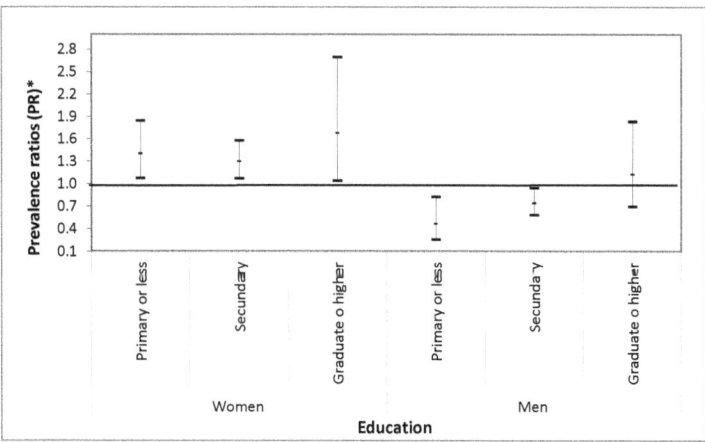

Figure 1. Prevalence ratios (PR) * and 95% confidence intervals of obesity for place of birth according to educational attainment in women and in men: Spanish National Health Survey 2011–2012, and European Health Survey in Spain 2014. * Adjusted for survey year, age, self-rated health, employment status, living arrangement, physical activity at work and at leisure time, smoking, alcohol consumption, daily consumption of fruits and vegetables and social class.

4. Discussion

We found a greater probability of obesity in immigrant women and a lower probability of obesity in immigrant men relative to their native counterparts, after adjusting for sociodemographic characteristics, self-rated health and health behaviors. In addition, this association depends on education in men with those with lower educational levels having a lower probability of obesity. Although we did not find heterogeneity of the association between place of birth and obesity according to education among women, immigrant women were more likely to be obese than the native regardless of their education, with the higher probability observed among women with the highest education.

For men, the finding of lower prevalence of obesity among immigrants from Africa, Asia and Latin America, relative to natives is consistent with studies conducted in Spain and in other countries of southern Europe [17,26,31]. However, the obesity inequalities between immigrants and native men are not conclusive and depend on the country of destination and the prevalence of obesity [15] of the home country [16,32], length of stay [31] or whether men are first or second generation in the host country [15,33]. For women, the highest prevalence of obesity among immigrants compared to natives is also consistent with previous studies in Europe regardless of the country of birth [14–16,26,32,34]. In addition, similarly to studies conducted in the Netherlands [16] and Sweden [14] with immigrants from Morocco, sub-Saharan Africa Central and South America, obesity inequalities between native and immigrant women, persist after adjusting for sociodemographic characteristics and health behaviors. Hence, place of birth in women may be considered a social determinant of obesity inequality. For women, factors associated with double discrimination, gender and immigration status, can explain their greater prevalence of obesity.

Despite the extant evidence on the protective effect of higher educational attainment on health status and specifically in obesity [18,19,21,22], we found a protective effect at lower educational levels in immigrant men relative to their native peers. This finding may be explained by the following reason: the health status before and after the migration process may help explain the different role of education on obesity for immigrant men. Before the migration process, evidence indicates that, even in their country of origin, the health status of immigrants is better than that of the rest of the population, a phenomenon known as healthy migrant effect [35]. Once in the host country, in this case Spain, regardless of education, immigrants are inserted in a precarious labor market segmented by place of birth and gender [36]. For immigrant men, the labor market includes construction, catering and agriculture requiring great physical effort and jobs in which discrimination attributable to obesity may be present [37]. This social reality may contribute to the lower prevalence of obesity among immigrant men with lower education, and thus, less chance to move into the labor market [38]. However, among immigrants with higher education, there is a mismatch between education and employment opportunities. This mismatch is referred in the literature as a determinant of health [39] and may explain the lack of a protective effect from education against obesity as we found in this study.

For immigrant women, as with immigrant men, the migration process is also triggered among those who are healthy [35]. However, in the host country, i.e., Spain, with the gender segmentation of the labor market, immigrant women are more likely to mainly hold domestic and care jobs, regardless of educational attainment [40]. This labor market is characterized by low-income, intense and long working hours, social isolation and poor opportunities for labor mobility leading to little control over schedules and to high level of stress [41]. The latter concurs with Sliwa et al. [42] findings of higher prevalence of obesity in immigrant women performing domestic work where strong physical demands are required. In addition, and as with immigrant men, the labor over-qualifications for immigrant women may explain the lack of a protective effect of education against obesity compared with native women. Thus, place of birth may affect how education related to health status among the immigrant population.

The study presents few limitations that deserve attention. First, this is a cross-sectional study and does not allow to establish a temporal relationship between exposure and outcome. Second, we could not present information according to country of birth for the immigrant population. The lack of this information may have masked greater obesity inequalities between the immigrant and the native populations. However, we repeated the analyses using region of birth (Europe, Latin America, Africa and Asia). Although not statistically significant, the results were consistent to the ones reported here for men (lower PR for immigrant relative to native) and women (higher PR for immigrant than native) with the exception of Asian women who exhibited lower prevalence of obesity than their native counterparts. Third, BMI was calculated using self-reported weight and height by the respondents. Evidence suggests that women may underestimate the body weight while men may overestimate their height. This misreporting may have biased the actual prevalence of obesity [43]. Finally, the proportion of missing values for BMI was higher for immigrants, with low education, especially in women. The latter may have underestimated our findings.

Despite the limitations, it is worth noting that this is the first study to examine obesity inequalities among a representative population of immigrants and natives in Spain. In addition, analyses were performed separately in women and in men to examine gender inequalities according to place of birth and further by educational attainment. Finally, we have access to a wide range of information collected through the surveys and a large sample size providing the power to examine interactions.

5. Conclusions

This study contributes to an understudied area, the investigation of obesity inequalities between immigrant and native populations. In addition, this study goes a step further by examining the joint effect of place of birth and education attainment. Our findings suggest that place of birth may affect obesity in both, women and men. However, this effect may be compounded with education differently for women and men. Thus, studies examining health outcome among immigrant populations relative to native populations should consider the inclusion of education as a potential partner for the effect of place of birth. A better understanding of how these factors work together is needed when designing strategies for health promotion to reduce obesity inequalities between immigrant and native populations regardless of gender. Furthermore, it is essential to develop gender-specific policies to promote equal opportunities in the labor market, especially among immigrant women with limited capacity to negotiate their working conditions.

Author Contributions: E.R.-A., N.L. and L.N.B. were responsible for the study concept and design. E.R.-A. wrote the first draft of the manuscript. N.L. and L.N.B. were responsible for conceptualizing and designing the analysis, interpreting the results and contribute to the writing of the manuscript. All authors critically reviewed and approved the final version of the manuscript.

Funding: This work was supported by the Basque Government's research fund to consolidate research groups. Ref. IT977-16.

Conflicts of Interest: The authors declare no conflict of interest. The results and opinions discussed in this article are the sole responsibility of the authors.

References

1. Afshin, A.; Forouzanfar, M.H.; Reitsma, M.B.; Sur, P.; Estep, K.; Lee, A.; Marczak, L.; Mokdad, A.H.; Moradi-Lakeh, M.; Naghavi, M.; et al. Health Effects of Overweight and Obesity in 195 Countries over 25 Years. *N. Engl. J. Med.* **2017**, *377*, 13–27. [CrossRef] [PubMed]
2. Flegal, K.M.; Kit, B.K.; Orpana, H.; Graubard, B.I. Association of all-cause mortality with overweight and obesity using standard body mass index categories: A systematic review and meta-analysis. *JAMA* **2013**, *309*, 71–82. [CrossRef] [PubMed]
3. James, W.P.T.; McPherson, K. The costs of overweight. *Lancet Public Health* **2017**, *2*, e203–e204. [CrossRef]
4. Cesare, M.D.; Bentham, J.; Stevens, G.A.; Zhou, B.; Danaei, G.; Lu, Y.; Cowan, M.J.; Riley, L.M.; Hajifathalian, K.; Fortunato, L.; et al. Trends in adult body-mass index in 200 countries from 1975 to 2014: A pooled analysis of 1698 population-based measurement studies with 19.2 million participants. *Lancet* **2016**, *387*, 1377–1396. [CrossRef]

5. Marques, A.; Peralta, M.; Naia, A.; Loureiro, N.; de Matos, M.G. Prevalence of adult overweight and obesity in 20 European countries, 2014. *Eur. J. Public Health* **2018**, *28*, 295–300. [CrossRef] [PubMed]
6. Webber, L.; Divajeva, D.; Marsh, T.; McPherson, K.; Brown, M.; Galea, G.; Breda, J. The future burden of obesity-related diseases in the 53 WHO European-Region countries and the impact of effective interventions: A modelling study. *BMJ Open* **2014**, *4*, e004787. [CrossRef] [PubMed]
7. Mackenbach, J.P.; Stirbu, I.; Roskam, A.J.; Schaap, M.M.; Menvielle, G.; Leinsalu, M.; Kunst, A.E. Socioeconomic inequalities in health in 22 European countries. *N. Engl. J. Med.* **2008**, *358*, 2468–2681. [CrossRef] [PubMed]
8. Thevenot, C. Inequality in OECD countries. *Scand. J. Public Health* **2017**, *45*, 9–16. [CrossRef] [PubMed]
9. Marmot, M.; Wilkinson, R.G. *Social Determinants of Health: The Solid Facts*, 2nd ed.; Oxford University Press: Oxford, UK, 2006; ISBN 978-92-890-1401-4.
10. Malmusi, D.; Borrell, C.; Benach, J. Migration-related health inequalities: Showing the complex interactions between gender, social class and place of origin. *Soc. Sci. Med.* **2010**, *71*, 1610–1619. [CrossRef] [PubMed]
11. Rodriguez-Alvarez, E.; Gonzalez-Rabago, Y.; Bacigalupe, A.; Martin, U.; Lanborena Elordui, N. Immigration and health: Social inequalities between native and immigrant populations in the Basque Country (Spain). *Gac. Sanit.* **2014**, *28*, 274–280. (In Spanish) [CrossRef] [PubMed]
12. Borrell, C.; Muntaner, C.; Sole, J.; Artazcoz, L.; Puigpinos, R.; Benach, J.; Noh, S. Immigration and self-reported health status by social class and gender: The importance of material deprivation, work organisation and household labour. *J. Epidemiol. Community Health* **2008**, *62*, e7. [CrossRef] [PubMed]
13. Ruiz-Perez, I.; Bermudez-Tamayo, C.; Rodriguez-Barranco, M. Socio-economic factors linked with mental health during the recession: A multilevel analysis. *Int. J. Equity Health* **2017**, *16*, 45. [CrossRef] [PubMed]
14. Carlsson, A.C.; Wandell, P.; Riserus, U.; Arnlov, J.; Borne, Y.; Engstrom, G.; Leander, K.; Gigante, B.; Hellenius, M.L.; de Faire, U. Differences in anthropometric measures in immigrants and Swedish-born individuals: Results from two community-based cohort studies. *Prev. Med.* **2014**, *69*, 151–156. [CrossRef] [PubMed]
15. Dijkshoorn, H.; Nicolaou, M.; Ujcic-Voortman, J.K.; Schouten, G.M.; Bouwman Notenboom, A.J.; Berns, M.P.; Verhoeff, A.P. Overweight and obesity in young Turkish, Moroccan and Surinamese migrants of the second generation in the Netherlands. *Public Health Nutr.* **2014**, *17*, 2037–2044. [CrossRef] [PubMed]
16. Ujcic-Voortman, J.K.; Bos, G.; Baan, C.A.; Verhoeff, A.P.; Seidell, J.C. Obesity and body fat distribution: Ethnic differences and the role of socio-economic status. *Obes. Facts* **2011**, *4*, 53–60. [CrossRef] [PubMed]
17. Toselli, S.; Gualdi-Russo, E.; Boulos, D.N.; Anwar, W.A.; Lakhoua, C.; Jaouadi, I.; Khyatti, M.; Hemminki, K. Prevalence of overweight and obesity in adults from North Africa. *Eur. J. Public Health* **2014**, *24*, 31–39. [CrossRef] [PubMed]
18. Devaux, M.; Sassi, F. Social inequalities in obesity and overweight in 11 OECD countries. *Eur. J. Public Health* **2013**, *23*, 464–469. [CrossRef] [PubMed]
19. Roskam, A.J.; Kunst, A.E.; Van Oyen, H.; Demarest, S.; Klumbiene, J.; Regidor, E.; Helmert, U.; Jusot, F.; Dzurova, D.; Mackenbach, J.P. Comparative appraisal of educational inequalities in overweight and obesity among adults in 19 European countries. *Int. J. Epidemiol.* **2010**, *39*, 392–404. [CrossRef] [PubMed]
20. Gallus, S.; Lugo, A.; Murisic, B.; Bosetti, C.; Boffetta, P.; La Vecchia, C. Overweight and obesity in 16 European countries. *Eur. J. Nutr.* **2015**, *54*, 679–689. [CrossRef] [PubMed]
21. Barrington, D.S.; Baquero, M.C.; Borrell, L.N.; Crawford, N.D. Racial/ethnic disparities in obesity among US-born and foreign-born adults by sex and education. *Obesity* **2010**, *18*, 422–424. [CrossRef] [PubMed]
22. Sanchez-Vaznaugh, E.V.; Kawachi, I.; Subramanian, S.V.; Sanchez, B.N.; Acevedo-Garcia, D. Differential effect of birthplace and length of residence on body mass index (BMI) by education, gender and race/ethnicity. *Soc. Sci. Med.* **2008**, *67*, 1300–1310. [CrossRef] [PubMed]
23. Rodriguez-Caro, A.; Vallejo-Torres, L.; Lopez-Valcarcel, B. Unconditional quantile regressions to determine the social gradient of obesity in Spain 1993–2014. *Int. J. Equity Health* **2016**, *15*, 175. [CrossRef] [PubMed]
24. National Institute of Statistics of Spain NIE. Population Figures at 1 January 2018. Available online: http://www.ine.es/prensa/pad_2018_p.pdf (In Spanish) (accessed on 15 March 2018).
25. Gutierrez-Fisac, J.L.; Marin-Guerrero, A.; Regidor, E.; Guallar-Castillón, P.; Banegas, J.R.; Rodríguez-Artalejo, F. Length of residence and obesity among immigrants in Spain. *Public Health Nutr.* **2010**, *13*, 1593–1598. [CrossRef] [PubMed]

26. Marín-Guerrero, A.C.; Gutiérrez-Fisac, J.L.; Guallar-Castillón, P.; Banegas, J.R.; Regidor, E.; Rodríguez-Artalejo, F. Prevalence of obesity in immigrants in Madrid. *Med. Clin.* **2010**, *134*, 483–485. (In Spanish) [CrossRef]
27. Eurostat. Migrant Integration Statistics-Education Statistics Explained [Internet]. Available online: http://ec.europa.eu/eurostat/statistics-explained/index.php?title=Migrant_integration_statistics_-_education (accessed on 8 February 2018).
28. World Health Organization (WHO). Global Database on Body Mass Index. 2013. Available online: http://www.who.int/bmi (accessed on 15 September 2017).
29. Domingo-Salvany, A.; Bacigalupe, A.; Carrasco, J.M.; Espelt, A.; Ferrando, J.; Borrell, C. Proposals for social class classification based on the Spanish National Classification of Occupations 2011 using neo-Weberian and neo-Marxist approaches. *Gac. Sanit.* **2013**, *27*, 263–272. (In Spanish) [CrossRef] [PubMed]
30. Rodriguez-Alvarez, E.; Gonzalez-Rábago, Y.; Borrell, L.N.; Lanborena, N. Perceived discrimination and self-rated health in the immigrant population of the Basque Country, Spain. *Gac. Sanit.* **2017**, *31*, 390–395. [CrossRef] [PubMed]
31. Da Costa, L.P.; Dias, S.F.; Martins, M.D. Association between length of residence and overweight among adult immigrants in Portugal: A nationwide cross-sectional study. *BMC Public Health* **2017**, *17*, 316. [CrossRef] [PubMed]
32. Kumar, B.N.; Meyer, H.E.; Wandel, M.; Dalen, I.; Holmboe-Ottesen, G. Ethnic differences in obesity among immigrants from developing countries, in Oslo, Norway. *Int. J. Obes.* **2006**, *30*, 684–690. [CrossRef] [PubMed]
33. Hosper, K.; Nicolaou, M.; van Valkengoed, I.; Nierkens, V.; Stronks, K. Social and cultural factors underlying generational differences in overweight: A cross-sectional study among ethnic minorities in the Netherlands. *BMC Public Health* **2011**, *11*, 105. [CrossRef] [PubMed]
34. Martin-Fernandez, J.; Grillo, F.; Tichit, C.; Parizot, I.; Chauvin, P. Overweight according to geographical origin and time spent in France: A cross sectional study in the Paris metropolitan area. *BMC Public Health* **2012**, *12*, 937. [CrossRef] [PubMed]
35. Kennedy, S.; Kidd, M.P.; McDonald, J.T.; Biddle, N. The Healthy Immigrant Effect: Patterns and Evidence from Four Countries. *J. Int. Migr. Integr.* **2014**, *16*, 317–332. [CrossRef]
36. Domingo, A.; Gil-Alonso, F. Immigration and changing labour force structure in the southern European Union. *Population* **2007**, *62*, 709–727. [CrossRef]
37. Averett, S. Obesity and labor market outcomes. *IZA World Labor* **2014**. [CrossRef]
38. King, G.A.; Fitzhugh, E.C.; Bassett, D.R., Jr.; McLaughlin, J.E.; Strath, S.J.; Swartz, A.M.; Thompson, D.L. Relationship of leisure-time physical activity and occupational activity to the prevalence of obesity. *Int. J. Obes.* **2001**, *25*, 606–612. [CrossRef] [PubMed]
39. Dunlavy, A.C.; Garcy, A.M.; Rostila, M. Educational mismatch and health status among foreign-born workers in Sweden. *Soc. Sci. Med.* **2016**, *154*, 36–44. [CrossRef] [PubMed]
40. Vidal-Coso, E.; Miret-Gamundi, P. The labour trajectories of immigrant women in Spain: Are there signs of upward social mobility? *Demogr. Res.* **2014**, *31*, 337–380. [CrossRef]
41. Ahonen, E.Q.; Lopez-Jacob, M.J.; Vazquez, M.L.; Porthe, V.; Gil-González, D.; García, A.M.; Ruiz-Frutos, C.; Benach, J.; Benavides, F.G. Invisible work, unseen hazards: The health of women immigrant household service workers in Spain. *Am. J. Ind. Med.* **2010**, *53*, 405–416. [CrossRef] [PubMed]
42. Sliwa, S.A.; Must, A.; Perea, F.C.; Boulos, R.J.; Economos, C.D. Occupational Physical Activity and Weight-Related Outcomes in Immigrant Mothers. *Am. J. Prev. Med.* **2016**, *51*, 637–646. [CrossRef] [PubMed]
43. Nyholm, M.; Gullberg, B.; Merlo, J.; Lundqvist-Persson, C.; Rastam, L.; Lindblad, U. The validity of obesity based on self-reported weight and height: Implications for population studies. *Obesity* **2007**, *15*, 197–208. [CrossRef] [PubMed]

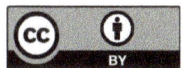

© 2018 by the authors. Licensee MDPI, Basel, Switzerland. This article is an open access article distributed under the terms and conditions of the Creative Commons Attribution (CC BY) license (http://creativecommons.org/licenses/by/4.0/).

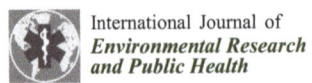

Article

Related Factors of Suicidal Ideation among North Korean Refugee Youth in South Korea

Subin Park [1], Soo Jung Rim [1] and Jin Yong Jun [2,*]

[1] Department of Research Planning, Mental Health Research Institute, National Center for Mental Health, Seoul 04933, Korea; subin-21@hanmail.net (S.P.); soojung0411@gmail.com (S.J.R.)
[2] Department of Psychiatry, National Center for Mental Health, Seoul 04933, Korea
* Correspondence: jjy826@naver.com; Tel.: +822-2204-0151

Received: 28 June 2018; Accepted: 7 August 2018; Published: 9 August 2018

Abstract: This study investigated the factors associated with suicidal ideation among 174 North Korean refugees (aged 13–27 years) residing in South Korea. Specifically, we compared sociodemographic, familial, social, and psychological characteristics between participants with and without suicidal ideation. Twenty-nine refugees (16.7%) had exhibited suicidal ideation in the past 12 months. These refugees had significantly lower levels of familial cohesion ($U = 1459.0$; $p < 0.001$), self-esteem ($U = 1032.0$; $p < 0.001$), and resilience ($U = 1190.0$; $p < 0.001$), as well as higher levels of expressional suppression ($U = 1202.5$; $p < 0.001$) and post-traumatic stress disorder symptoms ($U = 1303.0$; $p = 0.001$), (with Cohen's $d > 0.5$), compared to those without suicidal ideation. A multiple logistic regression analysis showed that the level of emotional suppression and familial cohesion were significantly associated with suicidal ideation, after controlling for the other variables. Familial and individual interventions, particularly those focused on encouraging emotional expression and familial cohesion, will be useful for North Korean refugee youth, who have a high risk of suicide.

Keywords: refugee; adolescent; risk factor; protective factor

1. Introduction

Almost half of the individuals who emigrate for reasons such as armed conflict, persecution, and economic pressure in their home countries are children and adolescents [1]. These children and youth not only suffer during their escape or displacement from their home country, but also after their arrival and during settlement in their new country [2]. Accordingly, researchers have been focusing greater attention on how to support their development following this rapid transition.

The number of North Korean refugees (NKRs) that settled in South Korea exceeded 30,000 in 2016, and around 40% of these were individuals aged 10–29 years [3]. Like other refugees, NKRs are exposed to traumatic events not only when residing in North Korea, but also during their escape [4]. Even after they have settled in South Korea, NKRs often struggle to adapt to their new culture [5]. NKR youths, in particular, face obstacles such as gaps in physical health, compared to same-age peers, perceived discrimination, culture shock, and low social support, all of which can lead to the high drop-out rates from school and unemployment after settling in South Korea [6,7]. Correspondingly, NKR youths often suffer from anxiety, depression, and post-traumatic stress disorder (PTSD) [8–10], all of which are associated with suicide ideation and attempts [11,12].

In 2009, suicide was reported as the leading cause of death among youth (i.e., 15–19 years old) in South Korea [13,14]. Since NKR youths are exposed to traumatic events and suffer in adapting to their new environment, they naturally require more clinical attention [15]; in fact, NKR youths appear to have a much higher prevalence of suicidal ideation compared to South Korean youths [16]. Since suicidal ideation is considered to have a strong association with suicidal behavior [17], it is important to investigate the factors related to suicidal ideation to prevent suicide. Klonsky and

May [18], proposed the Three Step Theory of Suicide. The first step states that for an individual to have suicidal ideation, pain and feeling of hopelessness are needed. Then, if an individual has a suicidal ideation and also feels unconnected to life, he or she will move on to the next step: strong ideation. Finally, if an individual is capable of making a suicide attempt, he or she will proceed to the final step, actual attempt. According to this theory, suicide happens in a stepwise manner, so finding factors that are related to suicidal ideation is important to prevent individuals from proceeding to the next step. Since NKR youths experience traumatic events, the factors that are related to suicidal ideation of this group could be different from the general public. Therefore, exploring which factors are associated with this vulnerable group's suicidal ideation is important. However, to our knowledge, there has been no study investigating the factors influencing the suicidal ideation of this vulnerable group.

This study investigated the factors associated with suicidal ideation among NKR youths to prevent them from proceeding to the next step of the Three Step Theory. When exploring factors related to suicidal ideation of NKR youths, we have referred to a conceptual framework used by Reed and colleagues [1], which is based on the ecological model by Bronfenbrenner [19]. This conceptual framework [1] is used to explain the risk and protective factors for mental health of refugees. In this framework, the protective and risk factors of mental health are divided into four levels: individual (e.g., physical, psychological, or developmental disorders, age, sex, and exposure to violence), family (e.g., family composition, bereavement, and functioning), community (community social support), and societal (for example, language or cultural differences). We concentrated on factors from individual, family, and community level that could influence NKR youth's mental health. Factors included in the societal level were not included in the present study, due to aspects of data availability. Specifically, we explored sociodemographic (individual level), psychological (individual level), familial (family level), and social (community level) factors that might influence suicidal ideation of NKR youths in South Korea.

2. Materials and Methods

2.1. Participants and Procedure

We recruited NKR youths between 2017 and 2018 from two alternative schools for NKRs who are preparing for qualification examinations for middle- or high-school graduation. NKR youths who settle in South Korea go through a mental health screening program, of which this study was a part. All individuals who participated in the program were selected for recruitment, and consequently, a total of 174 NKR youths aged 13–27 years participated in this study. Participants completed a self-report questionnaire on their sociodemographic, familial, social, and psychological characteristics, as well as whether they had ever seriously considered suicide in the last 12 months. Informed consent was obtained from all participants. Among 174 participants, 29 (16.7%) answered that they had seriously thought about suicide in the past 12 months. The study was reviewed and approved by the institutional review board of the National Center for Mental Health (No. 116271-2017-11).

2.2. Measurements

2.2.1. Sociodemographic Characteristics

Information on sociodemographic characteristics (i.e., age, sex, birthplace, parental educational levels, and type of residence), which is part of the individual level, was obtained.

2.2.2. Familial and Social Support

Familial (family level) and social support (community level) were assessed using the FACES III questionnaire [20,21], which comprises 20 items. There are two major parameters of family functioning that FACES III explores: cohesion and adaptability. Cohesion is assessed via statements such as "Family members know each other's close friends" and "Our family does things together". Adaptability is assessed via items such as "When problems arise we compromise" and "Family members say what they want". Each item is rated on a scale ranging from 1 ("almost never") to 5 ("almost always").

We also assessed participants' level of psychological support from others by asking participants "How much psychological support do you currently receive from your family, relatives, friends, and others around you?" Practical support was assessed by asking participants "How much practical support do you currently receive from your family, relatives, friends, and others around you?" For both questions, the responses were given on a 10-point Likert scale (1 = "not at all"; 10 = "receive enough support").

2.2.3. Psychological Characteristics

Psychological characteristics (i.e., resilience, self-esteem, cognitive style, impulsivity, and PTSD symptoms), which are included in the individual level, were assessed. We utilized the Brief Resilience Scale [22] to measure resilience (defined as the self-perceived ability to bounce back from stress). This scale contains three positive items (i.e., items 1, 3, and 5) and three negative items (i.e., items 2, 4, and 6). Each item is rated on a five-point scale (1 = "strongly disagree"; 5 = "strongly agree"). Negative items were reverse-scored. The total score ranges from 6 to 30, with higher scores indicating higher resilience.

The Rosenberg Self-Esteem Scale [23] was utilized to measure global self-worth. This scale contains ten items, and each rated on a 5-point Likert scale (1 = "strongly disagree" to 5 = "strongly agree"). The score ranges from 10 to 50, with higher scores indicating higher self-esteem.

The Emotion Regulation Questionnaire (ERQ) [24,25] was utilized to assess cognitive reappraisal (e.g., "When I'm faced with a stressful situation, I make myself think about it in a way that helps me stay calm") and expressive suppression (e.g., "I control my emotions by not expressing them"), which are two emotion regulation strategies. Each item was rated on a 7-point Likert scale (1 = "strongly disagree"; 7 = "strongly agree"). Higher scores on each subscale indicate the respondent's greater use of the corresponding emotion regulation strategy.

The Barratt Impulsivity Scale-Brief (BIS-Brief) was used to assess impulsivity [26]. This scale utilizes 8 items from the Korean version of the BIS-11, which has been evaluated for its validity and reliability [27]. Each item is rated on a 4-point Likert scale. Higher scores indicate higher impulsivity.

The Children's Revised Impact of Event Scale (CRIES) [28] was used to assess the degree of PTSD symptoms. The CRIES is a 13-item self-report scale adapted from the Impact of Event Scale [29]. Each item is scored on a four-point Likert scale (0 = "not at all"; 3 = "often"). Higher scores indicate higher PTSD symptoms.

2.2.4. Suicidal Ideation

Suicidal ideation was measured with a single question asking participants "Have you ever seriously considered suicide in the last 12 months?" Participants who stated that they had a suicidal ideation in the last 12 months were classified as high risk group and were consulted by a physician if needed.

2.3. Statistical Analyses

We compared the sociodemographic characteristics of individuals with and without suicidal ideation using the independent t-test for continuous variables and chi-square test for categorical variables. Then, we investigated the difference between familial, social, and psychological characteristics of those with and without suicidal ideation. According to the Kolmogorov–Smirnov normality test, none of these variables had a normal distribution. Therefore, the Mann–Whitney U test was performed. Also, the effect size for each factor was retrieved, and those with medium size effect (Cohen's $d > 0.5$) were accepted [30]. We then conducted a multiple binary logistic regression analysis with suicidal ideation as the main outcome variable, and the variables that significantly differed between suicidal and non-suicidal participants as the principal predictors. All statistical analyses were performed using SPSS Statistics 21.0 (IBM Corp, Armonk, NY, USA). Statistical significance was defined as an alpha of less than 0.05.

3. Results

Table 1 shows the sociodemographic characteristics of the NKR youths with and without suicidal ideation. We observed no significant group differences in terms of sex, age, parental origin, parental educational levels, or type of residence.

Table 2 shows the familial, social, and psychological characteristics of NKR youths with and without suicidal ideation. NKR youths with suicidal ideation reported lower familial cohesion compared to those without suicidal ideation. The former group also had lower resilience and self-esteem, higher PTSD symptoms, and used emotional suppression more frequently compared to the latter group. There was a difference between familial adaptability between NKR youths with and without suicidal ideation, however, the effect was small.

Table 1. Sociodemographic characteristics of North Korean refugee youths with and without suicidal ideation.

Characteristics	Without Suicidal Ideation (N = 145)	With Suicidal Ideation (N = 29)	χ^2/t	p
	N (%)	N (%)		
Sex, male	46 (31.7)	11 (37.9)	0.42	0.516
Age, mean (SD)	18.86 (2.86)	18.97 (3.41)	0.17	0.864
Birthplace			1.34	0.247
North Korea	82 (56.6)	13 (44.8)		
China	63 (43.4)	16 (55.2)		
Paternal educational level			0.04	0.851
High school degree or lower	97 (74.6)	16 (72.7)		
College degree or higher	33 (25.4)	6 (27.3)		
Maternal educational level			1.68	0.195
High school degree or lower	102 (73.9)	12 (60.0)		
College degree or higher	36 (26.1)	8 (40.0)		
Residence			0.10	0.752
With family	56 (38.9)	10 (35.7)		
With relatives/friends/alone or in a facility	88 (61.1)	18 (64.3)		

Table 2. Familial, social, and psychological characteristics of North Korean refugee youths with and without suicidal ideation.

Characteristics	Without Suicidal Ideation (N = 145)	With Suicidal Ideation (N = 29)	Mann-Whitney U	p	Cohen's d
	Mean Rank	Mean Rank			
Familial					
Familial adaptability	91.94	65.31	1459.0	0.009	0.40
Familial cohesion	93.51	57.47	1231.5	<0.001	0.55
Social					
Psychological support	90.28	73.62	1700.0	0.100	0.25
Practical support	90.25	73.76	1704.0	0.105	0.25
Psychological					
Resilience	93.79	56.03	1190.0	<0.001	0.58
Self-esteem	94.88	50.60	1032.0	<0.001	0.69
Cognitive reappraisal	90.29	73.57	1698.5	0.100	0.25
Emotional suppression	81.29	118.53	1202.5	<0.001	0.57
Impulsivity	85.86	95.71	1864.5	0.334	0.15
PTSD symptoms	81.55	114.07	1303.0	0.001	0.51

Abbreviations: PTSD, post-traumatic stress disorder.

Table 3 shows the results of the multiple regression analysis to identify the independent predictors of suicidal ideation. Only those factors with Cohen's $d > 0.5$ and $p < 0.05$ from Table 2 were included in the analysis. Emotional suppression and familial cohesion were significantly associated with suicidal ideation in this model.

Table 3. Variables associated with suicidal ideation in North Korean refugee youths.

Characteristics	AOR (95% CI)	p
Familial cohesion	0. 94 (0.89–0.99)	0.039
Resilience	0.88 (0.77–1.00)	0.053
Self-esteem	0. 93 (0.84–1.02)	0.111
Emotional suppression	1. 32 (1.08–1.60)	0.006
PTSD symptoms	1.02 (0.99–1.06)	0.183

Abbreviations: PTSD, post-traumatic stress disorder; AOR, adjusted odds ratio.

4. Discussion

This study explored the factors from the individual, family, and community level that are related to suicidal ideation of NKR youths. We found that NKR youths with suicidal ideation have lower level of familial cohesion, self-esteem, and resilience, with higher emotional suppression and PTSD symptoms than those without suicidal ideation. Moreover, according to the multiple regression analysis, emotional suppression and familial cohesion were associated with suicidal ideation. This shows that factors from individual and family level are associated with suicidal ideation of NKR youths.

In this study, 16.7% of the NKR youths reported having suicidal ideation in the past 12 months. According to our data, there were no significant differences in sociodemographic variables between youths with and without suicidal ideation. Past review studies [2,8] have found mixed results with regard to the associations between sociodemographic variables (e.g., sex, age, parental educational level, and residence) and the mental health of refugee youths. Obtaining a clear result is difficult, given the need to consider multiple potential confounders when investigating this association [2]. For instance, when investigating the association between age and mental health, confounders such as age at migration, age-related policies for education, age of first exposure to traumatic events, and many other factors must be considered.

As for familial factors, adolescents with suicidal ideation had significantly lower familial cohesion compared to those without suicidal ideation. Along with this result, multiple logistic regression analysis showed that familial cohesion was associated with lower odds of suicidal ideation, after controlling for other variables. The association between family cohesion and suicidal ideation might be explained by how family is a main source of emotional support [31], and the fact that family cohesion acts as a protective factor for mental problems (i.e., depressive symptoms) among NKRs [32]. NKR youths lose social connections by escaping from their country and settling to a new place. Accordingly, enhancing family cohesion might help adolescents endure traumatic experiences as well as adjust to their new environment, which in turn reduces their likelihood of suicide ideation. Interventions to help NKR youths to settle in Korea should include ways to build stronger familial cohesion.

As for the results concerning PTSD symptoms, these are in line with a case-control study [33] showing that NKRs tend to have more severe PTSD symptoms, on average, compared to South Koreans, and PTSD is known to be associated with suicide [11]. This finding highlights the importance of providing interventions aimed at preventing NKRs from developing PTSD symptoms after their exposure to traumatic events.

After arriving in South Korea, NKR youths must face another obstacle: acculturative stress. Acculturative stress manifests as homesickness, a sense of alienation, culture shock, feelings of marginalization, perceived discrimination, gaps in physical health, and problems in adjusting to their new education system [6,7], all of which lower NKRs' self-efficacy and self-esteem [6,33,34]. Moreover, various studies [6,34–37] have found that acculturative stress predicts psychiatric problems, including depression, anxiety, and PTSD. However, resilience might work as a buffer against these mental health problems—in other words, individual differences in resilience might help NKRs in dealing with environmental stress [8]. For instance, in one study [6], acculturative stress was related to greater depression and anxiety symptoms, while ego resiliency acted as a mediator in these relationships. Therefore, our findings that lower levels of self-esteem and resilience among NKRs exhibiting suicidal ideation are compatible with those of previous studies. This implies that programs that could improve NKR youths' self-efficacy and resilience need to be developed.

NKR youths with suicidal ideation exhibited lower emotional suppression compared to that of youths without suicidal ideation. Moreover, in the multiple regression analysis, emotional suppression was associated with higher odds of suicidal ideation of NKR youths. Alexithymia, defined as a difficulty in identifying, describing, and/or expressing emotions, has been suggested as a risk factor of psychiatric problems such as PTSD [38,39]. Indeed, Park, et al. [40] emphasized the important of expressing emotions among NKRs, stating that clearly identifying and expressing emotions alleviated PTSD symptoms among NKRs. Our result indicates that emotional suppression is not only associated with PTSD symptoms, but also suicidal ideation of NKR youths. This implies that helping NKR youths express their emotions after their traumatic experience is important for their mental health.

This study had several limitations. First, this study utilized a cross-sectional design. Therefore, we cannot infer any causal relationships between the studied variables and suicidal ideation among NKR youths. Next, the number of participants in our study was relatively small, with only 29 youths exhibiting suicidal ideation; this might influence the external validity of our results. For example, the small sample size might account for the negative results in the social support factor. Second, participants were students of only two schools, which mean that they were not likely drawn from a representative sample. Third, the data were collected through self-reports, and suicidal ideation was measured with a single question, which might have resulted in reporting bias [41]. Especially since suicidal ideation was measured with a single question, future studies need to use a validated scale to replicate our study. Fourth, we did not explore factors included in the societal level from the conceptual framework [1] we have referred to. Since NKR youths face various obstacles, including acculturative stress [6,7], factors included in the societal level need to be considered in future studies. Finally, the conceptual framework [1] that we have referred to was developed based on Bronfenbrenner's model [19]. Since we did not use the fundamental model, we may have missed some aspects from the model which could be associated with NKR youth's suicidal ideation.

Despite the aforementioned limitations, this study had several meaningful results. Specifically, NKR youths are at risk of suicide. To lower this risk, familial and individual interventions, particularly those focusing on emotional expression and familial cohesion, are essential. We believe that our results will help experts in related fields intervene in NKR youths' suicidal ideation. Further studies using a larger, more representative sample, and a longitudinal design, are needed to confirm our results. Additionally, future studies should aim to develop intervention programs for NKR youths and examine their effectiveness.

Author Contributions: Conceptualization, J.Y.J. and S.P.; Analysis, S.P.; Data collection, J.Y.J.; Writing-Original Draft Preparation, S.P.; Writing-Review and Editing, S.J.R.; Supervision, J.Y.J.; Funding Acquisition, S.P.

Funding: This work was supported by a National Research Foundation of Korea (NRF) grant funded by the Korean Government (NRF-2016R1D1A1B03931290).

Conflicts of Interest: The authors declare no conflict of interest.

References

1. Reed, R.V.; Fazel, M.; Jones, L.; Panter-Brick, C.; Stein, A. Mental health of displaced and refugee children resettled in low-income and middle-income countries: Risk and protective factors. *Lancet* **2012**, *379*, 250–265. [CrossRef]
2. Fazel, M.; Reed, R.V.; Panter-Brick, C.; Stein, A. Mental health of displaced and refugee children resettled in high-income countries: Risk and protective factors. *Lancet* **2012**, *379*, 266–282. [CrossRef]
3. Ministry of Unification. Number of North Korean Defectors by Age Group. Available online: http://www.unikorea.go.kr/eng-unikorea/relations/statistics/defectors/ (accessed on 3 January 2018).
4. Jeon, W.; Yu, S.; Cho, Y.; Eom, J. Traumatic experiences and mental health of North Korean refugees in South Korea. *Psychiatry Investig.* **2008**, *5*, 213–220. [CrossRef] [PubMed]
5. Jeon, W.; Min, S.; Lee, M.; Lee, E. A study on adaptation of North Koreans in South Korea. *J. Korean Neuropsychiatr. Assoc.* **1997**, *36*, 145–161.
6. Kim, Y.; Cho, Y.; Kim, H. A mediation effect of ego resiliency between stresses and mental health of North Korean refugee youth in South Korea. *Child Adolesc. Soc. Work J.* **2015**, *32*, 481–490. [CrossRef]
7. Sung, J.; Go, M. *Resettling in South Korea: Challenges for youth North Korean Refugees*; The Asan Institute for Policy Studies: Seoul, Korea, 2014; p. 18.
8. Lee, Y.; Lee, M.; Park, S. Mental health status of North Korean refugees in South Korea and risk and protective factors: A 10-year review of the literature. *Eur. J. Psychotraumatol.* **2017**, *8*, 1369833. [CrossRef] [PubMed]
9. Choi, S.K.; Min, S.J.; Cho, M.S.; Joung, H.; Park, S.M. Anxiety and depression among North Korean young defectors in South Korea and their association with health-related quality of life. *Yonsei Med. J.* **2011**, *52*, 502–509. [CrossRef] [PubMed]
10. Park, S.; Lee, M.; Jeon, J.Y. Factors affecting depressive symptoms among North Korean adolescent refugees residing in South Korea. *Int. J. Environ. Res. Public Health* **2017**, *14*, 912. [CrossRef] [PubMed]
11. Stevens, D.; Wilcox, H.C.; MacKinnon, D.F.; Mondimore, F.M.; Schweizer, B.; Jancic, D.; Coryell, W.H.; Weissman, M.M.; Levinson, D.F.; Potash, J.B. Posttraumatic stress disorder increases risk for suicide attempt in adults with recurrent major depression. *Depress. Anxiety* **2013**, *30*, 940–946. [CrossRef] [PubMed]
12. Sareen, J.; Cox, B.J.; Afifi, T.O.; de Graaf, R.; Asmundson, G.J.; ten Have, M.; Stein, M.B. Anxiety disorders and risk for suicidal ideation and suicide attempts: A population-based longitudinal study of adults. *Arch. Gen. Psychiatry* **2005**, *62*, 1249–1257. [CrossRef] [PubMed]
13. Statistics Korea. *Suicide Rates: Aged from 15 to 19 Years in Korea*; Statistics Korea: Daegeon, Korea, 2012.
14. Park, S. Brief report: Sex differences in suicide rates and suicide methods among adolescents in South Korea, Japan, Finland, and the U.S. *J. Adolesc.* **2015**, *40*, 74–77. [CrossRef] [PubMed]
15. Lee, Y.; Shin, O.; Lim, M. The psychological problems of North Korean adolescent refugees living in South Korea. *Psychiatry Investig.* **2012**, *9*, 217–222. [CrossRef] [PubMed]
16. Kim, M.J.; Yu, S.Y.; Kim, S.; Won, C.W.; Choi, H.; Kim, B.S. Health behavior and factors associated with depression in North Korean adolescent defectors in South Korea: The Korea Youth Risk Behavior Web-based Survey, 2011–2014. *Korean J. Fam. Med.* **2017**, *38*, 256–262. [CrossRef] [PubMed]
17. Lewinsohn, P.M.; Rohde, P.; Seeley, J.R. Adolescent suicidal ideation and attempts: Prevalence, risk factors, and clinical implications. *Clin. Psychol. Sci. Pract.* **1996**, *3*, 25–36. [CrossRef]
18. Klonsky, E.D.; May, A.M. The Three-Step Theory (3ST): A new theory of suicide rooted in the "Ideation-to-action" Framework. *Int. J. Cogn. Ther.* **2015**, *8*, 114–129. [CrossRef]
19. Bronfenbrenner, U. *The Ecological of Human Development: Experiments by Nature and Design*; Harvard University Press: Cambridge, MA, USA, 1979; pp. 16–44.
20. Yun, B.B.; Lee, H.L.; Kwak, K.W.; Oh, M.K.; Lim, J.H.; Lee, G.L. A study on reliability and validity of FACES 3. *Korean J. Fam. Med.* **1990**, *11*, 8–17.
21. Olson, D.H. *Family Adaptation and Cohesion Scales*; University of Minnesota: St. Paul, MN, USA, 1985.
22. Smith, B.W.; Dalen, J.; Wiggins, K.; Tooley, E.; Christopher, P.; Bernard, J. The brief resilience scale: Assessing the ability to bounce back. *Int. J. Behav. Med.* **2008**, *15*, 194–200. [CrossRef] [PubMed]
23. Lee, J.Y.; Nam, S.K.; Lee, M.K.; Lee, J.H.; Lee, S.M. The Rosenberg Self-esteem Scale: A validation study. *Korean J. Couns. Psychother.* **2009**, *21*, 73–89.
24. Gross, J.J.; John, O.P. Individual differences in two emotion regulation processes: Implications for affect, relationships, and well-being. *J. Pers. Soc. Psychol.* **2003**, *85*, 348–362. [CrossRef] [PubMed]

25. Han, S.H.; Hyun, O.K. Relationships of positive and negative emotion to cognitive reappraisal and expressive suppression emotional regulation strategies and self-control in adolescence. *Korean J. Child Stud.* **2006**, *27*, 1–11.
26. Steinberg, L.; Sharp, C.; Stanford, M.S.; Tharp, A.T. New tricks for an old measure: The development of the Barratt Impulsiveness Scale-Brief (BIS-Brief). *Psychol. Assess.* **2013**, *25*, 216–226. [CrossRef] [PubMed]
27. Heo, S.Y.; Oh, J.Y.; Kim, J.H. The Korean version of the Barratt Impulsiveness Scale, 11th version: Its reliability and validity. *Korean J. Psychol. Gen.* **2012**, *31*, 769–782.
28. Smith, P.; Perrin, S.; Dyregrov, A.; Yule, W. Principal components analysis of the impact of event scale with children in war. *Pers. Indiv. Differ.* **2003**, *34*, 315–322. [CrossRef]
29. Horowitz, M.; Wilner, N.; Alvarez, W. Impact of Event Scale: A measure of subjective stress. *Psychosom. Med.* **1979**, *41*, 209–218. [CrossRef] [PubMed]
30. Cohen, J. *Statistical Power Analysis for the Behavioural Sciences*, 2nd ed.; Earlbaum: Hillsdale, NJ, USA, 1988.
31. Schweitzer, R.; Greenslade, J.; Kagee, A. Coping and resilience in refugees from the Sudan: A narrative account. *Aust. N. Z. J. Psychiatry* **2007**, *41*, 282–288. [CrossRef] [PubMed]
32. Nam, B.; Kim, J.Y.; DeVylder, J.E.; Song, A. Family functioning, resilience, and depression among North Korean refugees. *Psychiatry Res.* **2016**, *245*, 451–457. [CrossRef] [PubMed]
33. Chang, M.; Son, E. Complex PTSD symptoms and psychological problems of the North Korean defectors. *Korean J. Health Psychol.* **2014**, *19*, 973–999. [CrossRef]
34. Lim, S.; Han, S. A predictive model on North Korean refugees' adaptation to South Korean society: Resilience in response to psychological trauma. *Asian Nurs. Res. (Korean Soc. Nurs. Sci.)* **2016**, *10*, 164–172. [CrossRef] [PubMed]
35. Kim, M.; Lee, D. Adaptation of North Korean adolescent refugees to South Korean society: A review of literature. *J. Rehabil. Psychol.* **2013**, *20*, 39–64. [CrossRef]
36. Kim, Y. Predictors for mental health problems among young North Korean refugees in South Korea. *Contemp. Soc. Multicult.* **2013**, *3*, 264–285.
37. Lee, K. A study on factors influencing on mental health in North Korean defector youth: The mediating effects of acculturative stress. *Contemp. Soc. Multicult.* **2011**, *1*, 157–180.
38. Bagby, R.M.; Parker, J.D.; Taylor, G.J. The twenty-item Toronto Alexithymia Scale—I. Item selection and cross-validation of the factor structure. *J. Psychosom. Res.* **1994**, *38*, 23–32. [CrossRef]
39. Bagby, R.M.; Taylor, G.J.; Parker, J.D. The twenty-item Toronto alexithymia scale—II. Convergent, discriminant, and concurrent validity. *J. Psychosom. Res.* **1994**, *38*, 33–40. [CrossRef]
40. Park, S.; Hatim Sulaiman, A.; Srisurapanont, M.; Chang, S.M.; Liu, C.Y.; Bautista, D.; Ge, L.; Choon Chua, H.; Pyo Hong, J.; Mood Disorders Research: Asian and Australian Network. The association of suicide risk with negative life events and social support according to gender in Asian patients with major depressive disorder. *Psychiatry Res.* **2015**, *228*, 277–282. [CrossRef] [PubMed]
41. Millner, A.J.; Lee, M.D.; Nock, M.K. Single-item measurement of suicidal behaviors: Validity and consequences of misclassification. *PLoS ONE* **2015**, *10*, e0141606. [CrossRef] [PubMed]

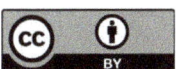

© 2018 by the authors. Licensee MDPI, Basel, Switzerland. This article is an open access article distributed under the terms and conditions of the Creative Commons Attribution (CC BY) license (http://creativecommons.org/licenses/by/4.0/).

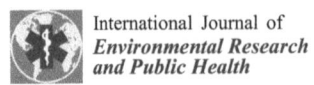

Review

The Effectiveness and Cost-Effectiveness of Screening for HIV in Migrants in the EU/EEA: A Systematic Review

Kevin Pottie [1,2,*], Tamara Lotfi [3,4], Lama Kilzar [3], Pamela Howeiss [5], Nesrine Rizk [5], Elie A. Akl [3,4,5], Sonia Dias [6], Beverly-Ann Biggs [7], Robin Christensen [8,9], Prinon Rahman [1], Olivia Magwood [1], Anh Tran [10], Nick Rowbotham [10], Anastasia Pharris [11], Teymur Noori [11], Manish Pareek [12] and Rachael Morton [10]

1. Bruyère Research Institute, 85 Primrose Ave, Annex E, Ottawa, ON K1R 7G5, Canada; prinon.rahman@dal.ca (P.R.); omagwood@bruyere.org (O.M.)
2. Departments of Family Medicine & Epidemiology and Community Medicine, University of Ottawa, Ottawa, ON K1N 6N5, Canada
3. Faculty of Health Sciences, American University of Beirut, Beirut 1107 2020, Lebanon; tamara_loutfi@hotmail.com (T.L.); lmk22@mail.aub.edu (L.K.); ea32@aub.edu.lb (E.A.A.)
4. AUB GRADE Center, Clinical Research Institute, American University of Beirut, Beirut 1107 2020, Lebanon
5. Department of Internal Medicine, American University of Beirut, Beirut 1107 2020, Lebanon; paa15@mail.aub.edu (P.H.); nr00@aub.edu.lb (N.R.)
6. National School of Public Health, Centro de Investigação em Saúde Pública & GHTM/IHMT, Universidade Nova de Lisboa, 2825-149 Caparica, Portugal; smfdias@yahoo.com
7. Department of Medicine/RMH at the Doherty Institute, The University of Melbourne Vic Australia, Parkville 3010, Australia; babiggs@unimelb.edu.au
8. Musculoskeletal Statistics Unit, The Parker Institute, Bispebjerg and Frederiksberg Hospital, 2000 Frederiksberg, Denmark; Robin.Christensen@regionh.dk
9. Department of Rheumatology, Odense University Hospital, 5000 Odense, Denmark
10. NHMRC Clinical Trials Centre, The University of Sydney, Campbell 2006, Australia; anh.tran@ctc.usyd.edu.au (A.T.); rowbothamn@gmail.com (N.R.); Rachael.morton@ctc.usyd.edu.au (R.M.)
11. European Centre for Disease Prevention and Control, 16973 Solna, Sweden; Anastasia.pharris@ecdc.europa.eu (A.P.); teymur.noori@ecdc.europa.eu (T.N.)
12. Department of Infection, Immunity and Inflammation, University of Leicester, Leicester LE1 7RH, UK; mp426@le.ac.uk
* Correspondence: kpottie@uottawa.ca

Received: 21 June 2018; Accepted: 1 August 2018; Published: 9 August 2018

Abstract: Migrants, defined as individuals who move from their country of origin to another, account for 40% of newly-diagnosed cases of human immunodeficiency virus (HIV) in the European Union/European Economic Area (EU/EEA). Populations at high risk for HIV include migrants, from countries or living in neighbourhoods where HIV is prevalent, and those participating in high risk behaviour. These migrants are at risk of low CD4 counts at diagnosis, increased morbidity, mortality, and onward transmission. The aim of this systematic review is to evaluate the effectiveness and cost-effectiveness of HIV testing strategies in migrant populations and to estimate their effect on testing uptake, mortality, and resource requirements. Following a systematic overview, we included four systematic reviews on the effectiveness of strategies in non-migrant populations and inferred their effect on migrant populations, as well as eight individual studies on cost-effectiveness/resource requirements. We assessed the certainty of our results using the Grading of Recommendations Assessment, Development, and Evaluation (GRADE) approach. The systematic reviews reported that HIV tests are highly accurate (rapid test >90% sensitivity, Western blot and ELISA >99% sensitivity). A meta-analysis showed that rapid testing approaches improve the access and uptake of testing (risk ratio = 2.95, 95% CI: 1.69 to 5.16), and were associated with a lower incidence of HIV in the middle-aged women subgroup among marginalised populations at a high risk of HIV exposure and HIV related stigma. Economic evidence on rapid counselling and testing identified strategic advantages with rapid tests. In conclusion, community-based rapid testing programmes may have the potential to improve uptake of HIV testing among migrant populations across a range of EU/EEA settings.

Keywords: HIV; AIDS; stigma; refugees; migrants

1. Introduction

Migrants, encompassing a broad range of subgroups (i.e., asylum seekers, refugees, undocumented and economic migrants, foreign students, etc.), are individuals who move from their country of residence to another. Populations at unique high risk for human immunodeficiency virus (HIV) include migrants from countries where HIV is prevalent, living in neighborhoods where HIV is prevalent, and participating in high-risk behaviour [1]. In 2016, 29,444 new HIV infections were diagnosed in the European Union/European Economic Area (EU/EEA) [2]. Although the overall number of HIV diagnoses in migrants from high-prevalence countries have declined in the EU/EEA over the past decade, migrants still accounted for 40% of the reported cases in 2016 (range 1–80%) [2]. HIV acquisition among migrants was thought to occur pre-migration, but recent EU/EEA evidence [3–6] suggests post-migration acquisition is also of concern and this suggests community based targeted interventions, including screening programmes, which may be needed many years after arrival to the EU/EEA. About 15% of all people living with HIV (n = 122,000) in the EU/EEA are unaware of their HIV positive status [7], making accurate data on HIV prevalence among migrant populations in the EU/EEA difficult. Those with an increased risk of HIV infection include migrants from HIV endemic regions, men who have sex with men (MSM), those with multiple sex partners, and injection drug users (IDU) [8].

In an effort to scale up diagnosis and treatment programmes, the Joint United Nations Programme on HIV/acquired immunodeficiency syndrome (AIDS) (UNAIDS) outlined the 90–90–90 treatment target to help end the AIDS epidemic. By 2020, 90% of those with HIV will know their status, 90% of all people with HIV will receive sustained antiretroviral therapy (ART), and 90% of all people receiving ART will have viral suppression [9]. In response to the variability in the testing and treatment approaches for HIV across EU/EEA countries, the European Centre for Disease Prevention and Control (ECDC) published guidelines on HIV testing [10]. Most countries have reported having guidance for HIV testing at the ational level [11,12]. At least 22 countries acknowledge that migrants are vulnerable to HIV infection, but six of these do not explicitly recommend HIV testing options for migrant populations [13]. Additionally, these testing options are often inconsistent between and within countries. Currently, there are no EU/EEA-wide HIV testing recommendations or strategies specifically tailored for migrant populations.

Conventional HIV testing is defined as traditional laboratory testing in healthcare settings, where patients have to wait days to weeks to receive their results; this testing approach includes an ELISA test followed by a Western blot. Rapid HIV testing refers to voluntary enrolment where results are obtained within hours, followed by a confirmatory test, and with links to outreach counselling for results and treatment options [14]. Rapid testing strategies are feasible for field settings, and the WHO recommends rapid testing as part of the community based testing strategy for communities with persistent HIV-related stigma [15].

In 2015, the World Health Organization (WHO) published consolidated guidelines on the use of antiretroviral drugs for treating and preventing HIV infection [15]. This public health approach advocated by the WHO considers the collective health status of a population, to ensure wide access to high quality services using simplified and standard HIV testing approaches, such as conventional, community-based, and other rapid testing techniques [15]. Migrants from Sub-Saharan Africa and

Latin America are more likely to be diagnosed late (defined as having a CD4 count of less than 350 CD4+ cells/mm^3) in comparison to non-migrant Europeans [2,8]. Late diagnosis increases the disease transmission rate, and increases the risk of morbidity and mortality [16]. The main reasons for late diagnosis among migrants are believed to include impaired access to testing as a result of HIV-related stigma, fear, guilt, economic difficulties, and difficulties accessing health care in Europe [8]. This review focuses on the newly arrived migrants to the EU/EEA, who migrated within the past five years, with consideration given to country and origin, circumstances of migration, gender, and age, where relevant. This group of migrants is often less well integrated into health systems because of a lack of reliable access to health services, poor information about healthcare, lack of supportive language provision, and inattention to the gender dimensions of healthcare [17]. While marginalized migrants were the specific focus, we recognize that other migrant populations may also benefit from this review. We conducted a systematic review on the effectiveness, as well as a second systematic review on the cost-effectiveness, of screening for HIV among migrants in the EU/EEA region, with the aim of informing the development of ECDC migrant screening guidance.

2. Methods

Using the Grading of Recommendations Assessment, Development, and Evaluation (GRADE) approach; the Campbell and Cochrane Collaboration Equity Methods Group; and a review team including clinicians, public health experts, and researchers from across the EU/EEA, to conduct the evidence syntheses. A detailed description of the methods can be found in the registered systematic review protocol [18].

The review group followed the PRISMA reporting guidelines [19] for the reporting of this systematic review (PROSPERO [CRD42016045798]). In summary, the review team developed key research questions (PICO: population, intervention, comparison, and outcome) and a logic model showing an evidence chain to identify key concepts, to consider potential role of indirect evidence related to populations and interventions, and to support the formulation of search strategies (see Appendices A and B) [18]. The review teams aimed to answer the following overarching questions.

- Should newly arrived migrants be screened for HIV? Who should be targeted and how?
- What implementation considerations should be considered when screening for HIV in newly arrived migrants to the EU/EEA?

'Migrants', a focus for the eligible evidence, included asylum seekers, refugees, undocumented migrants, and other foreign-born residents, with a focus on newly arrived migrants from HIV intermediate (>0.1%) and high (>1%) prevalence countries to EU/EEA in the last five years. Our analysis did not consider specific subgroups of migrants, but rather, it focused on those that were at high risk of exposure and facing poor access to testing and treatment. This review included various rapid testing approaches and provider-initiated testing approaches. Evidence was evaluated using a hierarchical approach, whereby systematic reviews/meta-analyses, and evidence based guidelines were given the most weight, followed by individual randomized controlled trials (RCTs), quasi-experimental studies, and observational studies [20,21]. The availability of existing high quality systematic reviews on these topics led us to follow a review of reviews methodology, thereby excluding all of the articles that were not systematic reviews. The team sought to build on existing high quality evidence and to identify gaps that may exist in the evidence-base.

Relevant search terms and strategies were used to search published literature in Ovid MEDLINE, Database of Abstracts of Reviews of Effects (DARE), Cochrane Database of Systematic Reviews (CDSR), and EMBASE from 2010 to December 2016, and NHS EED, CEA Registry (Tufts University), and Google Scholar from 1995 to 2016 (See Appendix B), and grey literature through Google, as well as the U.S. Centres for Disease Control and Prevention (CDC), ECDC, UNAIDS, and WHO websites. The general search terms used included "HIV", "AIDS", "screening", "early diagnosis", and "disease surveillance" (see Appendix B for complete search strategy). No language restrictions were applied to the searches.

Migrants and refugees were key populations of interest, but we also considered studies that included marginalised populations with a high prevalence of HIV.

Two independent team members (Tamara Lotfi and Lama Kilzar) manually reviewed the titles, abstracts, and full text of identified citations; selected evidence for inclusion; and compiled evidence reviews and PRISMA flow sheets. Disagreements were resolved by consensus or the involvement of a third reviewer. We assessed the methodological quality of the potentially included studies with AMSTAR [22] or Newcastle Ottawa Newcastle Scales [23]. For evidence of cost-effectiveness, we extracted data from relevant study designs (e.g., micro-costing studies, within-trial cost-utility analyses, and Markov models) for three specific questions, namely: the size of the resource requirements, the certainty of evidence around resource requirements, and whether the cost-effectiveness results favoured the intervention or comparator [24]. Finally, we assessed the certainty of the economic evidence in each study using the relevant items from the 1997 Drummond checklist [25]. The team created tables showing the characteristics of the included studies (see Tables 1 and 2), then rated the certainty of the effects for pre-selected outcome measures, and finally, conducted meta-analyses and created GRADE evidence profiles.

The final analysis report was on the GRADE synthesis. The certainty of the evidence rating reflects the level of confidence in an estimate of the desirable and undesirable effects. The implementation considerations were informed by exisiting literature.

3. Results

We retrieved 4241 articles on the effectiveness of HIV testing options. After the removal of duplicates, 3158 studies were screened by title and abstract for eligibility, based on our PICO criteria (see Table A1 in Appendix C). Of these, 34 studies were screened for full-text, and 30 studies were excluded at the full-text stage. The reasons for exclusion were that the intervention was not HIV testing ($n = 25$), conference abstract ($n = 1$), and not a systematic review ($n = 4$). Four systematic reviews were included in the end [26–29] (see Figure 1a). Additionally, 7346 economic studies were identified. After the removal of duplicates, we screened 6241 titles and abstracts for eligibility, and filtered the remaining records with "cost" and "review" in the title or abstract. Of the remaining 13 articles, 12 articles were selected for a full-text review. Eight studies were included [30–37] (see Figure 1b). Four studies were excluded, as a result of relevance to our PICO criteria.

Our systematic review evaluated voluntary HIV testing approaches among migrants from HIV intermediate (>0.1%) and high (>1%) prevalence countries arriving to the EU/EEA. This included various rapid testing approaches and provider-initiated testing approaches. Only one randomised-controlled trial (RCT), from the United States [38], explicitly identified migrants within their study population. This study was included in Pottie (2014). The GRADE methodology to assess the certainty of evidence considers differences in the study populations and interventions (indirectness) as a potential reason to downgrade the level of certainty (See Table 3), allowing us to interpret the findings consistently for the migrant populations [39]. None of the systematic reviews contained any RCTs or observational studies comparing clinical outcomes between indiviuals screened or not screened for HIV infection. No RCT or observational study evaluated the value of repeat HIV testing compared with one-time testing, or of different strategies for repeat testing. No studies compared the effects of different pre- or post-test HIV counselling methods on testing uptake or rates of follow up, and linkage to care.

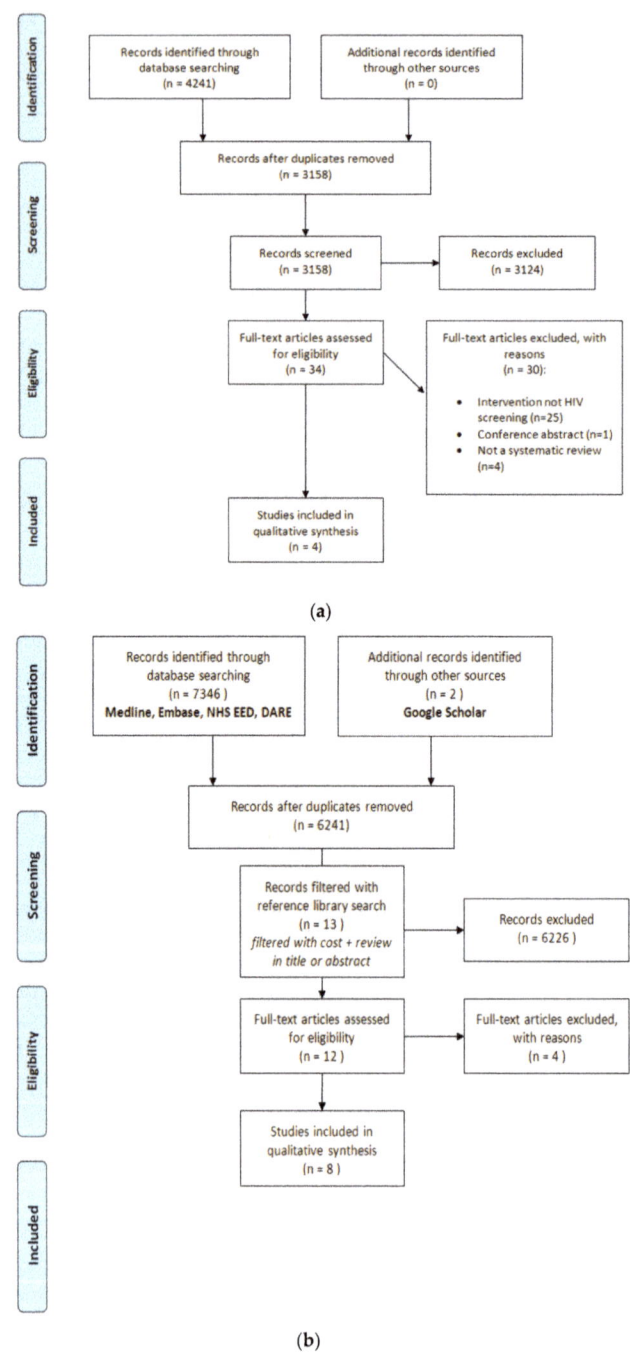

Figure 1. (a) Preferred reporting items for systematic review and meta-analysis protocols (PRISMA0 flow diagram (effectiveness); (b) PRISMA flow diagram (cost-effectiveness). HIV—human immunodeficiency virus.

Table 1. Characteristics of included studies (effectiveness). HIV—human immunodeficiency virus; EU/EEA—European Union/European Economic Area; RCT—randomised-controlled trial.; RR—relative risk; WHO—World Health Organization; CI—confidence interval; SMS—short message service.

Study	Design and Quality	Included Studies	Population	Intervention	Results/Outcomes
		Should Voluntary Testing for HIV Infection be Offered to all Recently Arrived Migrants to the EU/EEA?			
Pottie et al., 2014 [26]	Systematic review AMSTAR 9/11	$n = 13$ 1. Anaya et al. (RCT, $n = 251$, United States of America). 2. Coates et al. (cRCT, $n = 115,900$, Tanzania, Zimbabwe, Thailand, and South Africa). 3. Lugada et al. (cRCT, $n = 7184$, Uganda). 4. Malonza et al. (RCT, $n = 1249$, Kenya). 5. Read et al. (RCT, $n = 400$, Australia). 6. Spielberg et al. (cRCT, $n = 17,007$, United States of America). 7. Sweat et al. (cRCT, $n = 57,156$, Tanzania, Zimbabwe, and Thailand). 8. Walensky et al. (RCT, $n = 4855$, United States of America). 9. Appiah et al. (cross sectional, $n = $ Not reported Ghana). 10. Huebner et al. (Controlled before-after study $n = $ NR, United States of America). 11. Liang et al. (cohort, $n = $ not reported United States of America). 12. Shrestha et al. (cohort, $n = $ not reported United States of America). 13. White et al. (cohort, $n = $ not reported, United States of America).	Individuals at high risk of exposure	Facilitated voluntary enrolment; use of a rapid-testing approach (providing results within 24 h); outreach counselling, delivery of results and treatment options.	Receipt of HIV test results: Increased likelihood among participants randomized to the rapid approach study arms to receive test results (RR = 2.14, 95% CI 1.08 to 4.24) ($n = 3$; RCTs). Repeat HIV testing and test incidence rate: increased HIV repeat testing among those in the intervention arm (RR = 2.28, 95% CI 0.35 to 15.07) ($n = 1$; cluster RCT). HIV incidence 36-month period in five countries showed an 11% reduction in estimated incidence in intervention RR = 0.89, 95% CI = 0.63 to 1.24). Treatment program uptake: OR = 1.7, 95% CI 0.8 to 3.7 for the uptake of perinatal HIV-1 interventions between rapid VCT versus conventional VCT ($n = 1$)
Kennedy et al., 2013 [27]	Systematic Review AMSTAR 5/11	$n = 19$ 1. Allen et al. (time series, $n = 1458$, Rwanda). 2. Allen et al. (non-randomized trial, $n = $ not reported, Rwanda). 3. Allen et al. (time series, $n = 1438$, Rwanda). 4. Bentley et al. (time series, $n = 1628$, India). 5. Brou et al. (time series, $n = 980$, Cote d'Ivoire). 6. Chamdisarewa et al. (cross sectional, $n = 4872$, Zimbabwe). 7. Creek et al. (cross sectional, $n = 1456$, Botswana). 8. Desgrees-Du-Lou et al. (cohort, $n = 937$, Cote d'Ivoire). 9. Harris et al. (cross sectional, $n = $ not reported, Zambia). 10. Huerga et al. (cross sectional, $n = 409$, Kenya). 11. Khoshnood et al. (RCT, $n = 600$, China). 12. Kiene et al. (before-after, $n = 245$, Uganda). 13. Moses et al. (cross sectional, $n = $ not reported, Malawi). 14. Pang et al. (cross sectional, $n = 585$, China). 15. Stringer et al. (cRCT, $n = 246$, Zambia). 16. Van Rie et al. (nRCT, $n = 1238$, DRC). 17. Van't Hoog et al. (cross sectional, $n = 4142$, Kenya). 18. Wiktor et al. (time series, $n = 559$, Cote d'Ivoire). 19. Xu et al. (time series, $n = 779$, Thailand).	Low- and middle-income countries; health care setting where individuals were seeking health care services other than HIV testing. Individuals, couples, or groups had to receive pre- and post-test counseling about HIV and an HIV test	Provider-initiated testing and counseling (PITC) (aligned with the 2007 WHO).	The majority of studies were conducted before WHO PITC guidelines were developed, indicating that provider-initiated testing was occurring in many locations prior to global guidance. All studies included in this review that reported rates of HIV testing uptake showed increases associated with a PITC approach. Comparing behavior in the three months preceding PITC to behavior in the three months after PITC, the percentage of participants who reported engaging in risky sex decreased and knowing their partner's HIV status increased for both HIV-positive and HIV-negative participants.

229

Table 1. *Cont.*

Study	Design and Quality	Included Studies	Population	Intervention	Results/Outcomes
		Should Voluntary Testing for HIV Infection be Offered to all Recently Arrived Migrants to the EU/EEA?			
AHRQ 2012 [28]	Systematic Review AMSTAR 9/11	n = 42 1. Amaro et al. (before-after, n = 939, United States of America). 2. Anglemyer et al. (systematic review, n = 8). 3. Bedimo et al. (observational, n = 19,424, United States of America). 4. Brogly et al. (before-after, n = not reported, Canada). 5. Camoni et la (before-after, n = 487, Italy). 6. Cohen et al. (RCT, n = 1763, Botswana, Kenya, Malawi, South Africa, Zimbabwe, India, Brazil, Thailand, and United States of America). 7. Cunningham et al. (cross sectional, n = 300, United States of America). 8. Data collection on Adverse events of Anti-HIV Drugs (DAD) study group (observational, n = 33,308, North America, Europe, and Australia). 9. Das et al. (cohort, n = 12,512, United States of America). 10. Del Romero et al. (cross sectional, n = 625, Spain). 11. Donnell (pre-post, n = 3381, Botswana, Kenya, Rwanda, South Africa, Tanzania, Uganda, and Zambia). 12. Diamond et al. (cross sectional, n = 886, United States of America). 13. El-Bassel et al. (cRCT, n = 535, NR). 14. Elford et al. (cross sectional, n = 1687, United Kingdom). 15. Fidedi et al. (case control, n = 109, Zambia). 16. Fisher et al. (cohort, n = 859, United Kingdom). 17. Fox et al. (before-after, n = 98, United Kingdom). 18. Goncalyes Melo et al. (cohort, n = 93, Brazil). 19. Haukoos et al. (cohort, n = not reported, United States of America). 20. Hernando et al. (cohort, n = 399, Spain). 21. HIV-CAUSAL (cohort, n = 62,760, 12 European cohorts). 22. Kihata et al. (cohort, n = 17,517, North America). 23. May et al.; Lanoy et al.; Moore et al. (cohort, n = 20,379, Europe and North America). 24. Miguez-Burbbano et al. (cross sectional, n = 85, United States of America). 25. Montaner et al. (cohort, n = 5413, Canada). 26. Morin et al. (cross sectional, n = not reported, United States of America). 27. Musicco (cohort, n = 436, Italy). 28. Myers et al. (pre-post, n = not reported, United States of America). 29. Obel et al., Lohse et al, 2006 (observational, n = 2952, Denmark). 30. Reynolds et al. (cohort, n = 250, Uganda). 31. Ribaudo et al. (observational, n = 5056). 32. Severe et al. (RCT, n = 816, Haiti). 33. SMART (RCT, n = 477, USA/Europe). 34. Smit et al.; van Haastrecht et al. (cohort, n = 197, Amsterdam). 35. Sullivan et al. (cohort, n = 2993, Rwanda and Zambia). 36. Tun et al.; Vlahov et al. (before-after, n = 190, USA). 37. Wang et al. (cohort, n = 1927, China). 38. Weis et al. (corss sectional, n = not reported, United States of America). 39. When to Start Consortium (cohort, n = 45,691, Europe and North America). 40. White et al. (cohort, n-6479, United States of America). 41. Wood et al. (cohort, n = 2051, Canada). 42. Writing Committee for the CASCADE (Concerted Action on SeroConversion to AIDS and Death in Europe) Collaboration (cohort, n = 9455 Europe, Australia, and Canada).	Testing for asymptomatic HIV infection in Non-pregnant adults and adolescents.	Screening Strategies	No randomized trial or observational study compared clinical outcomes between adults and adolescents screened and not screened for HIV infection. Some modeling studies have estimated the cost-effectiveness of strategies involving repeat screening. No study directly evaluated the acceptability of universal versus targeted HIV screening. One study found universal, opt-out rapid screening associated with higher likelihood of testing compared with physician-directed, targeted rapid screening (25% vs. 0.8%; relative risk [RR], 30 [95% CI, 26 to 34]). One study found universal testing associated with a higher median CD4 count and lower likelihood of CD4 count <0.200 × 10⁹ cells/L at the time of diagnosis compared with targeted HIV screening, but these differences were not statistically significant.

Table 1. *Cont.*

Study	Design and Quality	Included Studies	Population	Intervention	Results/Outcomes
		Should Voluntary Testing for HIV Infection be Offered to all Recently Arrived Migrants to the EU/EEA?			
Desai et al., 2015 [29]	Systematic Review AMSTAR 6/11	$n = 17$ 1. Bloomfeild et al. (observational, $n = 399$, United States of America). 2. Bourne et al. (observational, $n = 3551$, Australia). 3. Burton et al. (observational, $n = 539$, United Kingdom). 4. Cameron et al. (observational, $n = 330$, United Kingdom). 5. Cook et al. (RCT, $n = 388$, United States of America). 6. Downing et al. (RCT, $n = 94$, Australia). 7. Gotz et al. (RCT, $n = 216$, The Netherlands). 8. Gotz et al. (observational, $n = 4191$, The Netherlands). 9. Guy et al. (observational, $n = 681$, Australia). 10. Harte et al. (observational, $n = 301$, United Kingdom). 11. La Montagne (observational, $n = 592$, United Kingdom). 12. Malotte et al. (RCT, $n = 499$, United States of America). 13. Paneth-Pollak et al. (observational, $n = 6220$, United States of America). 14. Sparks et al. (RCT, $n = 122$, United States of America). 15. Walker et al. (observational, $n = 1116$, Australia). 16. Xu et al. (RCT, $n = 1215$, United States of America). 17. Zou et al. (observational, $n = 4179$, Australia).	HIV-negative or unknown status in all countries; Hospitals, sexual health clinics, general practice, community venues, and home sampling/testing	Active recall	SMS: OR for retesting as compared to the control group ranged between 0.93 (95% CI 0.65 to 1.33) and 5.87 (95% CI 1.16 to 29.83). The pooled OR among the observational studies was 2.19 (95% CI 1.47 to 3.23). A pooled OR for retesting among SMS group is 5.66 (95% CI 1.78 to 17.99) among 126. Phone calls: phone calls and verbal advice and counseling had higher rates of retesting OR = 2.50 (95% CI 1.3 to 4.8) compared to phone calls only. Groups receiving phone calls and verbal advice had higher rates if retesting OR = 14.0 (95% CI 1.63 to 120.09) compared to phone calls only.

Table 2. Characteristics of included studies (cost-effectiveness). AIDS—acquired immunodeficiency syndrome.

Study	Quality/Drummond Score	Design	Population	Intervention	Cost Effectiveness	Resource Requirements
				What are the Cost-Effectiveness and Resource Requirements of HIV Testing?		
Farnham et al., 1996 [30]	Allowance was made for uncertainty; sensitivity analysis performed around a variety of model inputs. One-way sensitivity analysis in a decision analytic framework. Sensitivity analysis compares basic value with the breakeven value that makes the two strategies equally cost-effective. No range of values tested and no a priori justification for values tested in sensitivity analysis. There was no assumed range, as noted above, but results seem to be sensitive to plausible changes in some model inputs, especially waiting and counselling times.	Decision analytic model, societal perspective. Costs measured in 1992 U.S. dollars.	United States of America	ELISA test, and counselling and testing (C/T) vs. rapid C/T vs. no intervention	ELISA C/T: Average not incremental cost-effectiveness ratios: $1165 per correctly identified case vs. no intervention; rapid C/T $940 per correctly identified case Rapid vs. ELISA: $596 per correctly identified case	ELISA C/T: positive individual $103 per person, negative individual $33. Rapid C/T: positive individual $135 per person, negative individual $33 per person. Low to moderate costs of both strategies.
Kassler et al., 1997 [31]	No allowance was made of uncertainty. No sensitivity analyses.	Cost comparison, societal perspective. Comparison of testing strategies in an HIV clinic. Costs measured in 1993 U.S. dollars.	Individuals attending an anonymous testing clinic and a sexually transmitted disease (STD) clinic in Dallas, Texas	Standard C/T vs. rapid C/T	No incremental cost-effectiveness ratio calculated, not a full economic evaluation.	Cost per person receiving results and counselling: standard $151, rapid $131. Low to moderate cost savings of rapid C/T over standard C/T.
Wilkinson et al., 1997 [32]	No allowance was made for uncertainty. No sensitivity analyses.	Cost comparison, prospective comparison of testing strategies in a South African hospital. Costs measured in 1996 South African rand.	Resource-poor setting: adult inpatients of a rural South African district hospital	ELISA C/T vs. single rapid C/T vs. double rapid C/T. The double rapid strategy consists of two different rapid tests: a Capillus test and an Abbott test.	N/A	Cost per person counselled post-test: single rapid R 14–31.2, double rapid R 45.2, ELISA R 83.8. Cost savings of single rapid test.
Kallenborn et al., 2001 [33]	Some allowance made for uncertainty. Sensitivity analysis limited and discursive. Not statistically rigorous. No range of values for sensitivity analysis provided. Results overall not sensitive to whether basic or expanded regimen used, but as noted sensitivity analysis was incomplete.	Cost comparison study, retrospective chart review of Health Care Workers in an emergency department. Costs measured in 1999 U.S. dollars.	Healthcare workers	Rapid testing vs. ELISA testing	N/A. This is just a cost comparison	Total costs for 17 patients: ELISA $5966, Rapid test $466. Cost savings of switching from ELISA testing to rapid testing in health care workers.
Ekwueme et al., 2003 [34]	Allowance made for uncertainty. One-way sensitivity analysis performed in a cost analysis model. Range of sensitivity analysis is +/− 50% of the base value, or as wide as possible in the absence of hard data. Rank order of two-step rapid relative to standard C/T sensitive to the return rate for standard C/T, but one-step rapid consistently least expensive.	Cost analysis study using a decision analysis model, costs estimated from both societal and provider perspective, in 2000 U.S. dollars	United States of America	Standard ELISA C/T vs. both one-step (multiple rapid assays) and two-step rapid C/T (i.e., with a confirmatory Western blot test)	N/A	From both a provider and societal perspective, costs vary based on sero-status. However, one-step rapid testing is consistently the lowest cost option, and two-step rapid testing tends to be the highest cost. There appear to be cost savings of using a one-step rapid C/T protocol vs. standard ELISA testing or two-step rapid C/T.

Table 2. *Cont.*

Study	Quality/Drummond Score	Design	Population	Intervention	Cost Effectiveness	Resource Requirements
		What are the Cost-Effectiveness and Resource Requirements of HIV Testing?				
Doyle et al., 2005 [35]	Allowance made for uncertainty. One-way sensitivity analysis on "sensitivity, specificity, and positive predictive values of each screening test and confirmatory Western blot test, the costs of each test, and the costs of treatments" in a decision analytic model. Range of values tested in sensitivity analysis appears to be based on published estimates but this is not explicitly stated. The Oraquick rapid test is the dominant strategy over a wide range of assumptions. Results not sensitive to plausible changes.	Decision analysis techniques; decision tree	Low risk Mexican American population, incidence 0.05%	(1) testing with enzyme linked immunosorbent assay that was confirmed by Western blot (2) testing with Oraquick rapid testing that was confirmed by Western blot	Oraquick as the primary screening test for the unknown HIV status of women who were in labor was the most cost-effective at $217,718 per HIV case that was prevented. Assuming a 70-year lifespan, this equals $3111 per life-year gained.	Oraquick cost $98 spent for each child who was HIV negative, ELISA screening cost $491. High cost of ELISA screening in a low-prevalence Mexican American population were from unnecessary treatment of women and infants with false-positive test results. Oraquick has a relatively modest costs.
Paltiel et al., 2005 [36]	Allowance made for uncertainty One-way sensitivity analysis performed. Range of estimates seems to be derived from published estimates/a plausible a priori estimate. Not explicitly stated. Some sensitivity to assumptions regarding background therapy, adherence to ARV therapy, and rates of linkage to care. This does not significantly change the results, may simply whether screening every three or five years is preferable. Results regarding rapid vs. conventional testing are unclear and sensitive to plausible changes in background testing rates, acceptance and linkage to care, and rate of secondary transmission.	A stochastic model (individual model) of HIV screening and treatment: The cost-effectiveness of preventing AIDS, and a complications model (CEPAC model)	United States of America	(i) routine, voluntary HIV, CTR (counselling, testing and referral); (ii) current practice: background testing OR presentation with opportunistic infections in three target populations:	Compared to current practice, current practice plus one time ELISA costs $36,000 per Quality-Adjusted Life Year (QALY) gained; current practice plus ELISA every 5 years costs $50,000 per QALY gained; current practice plus ELISA every 3 years costs $63,000; current practices plus ELISA every year costs $100,000 per QALY gained	For HIV infected persons only: current practice costs: $78,100 lifetime cost per person; current practice plus one time ELISA costs $80,700; current practice plus ELISA every five years costs $89,000; current practice plus ELISA every 3 years costs $92,500; current practices plus ELISA every year costs $98,600 For general population: current practice costs $32,700 lifetime cost per person, current practice plus one-time ELISA costs $33,800; current practice plus ELISA every five years costs $37,300 current practice plus ELISA every three years costs $38,900; current practices plus ELISA every year costs $41,700. More frequent screening produced large costs, due to screening test cost plus the cost of managing false positives.
Vickerman et al., 2006 [37]	Allowance made for uncertainty. Univariate sensitivity analysis for a number of dimensions. Model input ranges derived from published estimates. The cost-effectiveness of the POC rapid test is sensitive to test cost.	Dynamic compartmental model	Female sex workers	A range of sensitivities of point of care (POC) tests.	If the POC test cost $2 per test (2004 $US), and was 70% sensitive, then POC test would cost $152 per additional HIV infection averted, which is cost-effective. If the cost of the POC test was $1 and the sensitivity was 80%, the cost per HIV infection averted would have been $58, which is cost-effective. When the POC test has a low sensitivity of 50%, POC is not cost-effective.	Possible cost savings from using POC tests include the reduction in the number of STI clinic attenders receiving treatment. Assuming each test takes an extra 0.3 h to undertake, POC testing costs for 4 years is $13,399 if the test cost $1 and $34,621 if the test cost $3 (in 2004 U.S.$). Moderate costs.

The U.S. Agency for Healthcare Research and Quality (AHRQ) systematic review reported that prior studies have shown that HIV testing was accurate (Rapid Test >90% sensitive, Western blot and ELISA >99% sensitive) [28]. However, the review found that targeted screening programmes, which test patients with identified risk factors, may still have missed a proportion of cases [28]. The universal opt-out rapid testing strategy was associated with a higher likelihood of testing compared with physician-directed, targeted rapid testing (25% vs. 0.8%; relative risk [RR] = 30 [95% CI: 26 to 34]), but not necessarily in marginalised populations [28]. Universal testing was also associated with a higher median CD4 count and lower likelihood of CD4 count <200 cells/mm^3 at the time of diagnosis, compared with targeted HIV testing, but these differences were not statistically significant [28].

New HIV diagnoses detected through universal testing in the United States had follow-up rates that were reported to be between 75–100% [28]. One study directly compared universal and targeted testing strategies [40]. Both the universal and targeted strategies resulted in very high rates of follow up (defined as attending at least one HIV clinic visit) between 97% and 100% [40]. The sample sizes of the included studies were small (range of 17–74 newly diagnosed HIV infections). The U.S. AHRQ review also reports that the treatment was very effective at improving clinical outcomes in adolescent and adult patients with advanced immunodeficiency [28]. The evidence indicates, from primary studies of included systematic reviews, that treatment reduced the risk of AIDS-defining events and mortality in persons with less advanced immunodeficiency and reduced sexual transmission in discordant couples [41].

In the EU/EEA, migrants from HIV-endemic countries were at a high risk of HIV infection [42]. The groups identified as having a high HIV prevalence were people originating from Sub-Saharan African, Latin America, Southeast Asia, and Eastern Europe [2,42]. These migrants had a higher frequency of delayed HIV diagnosis and are more vulnerable to the negative effects of the disclosure of their HIV status [42]. For migrants from countries where HIV prevalence is low, their socio-economic vulnerability put them at risk of acquiring HIV post-migration [42]. Migrants tended to report high-risk behaviour for HIV, such as multiple sexual partners, low and inconsistent condom use, high alcohol consumption, and drug use [42]. Men who have sex with men (MSM); sex workers, both male and female; and migrant women are considered particularly vulnerable populations within this group [42].

One systematic review and meta-analysis focused on the effectiveness of rapid tests for high-risk populations for HIV exposure. One of the RCTs included migrants-specific [38], and the others involved high-risk marginalised populations. The results of the included systematic review found that rapid voluntary counselling and testing was associated with a large increase in HIV-testing uptake and receipt of results in comparison to conventional testing (RR = 2.95, 95% CI: 1.69–5.16), but these studies did not report on uptake of HIV treatment [26]. The GRADE quality of the included studies was assessed to be low, because of the risk of bias and imprecision. All of the harms of rapid testing were not considered for the scope of the present review.

Repeat testing was found to be more likely among the individuals where rapid testing was performed (RR = 2.28, 95% CI 0.35 to 15.07) [26]. Retesting was also more likely for the individuals who were reminded to re-test by short message service (SMS) text messaging (pooled Odds ratio (OR) 2.19 [95% CI 1.46 to 3.29]) [29]. Receiving phone calls, verbal advice, and/or counselling also resulted in higher rates of retesting than phone calls alone (OR 2.50 [95% CI 1.3 to 4.8]) [29]. In the communities where rapid HIV testing was implemented, the HIV incidence decreased by 11% in comparison to the control arm communities [26]. The evidence for the uptake of HIV testing, receipt of results, and repeat testing were considered of moderate quality, because of randomisation and allocation concerns. In the review that addressed provider initiated treatment and counselling (PITC), nineteen studies were included, all from Sub-Saharan Africa (n = 15) or Asia (n = 4) [27]. The majority (13/19) of studies were conducted before the WHO PITC guidelines were developed in 2007, indicating that provider-initiated testing was occurring in many locations prior to the publication of global guidance. All of the studies that reported rates of HIV testing uptake showed increases in the HIV testing uptake associated with a PITC approach. The PITC's impact on other outcomes does not appear to be worse than voluntary counselling and testing (VCT).

Cost-Effectiveness

Three studies reported the cost-effectiveness of HIV testing strategies. Ekwueme [34] compared the costs of three HIV counselling and testing technologies, standard, one-step, and two-step rapid protocols. The standard protocol (i.e., ELISA) plus counselling and treatment, or one-step testing, was found to be less expensive than the third technology for all of the plausible ranges of HIV seroprevalence [34]. In low prevalence settings, a single rapid assay was cost-effective, as no follow-ups were required nor the use of the expensive Western blot confirmatory assay [34]. The second study, by Doyle [35], compared testing with an enzyme linked immunosorbent assay to rapid testing with Oraquick. In a low prevalence Mexican setting of 0.05%, rapid testing with Oraquick was the cost-effective strategy, at $217,718 per HIV case prevented. Assuming a 70-year lifespan, this equated to $3111 per life-year gained [35]. The third study, by Paltiel [36], compared testing with ELISA to the current practice (background testing OR presentation with opportunistic infections), in high (3%) prevalence, medium (1%) prevalence, and low (0.1%) prevalence settings. The addition of a one-off ELISA test was cost-effective compared to the current practice, for prevalence rates of 3% and 1%, but not cost-effective at a prevalence rate of 0.05% (incremental cost-effectiveness ratio: $113,000/QALY (Quality-adjusted Life Year) gained) [36].

The evidence supporting multiple rapid-tests, rather than a single rapid test followed by later confirmatory test if positive, were mixed. One study supported the use of a single rapid test [32], while another suggested possible cost savings with multiple rapid assays [34]. In this study, however, the cost advantage of multiple rapid assays was sensitive to HIV seroprevalence. In low prevalence settings (<0.1%), a single rapid assay was likely to be cost effective. The rapid tests evaluated in early economic studies were generally reported to have a lower sensitivity than ELISA tests [30,33]. Rapid testing is expanding to self-administered oral swabs. Of the limited economic evidence regarding rapid test false positives, one study [35] indicated a predictive value of 100% of the Oraquick rapid test, even in a low prevalence population (as low as 1 in 1000). Another study [36] assigned a loss of 14 quality-adjusted days to patients who received a false positive result from rapid testing.

Table 3. Recommendations Assessment, Development, and Evaluation (GRADE) evidence profile.

	Certainty Assessment						Effect				Certainty	Importance
No. of Studies	Study Design	Risk of Bias	Inconsistency	Indirectness	Imprecision	Other Considerations	Relative (95% CI)	Absolute (95% CI)				
Outcome: Testing Uptake (follow up: 7 to 24 months)												
								Without rapid testing for HIV	With rapid testing for HIV	Difference		
									General population			
3 (9745 participants)	Randomised trials	Serious concerns, allocation concealment was unclear, blinding of intervention not possible, and inability to determine blinding of researchers	No serious inconsistency	No serious indirectness	No serious imprecision	No other concerns	RR 2.95 (1.69 to 5.16)	0.1%	0.3% (0.2 to 0.5)	0.2% more (0.1 more to 0.4 more)	Moderate	Critical
									High risk population			
								2.0%	5.9% (3.4 to 10.3)	3.9% more (1.4 more to 8.3 more)		
Outcome: HIV incidence (follow up: 36 months)												
									Low risk population			
1 (8324 participants)	Randomised trial	Serious concerns Allocation concealment was unclear, blinding of intervention not possible and inability to determine blinding of researchers	No serious inconsistency	No serious indirectness	Serious imprecision	No other concerns	RR 0.89 (0.63 to 1.24)	7.2%	6.4% (4.5 to 8.9)	0.8% fewer (2.7 fewer to 1.7 more)	Low	Critical

The risk in the intervention group (and its 95% confidence interval) is based on the assumed risk in the comparison group and the relative effect of the intervention (and its 95% CI). CI—confidence interval; RR—risk ratio; GRADE working group grades of evidence: high quality: we are very confident that the true effect lies close to that of the estimate of the effect; moderate quality: we are moderately confident in the effect estimate, the true effect is likely to be close to the estimate of the effect, but there is a possibility that it is substantially different; low quality: our confidence in the effect estimate is limited: The true effect may be substantially different from the estimate of the effect; very low quality: we have very little confidence in the effect estimate, the true effect is likely to be substantially different from the estimate of effect. Interpreting relative values (e.g., uptake of testing) from the summary of findings table: relative risk: (RR 2.98; 95% CI: 1.69–5.16)-three RCTs included in the analysis provided consistent point estimates showing that the uptake of testing was 2.95 times better among participants randomized to rapid testing approaches.

4. Discussion

Our systematic review provides insight into HIV testing strategies to improve access and uptake in migrant populations in the EU/EEA, following the effectiveness and cost-effectiveness considerations.

In relation to our first research question, there were several HIV testing approaches. The literature showed three leading strategies, rapid testing, conventional testing, and universal testing approaches. Voluntary rapid tests improve HIV testing and uptake and have the potential to improve linkage to counselling and treatment for migrant populations. The universal opt-out testing approach has good intentions but lacks community outreach. Given the effectiveness of HIV treatment, measures and strategies are needed in order to increase the uptake of testing and to reduce the late diagnosis among migrant populations. However, heterogeneity between the results of the rapid testing approaches (I^2 of 93–99% in Figure 2) and limited EU/EEA-specific data suggest inconsistency between studies, thereby limiting our confidence in the transferability of these results across the EU/EEA migrant population contexts. The cost-effectiveness of the intervention, however, suggests that rapid testing is preferable to conventional testing in several contexts, due, in particular, to effective testing and counselling integration.

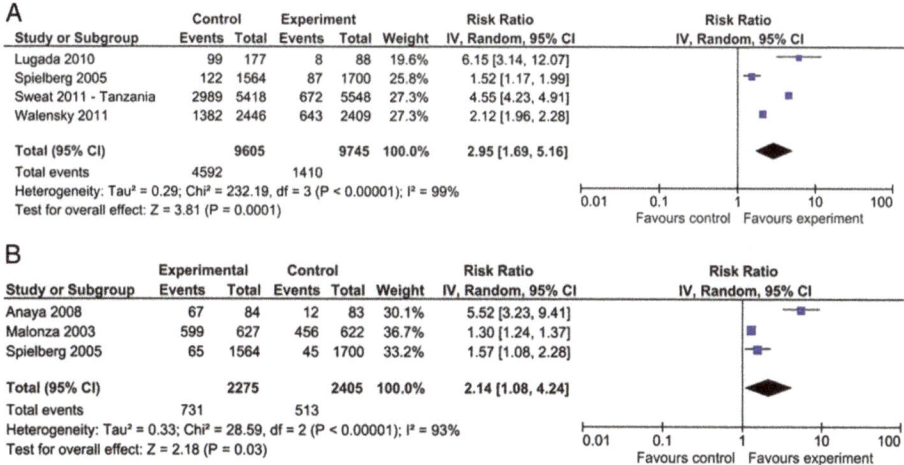

Figure 2. Meta-analysis (taken from Pottie et al., 2014 [26]). Forest plot of rapid HIV voluntary counselling and testing versus conventional care (**A**) on uptake of HIV testing and (**B**) on receipt of HIV results. Copyright received from BMJ. License Number 4403690523053.

There is no data on the cost-effectiveness and resource requirements of HIV testing in migrant populations in the EU/EEA. Indirect evidence from the United States and South Africa provide some insight into the resources required. We identified three studies on HIV testing strategies [34–36]. The economic evidence suggests that rapid testing is likely preferable to conventional testing across a range of contexts, largely due to the ability to more effectively integrate testing and counselling. One study supported the use of a single rapid test [32], while another suggested possible cost savings with multiple rapid assays [34]. The evidence supporting multiple rapid-tests, rather than a single rapid test followed by a later confirmatory test if positive, is mixed. In low prevalence settings (<0.1%), a single rapid assay may still be cost effective.

4.1. Implementation Issues

Identifying and addressing potential barriers to implementing effective and cost-effective HIV testing strategies can further promote access and uptake. Barriers to testing at organisational, provider (cultural competency), patient, and community levels in Europe include a perception of low risk, fear and stigma of the disease and disclosure, discrimination, financial limitations, poor access to care, lack of knowledge of where to obtain testing, and entitlement to medical care due to migration status [3,43,44]. The uncertain migration status among migrants to Europe is a barrier to preventive and health services in the EU/EEA [13,45]. This is especially true of undocumented migrants in the EU/EEA, as their uncertain legal status results in precarious living conditions, and discovery of their HIV status may risk deportation in certain countries [46]. HIV-related stigma is a significant barrier to HIV testing, in addition to challenges with socio-economic status, language barriers, and a poor understanding of European healthcare systems [44]. For many migrants, the barriers outweigh the advantages of testing and treatment [47], further perpetuating the HIV testing problem.

Migrant [13] populations in Sub-Saharan African [48] were more likely to be tested for HIV if they were of poor health, lost a child or sexual partner to HIV, ART was available, testing was a requirement for marriage preparation, enhanced confidentiality, had strong social networks and support [13,48], and had a history of sexually transmitted infections (STIs) [44]. Increasing cultural sensitivity and community engagement in counselling and in community-based approaches with outreach and mobilisation, were highlighted as ways to address and promote access and uptake [15], reflecting the WHO recommendations for vulnerable populations. More equity oriented research is needed to identify barriers to HIV testing in EU/EEA.

The ECDC antenatal screening for HIV, hepatitis B, syphilis, and rubella susceptibility highlights routine HIV testing for all pregnant women [49]. Certain high income countries such as the United States, Australia, Ireland, and Canada recommend testing refugees from HIV endemic areas within one month of arrival in primary health care settings. Such countries have national recommendations [50–53] for counselling and testing for refugee and migrant populations. Providing HIV testing during routine consultations was generally appreciated by users as an acceptable way to address user inhibitions in asking for it. Several Latin American migrants in Europe deemed compulsory testing as an acceptable public health measure, while healthcare practitioners reported feeling unprepared to communicate HIV positive results and adjust the flow of care [54]. Most migrants who reported knowing how to access HIV testing, preferred to receive information directly from community practitioners [55].

In general, HIV testing is cost-effective compared with no testing; the current focus is on which testing strategies are the most cost-effective in a migrant health context. The cost-effectiveness of rapid vs. conventional counselling and testing strengthens the need to increase access and uptake. The sensitivity analyses and analytic frameworks, however, were limited and demonstrate how this field is dynamic, as new rapid oral tests emerge. The cost-effectiveness data of rapid HIV testing in the EU/EEA were not available, but economic evidence about the integration of counselling, testing, and treatment was promising. The precise costs and benefits associated with rapid testing in a variety of EU/EEA member state contexts should be evaluated more closely in high-quality economic studies that directly compare various rapid testing assays to conventional testing with ELISA. Such research would need to provide quantitative evidence of the incremental cost-effectiveness of various strategies, including the uncertainty around these estimates.

4.2. Public Health Considerations

It is of particular importance to consider the challenges faced by undocumented migrants in order to increase the access and uptake of HIV testing and treatment programmes in the EU/EEA. We know from large clinical trials that treatment reduces onward transmission by 96% [56]. People living with undiagnosed HIV infection and those diagnosed with HIV but not yet on treatment contribute disproportionately to the number of new HIV infections [57]. Some of the contributing structural/organisational barriers to testing include a lack of migration status, lack of funding, availability of community based services, and discrimination in entitlement to care. More than half of the EU/EEA countries do not provide ART for undocumented migrants [12], further exacerbating the issue and reducing the likelihood that these individuals will come forward for testing. Certain

EU/EEA countries have initiated public health screening programmes for migrants at high risk for HIV infection. The benefits of HIV testing in migrants, at both individual and community levels are recognized by many EU/EEA countries, but developing suitable and comprehensive migrant screening programmes has been a challenge in many countries [13].

4.3. Strengths and Limitations

One of the strengths of this review is that it has used GRADE methodology to assess the certainty of the evidence of the included studies, including recent systematic reviews from the U.S. AHRQ and the WHO guidelines, in combination with recent reviews on rapid testing. This review's strengths lie in identifying barriers to accessing testing, and highlighting the cost-effectiveness of increasing the uptake of HIV testing for migrants. The barriers reported from Europe align with migrant HIV access barriers in other high-income countries.

We identified no migrant-specific HIV screening studies and therefore focused on studies that considered high HIV prevalence populations, many of which considered non EU/EEA migrants. This may limit the transferability of the findings to the EU/EEA context. We also acknowledge the lack of economic evidence for HIV testing approaches in migrants to the EU/EEA. The economic evidence is most relevant to the health system in which the study was undertaken, and therefore non-European studies may not be transferable. In addition, a few studies were more than twenty years old, and the costs may have changed since the resource use data was collected.

5. Conclusions

The migrants coming from countries with a high HIV prevalence often arrive with HIV related stigma and fear, and the screening and testing approaches need to address this challenge. HIV testing approaches that incorporate voluntary rapid testing programmes and primary care testing for high risk migrant populations may increase the uptake of testing, support timely diagnoses, and should provide more opportunities for linkage to effective treatment among migrant populations. All of the testing strategies may improve early diagnosis; treatment improves the individual's clinical outcomes, reduces AIDS-defining events' morbidity, and decreases mortality rates from HIV-related events, as well as having a clear public health benefit. Voluntary testing with rapid results offers an opportunity to overcome HIV related stigma in communities with high HIV prevalence compared to the conventional techniques for HIV testing alone.

Author Contributions: Conception and design, E.A.A., R.C., K.P., T.L., T.N., L.K. and R.M.; data acquisition, E.A.A., T.L., L.K., P.H., K.P., T.N., N.R. (Nesrine Rizk), S.D. and R.M.; data analysis, E.A.A., T.L., L.K., P.H., R.M., A.T., P.R. and K.P.; interpretation of results, E.A.A., R.C., T.L., L.K., P.H., R.M., N.R. (Nick Rowbotham), A.T., K.P. and S.D.; manuscript drafting, E.A.A., T.L., L.K., P.H., M.P., K.P., R.M., O.M., B.-A.B., A.P. and T.N.; critical revision of the manuscript and approval of the final version, all of the authors critically revised and approved the final version of the manuscript. T.L., L.K., P.H., N.R. (Nesrine Rizk) and E.A.A. conducted the overview of reviews on testing for HIV part of this paper (benefits, harms, barriers and enabling factors, and rapid VCT/community-based approaches).

Funding: European Centre for Disease Prevention and Control EHG Project No. 2169 "Evidence-based guidance on screening for infectious diseases among migrants to the EU/EEA".

Conflicts of Interest: Pareek is supported by the National Institute for Health Research (NIHR Post-Doctoral Fellowship, PDF-2015-08-102). The views expressed in this publication are those of the author(s) and not necessarily those of the NHS, the National Institute for Health Research or the Department of Health. Pareek reports an institutional grant (unrestricted) for project related to blood-borne virus testing from Gilead Sciences outside the submitted work. Pottie received a research contract from the Public Health Agency of Canada (2012) to prepare a report on migrants and HIV for the World AIDS Conference. Musculoskeletal Statistics Unit, The Parker Institute, Bispebjerg and Frederiksberg Hospital (R. Christensen) is supported by a core grant from the Oak Foundation (OCAY-13-309). RL Morton is supported by an Australian National Health and Medical Research Council, Sidney Sax Public Health Fellowship #1054216. All other authors report no conflicts of interest.

Appendix A

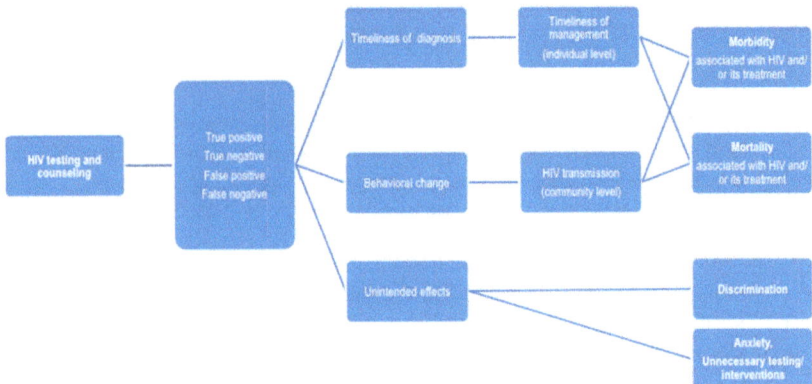

Figure A1. Logic Model.

Appendix B Search Strategy

Database: Ovid MEDLINE(R) 1946 to Present with Daily Update
Search Date: 8 April 2016

1. (hiv or hiv1$ or hiv2$).mp. (277,362)
2. (human adj (immunedeficienc$ or immune deficienc$ or immunodeficienc$ or immuno deficienc$)).tw. (72,052)
3. Acquired Immunodeficiency Syndrome/(74,163)
4. (acquired adj (immunedeficienc$ or immune deficienc$ or immunodeficienc$ or immuno deficienc$)).tw. (20,316)
5. aids.hw. (59,809)
6. (aids adj2 (infect$ or virus$)).tw. (5953)
7. or/1–6 (346,871)
8. exp Mass Screening/(107,701)
9. (screened or screening?).tw. (417,187)
10. Early Diagnosis/(18,989)
11. [or/8–15] (0)
12. [or/17–19] (0)
13. [remove duplicates from 24] (0)
14. (hiv or hiv1$ or hiv2$).mp. (277,362)
15. (human adj (immunedeficienc$ or immune deficienc$ or immunodeficienc$ or immuno deficienc$)).tw. (72,052)
16. Acquired Immunodeficiency Syndrome/(74,163)
17. (acquired adj (immunedeficienc$ or immune deficienc$ or immunodeficienc$ or immuno deficienc$)).tw. (20,316)
18. aids.hw. (59,809)
19. (aids adj2 (infect$ or virus$)).tw. (5953)
20. or/14–19 (346,871)
21. exp Mass Screening/(107,701)
22. (screened or screening?).tw. (417,187)

23. Early Diagnosis/ (18,989)
24. ((case? or early) adj2 (detected or detection? or diagnos$ or discover$)).tw. (149,145)
25. exp Population Surveillance/ (55,996)
26. (disease? adj2 surveillance).tw. (4047)
27. Contact Tracing/ (3517)
28. contact tracing.tw. (1151)
29. or/21–28 (646,541)
30. meta analysis.mp,pt. (90,987)
31. review.pt. (2,033,544)
32. search$.tw. (253,118)
33. or/30–32 (2,219,856)
34. animals/not (humans/and animals/) (4,191,261)
35. 33 not 34 (2,063,224)
36. 20 and 29 and 35 (3419)
37. 36 and (2010$ or 2011$ or 2012$ or 2013$ or 2014$ or 2015$ or 2016$).ed. (1178)
38. remove duplicates from 37 (1137)

****

Database: Embase <1980 to 7 April 2016>
Search Date: 8 April 2016

1. (hiv or hiv1$ or hiv2$).mp. (313,646)
2. exp Human immunodeficiency virus infection/ (322,600)
3. exp Human immunodeficiency virus/ (156,358)
4. (human adj (immunedeficienc$ or immune deficienc$ or immunodeficienc$ or immuno deficienc$)).tw. (81,168)
5. (acquired adj (immunedeficienc$ or immune deficienc$ or immunodeficienc$ or immuno deficienc$)).tw. (22,202)
6. aids.hw. (11,098)
7. (aids adj2 (infect$ or virus$)).tw. (6778)
8. or/1–7 (447,157)
9. exp mass screening/ (178,092)
10. (screened or screening?).tw. (612,553)
11. anonymous testing/ (221)
12. early diagnosis/ (82,014)
13. ((case? or early) adj2 (detected or detection? or diagnos$ or discover$)).tw. (223,587)
14. exp health survey/ (182,039)
15. (disease? adj2 surveillance).tw. (5133)
16. contact examination/ (2820)
17. contact tracing.tw. (1443)
18. or/9–17 (1,076,977)
19. meta analys$.mp. (166,352)
20. search$.tw. (360,207)
21. review.pt. (2,126,810)
22. or/19–21 (2,466,318)
23. animals/not (humans/and animals/) (1,150,973)
24. 22 not 23 (2,401,775)
25. 8 and 18 and 24 (5168)
26. 25 and (2010$ or 2011$ or 2012$ or 2013$ or 2014$ or 2015$ or 2016$).dd. (2136)

27. remove duplicates from 26 (2080)

****

Databases: Database of Abstracts of Reviews of Effects (DARE) and Cochrane Database of Systematic Reviews (CDSR)
Search Date: 20 March 2016
ID   Search
#1   (hiv or hiv1* or hiv2*) (15,056)
#2   human next (immunedeficienc* or immune deficienc* or immunodeficienc* or immuno deficienc*):ti,ab (2799)
#3   MeSH descriptor: [Acquired Immunodeficiency Syndrome] this term only (1248)
#4   acquired next (immunedeficienc* or immune deficienc* or immunodeficienc* or immuno deficienc*):ti,ab (646)
#5   aids:kw (2253)
#6   aids near/2 (infect* or virus*):ti,ab (457)
#7   #1 or #2 or #3 or #4 or #5 or #6 (16,330)
#8   MeSH descriptor: [Mass Screening] explode all trees (5443)
#9   (screened or screening*):ti,ab (22,416)
#10   MeSH descriptor: [Early Diagnosis] this term only (538)
#11   (case* or early) near/2 (detected or detection* or diagnos* or discover*):ti,ab (3639)
#12   MeSH descriptor: [Population Surveillance] explode all trees (709)
#13   disease* near/2 surveillance:ti,ab (30)
#14   MeSH descriptor: [Contact Tracing] this term only (96)
#15   contact tracing:ti,ab (30)
#16   #8 or #9 or #10 or #11 or #12 or #13 or #14 or #15 (27,248)
#17   #7 and #16 (1173)
#18   #17 in Other Reviews (27)
#19   #17 in Cochrane Reviews (Reviews and Protocols) (195)

****

Database: EBSCO CINAHL <1970 to April 2016>
Search Date: 8 April 2016
S27   S23 AND S26 297
S26   S24 OR S25 2,588,490
S25   EM 2010 or EM 2011 or EM 2012 or EM 2013 or EM 2014 or EM 2015 or EM 2016 2,411,599
S24   PY 2010 or PY 2011 or PY 2012 or PY 2013 or PY 2014 or PY 2015 or PY 2016 2,338,383
S23   S8 AND S16 AND S22 527
S22   S17 OR S18 OR S19 OR S20 OR S21 220,800
S21   (TI meta analy* or AB meta analy*) 29,599
S20   (MH "Meta Analysis") 24,899
S19   PT review 141,121
S18   PT systematic review 53,358
S17   (MH "Systematic Review") 37,370
S16   S9 OR S10 OR S11 OR S12 OR S13 OR S14 OR S15 154,560
S15   contact tracing 1457
S14   (disease* or population) N2 surveillance 18,647
S13   (MH "Population Surveillance+") 5939
S12   (case* or early) N2 (detected or detection* or diagnos* or discover*) 29,738
S11   (MH "Early Diagnosis") 4469
S10   TI ((screened or screening*)) OR AB ((screened or screening*)) 78,064

S9	(MH "Health Screening+") 62,689
S8	S1 OR S2 OR S3 OR S4 OR S5 S6 OR S7 108,656
S7	TX aids N2 (infect* or virus*) 10,961
S6	MW aids 22,515
S5	TX acquired N1 (immunedeficienc* or immune deficienc* or immunodeficienc* or immuno deficienc*) 21,283
S4	(MH "Acquired Immunodeficiency Syndrome") 13,583
S3	TX human N1 (immunedeficienc* or immune deficienc* or immunodeficienc* or immuno deficienc*) 23,570
S2	(hiv or hiv1* or hiv2*) 79,932
S1	(MH "Human Immunodeficiency Virus+") 6511

Appendix C

Table A1. Population, intervention, comparison, and outcome (PICO) inclusion criteria.

Population:	Migrants and refugees to EU/EEA countries (primary population of interest); will consider indirect evidence of marginalized groups in settings of high HIV prevalence
Intervention:	Voluntary testing for HIV
Outcome:	Testing outcomes: testing uptake, HIV incidence Treatment outcomes: Efficacy, withdrawals

References

1. Salama, P.; Dondero, T.J. HIV surveillance in complex emergencies. *AIDS* **2001**, *15*, S4–S12. [CrossRef] [PubMed]
2. Europe ECfDPaCWROf. *HIV/AIDS Surveillance in Europe 2017–2016 Data*; ECDC: Stockholm, Sweden, 2017.
3. Fakoya, I.; Reynolds, R.; Caswell, G.; Shiripinda, I. Barriers to HIV testing for migrant black Africans in Western Europe. *HIV Med.* **2008**, *9*, 23–25. [CrossRef] [PubMed]
4. Rice, B.D.; Elford, J.; Delpech, V.C. A new method to assign country of HIV infection among heterosexuals born abroad and diagnosed with HIV. *AIDS* **2012**, *26*, 1961–1966. [CrossRef] [PubMed]
5. Desgrées-du-Loû, A.P.J.; Ravalihasy, A.; Gosselin, A.; Supervie, V.; Panjo, H.; Bajos, N.; Lert, F.; Lydié, N.; Dray-Spira, R. Sub-Saharan African migrants living with HIV acquired after migration, France, ANRS PARCOURS study, 2012 to 2013. *Eurosurveillance* **2015**, *20*, 30065. [CrossRef] [PubMed]
6. Alvarez-del Arco, D.; Fakoya, I.; Thomadakis, C.; Pantazis, N.; Touloumi, G.; Gennotte, A.-F.; Zuure, F.; Barros, H.; Staehelin, C.; GÃpel, S.; et al. High levels of postmigration HIV acquisition within nine European countries. *AIDS* **2017**, *31*, 1979–1988. [CrossRef] [PubMed]
7. Pharris, A.; Quinten, C.; Noori, T.; Amato-Gauci, A.J.; van Sighem, A. Estimating HIV incidence and number of undiagnosed individuals living with HIV in the European Union/European Economic Area, 2015. *Eurosurveillance* **2016**, *21*, 30417. [CrossRef] [PubMed]
8. Hernando, V.; Alvárez-del Arco, D.; Alejos, B.; Monge, S.; Amato-Gauci, A.J.; Noori, T.; Pharris, A.; del Amo, J. HIV Infection in Migrant Populations in the European Union and European Economic Area in 2007–2012: An Epidemic on the Move. *JAIDS J. Acquir. Immune Defic. Syndr.* **2015**, *70*, 204–211. [CrossRef] [PubMed]
9. Joint United Nations Programme on HA. *90-90-90 An Ambitious Treatment Target to Help End the AIDS Epidemic*; UNAIDS: Geneva, Switzerland, 2014.
10. European Centre for Disease Prevention and Control. *HIV Testing: Increasing Uptake and Effectiveness in the European Union*; European Centre for Disease Prevention and Control: Stockholm, Sweden, 2010.
11. Mounier-Jack, S.; Nielsen, S.; Coker, R.J. HIV testing strategies across European countries. *HIV Med.* **2008**, *9*, 13–19. [CrossRef] [PubMed]
12. European Centre for Disease Prevention and Control. HIV and migrants. In *Monitoring Implementation of the Dublin Declaration on Partnership to Fight HIV/AIDS in Europe and Central Asia*; European Centre for Disease Prevention and Control: Stockholm, Sweden, 2017.

13. Alvarez-Del Arco, D.; Monge, S.; Caro-Murillo, A.M.; Ramirez-Rubio, O.; Azcoaga-Lorenzo, A.; Belza, M.J.; Rivero-Montesdeoca, Y.; Noori, T.; Del Amo, J. HIV testing policies for migrants and ethnic minorities in EU/EFTA Member States. *Eur. J. Public Health* **2014**, *24*, 139–144. [CrossRef] [PubMed]
14. Broeckaert, L.; Challacombe, L. *Rapid Point-of-Care HIV Testing: A Review of the Evidence*; Canadian AIDS Treatment Information Exchange (CATIE): Toronto, ON, Canada, 2015.
15. World Health Organization. *Consolidated Guidelines on the Use of Antiretroviral Drugs for Treating and Preventing HIV Infection*; World Health Organization: Geneva, Switzerland, 2016.
16. Mascolini, M. Late HIV diagnosis: Predictors, costs, consequences, and solutions. *Res. Initiat.* **2011**, *16*, 5.
17. Ager, A.; Strang, A. Understanding Integration: A Conceptual Framework. *J. Refug. Stud.* **2008**, *21*, 166–191. [CrossRef]
18. Pottie, K.; Mayhew, A.; Morton, R.; Greenaway, C.; Akl, E.; Rahman, P. Prevention and assessment of infectious diseases among children and adult migrants arriving to the European Union/European Economic Association: A protocol for a suite of systematic reviews for public health and health systems. *BMJ Open* **2017**. [CrossRef] [PubMed]
19. Moher, D.; Shamseer, L.; Clarke, M.; Ghersi, D.; Liberati, A.; Petticrew, M.; Shekelle, P.; Stewart, L.A. Preferred reporting items for systematic review and meta-analysis protocols (PRISMA-P) 2015 statement. *Syst. Rev.* **2015**, *4*, 1. [CrossRef] [PubMed]
20. Alahdab, F.; Alsawas, M.; Murad, M.H. Where should preappraised evidence summaries and guidelines place in a pyramid? *Evid. Based Med.* **2016**. [CrossRef] [PubMed]
21. Murad, M.H.; Asi, N.; Alsawas, M.; Alahdab, F. New evidence pyramid. *Evid. Based Med.* **2016**, *21*, 125–127. [CrossRef] [PubMed]
22. Shea, B.J.; Grimshaw, J.M.; Wells, G.A.; Boers, M.; Andersson, N.; Hamel, C.; Porter, A.C.; Tugwell, P.; Moher, D.; Bouter, L.M. Development of AMSTAR: A measurement tool to assess the methodological quality of systematic reviews. *BMC Med. Res. Methodol.* **2007**, *7*, 10. [CrossRef] [PubMed]
23. Wells, G.; Shea, B.; O'Connell, B. The Newcastle-Ottawa Scale (NOS) for Assessing the Quality of Nonrandomised Studies in Meta-Analyses. Available online: http://www.ohri.ca/programs/clinical_epidemiology/oxford.asp (accessed on 10 July 2017).
24. Alonso-Coello, P.; Schünemann, H.J.; Moberg, J.; Brignardello-Petersen, R.; Akl, E.A.; Davoli, M.; Treweek, S.; Mustafa, R.; Rada, G.; Rosenbaum, S.; et al. GRADE Evidence to Decision (EtD) frameworks: A systematic and transparent approach to making well informed healthcare choices. 1: Introduction. *Br. Med. J.* **2016**, *353*, i2016. [CrossRef] [PubMed]
25. National Information Center on Health Services Research and Health Care Technology. *Health Economics Information Resources: A Self-Study Course*; National Information Center on Health Services Research and Health Care Technology: Bethesda, MD, USA, 2016.
26. Pottie, K.; Medu, O.; Welch, V.; Dahal, G.P.; Tyndall, M.; Rader, T.; Wells, G. Effect of rapid HIV testing on HIV incidence and services in populations at high risk for HIV exposure: An equity-focused systematic review. *BMJ Open* **2014**, *4*. [CrossRef] [PubMed]
27. Kennedy, C.E.; Fonner, V.A.; Sweat, M.D.; Okero, F.A.; Baggaley, R.; O'Reilly, K.R. Provider-Initiated HIV Testing and Counseling in Low- and Middle-Income Countries: A Systematic Review. *AIDS Behav.* **2013**, *17*, 1571–1590. [CrossRef] [PubMed]
28. Chou, R.; Selph, S.; Dana, T.; Bougatsos, C.; Zakher, B.; Blazina, I.; Korthuis, P.T. *Screening for HIV: Systematic Review to Update the U.S. Preventive Services Task Force Recommendation*; Agency for Healthcare Research and Quality (US): Rockville, MD, USA, 2012.
29. Desai, M.; Woodhall, S.C.; Nardone, A.; Burns, F.; Mercey, D.; Gilson, R. Active recall to increase HIV and STI testing: A systematic review. *Sex. Transm. Infect.* **2015**, *91*, 314–323. [CrossRef] [PubMed]
30. Farnham, P.G.; Gorsky, R.D.; Holtgrave, D.R.; Jones, W.K.; Guinan, M.E. Counseling and testing for HIV prevention: Costs, effects, and cost-effectiveness of more rapid screening tests. *Public Health Rep.* **1996**, *111*, 44–54. [PubMed]
31. Kassler, W.J.; Dillon, B.A.; Haley, C.; Jones, W.K.; Goldman, A. On-site, rapid HIV testing with same-day results and counseling. *AIDS* **1997**, *11*, 1045–1051. [CrossRef] [PubMed]
32. Wilkinson, D.; Wilkinson, N.; Lombard, C.; Martin, D.; Smith, A.; Floyd, K.; Ballard, R. On-site HIV testing in resource-poor settings: Is one rapid test enough? *AIDS* **1997**, *11*, 377–381. [CrossRef] [PubMed]

33. Kallenborn, J.C.; Price, T.G.; Carrico, R.; Davidson, A.B. Emergency Department Management of Occupational Exposures: Cost Analysis of Rapid HIV Test. *Infect. Control Hosp. Epidemiol.* **2001**, *22*, 289–293. [CrossRef] [PubMed]
34. Ekwueme, D.U.; Pinkerton, S.D.; Holtgrave, D.R.; Branson, B.M. Cost comparison of three HIV counseling and testing technologies. *Am. J. Prev. Med.* **2003**, *25*, 112–121. [CrossRef]
35. Doyle, N.M.; Levison, J.E.; Gardner, M.O. Rapid HIV versus enzyme-linked immunosorbent assay screening in a low-risk Mexican American population presenting in labor: A cost-effectiveness analysis. *Am. J. Obstet. Gynecol.* **2005**, *193*, 1280–1285. [CrossRef] [PubMed]
36. Paltiel, A.D.; Weinstein, M.C.; Kimmel, A.D.; Seage, G.R.; Losina, E.; Zhang, H.; Freedberg, K.A.; Walensky, R.P. Expanded Screening for HIV in the United States—An Analysis of Cost-Effectiveness. *N. Engl. J. Med.* **2005**, *352*, 586–595. [CrossRef] [PubMed]
37. Vickerman, P.; Terris-Prestholt, F.; Delany, S.; Kumaranayake, L.; Rees, H.; Watts, C. Are targeted HIV prevention activities cost-effective in high prevalence settings? Results from a sexually transmitted infection treatment project for sex workers in Johannesburg, South Africa. *Sex. Transm. Dis.* **2006**, *33*, S122–S132. [CrossRef] [PubMed]
38. Walensky, R.P.; Reichmann, W.M.; Arbelaez, C.; Wright, E.; Katz, J.N.; Seage, G.R., 3rd; Safren, S.A.; Hare, A.Q.; Novais, A.; Losina, E. Counselor-Versus Provider-Based HIV Screening in the Emergency Department: Results From the Universal Screening for HIV Infection in the Emergency Room (USHER) Randomized Controlled Trial. *Ann. Emerg. Med.* **2011**, *58*, S126–S132. [CrossRef] [PubMed]
39. Schünemann, H.J.; Tugwell, P.; Reeves, B.C.; Akl, E.A.; Santesso, N.; Spencer, F.A.; Shea, B.; Wells, G.; Helfand, M. Non-randomized studies as a source of complementary, sequential or replacement evidence for randomized controlled trials in systematic reviews on the effects of interventions. *Res. Synth. Methods* **2013**, *4*, 49–62. [CrossRef] [PubMed]
40. Haukoos, J.S.; Hopkins, E.; Conroy, A.A.; Silverman, M.; Byyny, R.L.; Eisert, S.; Thrun, M.W.; Wilson, M.L.; Hutchinson, A.B.; Forsyth, J.; et al. Routine opt-out rapid hiv screening and detection of hiv infection in emergency department patients. *JAMA* **2010**, *304*, 284–292. [CrossRef] [PubMed]
41. Lundgren, J.D.; Babiker, A.G.; Gordin, F.; Emery, S.; Grund, B.; Sharma, S.; An-chalee, A. Initiation of Antiretroviral Therapy in Early Asymptomatic HIV Infection. *N. Engl. J. Med.* **2015**, *373*, 795–807. [PubMed]
42. Alvarez-del Arco, D.; Monge, S.; Azcoaga, A.; Rio, I.; Hernando, V.; Gonzalez, C.; Alejos, B.; Caro, A.M.; Perez-Cachafeiro, S.; Ramirez-Rubio, O.; et al. HIV testing and counselling for migrant populations living in high-income countries: A systematic review. *Eur. J. Public Health* **2013**, *23*, 1039–1045. [CrossRef] [PubMed]
43. Deblonde, J.; De Koker, P.; Hamers, F.F.; Fontaine, J.; Luchters, S.; Temmerman, M. Barriers to HIV testing in Europe: A systematic review. *Eur. J. Public Health* **2010**, *20*, 422–432. [CrossRef] [PubMed]
44. Blondell, S.J.; Kitter, B.; Griffin, M.P.; Durham, J. Barriers and Facilitators to HIV Testing in Migrants in High-Income Countries: A Systematic Review. *AIDS Behav.* **2015**, *19*, 2012–2024. [CrossRef] [PubMed]
45. Dias, S.; Gama, A.; Pingarilho, M.; Simões, D.; Mendão, L. Health Services Use and HIV Prevalence Among Migrant and National Female Sex Workers in Portugal: Are We Providing the Services Needed? *AIDS Behav.* **2017**, *21*, 2316–2321. [CrossRef] [PubMed]
46. Aids & Mobility Europe. *Sweden: Mikael's Testimony about His Friend Sebastian: Denied the Medication He Needed to Live*; Aids and Mobility Europe: Hanover, Germany, 2006; pp. 27–29.
47. Manirankunda, L.; Loos, J.; Alou, T.A.; Colebunders, R.; Nöstlinger, C. "It's Better Not To Know": Perceived Barriers to HIV Voluntary Counseling and Testing among Sub-Saharan African Migrants in Belgium. *AIDS Educ. Prev.* **2009**, *21*, 582–593. [CrossRef] [PubMed]
48. Musheke, M.; Ntalasha, H.; Gari, S.; McKenzie, O.; Bond, V.; Martin-Hilber, A.; Merten, S. A systematic review of qualitative findings on factors enabling and deterring uptake of HIV testing in Sub-Saharan Africa. *BMC Public Health* **2013**, *13*, 220. [CrossRef] [PubMed]
49. Control ECfDPa. *Antenatal Screening for HIV, Hepatitis B, Syphilis and Rubella Susceptibility in the EU/EEA*; Report No.: 9789291938445; ECDC: Stockholm, Sweden, 2017.
50. Australasian Society for Infectious Diseases. *Recommendations for Comprehensive Post-Arrival Health Assessment for People from Refugee-Like Backgrounds*; Australasian Society for Infectious Diseases: Surry Hills, Australia, 2016.
51. Centre HPS. *Infectious Disease Assessment for Migrants*; Health Protection Surveillance Centre, Committee MHASoHSA: Dublin, Ireland, 2015.

52. Pottie, K.; Greenaway, C.; Feightner, J. Evidence-based clinical guidelines for immigrants and refugees. *CMAJ* **2011**, *183*, E824–E925. [CrossRef] [PubMed]
53. Health USDo, Human Services/Centers for Disease Control and Prevention. *Screening for HIV Infection during the Refugee Domestic Medical Examination*; CDC: Atlanta, GA, USA, 2013.
54. Navaza, B.; Abarca, B.; Bisoffi, F.; Pool, R.; Roura, M. Provider-Initiated HIV Testing for Migrants in Spain: A Qualitative Study with Health Care Workers and Foreign-Born Sexual Minorities. *PLoS ONE* **2016**, *11*, e0150223. [CrossRef] [PubMed]
55. Dias, S.; Gama, A.; Severo, M.; Barros, H. Factors associated with HIV testing among immigrants in Portugal. *Int. J. Public Health* **2011**, *56*, 559–566. [CrossRef] [PubMed]
56. Cohen, M.S.; Chen, Y.Q.; McCauley, M.; Gamble, T.; Hosseinipour, M.C. Prevention of HIV-1 infection with early antiretroviral therapy. *N. Engl. J. Med.* **2011**, *365*, 493–505. [CrossRef] [PubMed]
57. Marks, G.; Crepaz, N.; Janssen, R.S. Estimating sexual transmission of HIV from persons aware and unaware that they are infected with the virus in the USA. *AIDS* **2006**, *20*, 1447–1450. [CrossRef] [PubMed]

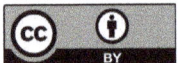

© 2018 by the authors. Licensee MDPI, Basel, Switzerland. This article is an open access article distributed under the terms and conditions of the Creative Commons Attribution (CC BY) license (http://creativecommons.org/licenses/by/4.0/).

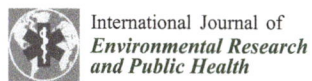

Review

Impact of the Refugee Crisis on the Greek Healthcare System: A Long Road to Ithaca

Ourania S. Kotsiou [1,*], Panagiotis Kotsios [2], David S. Srivastava [3], Vaios Kotsios [4], Konstantinos I. Gourgoulianis [1] and Aristomenis K. Exadaktylos [3]

1. Respiratory Medicine Department, Faculty of Medicine, University of Thessaly, Biopolis, 41500 Larissa, Greece; kgourg@med.uth.gr
2. International Business Department, Perrotis College, 57001 Thessaloniki, Greece; panagiotiskotsios@gmail.com
3. Inselspital, University Hospital Bern, 3010 Bern, Switzerland; DavidShiva.Srivastava@insel.ch (D.S.S.); Aristomenis.Exadaktylos@insel.ch (A.K.E.)
4. Metsovion Interdisciplinary Research Center, National Technical University of Athens, 44200 Athens, Greece; vaioskotsios@gmail.com
* Correspondence: raniakotsiou@gmail.com; Tel.: +30-241-350-2812

Received: 24 June 2018; Accepted: 20 August 2018; Published: 20 August 2018

Abstract: Greece is the country of "Xenios Zeus", the Ancient Greek god of foreigners and hospitality; however, it is also the main point of entry to Europe. Since the beginning of 2014, 1,112,332 refugees crossed the borders of Greece. Overall, 33,677 children and adolescent refugees sought asylum in Greece from 2013 to 2017, while 57,042 refugees are currently being hosted. The rapid entry of refugees into Greece raised the critical issue of health policy. The Greek National Health Service (NHS) faces many challenges. Adequate economic and human support is essential if this situation is to be managed successfully. However, Greece still bears the burden of the economic downturn since 2009. In fact, the crisis led to shortages in crucial equipment, and unmet health needs for both locals and refugees. The NHS deals with traumatic experiences, as well as cultural and linguistic differences. Overcrowded reception centers and hotspots are highly demanding and are associated with severe disease burden. This highlights the importance of guidelines for medical screening, healthcare provision, and a well-managed transition to definitive medical facilities. Furthermore, non-governmental organizations make an essential contribution by ensuring appropriate support to refugee minors, especially when they experience poor access to the NHS.

Keywords: economic crisis; Greece; migration; National Health System; refugee

1. Introduction

The refugee crisis resulted in journeys of despair to and throughout Europe and around the world. By the end of 2016, the number of forcibly displaced people reached a record of 65.6 million worldwide [1]. The estimates indeed reached the highest level since the end of World War II [1]. This population comprises refugees (22.5 million), persons internally displaced within their own countries (40 million), and asylum seekers (3.1 million) [1]. Based on the current world population of 7.4 billion, this would mean that one in every 113 people is either a refugee, an internally displaced person, or an asylum seeker [2]. More importantly, 10 million people around the world are stateless and denied access to mobility and fundamental rights, such as education, healthcare, and employment [1,2].

Over the two-year period of 2015 and 2016, 2.68 million refugees arrived in Europe [3,4]. The vast majority of them entered the European Union (EU) through a combination of land and sea routes [5]. Furthermore, 1,014,973 and 231,075 people in 2015 and in the first six months of 2016, respectively, who were seeking a better and safer life in Europe, risked their lives by attempting to cross the Mediterranean [3]. The majority of these entered Greece (1,015,100), and the rest reached Italy (224,064) and Spain (6884) by sea alone [3]. The year of 2016 was the deadliest for sea crossings, with 5096 deaths reported [4]. In the first half of 2017, over 105,000 people reached Europe [5], while over 2700 people were documented as having lost their lives while crossing the Mediterranean, with unconfirmed reports of many others perishing en route [5]. The ongoing refugee crisis challenges many countries to address the large number of significant political, economic, social, and health dimensions of this humanitarian crisis [6–8].

From 2015 to 2016, Greece experienced an unprecedented influx of refugees and migrants fleeing their home countries in the Middle East because of war [3,6–9]. Since the beginning of 2014, a total of 1,112,332 refugees arrived by sea in Greece [6]. Nearly 857,000 people arrived in Greece in 2015, a 750% increase from 2014 (41,038 arrivals) [3,6]. Approximately 16,000 sea arrivals were recorded in the first six months of 2018 [6]. The refugees mainly landed on Greek islands, which constitute a border with quick and easy access into Europe (Figure 1) [6,9]. From 2014 to 2017, the United Nations High Commissioner for Refugees (UNHCR) unfortunately recorded at least 1700 people dead or missing on the treacherous crossing from Turkey to Greece along the Eastern Mediterranean route [6–8]. Greece currently hosts approximately 57,000 refugees, 60% of whom are estimated to live on the mainland and the rest in the main reception centers in the islands of Lesvos, Chios, Kos, Samos, and Leros, or scattered throughout Greece [6]. More than 3000 are traveling alone [3].

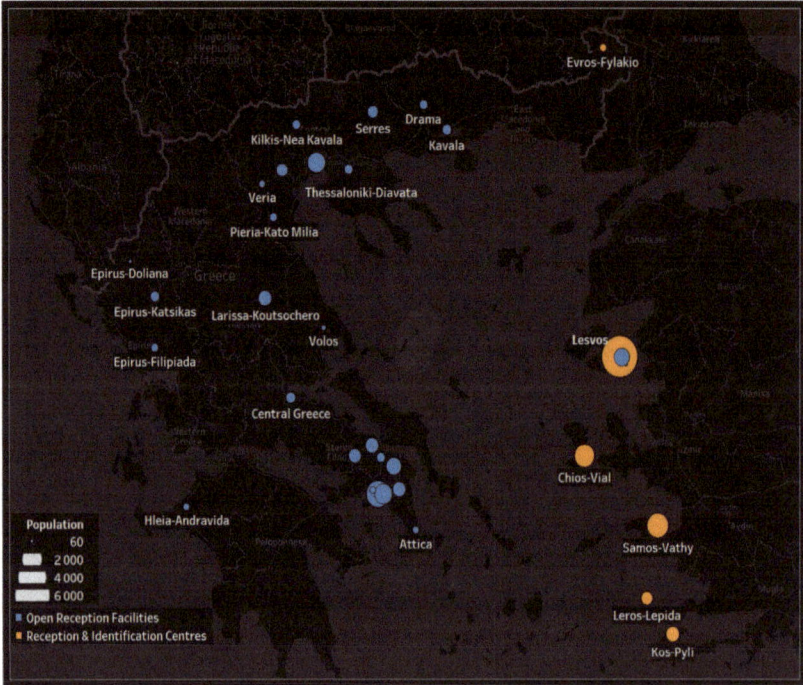

Figure 1. The main reception centers in Greece. Chios, Kos, Lesvos, Leros, Samos, and other Greek islands are rapidly and easily accessible points of entry into Europe. Notes: The orange circles represent the main reception and identification centers in Greek islands; the blue circles represent the open reception facilities (hotspots) on the mainland. The area of the circle depicts the size of the refugee population.

However, Greece is in the middle of a severe economic crisis and is struggling to pay for the migrant movement. A substantial part of the country was already profoundly affected by the economic downturn [10]. There are virtually no opportunities for employment that promise financial stability, which could then facilitate integration into the new country [11–13]. Pajic et al. recently highlighted the potentially adverse effect of social barriers in searching for a job [13]. Poor living conditions in Greece led the majority of refugees to travel deeper into Europe [14]. The main destination countries are Germany, Austria, and Sweden [2,4]. However, the barriers recently set up by many countries, notably the Former Yugoslav Republic of Macedonia (FYROM; soon to be Northern Macedonia), make migration much more difficult than in previous years [2,4,14]. In fact, it was documented that almost 60,000 asylum seekers are currently stuck in Greece due to closed European borders [2,14]. It is estimated that refugees now constitute nearly 10% of the Greek population [2,14].

Indeed, the pressure of migration waves became so great that the situation in Greece was described by the UNHCR as resembling a humanitarian crisis [9]. The unprecedented rise in the number of asylum seekers and migrants entering the country had major economic and social consequences for health outcomes [10,15–17], and created significant challenges for the Greek National Health Service (NHS) [10,15–17]. Public health risks arise both from health conditions during the journey and from health problems in the host country after arrival, along with the need to address the ongoing economic crisis and the fact that there is little pre-existing experience in Greece in the reception and integration of refugees [10,15–17]. The aim of the present manuscript is to provide a narrative review of the health conditions of arriving refugees, and the impact of both refugees and their diverse health conditions on the Greek healthcare system. A computer-based search of the English literature was performed in PubMed and Scopus. We limited our research in these databases to the English literature, since resources in other languages were limited. Google Scholar was also used to verify the results of the database searches. A considerable body of information examined in this article includes data that were largely, but not exclusively, presented in Greek studies and Greek gray literature. Key search terms included asylum seekers, children, crisis, Greece, healthcare system, health, immigrants, mental health, migration, National Health System, refugee, refugee crisis, and violence. No filters were applied for the article type and publication dates. Lastly, the reference lists of the retrieved articles were also reviewed for relevant articles, in order to assess whether database results were exhaustive. The literature search was conducted between 1 May and 4 August 2018.

2. Health Problems Facing Refugees

2.1. Health Problems Facing Adult Refugees

2.1.1. Mental Health and Deficiencies in Psychosocial Support

The refugees who reach resettlement countries were found to have experienced adverse events associated with forced migration, living in displacement under poor circumstances, legal insecurity, detention and deportation, financial privation, social isolation, racism, communication barriers, and employment difficulties, even after they obtained legal permission to remain in the host country [18,19]. These factors place them in jeopardy of mental illness, such as post-traumatic stress disorder (PTSD), depression, and anxiety disorders, which may be persistent [7,18–24]. It was recently reported that the vast majority of Syrian refugees (up to 92% of 728 individuals) screened positive for anxiety disorder that merited referral for a mental health evaluation [19]. According to Poole et al., a major depressive disorder is significantly over-expressed in female Syrian refugees in Greece, and is associated with large families and the extended asylum procedure [25]. Furthermore, refugees are at an elevated risk of psychopathology, psychosis, schizophrenia, and suicidal tendencies [7,18–24].

Moreover, there is drug abuse and alcoholism among refugees that can subsequently trigger aggressive behavior and exposure to violence [24,26]. Ben Farhat et al. reported that between 31% and 78% of refugees reported having experienced at least one incident of sexual or physical violence in Syria, 25–58% during the journey to Greece, and 5–8% in Greek holding centers [19]. More than three-quarters of the respondents aged over 15 years were diagnosed with an anxiety disorder and required referral for mental health evaluation [19]. However, only two-thirds of participants accepted a referral [19].

The importance of mental health services is underestimated throughout the EU [23–25,27–29]. As in Greece, the mental health of refugees receives little attention [15]. The reasons for this include poor finances and the failure to establish priorities. Screening for psychopathology is undoubtedly a neglected issue [15]. Most refugees claim that they had little or no access to information and assistance in relation to asylum procedures and mental health support [19]. Thus, a vicious cycle is established, since the uncertainty of their social economic and medical status exacerbates their anxiety [19]. As a consequence, many refugees do not want to stay in Greece and wish to continue migrating to Western Europe [19].

2.1.2. Physical Health and Immunization Status

Moreover, almost 40% of refugees contract diseases and illness in transit [16,17]. Many migrants face onerous conditions during migration, such as a lack of sufficient supplies and adequate shelter and hygiene, and this increases the risk of acquiring infectious diseases [16,17,30]. They present with dehydration and physical injuries, nutrition disorders, diarrhea, and tuberculosis, as well as scabies, one of the most prevalent communicable diseases [16,17,30]. There were many reports that refugees from eastern countries exhibit high rates of infection with hepatitis B virus (HBV) [31–34]. Handwritten notes by Off Track Health—a grassroots charity running Moria Medical Center in Lesvos—revealed that refugees' most common symptoms upon arrival in a reception center are fever, chills, sore throat, diarrhea, and chest or abdominal pain. Furthermore, a large number of refugees suffer from infections, asthma attacks, bronchiolitis, or trauma-related injuries [34].

Health screening in refugees arriving at the Greek border with Turkey showed that respiratory tract infections were the most common medical problem, diagnosed with a prevalence of 23% in 6899 migrants [35,36]. Another study detected respiratory tract infections in 41% of 33,331 patients who accessed care points of entry into Greece and Serbia [16,17,36,37]. Moreover, pregnancy-related issues are often mentioned [25,28,38]. In some cases, young mothers are too stressed to breastfeed their newborns. The nursing volunteers, such as volunteers of the "Save the Children" non-governmental organization (NGO), help these mothers [34]. As far as chronic disease is concerned, the most frequent condition is hypertension, followed by arthritis, diabetes, chronic respiratory diseases, and cardiovascular disease [16,17].

It is also known that immunization coverage is lower in migrants than in native populations [39–41]. It was demonstrated that diseases that can be prevented by vaccination cause flare-ups in reception and holding centers [39,42–48]. Outbreaks are generally more severe in refugee camps [48]. Sharing dormitories, a lack of accessible toilet facilities, poor hygiene conditions, undernourishment, and limited access to medical care were reported as factors contributing to the increased susceptibility to disease [35,49]. Children and the elderly are undoubtedly particularly vulnerable [50–52]. In addition, overcrowding in holding/detention centers or refugee camps may contribute to the rapid spread of communicable diseases, such as influenza, varicella, tuberculosis, measles, and meningococcal disease [16,17,39,42–49]. It is predicted that the complication rates for influenza in this setting will be double those in the general population [53]. However, this risk in refugee populations does not imply a risk of ongoing transmission to the hosting community [30,50].

The 2015 World Health Organization (WHO)/UNHCR/United Nations Children's Fund (UNICEF) joint statement recommended that refugees should be immediately immunized in accordance with the immunization schedule of the country in which they intend to stay for more than a week. Measles and polio vaccinations are generally awarded the highest priority [48,49,53,54]. In the same year, the European Centre for Disease Prevention and Control (ECDC) emphasized that assessment of vaccination status should be considered as a fundamental part of the general health assessment offered to asylum seekers upon arrival [48,50]. Until recently, there were no screening programs for asylum seekers arriving in Greece [32]. Medical screening was only offered to asylum seekers who applied for a work permit [32].

There was no decision by the Ministry of Health to apply mass screening [55]. By the late spring and summer of 2016, a mass vaccination campaign was finally organized by Médecins Sans Frontières (MSF) in collaboration with the Ministry of Health [55]. Greece now offers specific vaccinations according to the national guidelines for immunization, including those against diphtheria/tetanus/pertussis, poliomyelitis, and measles/mumps/rubella [47]. Vaccination services are provided in holding centers and/or community health services. Greece does not deliver vaccinations at the reception sites [47].

2.2. Health Problems Facing Refugee Children

2.2.1. Mental Health and Psychosocial Consequences of Child and Adolescent Refugees

From 2013 to 2017, 24,541 children and 9136 adolescent refugees sought asylum in Greece, the majority of whom were boys (50% and 66%, respectively) aged between 14 and 17 [56,57]. It is well established that more children from Middle Eastern countries, such as Syria, Iraq, and Iran, arrived in 2014–2015 than in 2011–2013. On the other hand, the absolute numbers of refugee children from Afghanistan and Pakistan decreased significantly within this period [56–61].

On the other hand, the actual number of child refugees who reach Greece may be wrongly estimated, as it is very difficult to verify the actual age of these minors, who are frequently not accompanied by their parents [59]. Young refugees in Greece may give their ages wrongly, depending on potential legal benefits [59].

In September 2017, there were almost 2850 unaccompanied children in Greece. Among these, 1096 children were accommodated in 50 shelters, and 240 in eight campuses nationwide [24,60]. Nowadays, more than half the refugee children are on a waiting list for accommodation, as there is a national lack of shelter capacity [62,63]. Many stay in closed reception facilities or police cells, or may be housed alongside adults in various sites, or in street encampments [62,63].

Children face family separation, detention, limited access to education and recreational activities, trafficking, and security problems [64]. Additionally, although exploitation of children is illegal in Greece, it is recognized that they are exposed to a wide range of risks, such as sexual violence, and physical and psychological harm [65]. In the capital of Greece, Athens, sexual exploitation is increasingly observed in many public places, such as parks, squares, and bars. In these places, particularly teenage boys are sexually abused by older men in exchange for money [63,66–70]. Children's exposure to violence is a critical public health issue, and is reported to be gender-based. Gender-based violence programming is justifiably focused on women and girls in light of their greater vulnerability; however, specific protection of boys must not be overlooked. In this context, females reported greater exposure to neglect, and males reported greater exposure to lifetime sexual violence [63].

Overall, these forms of harm are associated with a range of adverse health consequences among male and female survivors, including PTSD, depression, drug use, cutting behaviors, and suicidal ideation, along with human immunodeficiency virus (HIV) and other sexually transmitted infections [63]. Young refugees are documented with emotional, and cognitive social and behavioral problems, as well as many physical symptoms [24,56,71].

According to a study by Anagnostopoulos et al., no overall differences in frequency or type of psychiatric diagnosis were found between accompanied or unaccompanied refugee children and their Greek peers [72]; however, other studies found that refugee children are at elevated risk of mental health disorders [7,19,24,58]. It is interesting that no differences were found when a psychiatric assessment was made through a parent questionnaire, while in studies in which the educator was of the same nationality as the refugee, an increase in the rate of psychopathology was documented [72]. On the other hand, Hodes et al. supported the conclusion that the proportion of immigrants with a psychiatric diagnosis was higher than in both accompanied/unaccompanied refugees and groups of Greek children [73]. Specifically, 91% of the immigrant group received a psychosocial diagnosis, as opposed to 49% of the Greek group [72,73]. Economic migrants are reported to have low socioeconomic status, poor job status, bad living conditions, and only a low rate of health insurance coverage; these factors predispose children and adults to mental disorder [73]. However, as previously reported by Cortes, refugees lack the option of emigrating back to their homeland after prolonged periods of living in the host country, and hence, may be more inclined to invest in human capital [74]. This may take the form of becoming naturalized citizens, improving language skills, and being more likely to assimilate to the earnings growth path of the native-born population [74]. On this basis, the proportion of immigrants with a psychiatric diagnosis may be higher than currently accepted estimates among refugees [74]. However, different sources may provide conflicting data on the higher rate of psychopathology in immigrants [72,73]. Conversely, refugees report problems regarding their general health status, such as their difficulty in obtaining access to public healthcare services [72].

It is remarkable that many parents do not send their children to school, since they think that this could lead to permanent residence in Greece [72,75]. In 2017, the Ministry of Education, Research, and Religious Affairs, and the Greek mission of the International Organization for Migration (IOM) implemented a number of educational policies by supplying children with necessary school equipment [73]. According to the Ministry of Education, Research, and Religious Affairs, it was estimated that only 2500 of 12,000 school-age children enrolled in schools throughout Greece since the start of 2017, both in primary and secondary education [72,73,76].

2.2.2. Physical Health and Immunization Status of the Child and Adolescent Refugees

Furthermore, nearly one-third of the child population presented clinical laboratory abnormalities requiring intervention, which also varied by age and origin. Eosinophilia, anemia, and low ferritin are often observed in screening tests [77,78]. Dental problems are the most frequently reported health issue. In addition, skin, respiratory, and surgical diseases were reported in refugee children [77]. Moreover, various forms of malnutrition were recorded in children, particularly in infants, as breastfeeding is a challenge for mothers during their journey [79].

In addition to routine carrier testing, carrier screening for multi-drug resistant tuberculosis (MDR-TB) should be performed in refugees and migrants upon admission to a healthcare facility [80]. Greece is one of the EU countries that perform screening for active and latent TB, and TB prevalence is believed to be low [81].

It is most important that an increase in the mortality of unaccompanied children was reported in the peak migrant period of 2014–2015 compared to the previous years of 2009–2013, when no deaths were reported [58]. This rise results from children who were admitted to hospital for medical care and eventually died, or who were admitted dead in order to determine the cause of death [58]. This finding raises serious ethical and social questions.

The majority of refugee children lack proof of immunization [77]. For instance, 80% of individuals have unknown vaccination status and suboptimal serological protection against HBV. However, no child was reported to be suffering from chronic HBV or hepatitis C virus (HCV) infection. On the other hand, four-fifths of laboratory-confirmed symptomatic cases of hepatitis A virus (HAV) infection recorded in an eight-month period in 2016 were in Syrian children under 15 years in hosting facilities [82].

3. The Refugee Crisis Challenges the Greek Healthcare System

3.1. Barriers to Health System Access

Pursuant to Article 33 of the National Law 4368/2016, uninsured and vulnerable social groups, such as asylum seekers and members of their families, are entitled free of charge to necessary health, pharmaceutical, and hospital care. However, refugees face administrative barriers in access to healthcare, which are linked to the failure of the authorities to provide a Social Security Number (AMKA) [83–86]. Following a joint statement by 25 NGOs in August 2017 [85], a circular was issued on 13 February 2018 to clarify the process of issuing AMKA to beneficiaries of international protection and asylum seekers [85]. The Greek government currently provides NHS services free of charge for refugees [17,87–89].

Moreover, the economic crisis had a direct effect on the health sector [10]. Primary and secondary care are suffering from major shortages in crucial equipment and technically equipped staff, unmet health needs, and ineffective central coordination [10]. The ongoing refugee crisis poses additional threats to the NHS. Both natives and foreigners are facing barriers in using healthcare services [10].

3.1.1. Primary Healthcare Services for Refugees and Other Migrants

The Greek NHS was profoundly affected by the synergy of the economic and refugee crises, as reflected in the Aegean islands [35,90–92]. Without doubt, the reception centers in the Greek islands, already overstretched by the impact of the long-lasting economic crisis, witnessed the arrival of a large number of refugees; thus, they were then ill-prepared to cope with this influx and to address both locals' and refugees' needs [91,92]. According to a cohort study by Hermans et al. with 2291 patients, there is an urgent need for mental [35,90] and dental healthcare at Lesvos Island, which received almost half of the migrants who entered Europe [35]. More specifically, it was recently reported that most refugees (up to 80%) who were referred to a psychologist are enrolled in ongoing psychological care, and 30% of these need psychiatric support [91]. However, many patients on the islands wait three to six months for appointments with the psychiatrist, while, in some cases, patients with severe mental illness are detained at the police station's jail, where there are no equipped staff for emergency responses [92]. Blitz et al. reported that refugees have less access to necessary healthcare as only just over one-quarter of participants surveyed (26%) stated that they had access to psychological services [8,93,94].

Furthermore, there is evidence that medical assessment may be especially difficult to achieve in a refugee camp [95]. An investigation of a shigellosis outbreak in a refugee camp in Greece showed that the outbreak size was underestimated due to difficulties in language, under-diagnosis of cases with mild symptoms, or denial of symptoms from patients unwilling to risk a delay in departure [96]. In addition, it was reported that a full set of vital signs were measured in fewer than 5% of patients; thus, the severity of the disease remained largely unknown [28,76]. Moreover, the health services for infectious diseases that are provided to refugees and asylum seekers are highly fragmented [95]. Data collection is often missing or inefficient between or within countries, and this can directly impair the response to public health emergencies [79]. Records were only kept in 11% of consultations that met the case criteria for clinical surveillance reporting, as based on an independent assessment [79]. The Greek Ministry of Health is currently establishing a syndromic epidemiological surveillance system to detect potential health emergencies and infectious threats among refugees in accordance with experience from other European countries, such as Italy [97].

The lack of adequate cultural mediators is also a major factor hampering access to care. Interpreting was provided by volunteers; however, professional interpreters were demanded in order to enhance confidentiality [17,87]. Greek social workers are now added to primary healthcare (PHC) settings. Their role is to create an entry to secondary healthcare and Greek emergency medical services (EMS) [17,87]. Difficulties in the referral system were overcome when Greek-speaking social workers were employed. Their responsibility is to contact the social service of the hospitals and to promote the well-being of the refugees [88,89,95].

There are also transportation problems [88,89,95]. According to Greek law, refugees are not allowed to be transported by private transport until they are issued with international protection applicant cards; thus, no one takes the responsibility of driving them to hospitals [88,89,95]. A non-emergency medical carrier for transportation, such as a bus-based public transport system, is one possibility, although this is not available for every camp. After receiving an international protection applicant card, refugees are driven to the local hospitals by private cars and buses [88,89,95]. However, for emergencies, hospital ambulances are called by the doctor or the manager of a hotspot (often a military or police officer). There are evidently too many calls, and this may delay the delivery of service [88,89,95].

3.1.2. Secondary Healthcare Services for Refugees and Other Migrants

In addition, the sudden influx of refugees exposed critical public health issues, including ineffective emergency responses to address humanitarian needs, as well as the provision of health and social protection [88,89,95]. It was reported that Greek hospitals are struggling to meet the demands of both local people and migrants, mainly due to the lack of medical and human resources amid the economic crisis [10,16–18]. The health of refugees and migrants is jeopardized by barriers in access to Greek EMS [10,16–18]. Most of the barriers are related to language, culture, and lack of information about the healthcare system in the host country [10,16–18].

Linguistic and cultural differences make it more difficult to assess and manage these problems [10,16–18]. In consequence, migrants are often under time pressure [10,16–18]. Their care is often uncoordinated and they face difficulties in accessing proper specialized healthcare [10,16–18]. Frequent interruptions and multiple simultaneous consultations are likely to impair the quality of the consultations, but do reflect the reality of the working environment [18]. In all healthcare facilities, but especially in public hospitals, translation services and feedback mechanisms to enhance communication are urgently needed [10,16–18]. In addition, lack of continuity of care is a crucial issue (no personal hospitalization or medical history, or only in the local language), as well as difficulties in obtaining proper medication during the journey [10,16–18].

It is important that there was recently a shift of attention from the vulnerable victims of the Greek economic turmoil to the refugees, and this annoyed some members of the local population. In parallel with support for the refugees, it is essential to provide assistance to Greek citizens, thus developing a future balance between society's integration, humanity, and security [34].

3.2. Trends in Healthcare Resource Utilization

Although some refugees refused to receive any care because they wanted to continue their journey as soon as possible, the majority reported that they received inadequate information about the rules in the holding centers, as well as on the organization and location of health services [38].

Most of the barriers faced are related to cost, language, and lack of information about the healthcare system in the host country [32,38]. Cultural barriers to accessing healthcare were more rarely mentioned. This was predominantly by female participants, who preferred doctors of the same gender and geographical/cultural background [32,38]. However, in cases of emergencies, the gender of the doctor was considered less important [32,38].

It is apparent that differences in language are problematic in all settings for both healthcare professionals and refugees. It is too difficult to overcome this problem, even when interpreters are available.

Refugees also argued that they had difficulties in accessing medical care at busy border crossings and long-term reception centers [32,38], and the local customs and administrative problems of the healthcare system hampered accessibility. Furthermore, financial difficulties in making out-of-pocket payments for health and social care services are reported as an issue among refugees [34]. Additional barriers were linked to lack of time and continuity of care; this was related to the specific setting in hotspots, transit centers, and hospitals [32,38]. The bias of these groups toward the operation of public services may frighten some migrants [34,97,98].

3.3. Expenditure Data across the Health System

Since 2009, the Greek economy was severely harmed by a national debt crisis. The main causes of this debt crisis were related to continuous government deficits and inaccurate statistics, as well as to structural problems in the country's public and private sector [98–100]. The symptoms of the crisis were expressed through the risk of borrowing funds at very high interest rates, the possibility of debt default, and threats to the stability of the Eurozone. These symptoms were faced through a series of lending agreements (Memorandums of Understanding) with the so-called troika: the International Monetary Fund (IMF), the European Central Bank (ECB), and the European

Commission (EC) [101]. These agreements, however, included a series of harsh austerity measures, sudden reforms, deep budget cuts, large tax increases, and numerous privatizations that led to impoverishment for a large part of the population and loss of income and property [102,103].

Moreover, the country's gross domestic product (GDP) fell from 236 billion in 2008 to 184 billion in 2016, a value loss of 22%, while the unemployment rate of the workforce rose from 7.3% on 2008 to 20.1% in 2017 [104]. According to estimates made by Eurostat in 2015, 35.7% of the population was at risk of poverty or social exclusion [105]. The crisis also negatively affected health expenditure in Greece and the health status of the population. Total health expenditure in the country fell from €22.49 billion in 2009 to €14.73 billion in 2015, while the mean per capita healthcare expenditure declined from €2024 in 2009 to €1361 in 2015, an overall decrease of almost 33% [106]. The economic recession also negatively affected the health status of the population in Greece [100,107,108]. Finally, it must be mentioned that, whilst Greeks theoretically have access to healthcare and treatment in public hospitals, in reality, access is difficult and lengthy due to a general lack of infrastructure, equipment, and medical and human resources [16,17]. This is why high out-of-pocket private spending on health is a marked feature of the Greek healthcare system and continues to rise. In 2015, out-of-pocket payments comprised over one-third (35%) of total health spending, more than double the EU average (15%) [109].

A further burden put on to the already heavily loaded Greek health system comes from the thousands of refugees who pass the Greek borders. Even though most of the cost of refugees' healthcare is incurred by NGOs in order to permit primary healthcare in clinics in urban areas or in camps and reception centers, it is known that hundreds of refugees are transported to public hospitals [110]. Most refugees are now living in urban areas for extensive periods of time. Hence, this model can often lead to duplication of efforts through over-referral of patients by NGOs to public hospitals, and thus, to an increased burden on the health sector. Nevertheless, there is a lack of recorded data on the number of refugees who visit Greek hospitals to seek medical treatment [10].

According to the Ministry of Immigration Policy and a report from the Bank of Greece, the estimated cost of the refugee crisis to public expenditure for 2016 was about 0.3% of the country's GDP (i.e., about 600 million euros), and 35.7% of this sum was spent on open reception facilities, 26.3% on research and rescue operations, 20.6% on first reception facilities, 8.1% on transfers, 6.5% on asylum and relocation, and 2.8% on returns [111]. No exact cost for refugee health expenditure was made available by the Greek government. A report from the government's General Secretariat referred to 42,787 vaccinations of refugee children that took place from May 2016 to January 2017 with the collaboration of the Ministry of Health and various NGOs. The cost of these vaccinations, however, was at least partly covered by the NGOs [112].

There is still only limited information on the cost of refugees' healthcare in other countries. In comparison to the regularly insured, a study in Germany found that asylum seekers had more hospital and emergency department admissions that could be avoided through good outpatient care or prevention, and that their average expenditures were 10% higher. The authors concluded that access to the healthcare system, especially outpatient and mental healthcare, could improve asylum seekers' health status and integration, possibly at lower costs [113]. The lesson from past migrations is that restricting healthcare is economically counterproductive [114].

In conclusion, the economic effects of the recent refugee crisis on healthcare spending in Greece are not clear. Perhaps, however, someone should take into account the economic impact of refugees in the countries where they arrive. Importantly, even though in the short term they put extra weight on a country's budget, in the medium-to-long term, successful and timely integration of refugees into the labor market can contribute to greater flexibility, help address demographic challenges, and improve fiscal sustainability [109]. In this process, integration is the key. Nevertheless, what is clear from previous research and literature is that the earlier and better the integration, the more likely it is that legally residing, third-country nationals will make a positive contribution to growth and public finances [115]. However, the short-, medium-, and long-term impacts are bound to differ across countries, not only because of differences in the size of inflows, but also on whether or not a migrant passes through or stays, and on whether or not he is granted protection status or is rejected, together with the individual's profile, as well as the host country's economic structure and capacity to integrate those that will be granted protection [115].

3.4. The Role of Non-Governmental Organizations

As the broader Greek public healthcare sector cannot adequately handle the massive influx of refugees, a volunteer movement arose in order to help. This includes various NGOs, other social groups, and many individuals [116]. International organizations include the United High Commission for Refugees (UNHCR), the International Committee of the Red Cross (ICRC), the International Organization of Migration (IOM), and large international NGOs such as MSF, Médecins du Monde (MDM), and Save the Children, as well as many local ad hoc grassroots organizations, which quickly deployed staff and services to meet the needs of the refugees [117].

In fact, in most camps, primary healthcare (PHC) is generally ensured by army doctors and international and Greek NGOs, and these play a critical role in delivering healthcare services in all sites [17]. Since recently, medical services were provided mainly by a general practitioner and a nurse. Nursing, which is offered by NGOs and international establishments such as the Red Cross, provides basic services ranging from primary care to health promotion in the shelter camp [116]. Gynecologists (preferably female), midwives, dentists, psychologists, and psychiatrists were lately included in the camp clinics [17].

It is, therefore, important to consider the current roles of NGOs, which may have to be extended in order to provide appropriate healthcare services to migrants, refugees, and asylum-seekers, particularly when these groups are excluded from the public health system [88].

Access to specialist care or treatment in about half of all cases is offered by NGOs and not by the NHS [55]. NGOs also have a distinct role to play in emergency preparedness. Serving, negotiating, debating, monitoring, reporting, lobbying, or supporting NGOs are constantly seeking to achieve adequate and effective standards of law, policy, and practice [35]. In these terms, NGOs are key players in advocating adequate protection in the context of healthcare provision. Likewise, medical screening, and more research and systematic data collection by NGOs are needed to inform policies and to support the development of strategies for the specific humanitarian challenges posed by the recent refugee waves reaching Greece [55]. On the other hand, the existence of NGOs perpetuates the government's reliance on them, and this is a matter of great concern. The NHS should be able to integrate asylum seekers and refugees.

4. Impact of the Refugee Crisis on the Well-Being of Rescue Workers

"Rescue workers" or "rescuers" are defined as the professionals or volunteers who engage in stressful activities targeted at providing assistance to people in emergency circumstances [118]. It is totally clear that the refugee crisis had a negative impact on rescue workers' mental health. As with disaster victims and refugees, rescue and caregiving personnel may be at high risk of psychological impairment and PTSD, especially without adequate training or psychological support [118]. Many significant factors were identified as predictors for PTSD, perceived burnout, and well-being, including the family status (higher in single, divorced personnel) and increasing age, as well as the duration of demanding situations, such as gathering dead bodies. Female rescue workers were at significantly greater risk of PTSD [118].

PTSD is further accompanied by exhausting working conditions and lack of continuous psychological support. In other words, PTSD is positively correlated with burnout and inversely correlated with well-being.

Pre-departure psycho-educational training, as well as periodically organized psychological support sessions, might be essential for the prevention and mitigation of psychiatric morbidity in caregivers in refugee hotspots [119–121].

5. Conclusions

Greece is spoken of not only as a space of settlement and transit for refugees and immigrants, but also as a space for work and retirement. However, the refugee crisis had a major impact on the Greek NHS.

The recent steep influx of forcibly displaced people settling in Greece raised critical issues concerned with health policy. The health system must be ready to provide an effective response to the many challenges, especially in the prevention and control of the transmission of communicable diseases, and the treatment of acute infectious diseases by achieving effective health screening and vaccination coverage [95,122]. The results of medical screening can help identify health risk factors and epidemiological characteristics, and they should subsequently lead to more effective prevention and provision of healthcare services, and to guiding policy and interventions by authorities dealing with the specific needs. Therefore, it is important to establish a simple but accurate disease surveillance system [98].

Furthermore, the government should develop a strong NHS which can cater for the needs of populations facing distinct challenges, by empowering the NHS. The NHS in Greece must deal with traumatic experiences, and cultural and linguistic differences, as well as gaining trust, which requires more than basic care. Protection of fundamental human rights and refugee laws is urgently needed; this must offer a comprehensive approach combining a humanitarian and political response [123,124]. Furthermore, priorities include the provision of care for mental comorbidities via psychosocial training for healthcare providers, while people should be helped to retain their sympathetic approach to refugees.

Child-focused research could shed light on the multidimensional factors that contribute to children's mental illness [123,124]. Social intervention strategies to fight sexual exploitation of adolescents and children constitute a major social intervention. The prevalence of psychopathology is high, and it is certainly preferable to treat these not only on clinical and humanitarian grounds, but also on cost-effectiveness grounds [123,124].

Effective approaches are recommended to encourage young unaccompanied minors to speak about their difficulties and to support them [22]. In these terms, a collective narrative methodology called the "Tree of Life", originally developed by Ncube-Mlilo and Denborough, constitutes a culture-dependent eight-hour workshop as a paradigm to promote children's mental health [22].

The National and Kapodistrian University of Athens is developing the actions needed and the approach to meet the healthcare problems. This involves the participation of more than 100 doctors and scientific bodies in order to offer immediate and coordinated volunteer actions, including administrative support, healthcare services, and supplies [75]. More recently, Lionis et al. reported methods used for enhancing PHC for refugees in the context of a structured European project [49]. This work plan includes the assessment of the health needs of all the people reaching Europe, and it is anticipated to promote the working conditions and satisfaction of healthcare workers, as well as the interaction and collaboration between refugees, healthcare workers, and host communities [49].

As reception and holding centers are overcrowded, it is essential to have guidelines and instruments for accurate initial assessment (screening triage) and to provide transport to definitive care for refugees and other migrants [10,34,98]. For specialized human-centered, gender-specific care, it is essential to incorporate female healthcare providers and interpreters into medical teams [10,34,98]. To strengthen the referral mechanisms, NGOs and Greek health authorities should communicate strategically, in order to facilitate the transition of health service delivery to the Greek healthcare system [10,34,98]. Moreover, well-organized medical care adapted to the complex needs of populations should be flexible and cost-effective, and should protect local health structures from being overwhelmed at entry locations. Such an approach is essential for protecting social coherence by minimizing the impact on local public infrastructures [10,34,98].

On the other hand, Greek healthcare faces many severe challenges. The ability to deliver efficient management, adequate finances, and human resources is a pre-requisite. Greece is still bearing the brunt of the economic crisis. The economic downturn led to significant shortages in crucial equipment and unmet health needs due to economic limitations, which affected both locals and refugees. For this reason, wealthy nations should also push for measures to help the economically distressed countries of southern Europe to cope with the refugees that people in the north are not willing to accept.

Author Contributions: O.S.K. developed the layout of the manuscript, provided the literature review, and edited the content. P.K. critically evaluated the topics in the areas of economics. V.K. produced the draft figure with visualization Tableau software. D.S.S. and A.K.E. critically revised the draft. K.I.G. critically evaluated the draft. All authors approved the final manuscript.

Funding: This research received no external funding.

Conflicts of Interest: The authors declare no conflict of interest.

References

1. United Nations High Commissioner for Refugees (UNHCR), Figures at a Glance. Available online: http://www.unhcr.org/figures-at-a-glance.html (accessed on 5 June 2018).
2. United Nations High Commissioner for Refugees (UNHCR) Global Forced Displacement Hits Record High. Available online: http://www.unhcr.org/afr/news/latest/2016/6/5763b65a4/global-forced-displacement-hits-record-high.html (accessed on 5 June 2018).
3. United Nations High Commissioner for Refugees (UNHCR), Refugees and Migrants Sea Arrivals in Europe. Bur Eur. Available online: https://data2.unhcr.org/ar/documents/download/49921 (accessed on 5 June 2018).
4. United Nations High Commissioner for Refugees (UNHCR), Desperate Journeys. Bur Eur. Available online: http://www.unhcr.org/news/updates/2017/2/58b449f54/desperate-journeys-refugees-migrants-entering-crossing-europe-via-mediterranean.html (accessed on 5 June 2018).
5. United Nations High Commissioner for Refugees (UNHCR), Europe Situation. Available online: http://www.unhcr.org/europe-emergency.html (accessed on 24 June 2018).
6. Operational Portal Refugee Situations. Available online: http://data2.unhcr.org/en/situations/mediterranean/location/5179 (accessed on 24 June 2018).
7. Hodes, M.; Anagnostopoulos, D.S.; Kokauskas, N. Challenges and opportunities in refugee mental health: Clinical, service, and research considerations. *Eur. Child Adolesc. Psychiatry* **2018**, *27*, 385–388. [CrossRef] [PubMed]
8. Blitz, B.K.; d'Angelo, A.; Kofman, E.; Montagna, N. Health Challenges in Refugee Reception: Dateline Europe 2016. *Int. J. Environ. Res. Public Health* **2017**, *14*, 1484. [CrossRef] [PubMed]
9. United Nations High Commissioner for Refugees (UNHCR), Situation on Greek Islands Still Grim despite Speeded Transfers. Available online: http://www.refworld.org/docid/5a3cec6b4.html (accessed on 5 June 2018).
10. Kotsiou, O.S.; Srivastava, D.S.; Kotsios, P.; Exadaktylos, A.K.; Gourgoulianis, K.I. The Emergency Medical System in Greece: Opening Aeolus' Bag of Winds. *Int. J. Environ. Res. Public Health* **2018**, *15*, 745. [CrossRef] [PubMed]
11. Marmot, M.G.; Wilkinson, R.G. *Social Determinants of Health*, 2nd ed.; Oxford University Press: New York, NY, USA, 2006; pp. 6–30.
12. Bloch, A. *Refugees' Opportunities and Barriers in Employment and Training*; Corporate Document Services: Leeds, UK, 2002.
13. Pajic, S.U.; Ulceluse, M.; Kismihók, G.; Mol, S.T.; den Hartog, D.N. Antecedents of job search self-efficacy of Syrian refugees in Greece and the Netherlands. *J. Vocat. Behav.* **2018**, *105*, 159–172. [CrossRef] [PubMed]
14. Amnesty International, Trapped in Greece: An Avoidable Refugee Crisis. 2016. Available online: http://www.refworld.org/docid/571db6df4.html (accessed on 5 June 2018).
15. Christodoulou, G.N.; Abou-Saleh, M.T. Greece and the refugee crisis: Mental health context. *BJPsych Int.* **2016**, *13*, 89–91. [CrossRef] [PubMed]
16. Moris, D.; Kousoulis, A. Refugee crisis in Greece: Healthcare and integration as current challenges. *Perspect. Public Health* **2017**, *137*, 309–310. [CrossRef] [PubMed]
17. De Paoli, L. Access to health services for the refugee community in Greece: Lessons learned. *Public Health* **2018**, *157*, 104–106. [CrossRef] [PubMed]
18. Priebe, S.; Giacco, D.; El-Nagib, R. WHO Health Evidence Network Synthesis Reports. 2016. Public Health Aspects of Mental Health among Migrants and Refugees: A Review of the Evidence on Mental Health Care for Refugees, Asylum Seekers and Irregular Migrants in the WHO European Region. WHO Regional Office for Europe, Copenhagen. Available online: http://www.euro.who.int/__data/assets/pdf_file/0003/317622/HEN-synthesis-report-47.pdf?ua=1 (accessed on 5 June 2018).

19. Ben Farhat, J.; Blanchet, K.; Juul Bjertrup, P.; Veizis, A.; Perrin, C.; Coulborn, R.M.; Mayaud, P.; Cohuet, S. Syrian refugees in Greece: Experience with violence, mental health status, and access to information during the journey and while in Greece. *BMC Med.* **2018**, *16*, 40. [CrossRef] [PubMed]
20. Fazel, M.; Reed, R.V.; Panter-Brick, C.; Stein, A. Mental health of displaced and refugee children resettled in high-income countries: Risk and protective factors. *Lancet* **2012**, *379*, 266–282. [CrossRef]
21. Reed, R.V.; Fazel, M.; Jones, L.; Panter-Brick, C.; Stein, A. Mental health of displaced and refugee children resettled in low-income and middle-income countries: Risk and protective factors. *Lancet* **2012**, *379*, 250–265. [CrossRef]
22. Jacobs, S.F. Collective narrative practice with unaccompanied refugee minors: "The Tree of Life" as a response to hardship. *Clin. Child Psychol. Psychiatry* **2017**, *23*, 279–293. [CrossRef] [PubMed]
23. Pavli, A.; Maltezou, H. Health problems of newly arrived migrants and refugees in Europe. *J. Travel Med.* **2017**, *24*. [CrossRef] [PubMed]
24. Anagnostopoulos, D.C.; Giannakopoulos, G.; Christodoulou, N.G. The synergy of the refugee crisis and the financial crisis in Greece: Impact on mental health. *Int. J. Soc. Psychiatry* **2017**, *63*, 352–358. [CrossRef] [PubMed]
25. Poole, D.N.; Hedt-Gauthier, B.; Liao, S.; Raymond, N.A.; Bärnighausen, T. Major depressive disorder prevalence and risk factors among Syrian asylum seekers in Greece. *BMC Public Health* **2018**, *18*, 908. [CrossRef] [PubMed]
26. Arsenijevic, J.; Schillberg, E.; Ponthieu, A.; Malvisi, L.; Ahmed, W.A.E.; Argenziano, S.; Zamatto, F.; Burroughs, S.; Severy, N.; Hebting, C.; et al. A crisis of protection and safe passage: Violence experienced by migrants/refugees travelling along the Western Balkan corridor to Northern Europe. *Confl. Health* **2017**, *11*, 6. [CrossRef] [PubMed]
27. Shortall, C.K.; Glazik, R.; Sornum, A.; Pritchard, C. On the ferries: The unmet health care needs of transiting refugees in Greece. *Int. Health* **2017**, *9*, 272–280. [CrossRef] [PubMed]
28. Puchner, K.; Karamagioli, E.; Pikouli, A.; Tsiamis, C.; Kalogeropoulos, A.; Kakalou, E.; Pavlidou, E.; Pikoulis, E. Time to Rethink Refugee and Migrant Health in Europe: Moving from Emergency Response to Integrated and Individualized Health Care Provision for Migrants and Refugees. *Int. J. Environ. Res. Public Health* **2018**, *15*, 1100. [CrossRef] [PubMed]
29. Gray, B.H.; van Ginneken, E. Health care for undocumented migrants: European approaches. *Issue Brief* **2012**, *33*, 1–12. [PubMed]
30. Rojek, A.M.; Gkolfinopoulou, K.; Veizis, A.; Lambrou, A.; Castle, L.; Georgakopoulou, T.; Blanchet, K.; Panagiotopoulos, T.; Horby, P.W. Epidemic Diseases Research Group field team. Clinical assessment is a neglected component of outbreak preparedness: Evidence from refugee camps in Greece. *BMC Med.* **2018**, *16*, 43. [CrossRef] [PubMed]
31. Roussos, A.; Goritsas, C.; Pappas, T.; Spanaki, M.; Papadaki, P.; Ferti, A. Prevalence of hepatitis B and C markers among refugees in Athens. *World J. Gastroenterol.* **2003**, *9*, 993–995. [CrossRef] [PubMed]
32. Norredam, M.; Mygind, A.; Krasnik, A. Access to health care for asylum seekers in the European Union—A comparative study of country policies. *Eur. J. Public Health* **2006**, *16*, 286–290. [CrossRef] [PubMed]
33. Skliros, E.A.; Sotiropoulos, A.; Peppas, T.; Sofroniadou, K.; Lionis, C. High prevalence of HBV infection markers in refugees from eastern countries. *Ital. J. Gastroenterol. Hepatol.* **1999**, *31*, 84–85. [PubMed]
34. Kousoulis, A.A.; Ioakeim-Ioannidou, M.; Economopoulos, K.P. Access to health for refugees in Greece: Lessons in inequalities. *Int. J. Equity Health* **2016**, *15*, 122. [CrossRef] [PubMed]
35. Hermans, M.P.; Kooistra, J.; Cannegieter, S.C.; Rosendaal, F.R.; Mook-Kanamori, D.O.; Nemeth, B. Healthcare and disease burden among refugees in long-stay refugee camps at Lesbos, Greece. *Eur. J. Epidemiol.* **2017**, *32*, 851–854. [CrossRef] [PubMed]
36. Eonomopoulou, A.; Pavli, A.; Stasinopoulou, P.; Giannopoulos, L.A.; Tsiodras, S. Migrant screening: Lessons learned from the migrant holding level at the Greek-Turkish borders. *J. Infect. Public Health* **2017**, *10*, 177–184. [CrossRef] [PubMed]
37. Evlampidou, I. Refugee Crisis in Europe: Health Status, Life Experiences and Mental Health Problems of Transiting Refugees and Migrants on the Balkan Route in 2015. Available online: https://www.msf.org.uk/sites/uk/files/2._135_138_EVLAMPIDOU_Migrant_Health_COMBINATION_final.pdf (accessed on 5 June 2018).
38. van Loenen, T.; van den Muijsenbergh, M.; Hofmeester, M.; Dowrick, C.; van Ginneken, N.; Mechili, E.A.; Angelaki, A.; Ajdukovic, D.; Bakic, H.; Pavlic, D.R.; et al. Primary care for refugees and newly arrived migrants in Europe: A qualitative study on health needs, barriers and wishes. *Eur. J. Public Health* **2018**, *28*, 82–87. [CrossRef] [PubMed]

39. Williams, G.A.; Bacci, S.; Shadwick, R.; Tillmann, T.; Rechel, B.; Noori, T.; Suk, J.E.; Odone, A.; Ingleby, J.D.; Mladovsky, P.; et al. Measles among migrants in the European Union and the European Economic Area. *Scand. J. Public Health* **2016**, *44*, 6–13. [CrossRef] [PubMed]
40. Fabiani, M.; Riccardo, F.; Di Napoli, A.; Gargiulo, L.; Declich, S.; Petrelli, A. Differences in influenza vaccination coverage between adult immigrants and italian citizens at risk for influenza-related complications: A cross-sectional study. *PLoS ONE* **2016**, *11*, e0166517. [CrossRef] [PubMed]
41. Mipatrini, D.; Stefanelli, P.; Severoni, S.; Rezza, G. Vaccinations in migrants and refugees: A challenge for European health systems. A systematic review of current scientific evidence. *Pathog. Glob. Health* **2017**, *111*, 59–68. [CrossRef] [PubMed]
42. World Health Organization (WHO) Regional Office for Europe. Migration and Health: Key Issues. Available online: http://www.euro.who.int/en/health-topics/health-determinants/migration-and-health/migrant-health-in-the-european-region/migration-and-health-key-issues (accessed on 5 June 2018).
43. European Centre for Disease Prevention and Control. Epidemiological Update: Measles among Asylum Seekers in Germany, 2016. Available online: https://ecdc.europa.eu/en/news-events/epidemiological-update-measles-among-asylum-seekers-germany-10-august-2016 (accessed on 5 June 2018).
44. Jones, G.; Haeghebaert, S.; Merlin, B.; Antona, D.; Simon, N.; Elmouden, M.; Battist, F.; Janssens, M.; Wyndels, K.; Chaud, P. Measles outbreak in a refugee settlement in Calais, France: January to February 2016. *Eurosurveillance* **2016**, *21*, 30167. [CrossRef] [PubMed]
45. Haas, E.J.; Dukhan, L.; Goldstein, L.; Lyandres, M.; Gdalevich, M. Use of vaccination in a large outbreak of primary varicella in a detention setting for African immigrants. *Int. Health* **2014**, *6*, 203–207. [CrossRef] [PubMed]
46. Lesens, O.; Baud, O.; Henquell, C.; Lhermet, A.; Beytout, J. Varicella outbreak in Sudanese refugees from Calais. *J. Travel Med.* **2016**, *23*, taw042. [CrossRef] [PubMed]
47. Meinel, D.M.; Kuehl, R.; Zbinden, R.; Boskova, V.; Garzoni, C.; Fadini, D.; Dolina, M.; Blümel, B.; Weibel, T.; Tschudin-Sutter, S.; et al. Outbreak investigation for toxigenic Corynebacterium diphtheriae wound infections in refugees from Northeast Africa and Syria in Switzerland and Germany by whole genome sequencing. *Clin. Microbiol. Infect.* **2016**, *22*, 1003.e1–1003.e8. [CrossRef] [PubMed]
48. Giambi, C.; Del Manso, M.; Dalla Zuanna, T.; Riccardo, F.; Bella, A.; Caporali, M.G.; Baka, A.; Caks-Jager, N.; Melillo, T.; Mexia, R.; et al. National immunization strategies targeting migrants in six European countries. *Vaccine* **2018**. [CrossRef] [PubMed]
49. Lionis, C.; Petelos, E.; Mechili, E.A.; Pistolla, D.S.; Chatzea, V.E.; Angelaki, A.; Rurik, I.; Pavlic, D.R.; Dowrick, C.; Dückers, M.; et al. Assessing refugee healthcare needs in Europe and implementing educational interventions in primary care: A focus on methods. *BMC Int. Health Hum. Rights* **2018**, *18*, 11. [CrossRef] [PubMed]
50. European Centre for Disease Prevention and Control. ECDC Technical Document: Infectious Diseases of Specific Relevance to Newly-Arrived Migrants in the EU/EEA. Stockholm. 2015. Available online: https://ecdc.europa.eu/sites/portal/files/media/en/publications/Publications/Infectious-diseases-of-specific-relevance-to-newly-arrived-migrants-in-EU-EEA.pdf (accessed on 5 June 2018).
51. International Organization for Migration; World Health Organization. Tuberculosis Prevention and Care for Migrants. 2014. Available online: http://www.who.int/tb/publications/WHOIOM_TBmigration.pdf (accessed on 5 June 2018).
52. International Organization for Migration; World Health Organization. Health of Migrants: Resetting the Agenda. Report of the 2nd Global Consultation. Colombo, Sri Lanka. 2017. Available online: https://www.iom.int/sites/default/files/our_work/DMM/Migration-Health/GC2_SriLanka_Report_2017_FINAL_22.09.2017_Internet.pdf (accessed on 5 June 2018).
53. World Health Organization (WHO) Pandemic Influenza Preparedness and Mitigation in Refugee and Displaced Populations. 2008. Available online: http://www.who.int/diseasecontrol_emergencies/HSE_EPR_DCE_2008_3rweb.pdf (accessed on 5 June 2018).
54. World Health Organisation (WHO) Regional Office per Europe. WHO-UNHCR-UNICEF Joint Technical Guidance: General Principles of Vaccination of Refugees, Asylum-Seekers and Migrants in the WHO European Region. 2015. Available online: https://reliefweb.int/sites/reliefweb.int/files/resources/EuropeVaccinationPosition_WHO-UNHCR-UNICEFNov.pdf (accessed on 5 June 2018).

55. Kakalou, E.; Riza, E.; Chalikias, M.; Voudouri, N.; Vetsika, A.; Tsiamis, C.; Choursoglou, S.; Terzidis, A.; Karamagioli, E.; Antypas, T.; et al. Demographic and clinical characteristics of refugees seeking primary healthcare services in Greece in the period 2015–2016: A descriptive study. *Int. Health* **2018**. [CrossRef] [PubMed]
56. Giannakopoulos, G.; Anagnostopoulos, D.C. Child health, the refugees crisis, and economic recession in Greece. *Lancet* **2016**, *387*, 1271. [CrossRef]
57. The Lancet. Trauma for migrant children stranded in Greece. *Lancet* **2017**, *389*, 1166. [CrossRef]
58. Anagnostopoulos, D.C.; Triantafyllou, K.; Xylouris, G.; Bakatsellos, J.; Giannakopoulos, G. Migration mental health issues in Europe: The case of Greece. *Eur. Child Adolesc. Psychiatry* **2016**, *25*, 119–122. [CrossRef] [PubMed]
59. Ministry of Migration Policy. 2017. Available online: http://asylo.gov.gr/en/wp-content/uploads/2017/11/Greek_Asylum_Service_Statistical_Data_EN.pdf (accessed on 10 June 2018).
60. EKKA; National Center for Social Solidarity. Situation Update: Unaccompanied Children in Greece. Available online: http://www.ich-mhsw.gr/sites/default/files/Report.pdf (accessed on 5 June 2018).
61. ISSOP Migration Working Group. ISSOP position statement on migrant child health. *Child Care Health Dev.* **2018**, *44*, 161–170. [CrossRef] [PubMed]
62. United Nations High Commissioner for Refugees (UNHCR). Regional Refugee and Migrant Response Plan for Europe: January to December 2017. 2017. Available online: https://data2.unhcr.org/en/documents/download/52619 (accessed on 5 June 2018).
63. Freccero, J.; Biswas, D.; Whiting, A.; Alrabe, K.; Seelinger, K.T. Sexual exploitation of unaccompanied migrant and refugee boys in Greece: Approaches to prevention. *PLoS Med.* **2017**, *14*, e1002438. [CrossRef] [PubMed]
64. Pejovic-Milovancevic, M.; Klasen, H.; Anagnostopoulos, D. ESCAP for mental health of child and adolescent refugees: Facing the challenge together, reducing risk, and promoting healthy development. *Eur. Child Adolesc. Psychiatry* **2018**, *27*, 253–257. [CrossRef] [PubMed]
65. UN General Assembly. Optional Protocol to the Convention on the Rights of the Child on the Sale of Children, Child Prostitution and Child Pornography, 2000. International Documents on Corporate Responsibility. Available online: http://www.ohchr.org/EN/ProfessionalInterest/Pages/OPSCCRC.aspx (accessed on 5 June 2018).
66. Digidiki, V. *A Harsh New Reality: Transactional Sex among Refugee Minors as a Means of Survival in Greece*; FXB Center for Health and Human Rights, Harvard University: Boston, MA, USA, 2016; Available online: https://fxb.harvard.edu/a-harsh-new-reality-transactional-sex-among-refugee-minors-as-a-means-of-survival-in-greece/ (accessed on 5 June 2018).
67. Damon, A. *The Teenage Refugees Selling Sex on Athens Streets*; Cable News Network; CNN: Atlanta, GA, USA, 2016; Available online: http://www.cnn.com/2016/11/29/europe/refugees-prostitution-teenagers-athens-greece/ (accessed on 10 June 2018).
68. McGinnis, R.E. Sexual victimization of male refugees and migrants: Camps, homelessness, and survival sex. *Dignity* **2016**, *1*, 8. Available online: http://digitalcommons.uri.edu/cgi/viewcontent.cgi?article=1022&context=dignity (accessed on 5 June 2018). [CrossRef]
69. Karas, T. *Young, Alone, Abused: Unaccompanied Minors Wish They'd Never Come to Greece*; IRIN News: Nairobi, Kenya, 2016; Available online: https://www.irinnews.org/feature/2016/08/01/young-alone-abused (accessed on 5 June 2018).
70. Digidiki, V.; Bhabha, J. *Emergency within an Emergency: The Growing Epidemic of Sexual Abuse and Exploitation of Migrant Children in Greece*; FXB Center for Health and Human Rights at Harvard University: Boston, MA, USA, 2017; pp. 22–26.
71. Sanchez-Cao, E.; Kramer, T.; Hodes, M. Psychological distress and mental health service contact of unaccompanied asylumseeking children. *Child Care Health Dev.* **2012**, *39*, 651–659. [CrossRef] [PubMed]
72. Anagnostopoulos, D.; Vlassopoulou, M.; Rotsika, V.; Pehlivanidou, H.; Legaki, L.; Rogakou, E.; Lazaratou, H. Psychopathology and mental health service utilization by immigrants' children and their families. *Transcult. Psychiatry* **2004**, *41*, 465–486. [CrossRef] [PubMed]
73. Hodes, M.; Vasquez, M.M.; Anagnostopoulos, D.; Triantafyllou, K.; Abdelhady, D.; Weiss, K.; Koposov, R.; Cuhadaroglu, F.; Hebebrand, J.; Skokauskas, N. Refugees in Europe: National overviews from key countries with a special focus on child and adolescent mental health. *Eur. Child Adolesc. Psychiatry* **2018**, *27*, 389–399. [CrossRef] [PubMed]
74. Cortes, K. Are refugees different from economic immigrants? Some empirical evidence on the heterogeneity of immigrant groups in the United States. *Rev. Econ. Stat.* **2004**, *86*, 465–480. [CrossRef]

75. Moris, D.; Karamagioli, E.; Kontos, M.; Athanasiou, A.; Pikoulis, E. Refugee crisis in Greece: The forthcoming higher education challenge. *Ann. Transl. Med.* **2017**, *5*, 317. [CrossRef] [PubMed]
76. Ziomas, D.; Capella, A.; Konstantinidou, D.; European Social Policy Network. Integrating Refugee and Migrant Children into the Educational System in Greece. ESPN Flash Report 2017/67. Available online: file:///C:/Users/Rania/Downloads/ESPN%20-%20Flash%20Report%202017-67%20-%20EL%20-%20July%202017.pdf (accessed on 5 June 2018).
77. Pavlopoulou, I.D.; Tanaka, M.; Dikalioti, S.; Samoli, E.; Nisianakis, P.; Boleti, O.D.; Tsoumakas, K. Clinical and laboratory evaluation of new immigrant and refugee children arriving in Greece. *BMC Pediatr.* **2017**, *17*, 132. [CrossRef] [PubMed]
78. Tanaka, M.; Petsios, K.; Dikalioti, S.K.; Poulopoulou, S.; Matziou, V.; Theocharis, S.; Pavlopoulou, I.D. Lead Exposure and Associated Risk Factors among New Migrant Children Arriving in Greece. *Int. J. Environ. Res. Public Health* **2018**, *15*, 1057. [CrossRef] [PubMed]
79. Grammatikopoulou, M.G.; Theodoridis, X.; Poulimeneas, D.; Maraki, M.I.; Gkiouras, K.; Tirodimos, I.; Dardavessis, T.; Chourdakis, M. Malnutrition surveillance among refugee children living in reception centres in Greece: A pilotstudy. *Int. Health* **2018**. [CrossRef] [PubMed]
80. Dara, M.; Solovic, I.; Goletti, D.; Sotgiu, G.; Centis, R.; D'Ambrosio, L.; Ward, B.; Teixeira, V.; Gratziou, C.; Migliori, G.B. Preventing and controlling tuberculosis among refugees in Europe: More is needed. *Eur. Respir. J.* **2016**, *48*, 272–274. [CrossRef] [PubMed]
81. Dara, M.; Solovic, I.; Sotgiu, G.; D'Ambrosio, L.; Centis, R.; Tran, R.; Goletti, D.; Duarte, R.; Aliberti, S.; de Benedictis, F.M.; et al. Tuberculosis care among refugees arriving in Europe: A ERS/WHO Europe Region survey of current practices. *Eur. Respir. J.* **2016**, *48*, 808–817. [CrossRef] [PubMed]
82. Mellou, K.; Chrisostomou, A.; Sideroglou, T.; Georgakopoulou, T.; Kyritsi, M.; Hadjichristodoulou, C.; Tsiodras, S. Hepatitis A among refugees, asylum seekers and migrants living in hosting facilities, Greece, April to December 2016. *Eurosurveillance* **2017**, *22*, 30448. [CrossRef] [PubMed]
83. SolidarityNow, 'Issues in the Issuance of AMKA'. 2016. Available online: http://bit.ly/2ltg9Ql (accessed on 15 July 2018). (In Greek)
84. MSF, Greece in 2016: Vulnerable People Left Behind. 2016. Available online: http://bit.ly/2kPfBG1 (accessed on 15 July 2018).
85. SolidarityNow. Joint Report of 25 Organizations for Cases of Violation of Asylum Seekers' Rights. 2017. Available online: http://bit.ly/2oJxDs9 (accessed on 20 July 2018).
86. Circular 31547/9662 of 13 February 2018 «Σχετικά με την απόδοση ΑΜΚΑ σε δικαιούχουσ διεθνούσ προστασίασ και αιτούντεσ άσυλο». Available online: http://bit.ly/2H1ZCuE (accessed on 15 July 2018). (In Greek)
87. Tsiamis, C.; Terzidis, A.; Kakalou, E.; Riza, E.; Rosenberg, T. Is it time for a refugees' health unit in Greece? *Lancet* **2016**, *388*, 958. [CrossRef]
88. Tsitsakis, C.A.; Karasavvoglou, A.; Tsaridis, E.; Ramantani, G.; Florou, G.; Polychronidou, P.; Stamatakis, S. Features of public healthcare services provided to migrant patients in the Eastern Macedonia and Thrace Region (Greece). *Health Policy* **2017**, *121*, 329–337. [CrossRef] [PubMed]
89. Razum, O.; Kaasch, A.; Bozorgmehr, K. From the primacy of safe passage for refugees to a global social policy. *Int. J. Public Health* **2016**, *61*, 523–524. [CrossRef] [PubMed]
90. MSF, Confronting the Mental Health Emergency on Samos and Lesvos. 2017. Available online: http://bit.ly/2FUr5z4 (accessed on 15 July 2018).
91. Morgan, J. Disability-a neglected issue in Greece's refugee camps. *Lancet* **2017**, *389*, 896. [CrossRef]
92. Medecines Sans Frontieres. Confronting the Mental Health Emergency on Samos and Lesvos Why the Containment of Asylum Seekers on the Greek Islands Must End. 2017. Available online: https://www.msf.org/sites/msf.org/files/2018-06/confronting-the-mental-health-emergency-on-samos-and-lesvos.pdf (accessed on 3 August 2018).
93. Mock, C.N.; Donkor, P.; Gawande, A.; Jamison, D.T.; Kruk, M.E.; Debas, H.T. DCP3 Essential Surgery Author Group. Essential surgery: Key messages from Disease Control Priorities, 3rd edition. *Lancet* **2015**, *385*, 2209–2219. [CrossRef]
94. Moris, D.; Felekouras, E.; Linos, D. Global surgery initiative in Greece: More than an essential initiative. *Lancet* **2016**, *388*, 957. [CrossRef]

95. Bozorgmehr, K.; Samuilova, M.; Petrova-Benedict, R.; Girardi, E.; Piselli, P.; Kentikelenis, A. Infectious disease health services for refugees and asylum seekers during a time of crisis: A scoping study of six European Union countries. *Health Policy* **2018**. [CrossRef] [PubMed]
96. Georgakopoulou, T.; Mandilara, G.; Mellou, K.; Tryfinopoulou, K.; Chrisostomou, A.; Lillakou, H.; Hadjichristodoulou, C.; Vatopoulos, A. Resistant Shigella strains in refugees, August–October 2015, Greece. *Epidemiol. Infect.* **2016**, *144*, 2415–2419. [CrossRef] [PubMed]
97. European Centre for Disease Prevention and Control (ECDC). Technical Document on Implementing Syndromic Surveillance in Migrant Reception/Detention Centres and Other Refugee Settings. 2016. Available online: https://ecdc.europa.eu/sites/portal/files/media/en/publications/Publications/syndromic-surveillance-migrant-centres-handbook.pdf (accessed on 3 August 2018).
98. Hémono, R.; Relyea, B.; Scott, J.; Khaddaj, S.; Douka, A.; Wringe, A. *"The needs have clearly evolved as time has gone on"*: A qualitative study to explore stakeholders' perspectives on the health needs of Syrian refugees in Greece following the 2016 European Union-Turkey agreement. *Confl. Health* **2018**, *12*, 24. [CrossRef] [PubMed]
99. Kotsios, P. Structural Problems of the Greek Economy and Policy Recommendations. *Mod. Econ. Probl. Trends Prospect.* **2014**, *10*, 4–23.
100. Economou, C.; Kaitelidou, D.; Kentikelenis, A.; Sissouras, A.; Maresso, A. The Impact of the Financial Crisis on the Health System and Health in Greece, European Observatory on Health Systems and Policies, World Health Organization 2014. 2014. Available online: http://www.euro.who.int/__data/assets/pdf_file/0007/266380/The-impact-of-the-financial-crisis-on-the-health-system-and-health-in-Greece.pdf (accessed on 3 August 2018).
101. New York Times. Explaining Greece's Debt Crisis. Available online: https://www.nytimes.com/interactive/2016/business/international/greece-debt-crisis-euro.html (accessed on 30 July 2018).
102. Iefimerida, BBC: Greece Is under a Humanitarian Crisis-9 Revealing Graphs. 2015. Available online: http://www.iefimerida.gr/news/218032/bbc-i-ellada-vionei-anthropistiki-krisi-ennea-apokalyptika-grafimata-eikones (accessed on 30 July 2018).
103. Naftemporiki. Greece and Humanitarian Crisis. 2015. Available online: https://www.naftemporiki.gr/finance/story/928463/i-ellada-kai-i-anthropistiki-krisi (accessed on 30 July 2018).
104. Hellenic Statistical Authority. Greece in Figures July–September 2017. Available online: http://www.statistics.gr/en/greece-in-figures (accessed on 20 July 2018).
105. Eurostat. People at Risk of Poverty or Social Exclusion. Available online: http://ec.europa.eu/eurostat (accessed on 20 July 2018).
106. Eurostat. Health Statistics Database. Available online: http://ec.europa.eu/eurostat (accessed on 20 July 2018).
107. Kentikelenis, A.; Karanikolos, M.; Reeves, A.; McKee, M.; Stuckler, D. Greece's health crisis: From austerity to denialism. *Health Policy* **2014**, *383*, 748–753. [CrossRef]
108. Kotsiou, O.S.; Zouridis, Z.; Kosmopoulos, M.; Gourgoulianis, K.I. Impact of the financial crisis on COPD burden: Greece as a case study. *Eur. Respir. Rev.* **2018**, *27*, 170106. [CrossRef] [PubMed]
109. D'Kancs, A.; Lecca, P. Long-Term Social, Economic and Fiscal Effects of Immigration into the EU: The Role of the Integration Policy, JRC Working Papers in Economics and Finance, 2017/4. 2017. Available online: https://ec.europa.eu/futurium/sites/futurium/files/jrc107441_wp_kancs_and_lecca_2017_4.pdf (accessed on 20 August 2018).
110. European Commission, State of Health in the EU Greece Country Health Profile 2017. Available online: https://ec.europa.eu/health/sites/health/files/state/docs/chp_es_english.pdf (accessed on 20 August 2018).
111. Huffington Post. How Much Does the Refugee Crisis Cost to the Greek Economy. The Confidential Report of the Bank of Greece. Available online: https://www.huffingtonpost.gr/2016/02/04/ekthesi-tte-prosfygiko-stoixizei_n_9157364.html (accessed on 30 July 2018).
112. General Secretariat of the Greek Government. Vaccinations of Refugees and Immigrants in Hotspots. February 2017. Available online: https://government.gov.gr/wp-content/uploads/2017/02/Ekthesi-emvoliasmos-prosfygon-2017-02.pdf (accessed on 30 July 2018).
113. Bauhoff, S.; Göpffarth, D. Asylum-seekers in Germany differ from regularly insured in their morbidity, utilizations and costs of care. *PLoS ONE* **2018**, *13*, e0197881. [CrossRef] [PubMed]

114. Hunter, P. The refugee crisis challenges national health care systems: Countries accepting large numbers of refugees are struggling to meet their health care needs, which range from infectious to chronic diseases to mental illnesses. *EMBO Rep.* **2016**, *17*, 492–495. [CrossRef] [PubMed]
115. European Commission. An Economic Take on the Refugee Crisis. Institutional Paper 033. 2016. Available online: https://ec.europa.eu/info/sites/info/files/file_import/ip033_en_2.pdf (accessed on 30 July 2018).
116. Theofanidis, D.; Fountouki, A. Refugees and Migrants in Greece: An Ethnographic Reflective Case Study. *J. Transcult. Nurs.* **2018**, 1043659618781699. [CrossRef] [PubMed]
117. Kitching, G.T.; Haavik, H.J.; Tandstad, B.J.; Zaman, M.; Darj, E. Exploring the Role of Ad Hoc Grassroots Organizations Providing Humanitarian Aid on Lesvos, Greece. *PLoS Curr.* **2016**, *8*. [CrossRef] [PubMed]
118. Sifaki-Pistolla, D.; Chatzea, V.E.; Vlachaki, S.A.; Melidoniotis, E.; Pistolla, G. Who is going to rescue the rescuers? Post-traumatic stress disorder among rescue workers operating in Greece during the European refugee crisis. *Soc. Psychiatry Psychiatr. Epidemiol.* **2017**, *52*, 45–54. [CrossRef] [PubMed]
119. Psarros, C.; Malliori, M.; Theleritis, C.; Martinaki, S.; Bergiannaki, J.D. Psychological support for caregivers of refugees in Greece. *Lancet* **2016**, *388*, 130. [CrossRef]
120. Chatzea, V.E.; Sifaki-Pistolla, D.; Vlachaki, S.A.; Melidoniotis, E.; Pistolla, G. PTSD, burnout and well-being among rescue workers: Seeking to understand the impact of the European refugee crisis on rescuers. *Psychiatry Res.* **2018**, *262*, 446–451. [CrossRef] [PubMed]
121. Morgan, J. Frontline: Providing health care in Greece's refugee camps. *Lancet* **2016**, *388*, 748. [CrossRef]
122. ECDC. Expert Opinion on the Public Health Needs of Irregular Migrants, Refugees or Asylum Seekers across the EU's Southern and South-Eastern Borders. Stockholm: European Centre for Disease Prevention and Control. 2015. Available online: https://ecdc.europa.eu/sites/portal/files/media/en/publications/Publications/Expert-opinion-irregular-migrants-public-health-needs-Sept-2015.pdf (accessed on 5 June 2018).
123. Curtis, P.; Thompson, J.; Fairbrother, H. Migrant children within Europe: A systematic review of children's perspectives on their health experiences. *Public Health* **2018**, *158*, 71–85. [CrossRef] [PubMed]
124. Congress of Local and Regional Authorities. Unaccompanied Refugee Children: The Role and Responsibilities of Local and Regional Authorities. 34th Session. 2018. Available online: https://rm.coe.int/unaccompanied-refugee-children-current-affairs-committee-rapporteur-na/1680791c99 (accessed on 3 August 2018).

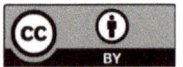

© 2018 by the authors. Licensee MDPI, Basel, Switzerland. This article is an open access article distributed under the terms and conditions of the Creative Commons Attribution (CC BY) license (http://creativecommons.org/licenses/by/4.0/).

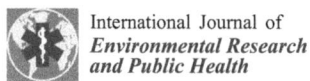

Article

Increased Urgent Care Center Visits by Southeast European Migrants: A Retrospective, Controlled Trial from Switzerland

Jolanta Klukowska-Röetzler [1,*], Maria Eracleous [2], Martin Müller [1,3], David S. Srivastava [1], Gert Krummrey [1], Osnat Keidar [1] and Aristomenis K. Exadaktylos [1]

1 Department of Emergency Medicine, University Hospital, 3010 Berne, Switzerland; martin.mueller@extern.insel.ch (M.M.); DavidShiva.Srivastava@insel.ch (D.S.S.); Gert.Krummrey@insel.ch (G.K.); osnatjacob@gmail.com (O.K.); Aristomenis.Exadaktylos@insel.ch (A.K.E.)
2 Department of Rheumatology, Immunology and Allergology, University Hospital, 3010 Bern, Switzerland; maria.eracleous@insel.ch
3 Institute of Health Economics and Clinical Epidemiology, University Hospital, 50935 Cologne, Germany
* Correspondence: jolanta.klukowska-roetzler@insel.ch; Tel.: +41-31-632-3396

Received: 25 July 2018; Accepted: 26 August 2018; Published: 28 August 2018

Abstract: We investigated whether immigrants from Southeast Europe (SE) and Swiss patients have different reasons for visiting the emergency department (ED). Our retrospective data analysis for the years 2013–2017 describes the pattern of ED consultations for immigrants from SE living in Switzerland (Canton Bern), in comparison with Swiss nationals, with a focus on type of referral and reason for admission. A total of 153,320 Swiss citizens and 12,852 immigrants from SE were included in the study. The mean age was 51.30 (SD = 21.13) years for the Swiss patients and 39.70 (SD = 15.87) years for the SE patients. For some countries of origin (Albania, Bosnia and Herzegovina, and Turkey), there were highly statistically significant differences in sex distribution, with a predominance of males. SE immigrants had a greater proportion of patients in the lower triage level (level 3: SE: 67.3% vs. Swiss: 56.0%) and a greater proportion of patients in the high triage level than the Swiss population (level 1: SE: 3.4% vs. Swiss: 8.8%). SE patients of working age (16–65 years) were six times more often admitted by ambulance than older ($\geq$65 years) SE patients, whereas this ratio was similar in the Swiss population. In both groups, the fast track service was primarily used for patients of working age (<65) and more than three times more often in the SE than the Swiss group (SE: 39.1%, Swiss: 12.6%). We identified some indications for access to primary care in emergency departments for immigrants and highlighted the need for attention to the role of organizational characteristics of primary health care in Switzerland. We highlighted the need for professional support to improve the quality of healthcare for immigrants. In the future, we will need more primary care services and general practitioners with a migrant background.

Keywords: Southeast Europe; immigrant; healthcare

1. Introduction

Switzerland is among the countries in Europe with the highest percentage of foreigners in its permanent population [1]. According to the information of the Swiss Federal Statistical Office (OFS) for the end of 2017, the Swiss population of 8,482,200 citizens included a high proportion of immigrants (2,108,001; 24.8%) [2]. The most common European country of origin was Italy (19.0%), followed by Serbia, Montenegro, and Kosovo (each 13.0%), Portugal (11.0%), and Germany (10.0%). Current immigration policy in Switzerland favors qualified workers from the European Union (EU) and particularly from Southeast Europe (SE) [3]. Most migrants from SE come from Kosovo (5.3%;

n = 112,233), Turkey (3.2%: n = 67,460), Macedonia (3.1%; n = 65,893), and Serbia (3.0%; n = 63,493) (Table 1).

Table 1. Number of Southeast Europe citizens (SE) in Switzerland and in Canton Bern and their percentage in comparison to the total number of immigrants [2].

Country	Switzerland	%	Canton Bern	%
Total number of immigrants	2,108,001		159,617	
Albania	1824	0.1	176	0.1
Bosnia and Herzegovina	30,282	1.4	1919	1.2
Bulgaria	9869	0.5	1145	0.7
Croatia	29,081	1.4	2419	1.5
Greece	13,684	0.7	616	0.4
Hungary	23,313	1.1	1846	1.2
Kosovo	112,233	5.3	8674	5.4
Macedonia	65,893	3.1	6378	4.0
Moldova	611	0.0	51	0.0
Montenegro	2517	0.1	0	0.0
Romania	18,092	0.9	1633	1.0
Serbia	63,493	3.0	4071	2.6
Slovenia	6753	0.3	408	0.3
Turkey	67,460	3.2	5392	3.4

Migration health is a specialized field of health sciences and focuses on the well-being of migrants. Migrants in a state of well-being are more receptive to education and employment [4]. They are not perceived to be a health threat to host societies, are less exposed to discrimination and are more likely to be accepted as equal citizens [4]. In various recent conventions and declarations (UN, WHO, EU), countries (including Switzerland) are called upon to work towards equality of opportunity in health. In order to improve the health status of the migrant population in Switzerland, the Confederation launched the "Migration and Public Health Strategy, 2008–2013", under the auspices of the FOPH. Various federal offices and federal agencies, as well as other organizations (Committee on the Elimination of Racial Discrimination, World Health Organization), have been involved in implementing the following strategy: "Everyone living in Switzerland shall be given a fair opportunity to develop their health potential. No-one will be disadvantaged by avoidable discrimination" [5].

In research on migration and health, questions about the health status and health-related behavior of the migrant population—and their causes and effects—are studied. However, there are gaps in current knowledge in this research area. A few publications have explored differences between immigrants and nationals [6–11], socioeconomic status [6], or general well-being and health of short- and long-term immigrants [7,12–14]. Some studies have found that immigrants attend EDs more often than host populations—but these findings have not been consistent [15,16]. Several studies have analyzed the health of immigrant patients in Switzerland and have reported specific health-related problems [6,8,9,17–20].

The first part of this study was aimed at describing the characteristics of SE immigrant patients admitted to our ED, in comparison to Swiss patients. The second part compared types of referral, reasons for admission, and triage of Swiss and SE patients.

2. Material and Methods

2.1. Setting

This study covers the city and canton of Bern, in central Switzerland. The study site is a level 1 interdisciplinary university ED, caring for more than 2 million people and treating about 42,000 patients (2017) of all social classes and insurance groups per year.

2.2. Study Design

This is a retrospective cohort study based on the demographic and health data of the patients admitted to the ED in Bern University Hospital from 1 January 2013 to 31 December 2017. Patients younger than 16 years are generally treated in the pediatric clinic and were therefore not included in this study.

2.3. Data Collection and Extraction

All data were extracted from the routine records of the digital data base system E.care (E.care BVBA, ED 2.1.3.0, Turnhout, Belgium). All patients were grouped according to nationality. Patients were classified into two groups: immigrants from SE without Swiss citizenship and Swiss citizens. Patients with other nationalities were excluded from this study. In these studies, we could not differentiate between native Swiss citizens and naturalized foreigners.

In accordance with the classification of SE by the European Travel Commission and the Danube-Sava definition [21,22], the SE immigrant group included all patients from: Albania, Bosnia and Herzegovina, Bulgaria, Croatia, Greece, Hungary, Kosovo, Macedonia, Moldova, Montenegro, Romania, Serbia, Slovenia, and Turkey. Although it is largely in Asia, we included Turkey in this study under SE. Relations between the European Union (EU) and Turkey were established in 1959 and Turkey is one of the EU's main partners in the southeast, and since 1987 Turkey has been an applicant to accede to EU.

Furthermore, demographic data (age, gender) and clinical data, including admission data, triage, reason for admission, and type of referral, were extracted from the ED's electronic database for patients.

The patients were classified into the following age classes: 16–25, 25–35, 35–45, 45–55, 55–65, 65–75, 75–85, 85–95, 95–105; genders (male, female); triage (1, 2, 3, 4, 5); type of referral (ambulance, air rescue, general practitioner, external hospital, walk-in, repatriation, military, police, and internal referral); and reason for admission (surgery, internal medicine, fast track, psychiatry). Fast track services are designed for patients seeking primary care services for less serious illnesses and injuries.

Patients in our ED are routinely triaged using an abbreviated version of the Manchester Triage System [23]. This triage system classifies the urgency of treatment for patients presenting to an ED in five levels: 1: acute life threating problem (immediate treatment required), 2: high urgency, 3: urgency, 4: less urgency, 5: no urgency. When a new patient presents to the ED, a specially trained nurse assigns the patient's reported complaints according to a defined algorithm and then determines the treatment priority with the aid of fixed rules that take into account the vital signs.

2.4. Definitions

In this study, 'immigrant' is defined as any foreign person according to the Swiss law on citizenship. A first-generation immigrant is someone who has moved to Switzerland after being born elsewhere. A second-generation immigrant is someone born to first-generation immigrants. Swiss citizenship is the status of being a citizen of Switzerland and can be obtained by birth or naturalization. People who are not born or naturalized in Switzerland were classified by their country of origin. The citizenship status is routinely assessed by our hospital administration system.

2.5. Ethical Considerations

This descriptive retrospective study was approved by the cantonal (district) ethics committee in Berne, (No. 2018-00198). No individual informed consent was obtained. The analysis was carried out with anonymized data.

2.6. Statistical Analysis

All data were presented as frequencies and percentages. The data were summarized using descriptive statistics. Data analysis was performed using Stata 13.1 (StataCorp, The College Station, TX, USA). Differences between patient groups were tested using the chi-square test.

3. Results

3.1. Demographic Distribution

A total of 12,852 immigrants from SE were admitted to the ED during the five-year study period. Over the same period, 153,320 Swiss citizens used our ED services (Table 2). Patients of other nationalities were excluded from this study (42,972). Some consultations were excluded from the analysis because key demographic information (nationality) was omitted in the patient information system ($n = 931$) or the patients were younger than 16 years old (SE immigrant patients: $n = 96$, Swiss: $n = 1869$). Thus, the total number of consultations included in the analysis was 166,172 (Figure 1).

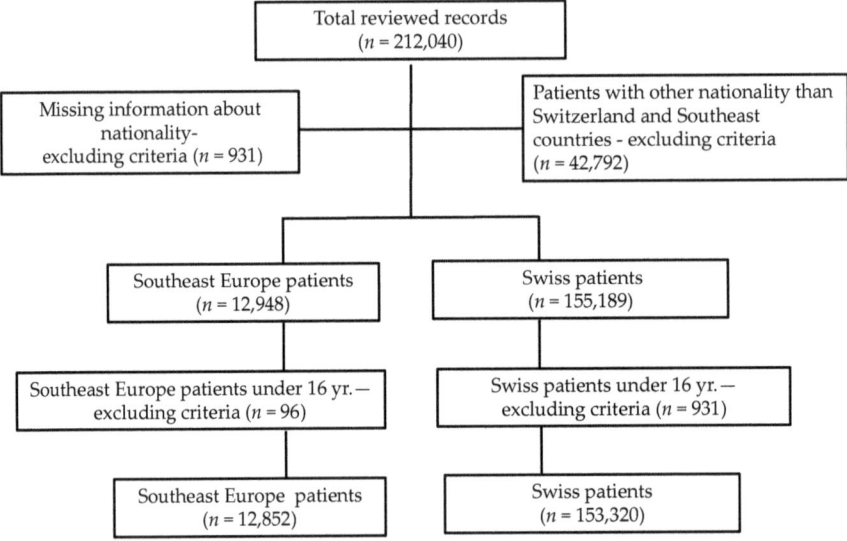

Figure 1. Flow chart of medical record selection.

Table 2. Comparison of the gender distribution in the Swiss and Southeast Europe groups and in the individual SE group countries.

Country of Origin	Male		Female		Total	
	n	%	n	%	n	%
Switzerland	85,195	55.6	68,125	44.4	153,320	100
Southeast Europe	6928	53.9	5924	46.1	12,852	100
Albania	672	61.9	414	38.1	1086	8.5
Bosnia and Herzegovina	455	59.4	311	40.6	766	6.0
Bulgaria	123	40.6	180	59.4	303	2.4
Croatia	379	51.8	353	48.2	732	5.7
Greece	115	58.7	81	41.3	196	1.5
Hungary	144	43	191	57.0	335	2.6
Kosovo	1011	49.7	1022	50.3	2033	15.8
Macedonia	1083	52.1	995	47.9	2078	16.2
Moldova	14	70.0	6	30.0	20	0.2
Montenegro	23	50.0	23	50.0	46	0.4
Romania	230	49.9	231	50.1	461	3.6
Serbia	959	52.7	861	47.3	1820	14.2
Slovenia	57	53.8	49	46.2	106	0.8
Turkey	1663	57.9	1207	42.1	2870	22.3

An increase in the annual number of patients was recorded in both analyzed groups over the study period: Swiss n = 33,074 and SE n = 3021 in 2017 compared to 27,218 (Swiss) and 2208 (SE) in 2013 (Figure 2). The largest group of SE patients were from Turkey (n = 2870, 22.3%), followed by Macedonia (n = 2078, 16.2%), and Kosovo (n = 2233, 15.8%) (Table 2).

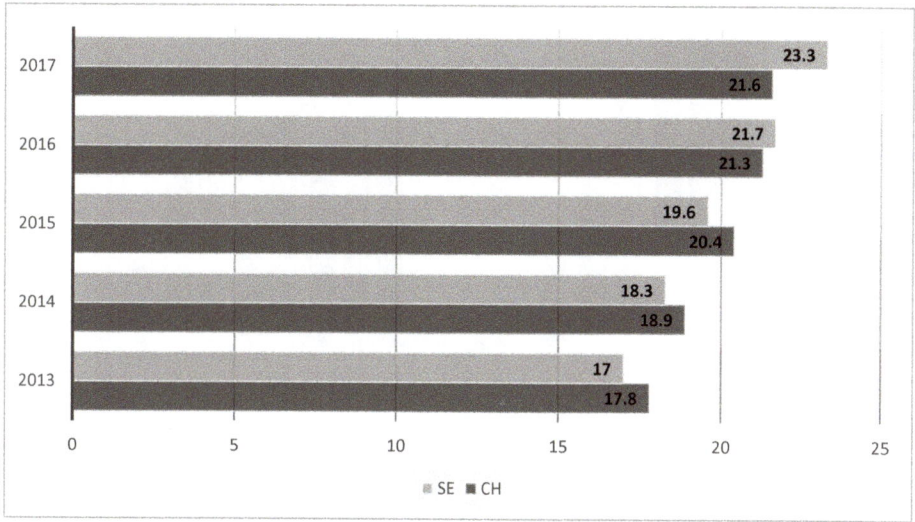

Figure 2. Percentage annual distribution of patients between 2013 and 2017 (SE: Southeast Europe; CH: Switzerland).

3.2. Gender Distribution

More than half of the Swiss patients were men (55.6%) and 44.4% were women. Similarly, 53.9% of the SE patients were men and 46.1% women. For most SE countries, most patients were male (max. Moldava: 70.0%). However, patients from some countries included many women (Bulgaria: 59.4%, Hungary 57.0%) (Table 2). There were highly significant differences ($p < 0.0001$) from the Swiss population in patients from Albania, Bosnia and Herzegovina, and Turkey and significant differences ($p < 0.05$) in patients from Bulgaria, Greece, Hungary, and Serbia.

3.3. Age Distribution

The mean age of the Swiss population was 51.30 (SD = 21.13), in comparison with 39.70 (SD = 15.87) in the SE population ($p < 0.0001$). Figure 3 highlights the age data of the cohort of ED patients studied. Between 2013 and 2017, 30.1% of the Swiss patients were older than 66 years, compared to 6.8% of the SE population (6.8%). Young adults of working age (16–65) were more common in the SE group (93.2% vs. 69.9% in the Swiss group). Very old patients (≥85) were represented only in the Swiss population (4.3%, n = 6655, including 26 centenarians, in contrast to only 29 patients (0.2%) in the SE group, including only six patients older than 90).

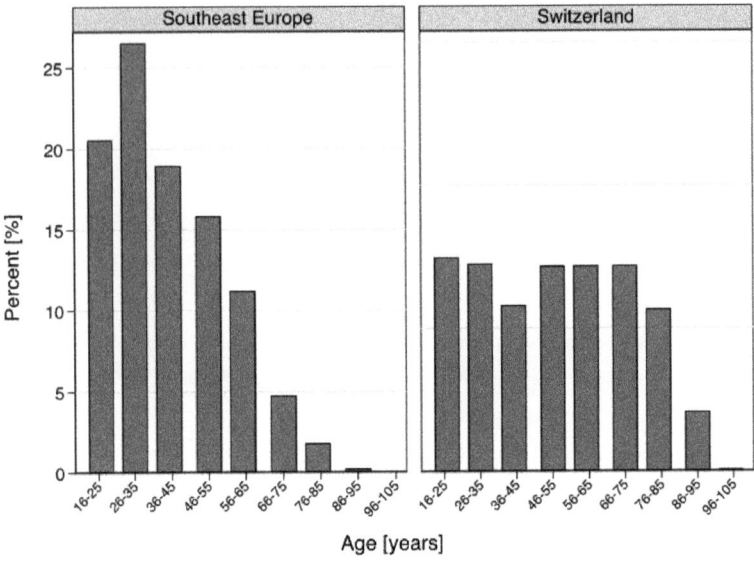

Figure 3. Comparison of the age distribution between Swiss and Southeast Europe patients.

3.4. Triage

The SE immigrant group exhibited different levels of triage, with a higher proportion in the lower triage level 3 (level 3: 67.3% vs. 56.0% in the Swiss group). Correspondingly, there were more patients in the high triage level in the Swiss group (level 1: Swiss: 8.8%, SE: 3.4%; level 2: Swiss 24.6%, SE: 17.6%) (Figure 4). There was a significant association between the triage level and immigration from SE ($p < 0.0001$). The mean triage level in patients from SE was 2.84 (95% CI: 2.82–2.85), but from Switzerland 2.61 (95% CI: 2.60–2.61) ($p < 0.001$).

Following the ED consultation, 65.5% of Swiss patients were treated as outpatients and 34.5% were hospitalized. SE immigrant patients were hospitalized less often (21.0%). There was a general trend that higher triage levels (1, 2) were associated with higher hospitalization rates (Swiss population: 48.9% vs. SE: 38.0%).

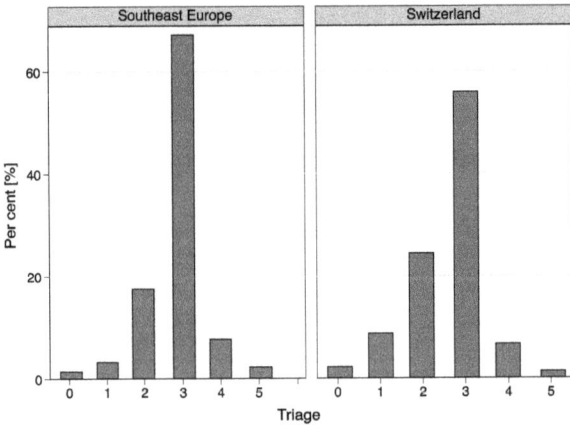

Figure 4. Comparison of triage distribution between Swiss and Southeast Europe immigrant groups.

3.5. Type of Referral

The main difference in the type of referral was observed in the self-referral group, which was more frequent with the SE immigrants (59.9%) than in the Swiss patient population (41.2%) (Figure 5). In contrast, referral by ambulance was more frequent in the Swiss patients than in the SE group (16.2% vs. 7.7%). SE patients of working age (16–65 years) were six times more often admitted by ambulance than were old ($\geq$66) SE patients (86.8% vs. 13.2%), whereas in the Swiss population this ratio was similar. Swiss patients were transferred twice more often from an external hospital or an external doctor than SE patients (external hospital, Swiss 7.0% vs. SE 3.6%; external doctor Swiss 7.0% vs. SE 3.0%).

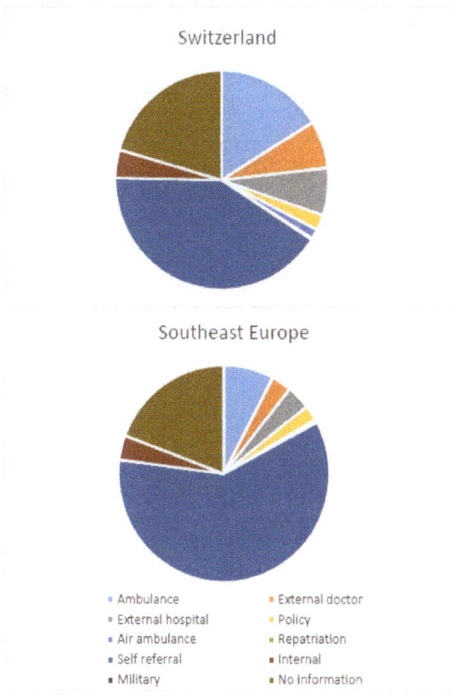

Figure 5. Comparison of type of referral between Swiss and Southeast Europe immigrant populations.

3.6. Reason for Admission

A highly significant association was found between 'reason for admission' and immigration from SE ($p < 0.001$). About 55.0% of Swiss patients (55.3%, n = 84,717) presented with internal medical complaints, 29.5% (n = 45,284) with surgical complaints, and 4.5% with psychiatric complaints. Almost 10.0% of Swiss patients (9.9%, n = 15,127) used a medical service in the fast track section of ED. These values differed significantly in the SE immigrant group: medical: 48.2% (n = 6326), surgery: 26.4% (n = 3388), psychiatry: 4.4% (n = 559), and fast track: 18.9% (n = 2423) (Figure 6).

In both groups, admission for internal medicine and surgical complaints increased steadily by about 3.0% during the five-year period. Within the same period, the total number of admitted patients increased from 38,027 in 2013 to 46,059 in 2017.

In the Swiss population, admission for internal medical and psychiatric complaints were predominant in Swiss patients between 16 and 65 years (working age population). In both study populations, the fast track service was used primarily by patients of 65 years and younger, corresponding to 12.6% of the Swiss population and 39.1% of SE immigrants. In patients aged >65, the use fast track was as follows: Swiss: 3.5% and SE immigrants 8.1%.

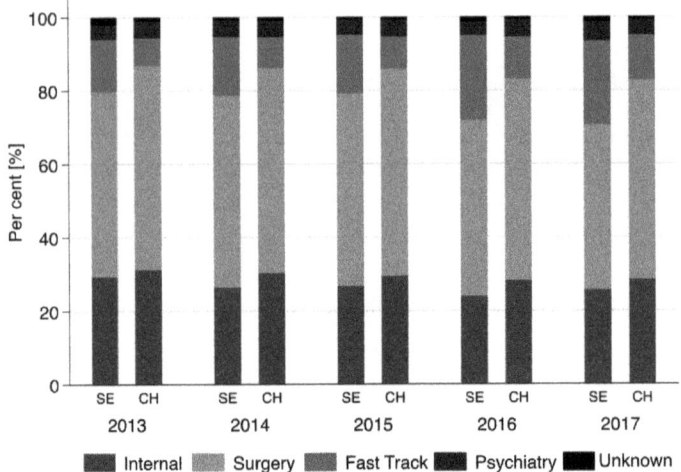

Figure 6. Reason for admission between 2013–2107 (SE: Southeast Europe; CH: Switzerland).

4. Discussion

4.1. Population of SE Immigrant Background in Switzerland

SE is a relatively new geopolitical denotation for the Balkan states, a region frequently regarded by Western countries as a heterogeneous set of countries with their own cultural specific features, dynamics, and an interconnected and complex modern history. There are many overlapping and conflicting definitions as to where exactly SE begins or ends or how it relates to other regions of the continent. The countries that form this part of Europe are Albania, Bosnia and Herzegovina, Bulgaria, Croatia, Kosovo, Macedonia, Moldova, Montenegro, Romania, Serbia, Slovenia, and—to some extent—Greece, Hungary, and Turkey [21].

After the Second World War, many refugees from countries involved in wars, including people from SE, found asylum in Switzerland. On the other hand, throughout the 20th century, immigration to Switzerland was organized around the needs of the domestic labor market and counteracted the shortage of (mostly unskilled) labor by hiring foreign workers.

For example, an anti-Communist revolt in Hungary started in 1956. Hundreds of thousands of people left the country, with around 14,000 seeking safety in Switzerland. The refugees were initially accommodated in army barracks, public buildings, hotels, and guesthouses. Over the following months, they were dispersed over all the Swiss cantons. Roughly 23,313 Hungarian citizens are now resident in Switzerland (2017) [2]. Most of these are former Hungarian refugees who chose to return to their country of origin after reaching retirement age in Switzerland. In comparison, Greece and Switzerland have a long relationship. During the rule of the military junta in Greece (1967–1974), many members of the opposition found protection in Switzerland. About 13,000 Greeks now live in Switzerland (2017); in 2010, there were 6808 [2]. Greeks who live permanently in Switzerland work in a variety of professions, such as medicine, banks, universities, organizations in the EU and the UN, where they excel and hold prominent and senior positions. The most numerous group of Southeast European immigrants (about 300,000 in 2017) arrived from the former Yugoslavia to live in Switzerland [2]. About half of these are Albanians (mostly Kosovar Albanians and to a lesser extent Albanians from Macedonia); the other half is made up of South Slavic groups (Serbs and Bosnians) and lower numbers of Croats, Macedonians, and Slovenes. Large numbers of workers obtained long-term permits between 1985 and 1998 and the subsequent inflow of family members generated the largest increase in the Yugoslav population in Switzerland.

Since immigration of skilled workers was initially promoted in the 1990s, and—as a result of the bilateral agreements with the EU—the proportion of well-educated and higher earning migrants has been increasing. At the same time, there are still high rates of immigration in industries with low levels of qualification (agriculture). Male and female foreign workers are very strongly represented in the construction sector and the hotel and restaurant industry, as well as in the healthcare sector. Foreign women are found in the sex industry and still often work illegally as domestics. Differences between Swiss citizens and SE immigrants are reflected in income. On average, the worst paid individuals in Switzerland are workers originating from the former Yugoslavia. The difference results from the individual level of education. Half of these immigrant workers from the Balkans did not receive any further training after completing obligatory school education. Unfortunately, that is also reflected in their quality of life and social status. Thirty percent of immigrants from the Balkans, Turkey, Romania, and Bulgaria are affected by poverty, whereas just under 20% from SE and only 7% from northern and western Europe are in poverty [5].

Many of the immigrants who arrived some time ago have stayed in Switzerland with their families, and these children born in Switzerland belong are now second-generation immigrants. On the one hand, there is an accumulation of risks and problems relating to the health; on the other hand, the second generation lives almost identically to the native population, with much better education and health conditions.

Immigrants may be very heterogeneous in some host countries and that the conventional Western conception of immigrants as vulnerable individuals characterized by low socio-economic status—working in unhealthy jobs, having poor health literacy and poor access to health services—may not necessarily be generalized [24]. Established theoretical explanations on migration and health can account for such differences: social and cultural patterns from the country of origin shape physical activity, body images, dietary intake, and food preferences [25,26]. Volhen and Rüesch reported that in the Switzlerland poor health and activities of daily living impairments were consistently associated with low socioeconomic status, low sense of mastery and little social support. Immigrant-specific preventive and health promotion initiatives should therefore target these immigrant groups [24].

As a result of their poorer overall socio-economic status compared with the native Swiss population, the migrant population has twice the rate of poverty (21.4%) and is also over-represented in the group of the working poor. A low level of education, unfavorable working conditions, or unemployment expose female foreigners to a particularly high risk of poverty. However, there are enormous differences in the poverty statistics depending on the country of origin. For instance, 30% of immigrants from the western Balkans—from Turkey, Romania, and Bulgaria—are affected by poverty, whereas just under 20% from southern Europe and only 7% from northern and western Europe are in poverty. It is hardly surprising that foreigners resident in Switzerland claim state benefits far more often than native Swiss men and women [5].

4.2. Health Care of SE Immigrants

In Switzerland, the foreign population is relatively young: for every 100 foreigners of working age (aged 20–65) there are only 11 aged 66 and over (compared with 36 among the Swiss) [27]. In our study, the mean age of SE immigrant patients was 39.7 (SD = 15.87) years, in contrast to the value for the Swiss group: 51.3 (SD = 21.13) years. The migrant groups from Turkey and former Yugoslavia contain a particularly high proportion of young people. Between 2013 and 2017, 1371 people from the 14 SE countries were awarded Swiss citizenship, mostly young people between 16–45 years (1207 applications) [2]. In the same time period, 1812 people decided for re-emigration. Some authors reported that people using the ED as their primary source of health care were significantly younger, which corresponds to our results [28]. Older patients more often favor the general practitioner for referral to the ED, rather than using the outpatient clinic [29]. This is consistent with our finding that younger patients of occupational age tend to visit the fast track.

Our data indicate that immigrants from SE to Switzerland—including both first- and second-generation immigrants—use the walk-in emergency services more often than Swiss patients. They tended to use the fast track (primary care) services in our emergency clinic, whereas the proportion of SE immigrants at the trauma clinic (internal medicine, surgery) was similar to the group's representation in the Swiss patient population. Between 2013 and 2017, the annual number of psychiatric emergencies among immigrants has tended to increase (by 70.0% in the five-year period). In the same period, the number of psychiatric cases in the native population increased by 17.8%. Similar findings have been seen in other studies on psychiatric problems among immigrants in ED [9,30]. As a comparison, other Swiss studies have found increasing numbers of psychiatric patients in ED (from 60 to 315 per year between 2007 and 2012) and the most common reasons for psychiatric presentation to ED were psychosis (20.3%), social problems (18.2%), auto-aggression (16.4%), and depression (16.2%) [9]. Cultural factors can play an important role in the psychological response to stress. The process of integration is certainly associated with stress and higher vulnerability for mental health problems [31,32]. Risk factors for mental health in the migration group are associated with living condition in the country of origin, duration of the migration, living condition in the country of immigration, sometimes with feelings of intolerance, the legal or social frameworks, and communications problems. Low social status (low incomes) are often associated with health-related behaviors like drinking and smoking and these may put physical and mental health at risk [31].

Previous publications on healthcare and migrants in Europe and Switzerland showed that migrants tend to have more contacts with general practitioners than the original population does [33,34]. In the present study, SE migrants more often carried out walk-in medical visits in ED than did the Swiss population. Walk-in SE patients more often use services in the fast track division (22.8% versus 15.8% in the Swiss population). Fast track services are designed for patients seeking primary care services (often without a general practitioner) for less serious illnesses and injuries. International studies have suggested that immigrants use emergency services more for non-urgent health care problems than do native populations [16,35,36]. A Norwegian study reported that a frequent reason for not contacting a general practitioner before the emergency department was because it was difficult to access him. In this study, 21% of the native Norwegians and 4% of the immigrants stated they had a general practitioner in another district and 33% of immigrants did not have their own general practitioner. In the same study, a high percentage of immigrants from Turkey (41.0%) and Africa (41.0%) had a problem in contacting any general practitioner [35]. Immigrant patients have frequently different reasons for underutilizing health services or the local health system, including poor education and lack of language skills. These impediments may lead to the wrong access to health care, so that immigrants may utilize ED services for non-urgent cases that can be treated in primary care settings [15]. This is consistent with our finding that the distribution of triage depends on the study population. During the analyzed period, immigrants were more likely to be frequent fast track users compared with Swiss population, although there were differences between immigrant groups. Older immigrants used fast track less often, whereas immigrants in the worked age were over-represented among frequent attenders.

The foreign population is on average younger than the Swiss population. Switzerland's population continues to age. 18.1% of the population is over 64, while there are 29 people over 64 for every 100 working-age people—those between the ages of 20 and 64 [34]. Taken as a whole, this may help to explain why most immigrants >65 years used their general practitioners less than younger immigrants and Swiss patients. As explained above, our study identifies the oldest immigrants as small group of patients in ED compared with numerous younger immigrants and Swiss patients. Although this could be partially explained by remigration to the country of origin after retirement. Our results are in contrast with other studies, where older immigrants used more health services than natives [35]. Thus, this group should be further studied, as a group with more access barriers to ED.

This group will probably increase in the future as second and subsequent generations of SE immigrants adapt to living conditions in Switzerland and are not motivated to return to their country of origin.

4.3. Limitations

Our study has some limitations. We decided to include all generation SE immigrants as one group in our study. As a result, we might have missed important differences between the first and second generations, who are generally better integrated and have a more similar lifestyle to the native population than did their parents. According information from the Federal Statistical Office FSO Section Population in District Bern for 2012–2016, ca. 96% of SE immigrants were first generation and only 7% second generation.

We only included data from an ED in central Switzerland, where the annual number of patients, including SE immigrants, is higher than in other emergency centers in private hospitals in Bern, or in the rest of the country. This might influence the choice of ED in case of an emergency. Other nationalities (except SE and Swiss) are excluded from the study, because Switzerland has a high percentage of immigrants and our goal was to characterize a SE patient population.

We restricted our analysis to adult patients. Thus, children (<16 years) were not included in the analysis. Furthermore, women with pregnancy- and delivery-related complications were not included in this study, as they were admitted directly to the Department of Obstetrics and Gynecology.

5. Conclusions

Between 2013 and 2007, SE immigrants used ED services differently than did Swiss citizens, depending on their nation of origin. Immigrants more often use the ED for low urgency complaints and this may suggest that barriers to primary healthcare may be driving the greater use of these services.

In Bern, immigrant subgroups use emergency services differently. Increased use was seen mostly at the fast track clinic, whereas the proportion of immigrants at the trauma and internal medicine was similar to the Swiss population. Immigrants of working age from SE used the fast track in the emergency department more frequently than the Swiss did. These different patterns of health-seeking behavior are important when planning and designing emergency and primary health care services for immigrants in large cities such as Bern.

We identified some differences in access to primary care in an emergency department for immigrants and emphasized the need for attention to the role of organizational characteristics of primary health care in the Switzerland. We highlighted the need for professional support to improve the quality of healthcare for immigrants. In the future, more primary care services and general practitioners with a migrant background must be provided.

Swiss primary health care needs to evolve to address the challenges of migrant populations. We hope that our results provide indications for practices and health systems interested in improving health care delivery for this vulnerable population. As numerous migrants with low income move to smaller cities, the primary health system must find ways to implement interpretation services, support comprehensive care and continuity of care, provide guidelines, and develop training for practitioners On the other hand, in the future access to preventive care will be particularly important for immigrant patients, as this is a determinant of the future risk of chronic disease, which in turn may lead to socioeconomic disadvantage.

Author Contributions: Conceptualization: J.K.-R., O.K., D.S.E., A.K.E.; Formal Analysis: J.K.-R., M.M., G.K., O.K.; Methodology: J.K.-R., M.E., M.M., D.S.E.; Project Administration: J.K.-R., O.K.; Validation: J.K.-R., M.E., M.M.; Writing-Original Draft: J.K.-R., M.E.; Writing-Review & Editing: J.K.-R., M.E., M.M.

Funding: This study was funded by the Bangerter Foundation and the Swiss Academy of Medical Sciences through the "Young Talents in Clinical Research" grant number (TCR 14/17).

Acknowledgments: We thank the Federal Statistical Office FSO Section Population POP for their data support.

Conflicts of Interest: The authors declare no conflict of interest.

References

1. Mahmoud, I.; Eley, R.; Hou, X.Y. Subjective reasons why immigrant patients attend the emergency department. *BMC Emerg. Med.* **2015**, *15*, 4. [CrossRef] [PubMed]
2. Johnson, T.; Gaus, D.; Herrera, D. Emergency Department of a Rural Hospital in Ecuador. *West. J. Emerg. Med.* **2016**, *17*, 66–72. [CrossRef] [PubMed]
3. Swiss Confederation Federal Department of Justice and Police. *Migration Report 2014*; Swiss Confederation Federal Department of Justice and Police: Berne, Switzerland, 2014.
4. Mahmoud, I.; Hou, X.Y. Immigrants and the utilization of hospital emergency departments. *World J. Emerg. Med.* **2012**, *3*, 245–250. [CrossRef] [PubMed]
5. Migration and Public Health. *Summary to the Federal Strategy Phase II (2008–2013)*; Federal Office of Public Health: Berne, Switzerland, 2008.
6. Pfortmueller, C.; Graf, F.; Tabbara, M.; Lindner, G.; Zimmermann, H.; Exadaktylos, A.K. Acute health problems in African refugees: Ten years' experience in a Swiss emergency department. *Wien. Klin. Wochenschr.* **2012**, *124*, 647–652. [CrossRef] [PubMed]
7. Tarraf, W.; Vega, W.; Gonzalez, H.M. Emergency department services use among immigrant and non-immigrant groups in the United States. *J. Immigr. Minority Health* **2014**, *16*, 595–606. [CrossRef] [PubMed]
8. Lay, B.; Lauber, C.; Nordt, C.; Rossler, W. Patterns of inpatient care for immigrants in Switzerland: A case control study. *Soc. Psychiatry Psychiatr. Epidemiol.* **2006**, *41*, 199–207. [CrossRef] [PubMed]
9. Chatzidiakou, K.; Schoretsanitis, G.; Schruers, K.; Mueller, T.; Ricklin, M.; Exadaktylos, A.K. Acute psychiatric problems among migrants living in Switzerland—A retrospective study from a Swiss University emergency department. *Emerg. Med. Open Access* **2016**, *6*. [CrossRef]
10. Beiser, M.; Wickrama, K.A. Trauma, time and mental health: A study of temporal reintegration and depressive disorder among Southeast Asian refugees. *Psychol. Med.* **2004**, *34*, 899–910. [CrossRef] [PubMed]
11. Beiser, M. The health of immigrants and refugees in Canada. *Can. J. Public Health Revue Can. Sante Publique* **2005**, *96* (Suppl. 2), S30–S44.
12. Zhao, X.; Yang, B.; Wong, C.W. Analyzing Trend for U.S. Immigrants' e-Health Engagement from 2008 to 2013. *Health Commun.* **2018**, 1–11. [CrossRef] [PubMed]
13. Giuntella, O.; Mazzonna, F. Do immigrants improve the health of natives? *J. Health Econ.* **2015**, *43*, 140–153. [CrossRef] [PubMed]
14. Gruer, L.; Millard, A.D.; Williams, L.J.; Bhopal, R.S.; Katikireddi, S.V.; Cezard, G.I.; Buchanan, D.; Douglas, A.F.; Steiner, M.F.C.; Sheikh, A. Differences in all-cause hospitalisation by ethnic group: A data linkage cohort study of 4.62 million people in Scotland, 2001–2013. *Public Health* **2018**, *161*, 5–11. [CrossRef] [PubMed]
15. Ruud, S.E.; Aga, R.; Natvig, B.; Hjortdahl, P. Use of emergency care services by immigrants—A survey of walk-in patients who attended the Oslo Accident and Emergency Outpatient Clinic. *BMC Emerg. Med.* **2015**, *15*, 25. [CrossRef] [PubMed]
16. Norredam, M.; Krasnik, A.; Moller Sorensen, T.; Keiding, N.; Joost Michaelsen, J.; Sonne Nielsen, A. Emergency room utilization in Copenhagen: A comparison of immigrant groups and Danish-born residents. *Scand. J. Public Health* **2004**, *32*, 53–59. [CrossRef] [PubMed]
17. Bosia, T.; Malinovska, A.; Weigel, K.; Schmid, F.; Nickel, C.H.; Bingisser, R. Risk of adverse outcome in patients referred by emergency medical services in Switzerland. *Swiss Med. Wkly.* **2017**, *147*, w14554. [CrossRef] [PubMed]
18. Pfortmueller, C.; Stotz, M.; Lindner, G.; Mueller, T.; Rodondi, N.; Exadaktylos, A.K. Multimorbidity in adult asylum seekers: A first overview. *PLoS ONE* **2013**, *8*, e82671. [CrossRef] [PubMed]
19. Bischoff, A.; Wanner, P. The self-reported health of immigrant groups in Switzerland. *J. Immigr. Minority Health* **2008**, *10*, 325–335. [CrossRef] [PubMed]
20. Grossmann, F.; Leventhal, M.E.; Auer-Boer, B.; Wanner, P.; Bischoff, A. Self-reported cardiovascular risk factors in immigrants and Swiss nationals. *Public Health Nurs.* **2011**, *28*, 129–139. [CrossRef] [PubMed]
21. Anton, J.I.; Munoz de Bustillo, R. Health care utilisation and immigration in Spain. *Eur. J. Health Econ. HEPAC Health Econ. Prev. Care* **2010**, *11*, 487–498. [CrossRef] [PubMed]

22. Shibusawa, T.; Mui, A.C. Health status and health services utilization among older Asian Indian immigrants. *J. Immigr. Minority Health* **2010**, *12*, 527–533. [CrossRef] [PubMed]
23. Mackway-Jones, K. *Emergency Triage: Manchester Triage Group*; BMJ Publishing Group: London, UK, 1997.
24. Volken, T.; Rüesch, P. Health Status Inequality among Immigrants in Switzerland. *Open J. Prev. Med.* **2014**, *4*, 459–469. [CrossRef]
25. Nicolaou, M.; Doak, C.M.; van Dam, R.M.; Brug, J.; Stronks, K.; Seidell, J.C. Cultural and social influences on food consumption in Dutch residents of Turkish and Moroccan origin: A qualitative study. *J. Nutr. Educ. Behav.* **2009**, *41*, 232–241. [CrossRef] [PubMed]
26. Kolcic, I.; Polasek, O. Healthy migrant effect within Croatia. *Coll. Antropol.* **2009**, *33* (Suppl. 1), 141–145. [PubMed]
27. Tiruneh, A.; Siman-Tov, M.; Radomislensky, I.; Itg Peleg, K. Characteristics and circumstances of injuries vary with ethnicity of different population groups living in the same country. *Ethn. Health* **2017**, *22*, 49–64. [CrossRef] [PubMed]
28. Clement, N.; Businger, A.; Martinolli, L.; Zimmermann, H.; Exadaktylos, A.K. Referral practice among Swiss and non-Swiss walk-in patients in an urban surgical emergency department. *Swiss Med. Wkly.* **2010**, *140*, w13089. [CrossRef] [PubMed]
29. Althaus, F.; Paroz, S.; Hugli, O.; Ghali, W.A.; Daeppen, J.B.; Peytremann-Bridevaux, I.; Bodenmann, P. Effectiveness of interventions targeting frequent users of emergency departments: A systematic review. *Ann. Emerg. Med.* **2011**, *58*, 41–52.e42. [CrossRef] [PubMed]
30. Mulder, C.; Koopmans, G.T.; Selten, J.P. Emergency psychiatry, compulsory admissions and clinical presentation among immigrants to the Netherlands. *Br. J. Psychiatry J. Ment. Sci.* **2006**, *188*, 386–391. [CrossRef] [PubMed]
31. Lindert, J.; Priebe, S.; Penka, S.; Napo, F.; Schouler-Ocak, M.; Heinz, A. Mental health care for migrants. *Psychother. Psychosom. Med. Psychol.* **2008**, *58*, 123–129. [CrossRef] [PubMed]
32. Hjern, A.; Wicks, S.; Dalman, C. Social adversity contributes to high morbidity in psychoses in immigrants—A national cohort study in two generations of Swedish residents. *Psychol. Med.* **2004**, *34*, 1025–1033. [CrossRef] [PubMed]
33. Norredam, M.; Nielse, S.S.; Krasnik, A. Migrants' utilization of somatic healthcare services in Europe—A systematic review. *Eur. J. Public Health* **2010**, *20*, 555–563. [CrossRef] [PubMed]
34. Alves, L.; Azevedo, A.; Barros, H.; Paccaud, F.; Marques-Vidal, P. Portuguese migrants in Switzerland: Healthcare and health status compared to Portuguese residents. *PLoS ONE* **2013**, *8*, e77066. [CrossRef] [PubMed]
35. Ruud, R.; Hjortdahl, P.; Natvig, B. Reasons for attending a general emergency outpatient clinic versus a regular general practitioner—A survey among immigrant and native walk-in patients in Oslo, Norway. *Scand. J. Prim. Health Care* **2017**, *35*, 35–45. [CrossRef] [PubMed]
36. Norredam, M.; Mygind, A.; Nielsen, A.S.; Bagger, J.; Krasnik, A. Motivation and relevance of emergency room visits among immigrants and patients of Danish origin. *Eur. J. Public Health* **2007**, *17*, 497–502. [CrossRef] [PubMed]

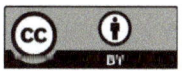

© 2018 by the authors. Licensee MDPI, Basel, Switzerland. This article is an open access article distributed under the terms and conditions of the Creative Commons Attribution (CC BY) license (http://creativecommons.org/licenses/by/4.0/).

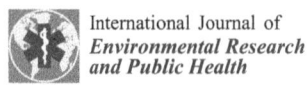

Review

The Effectiveness and Cost-Effectiveness of Screening for and Vaccination Against Hepatitis B Virus among Migrants in the EU/EEA: A Systematic Review

Daniel T Myran [1], Rachael Morton [2], Beverly-Ann Biggs [3], Irene Veldhuijzen [4], Francesco Castelli [5], Anh Tran [2], Lukas P Staub [2], Eric Agbata [6], Prinon Rahman [7], Manish Pareek [8], Teymur Noori [9] and Kevin Pottie [10],*

[1] University of Ottawa School of Epidemiology and Public Health, Ottawa, ON K1G 5Z3, Canada; dmyra088@uottawa.ca
[2] NHMRC Clinical Trials Centre, The University of Sydney, Sydney 2006, Australia; Rachael.morton@ctc.usyd.edu.au (R.M.); ahn.tran@ctc.usyd.edu.ar (A.T.); lukas.staub@ctc.usyd.edu.au (L.P.S.)
[3] Department of Medicine at the Doherty Institute, University of Melbourne, and Victorian Infectious Diseases Service, Royal Melbourne Hospital, Melbourne 3000, Australia; babiggs@unimelb.edu.au
[4] Centre for Infectious Disease Control, National Institute for Public Health and the Environment (RIVM), Bilthoven 3720, The Netherlands; irene.veldhuijzen@rivm.nl
[5] University Department of Infectious and Tropical Diseases University of Brescia and ASST Spedali Civili, Brescia 25123, Italy; francesco.castelli@unibs.it
[6] Department of Paediatrics, Obstetrics, Gynaecology and Preventive Medicine, Universität Autònoma de Barcelona, Barcelona 08193, Spain; ricagbata@yahoo.com
[7] C.T. Lamont Primary Health Care Research Centre, Bruyère Research Institute, Ottawa, ON K1R 7G5, Canada; prinon.rahman@dal.ca
[8] Department of Infection, Immunity and Inflammation, University of Leicester, Leicester LE1 7RH, UK; manish.pareek@leicester.ac.uk
[9] European Centre for Disease Prevention and Control, Stockholm 169 73, Sweden; Teymur.Noori@ecdc.europa.eu
[10] Bruyere Research Institute, School of Epidemiology and Public Health, University of Ottawa, Ottawa, ON K1R 7G5, Canada
* Correspondence: kpottie@uottawa.ca

Received: 28 June 2018; Accepted: 27 August 2018; Published: 1 September 2018

Abstract: Migrants from hepatitis B virus (HBV) endemic countries to the European Union/European Economic Area (EU/EEA) comprise 5.1% of the total EU/EEA population but account for 25% of total chronic Hepatitis B (CHB) infection. Migrants from high HBV prevalence regions are at the highest risk for CHB morbidity. These migrants are at risk of late detection of CHB complications; mortality and onwards transmission. The aim of this systematic review is to evaluate the effectiveness and cost-effectiveness of CHB screening and vaccination programs among migrants to the EU/EEA. We found no RCTs or direct evidence evaluating the effectiveness of CHB screening on morbidity and mortality of migrants. We therefore used a systematic evidence chain approach to identify studies relevant to screening and prevention programs; testing, treatment, and vaccination. We identified four systematic reviews and five additional studies and guidelines that reported on screening and vaccination effectiveness. Studies reported that vaccination programs were highly effective at reducing the prevalence of CHB in children (RR 0.07 95% CI 0.04 to 0.13) following vaccination. Two meta-analyses of therapy for chronic HBV infection found improvement in clinical outcomes and intermediate markers of disease. We identified nine studies examining the cost-effectiveness of screening for CHB: a strategy of screening and treating CHB compared to no screening. The median acceptance of HB screening was 87.4% (range 32.3–100%). Multiple studies highlighted barriers to and the absence of effective strategies to ensure linkage of treatment and care for migrants with CHB. In conclusion, screening of high-risk children and adults and vaccination of susceptible children, combined with treatment of CHB infection in migrants, are promising and cost-effective interventions, but linkage to treatment requires more attention.

Keywords: HBV; CHB; screening; vaccination; refugees; migrants

1. Introduction

Hepatitis B Virus (HBV) infection can cause acute and chronic hepatitis and lead to life threatening liver complications including cirrhosis and hepatocellular carcinoma (HCC) [1]. Infection with chronic hepatitis B (CHB) is typically asymptomatic until health complications develop. However, individuals with CHB, including asymptomatic cases, can spread the virus through sexual contact, blood-blood contact, and mother to child transmission [1]. Six percent of the world's population, approximately 248 million people, are infected with CHB [2]. The global distribution of HBV is highly variable and regions are characterized by the prevalence of Hepatitis B surface Antigen (HBsAg) as low (<2%), or endemic (≥2%) [2]. In the European Union/European Economic Area (EU/EEA) an estimated 4–7.5 million people are chronically infected with HBV, with an overall prevalence of 1.12% [3,4]. The majority of countries in the EU/EEA have a low prevalence of HBV infection, although in 2013 five countries had a prevalence >2% [3]. However, CHB infection remains a leading cause of chronic liver disease and liver cancer in the EU/EEA, and results in significant economic burden and lost productivity [5,6].

Migrants to the EU/EEA originating from endemic countries suffer a disproportionate burden of CHB, constituting 5.1% of the population but comprising an estimated 25% (range 14–47%) of total CHB cases [3]. Antenatal screening programs in the EU/EEA report that migrant women account for 1.0% to 15.4% of diagnoses of CHB, on average, six times higher than in the general female population [7]. The risk of CHB infection varies amongst different migrant groups. A systematic review of migrants throughout the world found higher prevalence of CHB in refugees, asylum seekers and migrants originating from HBV endemic countries [8].

As the majority of cases of CHB are asymptomatic, screening is important to identify individuals at risk of progression to complications and who are at risk of transmitting the virus. In addition, screening can identify individuals who are susceptible to infection and would benefit from vaccination. An effective HB vaccine has been available for nearly four decades and has reduced the incidence of new infections in the EU/EEA and globally [1,6,9,10]. Universal childhood vaccination against HB is recommended in 27/31 EU/EEA countries, and all countries recommend vaccination for children in high-risk groups, including migrants [11]. However, identification of migrants susceptible to HB infection and delivery of vaccination can be complicated. Internationally, several strategies for vaccination programs exist including universal childhood vaccination, targeted vaccination of individuals found to be susceptible to HB, and ring vaccination strategies that prevent the spread of disease by vaccinating close contacts of known HBV cases [1,12]. Individuals infected during childhood are at higher risk of developing CHB infection and complications than individually infected later in life [1,13]. Consequently, prevention of childhood HB infection in migrant communities is a public health priority.

The World Health Organization (WHO) has set the goal of eliminating CHB as a major public health threat by 2030 with targets to reduce the incidence of chronic infection by 90% and mortality by 65% [14]. National programs should include migrants from endemic countries as an important component of this global strategy. Screening programs for CHB vary by country; at present the majority of EU/EEA countries do not recommend screening for CHB in migrants [15]. Detecting CHB infections in migrants from endemic countries and subsequent management including treatment and behavioral change counselling is likely to decrease the burden of disease in the EU/EEA. In this systematic review, we aim to evaluate the effectiveness, costs (resource requirements), and cost-effectiveness of CHB screening and vaccination programs for migrants to the EU/EEA.

2. Materials and Methods

The Campbell and Cochrane Collaboration Equity Methods Group and review team including clinicians, public health experts, and researchers from across the EU/EEA used the Grading of Recommendations Assessment, Development and Evaluation (GRADE) approach to conduct evidence reviews. Additional details of the methods can be found in registered systematic review protocol published in BMJ Open [16].

HBV was selected as a key infectious disease by the review team. The review group followed the PRISMA reporting guidelines [17] for the reporting of this systematic review. In summary, the review team developed key research questions (PICO: Population, Intervention, Comparison, Outcome) and a logic model showing an evidence chain to identify key concepts, to consider the potential role of indirect evidence related to populations and interventions and to support the formulation of search strategies [16].

The review teams aimed to answer the following overarching questions:

- Is screening for HBV infection (and subsequent management) associated with decreased morbidity and mortality in migrant populations?
- What is the effectiveness of HBV vaccination programs in migrant populations?
- What is the cost-effectiveness of screening and vaccination programs for HBV?

We used a combination of key terms including "hepatitis B", "prevalence", "screening", "cost", "efficacy", and "harms". See Appendix A for the complete list of search terms. Evidence specific to migrants and the EU/EEA was prioritized, but evidence was considered regardless of the population. In particularly whenever possible, we sought to include studies examining marginalized communities, or those with limited health care access, which may be more comparable to migrants than the general population. Migrants included asylum seekers, refugees, undocumented migrants, and other foreign-born residents with a focus on those recently arrived.

We searched MEDLINE via OVID and EMBASE, and NHS EED for evidence on the effectiveness of screening and the cost-effectiveness of screening between 1 January 2010 and 31 December 2016. Finally, we searched the CEA Registry (Tufts University) and Google Scholar databases for additional evidence on cost-effectiveness. For the purpose of this review we considered English language systematic reviews, randomized control trials, and economic studies, evaluating testing, vaccination, and treatment.

Two independent team members (DM & EA) reviewed the titles and abstracts identified by the search. Disagreements were resolved by consensus. The full text of identified citations was then screened for inclusion (DM & EA) with disagreements resolved by consensus. One reviewer (DM) extracted the data from the included study and a second reviewer (EA) verified the data. The methodological quality of included studies was assessed using AMSTAR (Assessing the Methodological Quality of Systematic Reviews) [18].

For evidence around cost-effectiveness, we independently screened and extracted relevant data from the primary studies including economic study design (e.g., micro-costing study, within-trial cost-utility analysis, decision-analytic model); the intervention and comparator, the difference in resource use, costs and cost-effectiveness (e.g., incremental net benefit or incremental cost-effectiveness ratio), and three specific questions for the GRADE Evidence to Decision table: the size of the resource requirements, the certainty of evidence around resource requirements, and whether the cost-effectiveness results favored the intervention or comparison [19]. Finally, we assessed the certainty of economic evidence in each study using the relevant items from the 1997 Drummond checklist [20].

We assessed the certainty of the quantitative evidence using the GRADE approach. We incorporated evidence from a review of qualitative studies relating to hepatitis B and migrants.

On 5 June 2018, we did a pre-publication rapid update search for new high-quality evidence pertaining to our PICO questions.

3. Results

The search for evidence on effectiveness of screening and vaccination for CHB identified a total of 1829 results. After full text screening, we included four systematic reviews, three guidelines, and two studies, which met our inclusion criteria. See Figure 1 (PRISMA flow chart) and Table 1. List of included studies. Studies were excluded for the following reasons: focus on hepatitis C and not hepatitis B, HCC screening, animal studies and screening for HBV before starting immunosuppressive therapies.

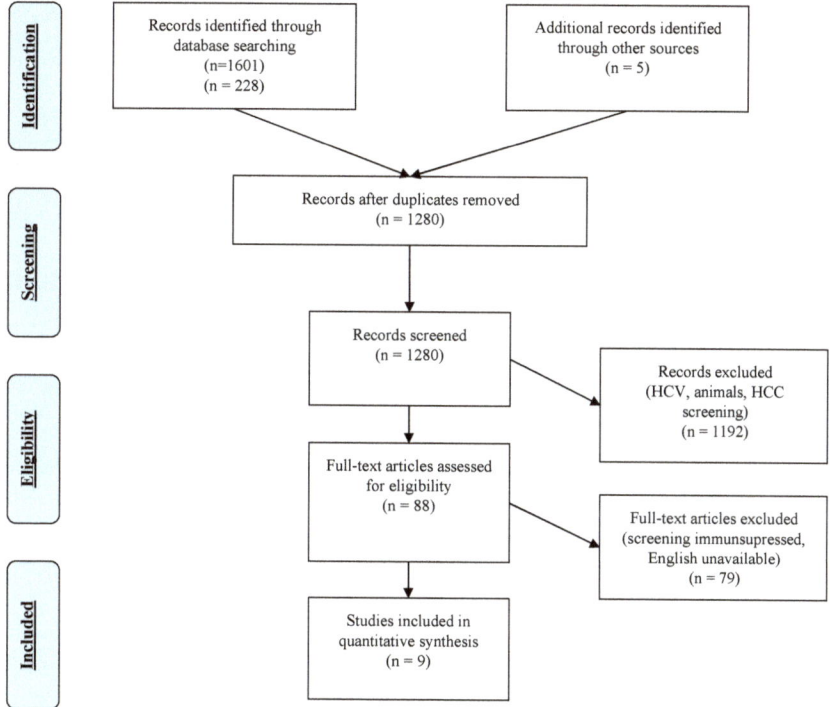

Figure 1. PRISMA Flow Diagram for Effectiveness of HBV screening and vaccination programs * No randomized control studies on screening were identified. Included studies were on topics relevant to the evidence chain (testing, prevalence, vaccination, and treatment).

Table 1. (a) Characteristics of included studies for screening and vaccine program effectiveness for Hepatitis B Virus.

Study	Quality	Type of Study	Population	Intervention	Results/Outcomes
		Should Hepatitis B Virus (HBV) screening be offered to recently arrived migrants to the EU/EEA?			
Choi et al. 2014 [21]	AMSTAR * 9/11	Systematic Review	12 RCTs	Treatment with Nucleos(t)ide Analogues (NAs) compared to placebo	Reduced rate of intermediate outcomes in NA group (HBV DNA loss, HBeAg loss, Histologic improvement, HBsAg loss). No significant decrease in HCC incidence. No increase in significant adverse events in NA group but higher rates of study withdrawal
Wong et al. 2010 [22]	AMSTAR 7/11	Systematic Review	11 RCTs	Treatment with pegylated interferon alpha compared to placebo	Decreased rate of Hepatic Events (RR 0.55 95% CI 0.43 to 0.70), cirrhotic complications (RR 0.46 95% CI 0.32 to 0.67) and liver related mortality (RR 0.63 95% CI 0.42 to 0.96) for treatment group
EASL 2017 [23]	NA	Guideline			Current Treatment Guidelines for acute and chronic infection with hepatitis B for the EU/EEA
ECDC 2016 [3]	NA	Technical Document	EU/EEA Migrants/General Population	No intervention	5.5% of migrants born in intermediate/high prevalence countries infected with CHB infection compared to 1.12% in the general population of EU/EEA Migrants from HBV endemic countries 5.1% of population of the EU/EEA but 25% (range 14–47%) of the total number of CHB cases
WHO 2017 [2]	NA	Guideline			Guidelines on hepatitis B testing including information on implementation of screening programs.
WHO 2015 [1]	NA	Guideline			Guidelines for the prevention, care and treatment of persons with chronic hepatitis B infection.
		What is the effectiveness of vaccination programs against HBV?			
Graham et al. 2013 [24]	AMSTAR 4/11	Systematic Review	Australia; Aboriginal population/general population	Vaccination with HBV vaccine compared to no vaccine	Reduced rate of positive HBeAg in post vaccination cohort 3.96% (95% CI: 3.15-4.77) compared to pre-vaccination cohort 16.72 (95% CI: 7.38–26.06).
Chang et al. 2009 [25]	NA	Individual Study	Endemic Country Taiwan (Republic of China)	Vaccination with HBV vaccine compared to no vaccine	Reduced rate of positive HBsAg (RR 0.07 95% CI 0.04 to 0.13) and chronic liver disease mortality (RR 0.34 95% CI 0.25 to 0.45) in post vaccination cohort
Rossi et al. 2012 [8]	AMSTAR 6/11	Systematic Review	Global Migrant Population	No intervention	Prevalence of CHB higher in refugees and asylum seekers compared to immigrants (9.6% vs. 5.1%). 39.7% of migrants demonstrated prior immunity to HBV either through prior infection or vaccination (95% CI: 35.7–43.9%).

* A Measurement Tool to Assess Systematic Reviews (AMSTAR).

Table 1. (b) Characteristics of included studies cost-effectiveness of screening for HBV.

Study	Certainty of Economic Evidence (Quality)	Design	Population	Intervention	Cost-Effectiveness	Resource Requirements
What is the cost-effectiveness of screening (and subsequent management) migrants for chronic hepatitis B (CHB)?						
Rossi et al. 2013 [26]	Allowance was made for uncertainty in the estimates of costs and consequences across plausible ranges. Appropriate statistical analyses: probabilistic sensitivity analyses (PSA) were performed for costs and consequences. Justification was provided for key study parameters and some upper and lower range estimates. Some ranges cited the data sources; other ranges provided an assumption for upper and lower limits but no further justification. The cost-effectiveness results were not very sensitive to changes in the values. Most of the time, the intervention was still cost-effective. At a standard willingness to pay threshold, the probability of being cost-effective was 78% (high).	Decision-analytic Markov model, results presented in Canadian dollars.	Vaccination strategies for newly arrived adult Canadian immigrants and refugees	(i) universal vaccination, (ii) screening + vaccination (iii) screening+ treatment (iv) screening +treatment + vaccination	(i) and (ii) were dominated by no intervention (iii) screening and treatment: CAN$40,880 per QALY gained vs no intervention (iv) screen, treatment, vaccination: CAN$437,335 per QALY gained vs no intervention	The intervention has moderate costs. Categories and volumes of resource use were not reported separately.
Wong et al. 2011 [27]	All the ranges were provided. Both one way, and probabilistic sensitivity analyses were performed. All data sources for model inputs were provided, with the exception of reference years for all costs. The results were sensitive to the progression rate and discount rate used. The intervention had a 55% probability of being cost-effective compared to a no screening strategy. Certainty in the results was deemed to be moderate overall.	Decision-analytic Markov model; reported in Canadian dollars	Immigrants to Canada	(i) 'No screening'; (ii) 'Screen and Treat' (iii) 'Screen, Treat and Vaccinate'	ICER for Screen and treat ranged from CAN$45,221 (Tenofovir, 3% discount) per QALY gained to CAN$101,513 (Entecavir, 5% discount) ICER for Screen, treat and vaccinate ranged from CAN$96,523 (Entecavir, 3% discount) to CAN$3,648,123 per QALY gained (Tenofovir, 5% discount) Favours intervention (ii): screen and treat, CAN$69,209/QALY gained (cost-effective) A vaccination program following the screening program was not cost-effective compared with the screen and treat strategy.	Large costs for strategy ii: screen and treat if using either Entecavir or Tenofovir. Large costs for strategy iii: screen, treat and vaccinate using Entecavir. Other interventions had moderate costs. Resource use was not quantified separately.
Hutton et al. 2007 [12]	Allowance for uncertainty was accommodated. Both one way and PSA were conducted. All the data sources were provided for ranges used in sensitivity analyses. The probability of being cost-effective was 82–85% when the values of key variables were changed. Therefore the certainty of the intervention being cost-effective was deemed high.	Decision-analytic Markov model; results in US dollars	Asian and Pacific Islander adult immigrants to the US	(i) No Screening: universal vaccination strategy for all individuals (ii) Screen, Treat and No Vaccination: a screen-and-treat strategy: screen individuals and treat infected persons; (iii) Screen, Treat and Vaccinate: vaccine for non-infected persons (iv) Screen, Treat and Ring Vaccinate: screen for close contacts and vaccinate non-infected persons	The screen-and-treat strategy, intervention (ii) has an incremental cost-effectiveness ratio of US$36,088 per QALY gained compared with the status quo. Screen and treat and ring vaccinate strategy, intervention (iv) has a cost-effectiveness ratio of US$39,903 per QALY gained compared with the screen-and-treat strategy. Universal vaccination, intervention (i) and screen and treat and vaccine were dominated.	Costs were moderate, ranging from US$85,000 per person per lifetime with universal vaccination to US$87,000 per person per lifetime to screen, treat and ring vaccinate.

283

Table 1. (b) Cont.

Study	Certainty of Economic Evidence (Quality)	Design	Population	Intervention	Cost-Effectiveness	Resource Requirements
What is the cost-effectiveness of screening (and subsequent management) migrants for chronic hepatitis B (CHB)?						
Veldhuijzen et al. 2010 [28]	Uncertainty was tested and all ranges were provided. Univariate, multivariate, PSA were conducted. Data sources for all the ranges were provided. Cost-effectiveness results were robust to changes in model parameters. The probability of being cost-effective was 72%; the certainty was deemed moderate.	Decision-analytic Markov model; results reported in Euros	Migrants to the Netherlands from intermediate and high HBV endemic areas	One-off systematic screening and subsequent treatment of eligible patients, compared with the status quo: i.e., existing pregnancy screening, testing due to medical complaints, contact tracing, and checkup for STIs.	Incremental cost-effectiveness ratio (ICER) of €8966 per QALY gained. Discounted costs at 4% and effects at 1.5%, resulted in a slightly lower ICER of €8823 per QALY gained.	Status quo had low test costs at €458 while the screen and treat strategy had a test cost of €15,954. Referral and follow up costs for the status quo strategy was €838; while the screen and treat strategy had a follow up cost of €3074. i.e., a large difference. Screening and treatment costs per person were ~€130 per person.
Rein et al. 2011 [29]	Standard deviations were provided for costs.	Costing study (exploratory, pilot study)	Overseas-born community living in the US	Screening models: (i) Community Clinic (ii) Community Outreach (iii) Outreach partnership (iv) Partnership contract	Cost-effectiveness was not reported	Cost per complete screen ranged from US$640 for the Community Clinic to US$280 for the Partnership Contract model. Low costs for Community based but higher costs for Partnership model. The costs per positive person identified varied from US$609 in the Community model to US$4657 in the Partnership model. Cost per complete screen/cost per newly identified positive case (adj. for prevalence): 1) US$40/$854 ($895) 2) US$102/$2641 ($2698) 3) US$280/$6300 ($6013) 4) US$176/$5709 ($5063)
Jazwa et al. 2015 [30]	Allowance was made for uncertainty, all the ranges were provided. Not all statistical tests were reported. Univariate sensitivity analysis was conducted, which is consistent with the study design (cost benefit study, not cost-effectiveness). All the data sources and assumptions were provided. Not applicable.	Cost-benefit analysis	Refugees to the US; costs reported in US dollars	(i) Vaccinate only without HBV screening (ii) Screen, then vaccinate or initiate management	The net benefits of the screen and vaccinate strategy ranged from US$24 million to US$130 million after 5 years from program initiation	The cost per refugee for the vaccination only strategy was low if the screen rate <70%, however after 10 years, if the screening rate was more than 70%, the cost of the vaccination only strategy was moderate: US$706–$968 per person.
Ruggeri et al. 2011 [31]	Allowance was made for uncertainty, all the ranges were provided. Both one way and PSA were conducted. All the data sources and assumptions were provided. The results were not sensitive to changes in the model values. The probability of being cost-effective was 70–98%; the certainty of the results was deemed high.	Decision-analytic Markov model; results reported in Euros	Residents of Italy	(i) Screening of Italian patients at risk (assumed prevalence of 7%) and treatment of cases according to protocol; (ii) compared with no screening and treatment of patients with cirrhosis or HCC	ICER of €18,256 per QALY gained (±€367) for screening compared to no screening	High costs for the screening strategy: €67,008 (±€515) per person per year; Low cost for no screening strategy, but moderate costs for the screen and treat strategy. Moderate cost for no screening strategy: €7939 (±€1679) per person per year

Table 1. (b) Cont.

Study	Certainty of Economic Evidence (Quality)	Design	Population	Intervention	Cost-Effectiveness	Resource Requirements
	What is the cost-effectiveness of screening (and subsequent management) migrants for chronic hepatitis B (CHB)?					
Eckman et al. 2011 [32]	Allowance was made for uncertainty, all the ranges were provided. PSA was conducted. All the data sources and assumptions were provided. The cost-effectiveness results were sensitive to model parameters including cost of treatment, drug resistance, and disease prevalence. The probability of the intervention being CE was 49%; certainty was deemed moderate.	Decision-analytic Markov model; results reported in US dollars.	Asymptomatic outpatients in the US	Screening for Hepatitis B surface antigen followed by treatment of appropriate patients with (i) pegylated interferon-a2a for 48 weeks, (ii) a low-cost nucleoside or nucleotide agent with a high rate of developing viral resistance for 48 weeks, (iii) prolonged treatment with low-cost, high-resistance nucleoside or nucleotide, (iv) prolonged treatment with a nucleotide with a low rate of developing viral resistance; compared with no screening	Intervention (iii) was dominated by the no screening intervention; Intervention (ii) and intervention (v) were dominated by intervention (iv). Intervention (iv) was cost-effective with an ICER of US$29,232 per QALY gained.	Low cost for no screening strategy US$915 per person per year. Moderate cost for screen and treat, ranging from US$1170 (treat with low cost, high resistance nucleoside) to US$1286 (treat with high cost, low resistance nucleoside). Resource use was not reported separately.
Li et al. 2013 [33]	Allowance was made for uncertainty. All upper bound and lower bound limits were provided. Only univariate sensitivity analysis was conducted. No justification was provided for the ranges tested for price of treatment, or probability of disease progression. The cost-effectiveness results were not sensitive (i.e., remained robust) to changes in the values of variables. Moderate certainty.	Decision-analytic Markov model; results reported in US dollars.	Residents of Zhoushan Island in mainland China.	Monitor and treat scenarios in 3 patient groups according to treatment eligibility. (1) ineligible (2) borderline (3) eligible compared with natural history (no screening and no antiviral treatment of patients with cirrhosis or HCC)	ICER of the monitor and treat strategy compared to the natural history was US$97 per QALY gained for the ineligible group, US$500/QALY for the borderline group, US$1131/QALY for the eligible group. With a 5% reduction in Entecavir price: the monitor and treat strategy becomes cost saving (ICER < 0) in the ineligible group; the ICER was US$254 for the eligible group, and US$860 for the eligible group. With a 50% reduction in Entecavir price: the monitor and treat strategy was cost saving for all sub groups: (ICER < 0).	For the ineligible group: Difference in costs was small. For example, total costs per patient per lifetime was US$21,229 for natural history strategy, and US$21,530 for Monitor and Treat. For the borderline group: The difference in costs was larger. For natural history strategy, the total costs = per patient lifetime was US$33,280 while the total cost per patient lifetime for the monitor and treat strategy was US$37,043. For the eligible group: The difference in costs was largest. With natural history strategy, total cost per patient lifetime was US$32,430 while total cost per patient lifetime for monitor and treat strategy was US$42,711.

In a rapid update prior to publication, we identified one additional systematic review examining the uptake of screening for HBV in migrant communities.

3.1. Effectiveness of Screening for CHB

Screening tests involving serologic markers are considered to have high validity (sensitivity and specificity of greater than 98% for detecting HBsAg) for the detection of CHB infection [2]. Our review found evidence of effective treatment options for CHB that reduced disease morbidity and mortality in specific subsets of patients [22,23]. Treatment guidelines, including whom to treat, when to initiate therapy and the first line agents vary across the EU/EEA [22]. Addressing optimal treatment for CHB was outside the scope of this review. However, the presence of effective treatment options including pegylated IFNα [22] and nucleos(t)ide analogues [21,23] provide indirect evidence that suggests screening is likely to be worthwhile, at least for high-risk populations.

We identified an additional systematic review examining the uptake of screening for CHB among migrants [34]. The review identified four studies examining CHB screening in migrants to the EU/EEA. The median acceptance of HB screening was 87.4% (range 32.3–100%), and 7.3% of migrants were found to have CHB infection (range 0.35–31.8%). The review identified no studies that had examined what percent of migrants identified with CHB were linked to follow up and ongoing care.

3.2. Vaccination Against HBV

Despite the inclusion of HB vaccine in many EU/EEA countries National Immunization Programs (NIP), migrant populations may not have access to vaccines due to arrival after the age of vaccination in the general population. Our search and selection did not identify studies examining vaccination programs in migrant populations. However, we did identify evidence from two childhood vaccination programs, one involving marginalized sub populations, within endemic HB communities, demonstrating that childhood vaccination programs were effective at preventing infection. Evidence from a universal infant and childhood vaccination program in Taiwan showed a dramatic decrease in HBsAg seropositivity (9.8–0.7%) between 1984 and 1999 [35,36]. Similarly, a review examining the prevalence of HBV in indigenous and non-indigenous people in the Torres Strait Islands (which is off the coast of mainland Australia) following the implementation of a universal vaccination program for infants and adolescents in 2000 showed a decrease in prevalence of HB infection (6.47% overall prevalence pre 2000 to 2.25%). The impact was particularly pronounced for the indigenous populations who also faced access barriers to health care (16.72% prevalence pre 2000 to 3.96%) [24]. See Table 2 for a summary of evidence for HB vaccination strategies and Box 1 for the GRADE grades of evidence.

Box 1. GRADE Working Group grades of evidence.

High quality: We are very confident that the true effect lies close to that of the estimate of the effect
Moderate quality: We are moderately confident in the effect estimate: The true effect is likely to be close to the estimate of the effect, but there is a possibility that it is substantially different
Low quality: Our confidence in the effect estimate is limited: The true effect may be substantially different from the estimate of the effect
Very low quality: We have very little confidence in the effect estimate: The true effect is likely to be substantially different from the estimate of effect

Table 2. GRADE Evidence Profile: Effect of HBV vaccination on preventing HBV infection, chronic liver disease and HCC.

No of participants (studies) Follow-up	Certainty Assessment						Study event rates (%)		Summary of Findings	Anticipated absolute effects	
	Risk of bias	Inconsistency	Indirectness	Imprecision	Publication bias	Overall certainty of evidence	With no vaccine	With HBV vaccine	Relative effect (95% CI)	Risk with no vaccine	Risk difference with HBV vaccine
HCC mortality											
54289638 (1 observational study)	serious [a]	not serious [b]	not serious	serious [c]	none	Very Low	135/27144819 (0.0%)	20/27144819 (0.0%)	RR 0.90 (0.75 to 1.09)	0 per 100,000	0 fewer per 100,000 (0 fewer to 0 fewer)
Liver cancers (except non-hepatocellular carcinoma)											
6898803 (1 observational study)	serious [a]	serious [b]	not serious	serious [c]	none	Very Low	24/3381519 (0.0%)	20/3517284 (0.0%)	RR 0.80 (0.42 to 1.48)	1 per 100,000	0 fewer per 100,000 (0 fewer to 0 fewer)
HBsAg carriage											
1916 (1 observational study)	serious [d]	not serious	not serious	not serious	strong association [e]	Low	39/559 (7.0%)	9/1357 (0.7%)	RR 0.07 (0.04 to 0.13)	6977 per 100,000	6488 fewer per 100,000 (6698 fewer to 6070 fewer)
Anti-HBc											
1916 (1 observational study)	serious [d]	not serious	not serious	not serious	strong association [e]	Low	115/559 (20.6%)	39/1357 (2.9%)	RR 0.11 (0.08 to 0.16)	20,572 per 100,000	18,309 fewer per 100,000 (18,927 fewer to 17,281 fewer)
Chronic Liver Disease											
54289638 (1 observational study)	serious [a]	not serious	not serious	not serious	strong association	Low	407/36702888 (0.0%)	55/15586750 (0.0%)	RR 0.34 (0.25 to 0.45)	1 per 100,000	1 fewer per 100,000 (1 fewer to 1 fewer)
HCC Incidence											
54289638 (1 observational study)	serious [a]	not serious	not serious	not serious	none	Very Low	712/36702888 (0.0%)	191/15586750 (0.0%)	RR 0.89 (0.75 to 1.04)	2 per 100,000	0 fewer per 100,000 (0 fewer to 0 fewer)
HBsAg (continuous)											
1–12 8545 (8 observational studies)	serious [a]	serious [f]	not serious	not serious	none	Very Low	5516 (Number of Events)	3029 (Number of Events)	N/A	The mean HBsAg (continuous) ranged from 5.19–25.99 %	3.96 % lower (3.15 lower to 4.17 lower)

[a] Cohort Study, downgraded due to risk of bias; [b] Heterogeneity is not reported; [c] Large confidence intervals; [d] Cohort Study, risk of bias was not assessed; [e] Large effect; [f] Hetegeniety (I-squared: 94.9%); **CI:** Confidence interval; **RR:** Risk retio.

Bibliography: Ni YH, Chang MH, Huang LM, et al. Hepatitis B virus infection in children and adolescents in a hyperendemic area: 15 years after mass hepatitis B vaccination. Ann Intern Med 2001;135:796–800 Chang M-H, Chen C-J, Lai V-S, et al. Universal hepatitis B vaccination in Taiwan and the incidence of hepatocellular carcinoma in children. NEngl J Med 1997;336:1855-9. Graham S, Guy RJ, Cowie B, Wand HC, Donovan B, ALre SP, et al. Chronic hepatitis B prevalence among Aboriginal and Torres Strait Islander Australians since universal vaccination: a systematic review and meta-analysis. BMC Infect Dis. 2013 Dec;13(1):403. Chang MH, You SL, Chen CJ, Liu CJ, Lee CM, Lin SM, et al. Decreased incidence of hepatocellular carcinoma in hepatitis B vaccines: A 20-year follow-up study. J Natl Cancer Inst. 2009;101 19;1348–55.

Analysis of children vaccinated against HBV in Taiwan demonstrated a decline in the annual incidence of HCC in children 6 to 14 years of age from 0.70 per 100,000 children between 1981 and 1986 to 0.57 between 1986 and 1990, and to 0.36 between 1990 and 1994 ($P < 0.01$). The corresponding rates of mortality from HCC also decreased [25]. We found no studies directly examining the impact of vaccinating susceptible adult migrants against HB.

Surveillance data following vaccination with HBV have not demonstrated significant adverse events [37,38]. In 43,618 Alaskan Natives who received 101,360 doses of HB vaccine, possible adverse reactions occurred in 39 persons and none of the adverse reactions were considered severe [38].

3.3. Cost-Effectiveness of Screening and Subsequent Management for Hepatitis B

We retrieved a total of 228 articles from the National Health System Economic Evaluation Database (NHS EED) and the Cost-Effectiveness Analysis Registry at Tufts University (CEA Tufts), and a further ten studies from the effectiveness search from the title and abstract screening. After full text review, we included nine primary studies from our search, see Figure 2 (PRISMA flow chart). Six of the included studies were specific to migrant populations, one of which was conducted in The Netherlands [28], while three were from the USA and two from Canada. Nine primary studies compared the costs and benefits of different strategies including no screening (n = 6); screening and treating (n = 6); screening, treating, and vaccinating (n = 4); universal vaccination (n = 3), and ring vaccination (n = 1).

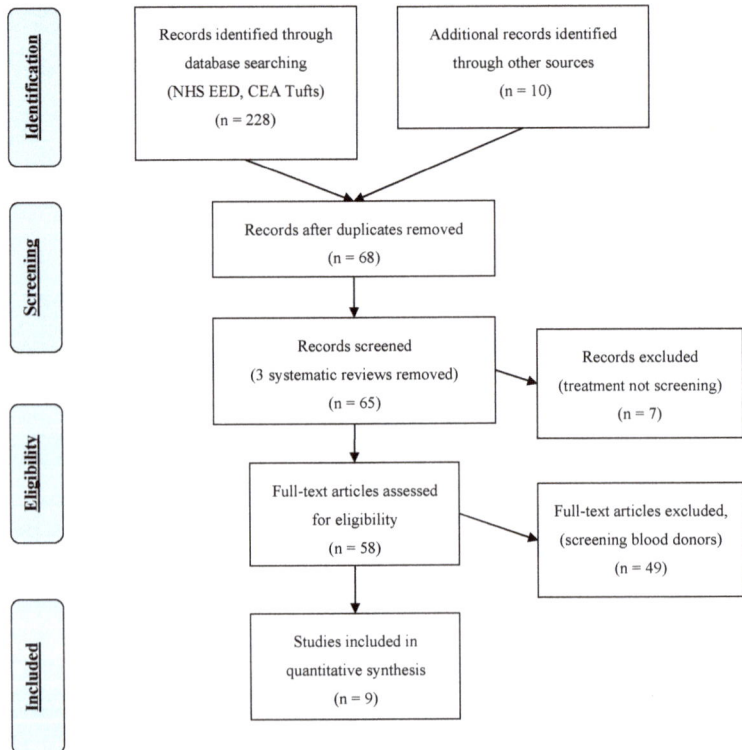

Figure 2. PRISMA Flow Diagram for Cost-Effectiveness of HBV screening.

The review identified one modelling study from the EU/EEA conducted in the Netherlands. The study modelled a cohort of people who either experienced the natural history of HBV infection or received antiviral treatment reported that one-off screening for HBsAg and treating active cases of CHB with Entecavir, resulted in an incremental cost-effectiveness ratio (ICER) of screening and treatment compared with no formal screening, of €8966 per quality-adjusted life year (QALY) gained, with the range of €7222 to €15,694 in sensitivity analysis. These values are below the commonly-used Dutch cost-effectiveness threshold of €20,000 per QALY gained [28].

Among the five studies of migrants to North America, the costs ranged from CAN$6077 [26] to US$86,620 [12] per person screened (and treated in the event of a positive result), with the majority of studies estimating program costs of >$20,000 per person per year. Thus, the costs of these interventions were generally considered moderate. The ICER of screening and treatment for HBV, compared to no screening, ranged from US$36,088 [12] to CAN$40,880 [28] and CAN$101,513 (€72,508) [27] per quality-adjusted life year (QALY) gained. Screening was cost-effective at the host countries' commonly accepted willingness to pay thresholds. Therefore, all included studies favored screening and treatment for HBV over the status quo of no (or voluntary) screening. Two studies found that HBV screening was likely cost-effective for populations with a prevalence of CHB $\geq$2% [27]. One study of outpatients to US hospitals found that screening may be cost-effective even in populations with lower than 2% prevalence (i.e., 0.3%) [28].

3.4. Cost-Effectiveness of Vaccination

Three studies from North America reported the cost-effectiveness of HBV vaccination, either as a universal strategy or in addition to screening and treatment in mostly migrant populations with the majority arriving from South Asia and Sub-Saharan Africa. The universal vaccination strategy was dominated (i.e., slightly more expensive and slightly less effective) than a no screening intervention in two studies [12,39]. When examining screening for prior immunity and vaccination, all three studies found that strategies adding vaccination of susceptible migrants were not cost-effective or were dominated by the screen and treat strategy [12,26,27]. One of the studies, a US study of Asian and Pacific Islander adult migrants, found that including screening close contacts of infected persons and vaccinating susceptible contacts was cost-effective with an ICER of $39,903 per QALY gained, compared to a screen-and-treat strategy (ICER $36,088/QALY) [12].

4. Discussion

Our review found evidence of effective HB vaccination programs for children and adolescents in endemic communities with limited access to care. In addition, we found evidence for effective treatments for cases of CHB that decrease long-term complications in a subset of patients with CHB. A high percentage of migrants to the EU/EEA accept screening for CHB when offered, and this screening successfully identifies cases. Our review found cost-effectiveness studies examining the effect of screening migrants and other populations for HBV infection versus no screening on clinical outcomes.

Our study did not identify any studies examining the impact of vaccination programs on migrant populations. However, we found evidence that vaccination programs are highly effective at reducing disease prevalence and some complications in the general population [35]. In addition, evidence from New Zealand demonstrated that individuals with access barriers to care gain the most from vaccination programs [24]. Vaccination programs targeting migrant children and adolescents and efforts to link migrants to existing national vaccination programs would likely confer similar reductions in disease burden.

More community based and integrated multi-disease screening studies and related cost-effectiveness studies on migrant populations are required to determine the optimal approach to improve uptake and linkage to care. Studies in the EU/EEA on migrant groups with a high prevalence of CHB infection are needed to build trust and knowledge to support the testing approach. Research is needed to ensure vaccination programs reach all migrant children and youth.

The economic literature suggests that screening programs for HBV to identify susceptible individuals or cases and provide treatment are highly likely to be cost-effective in populations with a prevalence of HBV ≥2%, and may be cost-effective at a prevalence as low as 0.3% [27,28]. This finding aligns with studies that support screening for Hepatitis C virus. The evidence for cost-effectiveness of ring vaccination for close contacts is limited, with one study suggesting cost-effectiveness [12].

4.1. Implementation Considerations

Qualitative evidence suggests that implementing screening programs and ensuring linkage to treatment and care for migrants presents a number of challenges including: limited access to health care, inability to navigate a complex health care system and cultural and linguistic barriers [40,41]. Migrant populations have identified stigma, lack of access to primary care or testing, and false and confusing information regarding testing and treatment eligibility as significant barriers to accessing screening, vaccination, and treatment [42,43]. For example, a study of predominantly Turkish migrants in the Netherlands found that those who did not speak Dutch were less likely to attend follow up appointments [41]. Nevertheless, the majority of migrants appear to accept screening when offered and studies have suggested they would prefer an integrated screening program to test for multiple diseases simultaneously [43–45].

Migrants and other populations from high CHB prevalence countries would potentially benefit from CHB screening in opportunistic facility and community based settings [46]. Facility-based testing occurs when screening is offered to individuals accessing health care for reasons unrelated to HBV. Two examples of offering opportunistic HBV screening for migrants presenting for unrelated reasons to primary health care clinics in Italy found that greater than 90% of migrants accepted screening for HB when offered [47,48]. Community-based screening, in which screening occurs outside health care facilities and community members participate in the programs design and implementation, offers an opportunity to screen patients who may not otherwise present for health care, but this approach is more resource intensive than facility-based testing [46]. A study of Chinese migrants in the Netherlands offered screening in schools, community centers and churches or at the local public health clinic. The study screened 1090 of the estimated 8000 Chinese individuals living in Rotterdam over a 3-month period with the majority preferring to be screened in a community setting [49]. However, in a community based mosque screening program in UK without Pakistani community engagement, no patients presented for screening [50]. Approaches resulting in low uptake raise concerns about missing marginalized populations, such as migrants. Strategies to promote successful linkage of cases to care for migrants with CHB should be a priority for all programs [41,51]. Successful implementation of HBV screening depends on factors relevant to the local health systems and population. Deciding on the best way to implement screening programs may fall to local public health officials and health systems planners.

4.2. Strengths and Weaknesses

Our review has several strengths: the use of a systematic review with a GRADE approach allows for evaluation of the certainty and strength of the best available evidence. In addition, the vaccination studies included both CHB prevalent and marginalized populations, such as an indigenous population in New Zealand.

Our review also has several limitations: we found no systematic reviews or RCTs that directly examined the efficacy of screening migrants for HBV. Instead, we followed an evidence chain approach to estimate the effectiveness of testing and the effectiveness of treatment. The evidence for linkage to HBV care and treatment and existing screening programs for migrants in the EU/EEA was also very limited. There are evidence gaps within the screening and vaccination programs. While testing and treatment for CHB were promising, there is an undeniable evidence gap between linkage to care and treatment for migrants. The vaccination programs that we identified targeted various high-risk and sometimes marginalized children. Studies on high-risk migrant populations were limited.

The number of cost-effectiveness studies identified was limited and mostly related to migrants in North America. Economic evidence is most relevant to the health system in which the study was undertaken, and therefore, certain economic evidence may not be transferable to EU/EEA. It was not possible to accurately convert from US or Canadian dollars to Euros, as the reference year for costs was not adequately reported in all primary studies. In addition, costs may change over time. Not all economic studies assessed the levels of seroprevalence across plausible ranges in their sensitivity analyses, limiting the generalizability of the cost-effectiveness results. Furthermore, most studies used static decision tree models, which assume a constant probability of acquiring an HBV infection, limiting the model's ability to accurately predict cost-effectiveness. Test sensitivity and specificity was not clearly described in some studies. Definitive economic analysis was limited as most included studies only considered screening for HBV in isolation rather than an integrated multi-disease screening program for HBV, HCV, and HIV.

5. Conclusions

Migrants arriving or living in the EU/EEA who originate from HBV endemic countries, have an increased burden of CHB compared to the general population. Screening high-risk migrants for HBV and offering monitoring and treatment to those found to be chronically infected will offer clinical benefits. HBV vaccination programs targeting marginalized and high-risk children and adolescents significantly reduces the prevalence of CHB. A strategy of screening and treating CHB compared to no screening is likely to be cost-effective. Cost-effectiveness of screening increases with increasing HB seroprevalence and uptake, but programs may be cost-effective even in lower seroprevalence groups (<2%). Qualitative evidence suggests that developing screening approaches for migrants will be challenging as migrants often lack access to primary health care and may face additional barriers to care. A mixture of vaccination and testing programs, in a variety of settings, with an emphasis on the linkage of positive cases to care will most likely have the greatest impact.

Author Contributions: Conception and design: D.M., R.M., K.P., M.P., T.N., I.V., B.-A.B. Data acquisition: D.M., E.A., L.S., A,T., K.P., R.M. Data analysis: D.M., R.M., E.A., P.R., A.T., L.S., K.P. Interpretation of results: D.M., R.M., B.-A.B., I.V., F.C., A.T., P.R., L.S., M.P., T.N., K.P. Manuscript drafting: D.M., R.M., B.-A.B., I.V., F.C., M.P., T.N., K.P. Critical revision of the manuscript and approval of the final version: All authors critically revised and approved the final version of the manuscript.

Funding: European Centre for Disease Prevention and Control—EHG Project No. 2169 "Evidence-based guidance on screening for infectious diseases among migrants to the EU/EEA".

Acknowledgments: We would like to acknowledge the expert librarian support of Doug Salzwedel and technical support of Oliva Magwood.

Conflicts of Interest: Dr. Pareek is supported by the National Institute for Health Research (NIHR Post-Doctoral Fellowship, PDF-2015-08-102). The views expressed in this publication are those of the author(s) and not necessarily those of the NHS, the National Institute for Health Research or the Department of Health. Dr Pareek reports an institutional grant (unrestricted) for project related to blood-borne virus testing from Gilead Sciences outside the submitted work. RL Morton is supported by an Australian National Health and Medical Research Council, Sidney Sax Public Health Fellowship #1054216. All other authors report no conflicts of interest. Dr Pottie led the consultant team that received funding from the European Centre for Disease Control to conduct systematic reviews for the Guidelines for Newly Arriving Migrants to EU/EEA. Francesco Castelli is a UNESCO Chair and the choice and presentation of views contained in this article and for opinions expressed therein, are not necessarily those of UNESCO and do not commit the Organization.

Appendix A. Search Terms

Database: Ovid MEDLINE(R) Epub Ahead of Print <May Week 3 2016>, Ovid MEDLINE(R) 1946 to Present with Daily Update.
Search Date: 26 May 2016

1 exp Hepatitis B/ (49954)
2 (CHB or HBV or HepB).mp. (32246)
3 ((hep or hepatitis) adj3 B).mp. (82681)
4 hbsag.tw. (16191)
5 (hbs adj2 ag).tw. (720)
6 hb-s-ag.tw. (24)
7 ((serum or type b) adj2 hepatitis).tw. (3299)
8 or/1–7 (86774)
9 exp Mass Screening/ (108496)
10 (screened or screening? or tested or testing or tests).tw. (1733475)
11 Early Diagnosis/ (19328)
12 ((case? or early) adj2 (detected or detection? or diagnos$ or discover$)).tw. (153478)
13 exp Population Surveillance/ (56663)
14 (disease? adj2 surveillance).tw. (4191)
15 Contact Tracing/ (3561)
16 contact tracing.tw. (1176)
17 or/9–16 (1940435)
18 meta analysis.mp,pt. (96656)
19 review.pt. (2060002)
20 search$.tw. (266555)
21 guideline.pt. (15761)
22 guideline/ (15761)
23 guidelines as topic/ (34049)
24 practice guideline.pt. (21200)
25 practice guideline/ (21200)
26 practice guidelines as topic/ (91709)
27 (CPG or CPGs or guidance or guideline? or recommend$ or standard?).ti. (147079)
28 exp clinical pathway/ (5268)
29 exp clinical protocol/ (139279)
30 ((care or clinical) adj2 pathway?).tw. (5122)
31 or/18-30 (2570832)
32 8 and 17 and 31 (2192)
33 animals/ not (humans/ and animals/) (4214239)
34 32 not 33 (2176)
35 34 and (2010$ or 2011$ or 2012$ or 2013$ or 2014$ or 2015$ or 2016$).ed. (675)
36 remove duplicates from 35 (reviews and guidelines) (652)
37 exp "costs and cost analysis"/ (197842)
38 cost$.mp. (467557)
39 cost effective$.tw. (83015)
40 cost benefit analys$.mp. (67281)
41 health care costs.mp. (37134)
42 or/37–41 (476890)
43 8 and 17 and 42 (888)
44 animals/not (humans/and animals/)(4214239)
45 43 not 44 (883)
46 45 and (2010$ or 2011$ or 2012$ or 2013$ or 2014$ or 2015$ or 2016$).ed. (266)
47 remove duplicates from 46 (costing) (254)

Database: Embase <1974 to 2016 May 26>
Search Date: 26 May 2016

1 exp hepatitis B/(79653)
2 (CHB or HBV or HepB).mp. (53611)
3 ((hep or hepatitis) adj3 B).mp. (132717)
4 hbsag.tw. (24116)
5 (hbs adj2 ag). tw. (1126)
6 hb-s-ag.tw (626)
7 ((serum or type b) adj2 hepatitis).tw. (4201)
8 or/1–7 (140818)
9 exp mass screening/(182894)
10 (screened or screening? or tested or testing or tests).tw. (2429779)
11 anonymous testing/(223)
12 early diagnosis/(83109)
13 ((case? or early) adj2 (detected or detection? or diagnos$ or discover$)).tw. (235744)
14 exp health survey/(184232)
15 (disease? adj2 surveillance).tw. (5252)
16 contact examination/(2867)
17 contact tracing.tw. (1512)
18 or/9-17 (2853474)
19 meta analysis.mp,pt. (163362)
20 review.pt. (2163167)
21 search$.tw. (371891)
22 guideline.pt. (0)
23 guideline/(144)
24 guidelines as topic/(229891)
25 practice guideline.pt. (0)
26 practice guideline/(275498)
27 practice guidelines as topic/(171087)
28 (CPG or CPGs or guidance or guideline? or recommend$ or standard?).ti. (203281)
29 exp clinical pathway/(6983)
30 exp clinical protocol/(75932)
31 ((care or clinical) adj2 pathway?).tw. (9455)
32 or/19-31 (2897811)
33 8 and 18 and 32 (3886)
34 (exp animal/ or animal.hw. or nonhuman/) not (exp human/ or human cell/ or (human or humans).ti.) (5865316)
35 33 not 34 (3822)
36 (immigra$ or migrant$ or migration$ or refugee$).mp. (337937)
37 35 and 36 and (2010$ or 2011$ or 2012$ or 2013$ or 2014$ or 2015$ or 2016$).dd. (68)
38 remove duplicates from 37 (reviews and guidelines) (67)
39 cost effectiveness analysis/(114261)
40 cost.tw. (387424)
41 costs.tw. (208729)
42 or/39-41 (544762)
43 8 and 18 and 42 (1580)
44 (exp animal/ or animal.hw. or nonhuman/) not (exp human/ or human cell/ or (human or humans).ti.) (5865316)
45 43 not 44 (1556)
46 (immigra$ or migrant$ or migration$ or refugee$).mp. (337937)
47 45 and 46 and (2010$ or 2011$ or 2012$ or 2013$ or 2014$ or 2015$ or 2016$).dd. (59)

References

1. World Health Organization (WHO). *Guidelines for the Screening, Care and Treatment of Persons with Chronic Hepatitis C Infection*; WHO: Geneva, Switzerland, 2015.

2. World Health Organization. *WHO Guidelines on Hepatitis B and C Testing*; World Health Organization: Geneva, Switzerland, 2017.
3. European Centre for Disease Prevention and Control (ECDC). *Epidemiological Assessment of Hepatitis B and C among Migrants in the EU/EEA*; ECDC: Stockholm, Sweden, 2016.
4. Hatzakis, A.; Wait, S.; Bruix, J.; Buti, M.; Carballo, M.; Cavaleri, M.; Colombo, M.; Delarocque-Astagneau, E.; Dusheiko, G.; Esmat, G.; et al. The State of Hepatitis B and C in Europe: Report from the Hepatitis B and C Summit Conference. *J. Viral Hepat.* **2011**, *18* (Suppl. 1), 1–16. [CrossRef] [PubMed]
5. European Centre for Disease Prevention and Control. *Hepatitis B and C in the EU Neighbourhood: Prevalence, Burden of Disease and Screening Policies*; ECDC: Stockhlom, Sweden, 2010.
6. Blachier, M.; Leleu, H.; Peck-Radosavljevic, M.; Valla, D.C.; Roudot-Thoraval, F. The Burden of Liver Disease in Europe: A Review of Available Epidemiological Data. *J. Hepatol.* **2013**, *58*, 593–608. [CrossRef] [PubMed]
7. European Centre for Disease Prevention and Control. *Antenatal Screening for HIV, Hepatitis B, Syphilis and Rubella Susceptibility in the EU/EEA*; ECDC: Stockholm, Sweden, 2016.
8. Rossi, C.; Shrier, I.; Marshall, L.; Cnossen, S.; Schwartzman, K.; Klein, M.B.; Schwarzer, G.; Greenaway, C. Seroprevalence of Chronic Hepatitis B Virus Infection and Prior Immunity in Immigrants and Refugees: A Systematic Review and Meta-Analysis. *PLoS ONE* **2012**, *7*, e44611. [CrossRef] [PubMed]
9. Duffell, E.F.; Hedrich, D.; Mardh, O.; Mozalevskis, A. Towards Elimination of Hepatitis B and C in European Union and European Economic Area Countries: Monitoring the World Health Organization's Global Health Sector Strategy Core Indicators and Scaling up Key Interventions. *Eurosurveillance* **2017**, *22*, 30476. [CrossRef] [PubMed]
10. LeFevre, M.L. Screening for Hepatitis B Virus Infection in Nonpregnant Adolescents and Adults: U.S. Preventive Services Task Force Recommendation Statement. *Ann. Intern. Med.* **2014**, *161*, 58–66. [CrossRef] [PubMed]
11. European Centre for Disease Prevention and Control. Vaccine Schedule. Available online: https://vaccine-schedule.ecdc.europa.eu/ (accessed on 17 August 2018).
12. Hutton, D.W.; Tan, D.; So, S.K.; Brandeau, M.L. Cost-Effectiveness of Screening and Vaccinating Asian and Pacific Islander Adults for Hepatitis B. *Ann. Intern. Med.* **2007**, *147*, 460–469. [CrossRef] [PubMed]
13. Edmunds, W.J.; Medley, G.F.; Nokes, D.J.; Hall, A.J.; Whittle, H.C. The Influence of Age on the Development of the Hepatitis B Carrier State. *Proc. R. Soc. B Biol. Sci.* **1993**, *253*, 197–201. [CrossRef] [PubMed]
14. World Health Organisation. *Global Health Sector Strategy on Viral Hepatitis 2016–2021. Towards Ending Viral Hepatitis*; WHO: Geneva, Switzerland, 2016.
15. European Centre for Disease Prevention and Control. *Hepatitis B and C Testing Activities, Needs, and Priorities in the EU/EEA*; ECDC: Stockholm, Sweden, 2017.
16. Pottie, K.; Mayhew, A.; Morton, R.; Greenaway, C.; Akl, E.; Rahman, P. Prevention and Assessment of Infectious Diseases among Children and Adult Migrants Arriving to the European Union/European Economic Association: A Protocol for a Suite of Systematic Reviews for Public Health and Health Systems. *BMJ Open* **2017**, *7*, e014608. [CrossRef] [PubMed]
17. Moher, D.; Liberati, A.; Tetzlaf, J.; Altman, D.G.; Group, T.P. Preferred Reporting Items for Systematic Reviews and Meta-Analyses: The PRISMA Statement. *PLoS Med.* **2009**, *6*, e1000097. [CrossRef] [PubMed]
18. Shea, B.J.; Grimshaw, J.M.; Well, G.A.; Boers, M.; Andersson, N.; Hamel, C.; Porter, A.C.; Tugwell, P.; Moher, D.; Bouter, L.M. Development of AMSTAR: A Measurement Tool to Assess the Methodological Quality of Systematic Reviews. *BMC Med. Res. Methodol.* **2007**, *7*, 10. [CrossRef] [PubMed]
19. Schünemann, H.J.; Wiercioch, W.; Brozek, J.; Etxeandia-Ikobaltzeta, I.; Mustafa, R.A.; Manja, V.; Brignardello-Petersen, R.; Neumann, I.; Falavigna, M.; Alhazzani, W.; et al. GRADE Evidence to Decision (EtD) Frameworks for Adoption, Adaptation, and de Novo Development of Trustworthy Recommendations: GRADE-ADOLOPMENT. *J. Clin. Epidemiol.* **2017**, *81*, 101–110. [CrossRef] [PubMed]
20. Larsson, L.; Hendricksen, C. *Health Economics Information Resources: A Self-Study Course: Module 4*; U.S. National Library of Medicine: Bethesda, MD, USA, 2014.
21. Chou, R.; Dana, T.; Bougatsos, C.; Blazina, I.; Khangura, J.; Zakher, B. Screening for Hepatitis B Virus Infection in Adolescents and Adults: A Systematic Review to Update the U.S. Preventive Services Task Force Recommendation. *Ann. Intern. Med.* **2014**, *161*, 31–45. [CrossRef] [PubMed]

22. Wong, G.L.H.; Yiu, K.K.L.; Wong, V.W.S.; Tsoi, K.K.F.; Chan, H.L.Y. Meta-Analysis: Reduction in Hepatic Events Following Interferon-Alfa Therapy of Chronic Hepatitis B. *Aliment. Pharmacol. Ther.* **2010**, *32*, 1059–1068. [CrossRef] [PubMed]
23. EASL. EASL 2017 Clinical Practice Guidelines on the Management of Hepatitis B Virus Infection. *J. Hepatol.* **2017**, *67*, 370–398. [CrossRef] [PubMed]
24. Graham, S.; Guy, R.J.; Cowie, B.; Wand, H.C.; Donovan, B.; Akre, S.P.; Ward, J.S. Chronic Hepatitis B Prevalence among Aboriginal and Torres Strait Islander Australians since Universal Vaccination: A Systematic Review and Meta-Analysis. *BMC Infect. Dis.* **2013**, *13*, 403. [CrossRef] [PubMed]
25. Chang, M.H.; You, S.L.; Chen, C.J.; Liu, C.J.; Lee, C.M.; Lin, S.M.; Chu, H.C.; Wu, T.C.; Yang, S.S.; Kuo, H.S.; et al. Decreased Incidence of Hepatocellular Carcinoma in Hepatitis B Vaccinees: A 20-Year Follow-up Study. *J. Natl. Cancer Inst.* **2009**, *101*, 1348–1355. [CrossRef] [PubMed]
26. Rossi, C.; Schwartzman, K.; Oxlade, O.; Klein, M.B.; Greenaway, C. Hepatitis B Screening and Vaccination Strategies for Newly Arrived Adult Canadian Immigrants and Refugees: A Cost-Effectiveness Analysis. *PLoS ONE* **2013**, *8*, e78548. [CrossRef] [PubMed]
27. Wong, W.W.L.; Woo, G.; Heathcote, E.J.; Krahn, M. Cost Effectiveness of Screening Immigrants for Hepatitis B. *Liver Int.* **2011**, *31*, 1179–1190. [CrossRef] [PubMed]
28. Veldhuijzen, I.K.; Toy, M.; Hahné, S.J.M.; De Wit, G.A.; Schalm, S.W.; de Man, R.A.; Richardus, J.H. Screening and Early Treatment of Migrants for Chronic Hepatitis B Virus Infection Is Cost-Effective. *Gastroenterology* **2010**, *138*, 522–530. [CrossRef] [PubMed]
29. Rein, D.B.; Lesesne, S.B.; Smith, B.D.; Weinbaum, C.M. Models of Community-Based Hepatitis B Surface Antigen Screening Programs in the U.S. and Their Estimated Outcomes and Costs. *Public Health Rep.* **2011**, *126*, 560–567. [CrossRef] [PubMed]
30. Jazwa, A.; Coleman, M.S.; Gazmararian, J.; Wingate, L.T.; Maskery, B.; Mitchell, T.; Weinberg, M. Cost-Benefit Comparison of Two Proposed Overseas Programs for Reducing Chronic Hepatitis B Infection among Refugees: Is Screening Essential? *Vaccine* **2015**, *33*, 1393–1399. [CrossRef] [PubMed]
31. Ruggeri, M.; Cicchetti, A.; Gasbarrini, A. The Cost-Effectiveness of Alternative Strategies against HBV in Italy. *Health Policy* **2011**, *102*, 72–80. [CrossRef] [PubMed]
32. Eckman, M.H.; Kaiser, T.E.; Sherman, K.E. The Cost-Effectiveness of Screening for Chronic Hepatitis B Infection in the United States. *Clin. Infect. Dis.* **2011**, *52*, 1294–1306. [CrossRef] [PubMed]
33. Li, S.; Xie, Q.; Liu, Y.; Toy, M.; Onder, F.O. Cost-Effectiveness of Early Detection of Inactive and Treatment of Active Cases in a High Endemic Chronic Hepatitis B Region. *J. Antivir. Antiretrovir.* **2013**, *5*, 154–159. [CrossRef]
34. Seedat, F.; Hargreaves, S.; Nellums, L.B.; Ouyang, J.; Brown, M.; Friedland, J.S. How Effective Are Approaches to Migrant Screening for Infectious Diseases in Europe? A Systematic Review. *Lancet Infect. Dis.* **2018**, *18*, e259–e271. [CrossRef]
35. Chang, M.-H.; Chen, C.-J.; Lai, M.-S.; Hsu, H.-M.; Wu, T.-C.; Kong, M.-S.; Liang, D.-C.; Shau, W.-Y.; Chen, D.-S. Universal Hepatitis B Vaccination in Taiwan and the Incidence of Hepatocellular Carcinoma in Children. *N. Engl. J. Med.* **1997**, *336*, 1855–1859. [CrossRef] [PubMed]
36. Ni, Y.H.; Chang, M.H.; Huang, L.M.; Chen, H.L.; Hsu, H.Y.; Chiu, T.Y.; Tsai, K.S.; Chen, D.S. Hepatitis B Virus Infection in Children and Adolescents in a Hyperendemic Area: 15 Years after Mass Hepatitis B Vaccination. *Ann. Intern. Med.* **2001**, *135*, 796–800. [CrossRef] [PubMed]
37. Brown, R.S.; Mcmahon, B.J.; Lok, A.S.F.; Wong, J.B.; Ahmed, A.T.; Mouchli, M.A.; Wang, Z.; Prokop, L.J.; Murad, M.H.; Mohammed, K. Antiviral Therapy in Chronic Hepatitis B Viral Infection during Pregnancy: A Systematic Review and Meta-Analysis. *Hepatology* **2016**, *63*, 319–333. [CrossRef] [PubMed]
38. McMahon, B.J.; Helminiak, C.; Wainwright, R.B.; Bulkow, L.; Trimble, B.A.; Wainwright, K. Frequency of Adverse Reactions to Hepatitis B Vaccine in 43,618 Persons. *Am. J. Med.* **1992**, *92*, 254–256. [CrossRef]
39. Hahné, S.J.; Veldhuijzen, I.K.; Wiessing, L.; Lim, T.-A.; Salminen, M.; van de Laar, M. Infection with Hepatitis B and C Virus in Europe: A Systematic Review of Prevalence and Cost-Effectiveness of Screening. *BMC Infect. Dis.* **2013**, *13*, 181.
40. Hacker, K.; Anies, M.; Folb, B.L.; Zallman, L. Barriers to Health Care for Undocumented Immigrants: A Literature Review. *Risk Manag. Healthc. Policy* **2015**, *8*, 175–183. [CrossRef] [PubMed]
41. Mostert, M.C.; Richardus, J.H.; De Man, R.A. Referral of Chronic Hepatitis B Patients from Primary to Specialist Care: Making a Simple Guideline Work. *J. Hepatol.* **2004**, *41*, 1026–1030. [CrossRef] [PubMed]

42. Jones, L.; Bates, G.; McCoy, E.; Beynon, C.; McVeigh, J.; Bellis, M. *A Systematic Review of the Effectiveness and Cost-Effectiveness of Interventions Aimed at Raising Awareness and Engaging with Groups Who Are at an Increased Risk of Hepatitis B and C Infection—Final Report*; Liverpool John Moores University: Liverpool, UK, 2012.
43. Seedat, F.; Hargreaves, S.; Friedland, J.S. Engaging New Migrants in Infectious Disease Screening: A Qualitative Semi-Structured Interview Study of UK Migrant Community Health-Care Leads. *PLoS ONE* **2014**, *9*, e108261. [CrossRef] [PubMed]
44. Hargreaves, S.; Seedat, F.; Car, J.; Escombe, R.; Hasan, S.; Eliahoo, J.; Friedland, J.S. Screening for Latent TB, HIV, and Hepatitis B/C in New Migrants in a High Prevalence Area of London, UK: A Cross-Sectional Study. *BMC Infect. Dis.* **2014**, *14*, 657. [CrossRef] [PubMed]
45. O'Connell, S.; Lillis, D.; Cotter, A.; O'Dea, S.; Tuite, H.; Fleming, C.; Crowley, B.; Fitzgerald, I.; Dalby, L.; Barry, H.; et al. Opt-out Panel Testing for HIV, Hepatitis B and Hepatitis C in an Urban Emergency Department: A Pilot Study. *PLoS ONE* **2016**, *11*, e0150546. [CrossRef] [PubMed]
46. Robotin, M.C.; George, J. Community-Based Hepatitis B Screening: What Works? *Hepatol. Int.* **2014**, *8*, 478–492. [CrossRef] [PubMed]
47. Coppola, N.; Alessio, L.; Gualdieri, L.; Pisaturo, M.; Sagnelli, C.; Caprio, N.; Maffei, R.; Starace, M.; Angelillo, I.F.; Pasquale, G.; et al. Hepatitis B Virus, Hepatitis C Virus and Human Immunodeficiency Virus Infection in Undocumented Migrants and Refugees in Southern Italy, January 2012 to June 2013. *Eurosurveillance* **2015**, *20*, 30009. [CrossRef] [PubMed]
48. El-Hamad, I.; Pezzoli, M.C.; Chiari, E.; Scarcella, C.; Vassallo, F.; Puoti, M.; Ciccaglione, A.; Ciccozzi, M.; Scalzini, A.; Castelli, F. Point-of-Care Screening, Prevalence, and Risk Factors for Hepatitis B Infection among 3728 Mainly Undocumented Migrants from Non-EU Countries in Northern Italy. *J. Travel Med.* **2015**, *22*, 78–86. [CrossRef] [PubMed]
49. Veldhuijzen, I.K.; Wolter, R.; Rijckborst, V.; Mostert, M.; Voeten, H.A.; Cheung, Y.; Boucher, C.A.; Reijnders, J.G.P.; De Zwart, O.; Janssen, H.L.A. Identification and Treatment of Chronic Hepatitis B in Chinese Migrants: Results of a Project Offering on-Site Testing in Rotterdam, the Netherlands. *J. Hepatol.* **2012**, *57*, 1171–1176. [CrossRef] [PubMed]
50. Lewis, H.; Burke, K.; Begum, S.; Ushiro-Limb, I.; Foster, G. What is the best method of case finding for chronic viral hepatitis in at-risk migrant communities? *J. Hepatol.* **2012**, *56*, S351. [CrossRef]
51. Gish, R.G.; Cooper, S. Hepatitis B in the Greater San Francisco Bay Area: An Integrated Programme to Respond to a Diverse Local Epidemic. *J. Viral Hepat.* **2011**, *18*, e40–e51. [CrossRef] [PubMed]

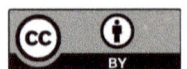

© 2018 by the authors. Licensee MDPI, Basel, Switzerland. This article is an open access article distributed under the terms and conditions of the Creative Commons Attribution (CC BY) license (http://creativecommons.org/licenses/by/4.0/).

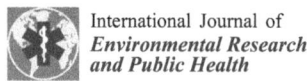

Article

Pregnancy Related Health Care Needs in Refugees—A Current Three Center Experience in Europe

Christian Dopfer [1,2,†], Annabelle Vakilzadeh [3,†], Christine Happle [1,2], Evelyn Kleinert [4], Frank Müller [4], Diana Ernst [5,6], Reinhold E. Schmidt [5,6], Georg M. N. Behrens [5,6], Sonja Merkesdal [5], Martin Wetzke [1,6,†] and Alexandra Jablonka [5,6,*,†]

1. Department of Pediatric Pneumology, Allergology, and Neonatology, Hannover Medical School, 30625 Hannover, Germany; dopfer.christian@mh-hannover.de (C.D.); happle.christine@mh-hannover.de (C.H.); wetzke.martin@mh-hannover.de (M.W.)
2. German Center for Lung Research, Biomedical Research in End Stage and Obstructive Lung Disease/BREATH Hannover, 30625 Hannover, Germany
3. Hannover Medical School, 30625 Hannover, Germany; annabelle.schaell@stud.mh-hannover.de
4. Department of General Practice, University Medical Center Göttingen, 37073 Göttingen, Germany; evelyn.kleinert@med.uni-goettingen.de (E.K.); frank.mueller@med.uni-goettingen.de (F.M.)
5. Department of Clinical Immunology and Rheumatology, Hannover Medical School, 30625 Hannover, Germany; ernst.diana@mh-hannover.de (D.E.); schmidt.reinhold.ernst@mh-hannover.de (R.E.S.); behrens.georg@mh-hannover.de (G.M.N.B.); merkesdal.sonja@mh-hannover.de (S.M.)
6. German Center for Infection Research (DZIF), Partner Site Hannover-Braunschweig, 38124 Braunschweig, Germany
* Correspondence: jablonka.alexandra@mh-hannover.de; Tel.: +49-511-532-5337; Fax: +49-511-532-5324
† These authors contributed equally to this work.

Received: 30 June 2018; Accepted: 28 August 2018; Published: 5 September 2018

Abstract: *Background:* Immigration into Europe has reached an all-time high. Provision of coordinated healthcare, especially to refugee women that are at increased risk for adverse pregnancy outcomes, is a challenge for receiving health care systems. *Methods:* We assessed pregnancy rates and associated primary healthcare needs in three refugee cohorts in Northern Germany during the current crisis. *Results:* Out of $n = 2911$ refugees, 18.0% were women of reproductive age, and 9.1% of these were pregnant. Pregnancy was associated with a significant, 3.7-fold increase in primary health care utilization. Language barrier and cultural customs impeded healthcare to some refugee pregnant women. The most common complaints were demand for pregnancy checkup without specific symptoms (48.6%), followed by abdominal pain or urinary tract infections (in 11.4% of cases each). In 4.2% of pregnancies, severe complications such as syphilis or suicide attempts occurred. *Discussion:* We present data on pregnancy rates and pregnancy associated medical need in three current refugee cohorts upon arrival in Germany. Healthcare providers should be particularly aware of the requirements of pregnant migrants and should adapt primary caretaking strategies accordingly.

Keywords: pregnancy; migration; refugees; health care provision; reception center

1. Introduction

Currently, migration towards Europe is at an all-time high, and receiving countries are struggling with the task of coordinated and appropriate care provision [1]. In this situation, medical care should be adapted to the specific requirements of migrants as they represent a population with increased risk for overall morbidity and mortality [2]. This particularly holds true for pregnant women among them [3].

Pregnant refugee women show higher rates of adverse pregnancy outcomes, including caesarean section, stillbirth, and other maternal and perinatal morbidities [4–10].

The majority of women on the move have no access to appropriate antenatal care [11]. No or late access to antenatal care is associated with poor pregnancy outcomes [12]. Optimized maternal healthcare significantly improves pregnancy outcomes; hence, a targeted outreach to pregnant refugees may be needed to improve healthcare utilization in this patient group [3,13]. For example, refugees may carry an increased risk for intrauterinely transmitted diseases such as hepatitis, syphilis, and HIV [14,15]. Furthermore, they are at risk for insufficient vaccination against diseases such as rubella and varicella which can lead to profound and fatal outcome in their offspring [16,17].

Data on pregnancy associated health in the migrating population currently entering Europe is scarce. Analyzing pregnancy related health care utilization in current and representative refugee cohorts may facilitate identifying the particular needs of this vulnerable population and adapt care taking strategies accordingly. Therefore, we here analyzed pregnancy rates and healthcare utilization behavior in three representative cohorts of newly arriving refugees in Germany during the current crisis.

2. Methods

2.1. Study Population

Data from three independent cohorts was included in the study. In total $n = 1533$ refugees residing at a reception center in Celle, Northern Germany in Summer of 2015 (from now on referred to as "cohort one"), $n = 1220$ refugees residing in 6 locations in Wolfsburg, Northern Germany in autumn 2015 (from now on referred to as "cohort two") and $n = 158$ refugees living in a reception center in Harsefeld, Northern Germany in winter and spring 2016 (from now on referred to as "cohort three") were included into the analysis. All three cohorts contained refugees that were allocated to a designated reception center in Lower Saxony based on a federal state-specific allocation key (Königssteiner Schlüssel). Cohorts or asylum seekers within each cohort were not preselected in any way, and data sets were chosen based on data availability and harmonization of data collection. For localization and age and gender distribution within the three reception centers, please refer to Supplementary Figure S1. Please note that part of the cohort in Celle were previously described [16,18,19]. Migrants were registered upon arrival, and their departure date was documented. For refugees leaving the center without notice to camp authorities, last contact documentation of the camp staff (medical service, food service, transportation, etc.) was used as date of departure.

2.2. Collection of Medical Data

A full-time medical ward offering primary medical care to all residents was erected at the center in Celle, including a medical team offering full medical services at primary care level and visiting services by a midwife. In Wolfsburg, paramedic care was offered at one of the sites and a visiting physician was available an average 2 times a week. For differences in health care utilization, only $n = 309$ refugees with on-site healthcare were included in the analysis. In the center of Harsefeld, only paramedic care was offered on site, and all other healthcare needs were referred to local physicians. For differences in health care utilization pregnant women were compared to the age matched mean of controls (refugees residing at the camp for 1 day or less were excluded from the analysis). All refugee women were asked whether they were pregnant at arrival. All refugees underwent an off-site mandatory checkup within their first weeks of residence. Prenatal care was offered to all pregnant refugees based on the standardized prenatal care guidelines [20]. All information was collected in routine clinical care. Sociodemographic information and health care data including complaints, diagnoses and prescribed medication was documented in an electronic filing system. For analysis of pregnancy associated health care utilization, the data was fully pseudonymized by the Order of Malta before scientific analysis.

2.3. Serological Analysis

IgG levels against varicella, measles and rubella were analyzed by Chemiluminescence Immunoassays according to the manufacturer's recommendations (LIAISON XL, Fa. DiaSorin, Saluggia, Italy) in a diagnostic laboratory certified for routine testing (DIN ENISO 15189:2014). Threshold for protective immunity levels were: >100 IU/L for varicella (borderline 50–100 IU/L; limit of detection 10.0 IU/L), >13.4 AU/mL for measles (limit of detection 5.0 AU/mL) and >11 IE/mL (borderline 9–11 IE/mL; limit of detection 3.0 IE/mL) for rubella.

2.4. Statistics

For statistical analyses, Graphpad Prism version 5.02 in combination with SPSS version 24.0 (IBM, Armonk, NY, USA) was used. To assess group differences in not normally distributed data, Mann-Whitney-U testing was applied, and p values below 0.05 were considered significant.

2.5. Ethics Compliance

All analyses were approved by local authorities (Institutional Review Board of Hannover Medical School approval # 2972-2015). All patient information was pseudonymized prior to analysis. All procedures followed were in accordance with the ethical standards of the responsible committee on human experimentation and with the Helsinki Declaration of 1964, as revised in 2013.

3. Results

Data on pregnancy associated health care utilization in n = 2911 refugees from three cohorts was included into the analysis. In all three cohorts, the majority of refugees were of male gender (Supplementary Figure S1) with 71.8% of men in the largest cohort one with n = 1533 refugees, 65.2% of men in the large cohort two with n = 1220 migrants, and 63.3% of men in the smallest cohort three with n = 158 refugees. The proportion of women of childbearing age was 18.0% (n = 524; 16.3% in cohort one, 19.3% in cohort two, and 23.4% in cohort three). The frequency of women reporting to be pregnant among all refugees was 1.6% (n = 47), 1.3% in cohort one, 2.0% in cohort two and 1.8% in cohort three (Figure 1A–C). When we analyzed the frequency of pregnant migrants among all women of fertile age in all three cohorts (15–49 years as previously defined [21,22]), we observed a rate of 9.1 ± 0.8%, with most pregnant women in the age group 25–29 years (17.0 ± SD 7.0%, Figure 1D). Mean age of all pregnant refugees was 27.1 ± SD 5.3 years, with the youngest childbearing refugee being 16 years and the oldest one 38 years old (cohort one: mean age 27.2 ± SD 5.7 years, cohort two: mean age 25.8 ± SD 5.4 years, cohort three mean age 27.7 ± SD 3.8 years).

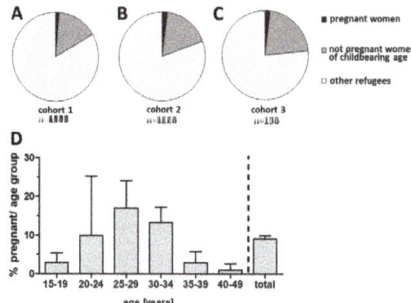

Figure 1. Proportion of women of childbearing age and pregnant refugees in cohort 1 (**A**) and cohort 2 (**B**), and cohort 3 (**C**). (**D**) Frequency of pregnant women among women of respective age groups and overall pregnancy rate among women of childbearing age in all three cohorts (total; bars display mean plus SD from all cohorts).

Most women of reproductive age (53.2%) came from Syria (61.2% in cohort one, 47.7% in cohort two and 35.1% in cohort three, Table 1). Syria was also the top country of origin of pregnant refugees (51.1%). In cohort one 60.0%, and in cohort two 45.4% of pregnant women came from this country, whereas two out of three pregnant women in cohort three came from Afghanistan and only one from Syria. Most females of reproductive age and most pregnant women were Muslims: overall, 86.1% of all females at childbearing age and 89.4% of all pregnant migrants were Muslim, 10.1% of all women at fertile age and 4.3% of pregnant females were of Christian, and 3.8% of all women at childbearing age and 6.3% of pregnant migrants in the three cohorts belonged to other religious groups or reported no belief (Table 1). Most pregnant women arrived with their husbands (85% in cohort one, 83.3% in cohort two and all pregnant women in cohort three). Overall, pregnant refugees reported no previous children in 42.6%, one in 29.8%, two in 17.0%, three in 2.1%, four in 6.4% and eight in 2.1% of cases (cohort one: 45.0% ($n = 9$) no children, 20% ($n = 4$) one, 20% ($n = 4$) two, 10% ($n = 2$) four, 5% ($n = 1$) eight children; cohort two: 33.3% ($n = 8$) no previous children, 41.7% ($n = 10$) one child, 16.7% ($n = 4$) two, 4.2% ($n = 1$) three and another 4.2% ($n = 1$) four children; cohort three: all women reported to have had no previous children, but one pregnant woman reported that she had lost one child about one year before her current pregnancy).

The majority of women of childbearing age, as well as most pregnant women, spoke Arabic, Kurdish or Persian languages (in total 60.5%, 22.2% and 19.6%, respectively, Table 2). Language barriers may have impacted the opportunities to comprehend the pregnant women's complaints, as only 21.3% of pregnant women spoke English (15% in cohort one, 29.3% in cohort two and none in cohort three) and none reported to speak German. Lay-interpreters were available for most consultations, but not all. 35.6% of women at childbearing age in cohort one, 84% in cohort two and 97.3% in cohort three reported a profession. Of these, the occupation most reported by pregnant women as well as their non-pregnant counterparts of fertile age was housewife, followed by reported occupations as students or teachers (Table 2).

In cohort one, $n = 14$ pregnant women reported their pregnancy during initial registration in the camp, one woman was unsure and five did not initially report or were primarily unaware of their pregnancy upon arrival at the reception center. In cohort two, one woman received test results as first confirmation of her pregnancy during camp inhabitance. In cohort three, one woman had already reported her pregnancy upon center entrance, and two early pregnancies were first detected during residence at the respective reception center. In 68.1% of pregnancies, the month of pregnancy upon first contact with the onsite medical personnel was known. Of these cases, 21.9% of women reported to be in their first, 43.8% in their second and 34.4% in their third trimester.

Table 1. Cohort-specific characteristics of women of childbearing age and pregnant refugees, country of origin and religion.

	Total		Cohort 1		Cohort 2		Cohort 3	
	Women of Child-Bearing Age $n = 524$	Pregnant Women $n = 47$	Women of Child-Bearing Age $n = 250$	Pregnant Women $n = 20$	Women of Child-Bearing Age $n = 237$	Pregnant Women $n = 24$	Women of Child-Bearing Age $n = 37$	Pregnant Women $n = 3$
	%	%	%	%	%	%	%	%
country of origin (Top 10)								
Syria	53.2	51.1	61.2	60.0	47.7	45.4	35.1	33.3
Afghanistan	17.7	21.3	7.2	5.0	26.6	27.3	29.7	66.6
Iraq	13.5	14.9	6.4	5.0	20.3	27.3	18.9	0
Iran	3.4	0	1.6	0	3.8	0	13.5	0
Eritrea	2.5	0	4.8	0	0	0	2.6	0
Albania	1.9	2.1	4.0	5.0	0	0	0	0
Serbia	1.1	0	2.8	0	0	0	0	0
Azerbaijan	1.0	4.1	2.0	10.0	0	0	0	0
Bosnia	0.4	2.1	0.8	5.0	0	0	0	0
Montenegro	0.4	2.1	0.8	5.0	0	0	0	0
Nigeria	0.2	2.1	0.4	5.0	0	0	0	0
religion								
Muslim	86.1	89.4	85.6	90.0	88.6	91.7	73.0	66.7
Christian	10.1	4.3	10.8	5.0	8	0.0	18.9	33.3
Others/unknown	3.8	6.3	3.6	5.0	3.4	8.3	8.1	0

Table 2. Cohort-specific characteristics of women of childbearing age and pregnant refugees, language skills and profession.

	Total		Cohort 1		Cohort 2		Cohort 3	
	Women of Child-Bearing Age $n = 524$	Pregnant Women $n = 47$	Women of Child-Bearing Age $n = 250$	Pregnant Women $n = 20$	Women of Child-Bearing Age $n = 237$	Pregnant Women $n = 24$	Women of Child-Bearing Age $n = 37$	Pregnant Women $n = 3$
	%	%	%	%	%	%	%	%
Languages (Top 5)								
Arabic	60.5	59.6	62.4	55.0	61.1	66.7	43.2	33.3
English	16.1	21.3	20.4	15.2	13.2	29.3	5.4	0
Kurdish	22.2	14.9	16.4	10.0	26.7	20.9	32.4	0
Persian languages	19.6	10.0	8.8	5.0	27.4	7.0	43.2	66.6
Albanian	1.9	2.1	4.0	5.0	0	0	0	0
Profession (top 5)								
None/unknown	38.2	36.2	64.4	65.0	16.0	16.7	2.7	0
Housewife	29.9	34.1	9.6	20.0	46.7	41.7	59.5	0
Student	13.8	8.5	8.8	5.0	19	12.5	13.	66.6
Teacher	5.1	4.3	4.0	0	5.8	4.2	8.1	33.3
Tailor	1.9	2.1	2.0	0	1.7	4.2	2.7	0
IT specialist	0.4	2.1	0.8	5.0	0	0	0	0
Hairdresser	1.7	4.3	0.8	5.0	3	4.2	0	0

With regard to healthcare utilization, pregnant refugees of all three cohorts displayed a significantly higher demand for medical care compared to non-pregnant women. As shown in Figure 2, pregnant women displayed a 3.7-fold higher frequency of visits to the onsite medical unit compared to their non-pregnant female counterparts (one-tailed, $t = 1.84$, DF 52, $p = 0.036$). While pregnant women consulted the medical team at the reception center a mean of $0.16 \pm \text{SD } 0.32$ times per day of refugee center residence, age- and gender-matched non-pregnant women spent a mean of only $0.04 \pm \text{SD } 0.05$ visits to the medical unit per day of stay at the camp.

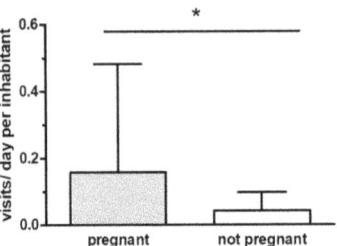

Figure 2. Healthcare utilization of pregnant women of the three cohorts versus the mean of the age- and gender-matched subgroup within the respective refugee cohort (bars display mean plus SD from both cohorts, * $p < 0.05$).

Pregnant refugees spent between 0 and 9 visits to the medical unit during a mean duration of residence of $38.8 \pm \text{SD } 24.9$ (mean of $2.75 \pm \text{SD } 2.6$ during a mean duration of stay of $31.8 \pm \text{SD } 18.8$ in cohort one, mean of $1.25 \pm \text{SD } 1.5$ during a mean duration of stay of $49.1 \pm \text{SD } 39.8$ in cohort two and $4.0 \pm \text{SD } 2.2$ during a mean duration of stay of 78.3 ± 17.1 SD in cohort three). When analyzing all visits to the onsite medical units in both camps, the reason of consultation was reported in 96.8% of visits. The most frequent demand in all consultations of pregnant refugees was to receive a general checkup by a specialized obstetrician or midwife without specific complaints (48.6% of consultations). The most frequent specific symptoms or diagnoses pregnant women presented with were abdominal pain (11.4%) or urinary tract infections (11.4%), followed by symptoms such as skin rash and itching (8.6%). Overall, 54.4% of consultations were because of general pregnancy-related medical demands for checkups or nutritional supplements, 25.7% because of pain-related problems, 20% because of infections, and another 20% because of other, less frequent complaints or diagnoses (Table 3). No woman asked for abortion.

Out of all pregnant migrants in the three cohorts, in two pregnant women (4.2% of all pregnancies), severe complications were diagnosed, necessitating immediate expert care: one pregnant migrant in cohort one had a positive syphilis serology during routine testing and was treated with antibiotics. In cohort three, one depressed refugee attempted to commit suicide during her second month of pregnancy and was admitted to the hospital for five days. After hospitalization, this woman was closely monitored with weekly gynecologist checkups and psychological support until she moved out of the reception center.

In nine pregnant women from cohort one, information on serological screening for immunoglobulins (Ig) against infectious diseases was available. One woman tested positive for anti-hepatitis B core antigen, as well as anti-hepatitis B surface antibodies, but negative for hepatitis B surface antigen. None of the pregnant refugees had positive screening results for hepatitis C, D, or E. All tested pregnant migrants were seropositive for IgG against varicella, and 89% of them were seropositive for measles-IgG. However, with regard to anti-rubella IgG, only 44% of pregnant refugees had protective titers, and an additional 22% had borderline protective levels of IgG against this vaccine preventable disease.

The onsite medical ward in cohort one, which offered daily physician attendance and regular midwife consultations, provided medical care for most of the problems that occurred during consultations. Cohort two had regular access to an attending physician (average 2 times a week) and cohort three had unrestricted access to a close by general practitioner that provided medical care for most of the acute problems. However, thorough obstetric checkups that were requested by 48.6% of pregnant women, as well as the suicidal female refugee had to be referred to specialized physicians as their problems exceeded the level of primary onsite care. Of note, one pregnant Muslim wanted to only be examined by female doctors and preferred not to be treated over being examined by a male physician, who was the only available doctor at the onsite ward on that day.

Table 3. Overview on pregnancy associated medical complaints and requests (proportion of all consultations in all three cohorts).

Complaints	% of Cases	Complaints	% of Cases
pregnancy related. no acute complaints	54.3	infections	20.0
demand for obstetric checkup	48.6	urinary tract infection	11.4
demand for pregnancy supplements	5.7	syphilis	2.9
iron deficiency	iron deficiency	respiratory infection	5.7
pain	25.7	others	20.0
abdominal pain	11.4	skin rash/ pruritus	8.6
toothache	2.9	hyperventilation	2.9
backpain	2.9	dyspnea	2.9
headache	5.7	weakness	2.9
physical trauma	2.9	depression. suicide attempt	2.9

4. Discussion

Immigration into Europe has reached an all-time high, and provision of coordinated healthcare poses an enormous challenge for receiving communities [1,23,24]. Medical care is key in management during humanitarian crises as the current, and especially for refugee woman, that are at increased risk for adverse pregnancy outcomes, caretaking strategies need to be adapted [3,25,26]. Accordingly, we analyzed pregnancy rates and pregnancy-associated primary healthcare utilization in three representative cohorts of newly arriving migrants in Western Europe.

In total, healthcare utilization data of n = 2911 refugees from three cohorts was included into the analysis. Both cohorts contained large proportions of young adult males and the majority of refugees came from the Eastern Mediterranean region, both typical demographic characteristics of current European immigration statistics [17,27–29]. In these representative cohorts, 18% of refugees were females of fertile age, and 9.1% of these women were pregnant. These pregnancy rates are comparable with previous publications. While it is challenging to obtain accurate statistics on the exact frequency of pregnancies among female migrants, the women's refugee commission reports that at any given time 0.6 to 14 percent of all displaced women between 15 and 49 years could be pregnant, and other authors estimate that, depending on country of origin, even higher proportions of up to 25% of female refugees of fertile age could be pregnant [22,26,30].

Refugees are at particular risk for infectious diseases, for physical and psychological trauma, sexual violence and for insufficient access to healthcare and prevention programs, as well as contraception [1,11,17,31]. This particularly holds true for pregnant migrants [3,25,26]. Up to 15% of women who are pregnant while fleeing their homelands experience life-threatening obstetric complications, and Simsek et al. recently reported a frequency as high as 47.7% of pregnancy losses among Syrian refugee women living in Turkey [22,26]. Multiple studies have confirmed increased rates of adverse pregnancy outcomes in migrants, including reduced fetal growth, caesarean section, stillbirth, maternal depression and other maternal and perinatal morbidities [4–10].

Consequently, pregnant refugees should receive particular medical attention, especially when arriving in a country with high economic and healthcare standards such as Germany. Indeed, in our observations of newly arriving refugees, pregnancy was associated with a significant, 3.7-fold increase in primary health care utilization. The most common reasons for medical consultations by pregnant refugees in our cohorts were the demand for pregnancy checkups or prescription of nutritional supplements without acute symptoms, followed by abdominal pain or other pain related issues and less frequent problems such as headache or infections.

One pregnant woman in our cohorts tested positive for hepatitis B core antigen without presence hepatitis B surface antigen. Another pregnant refugee suffered from syphilis and was treated immediately to prevent vertical transmission. Even though, in the first case, test results suggested no immediate threat to the offspring, and treatment was successful in the second case, both observations illustrate the importance infectious disease screening in migrants, especially in pregnant refugees, as the prevalence of severe, vertically transmittable diseases is higher in migrants than in the general population [14,32]. Also, we observed an alarmingly low rate of anti-rubella seropositivity in the small specimen of serologically tested pregnant refugees: only 44% of the expecting mothers had protective anti-rubella IgG-levels. Even though seroprevalences do not necessarily reflect immunity acquired by vaccination, this observation is in line with previous reports by us and others and illustrates a significant gap in rubella immunity in young female refugees [16,17,33–35].

One woman within our cohorts attempted to commit suicide while being pregnant. Although this is just a single observation, it is in line with the results of multiple observational studies reporting on the increased burden of mental diseases and depression in refugee women during pregnancy and the perinatal phase [36–38]. Factors such as social isolation, poverty, lack of host language skills and belonging to an ethnic minority have been described to put pregnant refugees at increased risk of mental disorders [37]. Especially for pregnant women prone to depression, access to psychological help and appropriate support programs should be facilitated, as at least preliminary data shows that the latter measure reduces the rate of mental disorders in Syrian refugee mothers arriving in Canada [26].

Pregnancy outcomes in migrants are influenced by several factors such as country of origin, race and destination country [39]. During their migration, pregnant women only rarely have access to appropriate health care services along the way [22]. Healthcare provision in the receiving country is a main factor in maternal health. For example, Syrian refugees in Jordan experience significantly higher rates of perinatal complications, including iron deficiency, caesarian section, and low birth weight than Jordanian women, but Turkish and Syrian refugee women in Turkey have been reported to show similar pregnancy outcomes [40–42]. In Lebanon, the United Nations High Commissioner for Refugees covers 75% of the cost of life-saving, obstetric, and emergency hospital care for migrants, but the remaining 25% is oftentimes unaffordable for refugees, leading to high morbidity and mortality, particularly in pregnant migrants [43].

Besides structural and organizational barriers, social, personal and cultural factors may significantly impact healthcare utilization in pregnant migrants. Language barriers and cultural customs can significantly impede healthcare to some pregnant refugee women. For example, only the minority of pregnant women in the here-analyzed cohorts spoke English, and none of them spoke the host language, German; thus, without interpreters, medical problems could not be fully communicated between patient and doctor. Furthermore, cultural customs may have impacted healthcare utilization in our observation. In both cohorts, most of the pregnant women were Muslims, and one of them refused to be examined by a male doctor. Cultural background has been previously described to significantly impact peripartum care and well-being in refugee women. In general, medical staff taking care of newly arriving refugees should consider the probability of a limited understanding of Western medicine in refugee women, and avoid them feeling forced to adapt, being labelled as non-compliant if they resist Western approaches [3]. Our experience supports the notion that appropriate language interpretation and the availability of female medical staff could facilitate healthcare utilization for pregnant refugees.

Our study has important limitations. Although the demographics of our cohorts mirror current migration statistics, they can only represent a small specimen of refugees entering Europe during the current crisis. Especially in the smaller cohort and in specific demographic subgroups of the larger cohort, the low number of subjects needs to be taken into account when interpreting our data. Another limitation may lie in the fact that we could only analyze self-reported pregnancies and, due to the fact that our data collection was conducted during routine clinical care, it could not be controlled for language or cultural barriers that may have impacted the refugees answer to the question of pregnancy upon entrance into the reception center or at health care encounters. The same limitation may also have impacted the documentation of complaints. Furthermore, we were unfortunately unable to follow-up on pregnancy outcomes, as all women were moved to their permanent location of residence after registration by the German asylum agency.

5. Conclusions

Optimized maternal healthcare is an effective method to improve pregnancy outcomes as well as lifelong maternal and offspring health, and a targeted outreach to pregnant refugees may be needed to improve utilization of beneficial care [3,13].

The here presented data may facilitate the setup of an appropriate outreach of this kind. It confirms that pregnant migrants are a patient group with increased healthcare utilization and particular medical needs. Primary care providers offering medical help during the current crisis should be aware of the high demand for obstetric checkups in pregnant migrants and ideally be supported by interpreters capable of speaking Arabic and Persian languages. Furthermore, they should consider religious and cultural customs of arriving pregnant migrants, for example female staff could be preferred over male doctors offering obstetric care. Moreover, an increased burden of psychological stress during escape should be considered in pregnant women compared to their non-pregnant counterparts. Also, it should be kept in mind that effective reproductive healthcare starts well before pregnancy, when preventive measures such as screening for infectious diseases, rubella vaccination, or alimentary supplementation need to be commenced.

We hope that our data on the particular healthcare demands of pregnant refugees may help to adapt care-taking strategies in this particularly vulnerable patient group.

Supplementary Materials: The following are available online at http://www.mdpi.com/1660-4601/15/9/1934/s1.

Author Contributions: Research design: A.J., G.M.N.B., R.E.S. Sample collection and analyses: Routine clinical care. Data analysis: C.D., A.V., C.H., D.E., E.K., F.M., S.M., M.W., A.J., Writing and contributing to writing of the manuscript: All authors.

Funding: Christine Happle received funding from the Young Academy Clinician/Scientist foundation and HiLF funding of Hannover Medical School, Germany. Martin Wetzke received funding from the Young Academy Clinician/Scientist foundation Hannover Medical School, Germany and the Clinical Leave Clinician/Scientist program of the German Center for Infection Research (DZIF). Alexandra Jablonka was funded by the Young Academy Clinician Scientist program of Hannover Medical School, Germany. This project was supported by the German Center for Infection Research by funding of infrastructure.

Acknowledgments: The authors would like to thank all doctors and medical personnel involved in medical care of the refugees for their exceptional work. Furthermore, the authors thank the Order of Malta (Malteser Hilfsdienst) of Lower Saxony for their kind help with data provision.

Conflicts of Interest: The authors declare no conflict of interest.

References

1. Puchner, K.; Karamagioli, E.; Pikouli, A.; Tsiamis, C.; Kalogeropoulos, A.; Kakalou, E.; Pavlidou, E.; Pikoulis, E. Time to Rethink Refugee and Migrant Health in Europe: Moving from Emergency Response to Integrated and Individualized Health Care Provision for Migrants and Refugees. *Int. J. Environ. Res. Public Health* **2018**, *15*. [CrossRef] [PubMed]
2. Castelli, F.; Sulis, G. Migration and infectious diseases. *Clin. Microbiol. Infect.* **2017**, *23*, 283–289. [CrossRef] [PubMed]

3. Heslehurst, N.; Brown, H.; Pemu, A.; Coleman, H.; Rankin, J. Perinatal health outcomes and care among asylum seekers and refugees: A systematic review of systematic reviews. *BMC Med.* **2018**, *16*, 89. [CrossRef] [PubMed]
4. Gibson-Helm, M.; Teede, H.; Block, A.; Knight, M.; East, C.; Wallace, E.M.; Boyle, J. Maternal health and pregnancy outcomes among women of refugee background from African countries: A retrospective, observational study in Australia. *BMC Pregnancy Childbirth* **2014**, *14*, 392. [CrossRef] [PubMed]
5. Gissler, M.; Alexander, S.; MacFarlane, A.; Small, R.; Stray-Pedersen, B.; Zeitlin, J.; Zimbeck, M.; Gagnon, A. Stillbirths and infant deaths among migrants in industrialized countries. *Acta Obstet. Gynecol. Scand.* **2009**, *88*, 134–148. [CrossRef] [PubMed]
6. Flynn, M.P. Obstetric profiles and pregnancy outcomes of immigrant women with refugee status. *Ir. Med. J.* **2001**, *94*, 79–80.
7. Essen, B.; Hanson, B.S.; Ostergren, P.O.; Lindquist, P.G.; Gudmundsson, S. Increased perinatal mortality among sub-Saharan immigrants in a city-population in Sweden. *Acta Obstet. Gynecol. Scand.* **2000**, *79*, 737–743. [CrossRef] [PubMed]
8. Small, R.; Gagnon, A.; Gissler, M.; Zeitlin, J.; Bennis, M.; Glazier, R.; Haelterman, E.; Martens, G.; McDermott, S.; Urquia, M.; et al. Somali women and their pregnancy outcomes postmigration: Data from six receiving countries. *BJOG* **2008**, *115*, 1630–1640. [CrossRef] [PubMed]
9. Gagnon, A.J.; Zimbeck, M.; Zeitlin, J.; Collaboration, R.; Alexander, S.; Blondel, B.; Buitendijk, S.; Desmeules, M.; Di Lallo, D.; Gagnon, A.; et al. Migration to western industrialised countries and perinatal health: A systematic review. *Soc. Sci. Med.* **2009**, *69*, 934–946. [CrossRef] [PubMed]
10. Zanconato, G.; Iacovella, C.; Parazzini, F.; Bergamini, V.; Franchi, M. Pregnancy outcome of migrant women delivering in a public institution in northern Italy. *Gynecol. Obstet. Investig.* **2011**, *72*, 157–162. [CrossRef] [PubMed]
11. World Health Organization. WHO Recommendations on Antenatal Care for a Positive Pregnancy Experience. Sexual and Reproductive Health. 2016, pp. 13–105. Available online: http://apps.who.int/iris/bitstream/handle/10665/250796/9789241549912-eng.pdf (accessed on 28 June 2018).
12. Gibson-Helm, M.E.; Teede, H.J.; Cheng, I.H.; Block, A.A.; Knight, M.; East, C.E.; Wallace, E.M.; Boyle, J. Maternal health and pregnancy outcomes comparing migrant women born in humanitarian and nonhumanitarian source countries: A retrospective, observational study. *Birth* **2015**, *42*, 116–124. [CrossRef] [PubMed]
13. Kentoffio, K.; Berkowitz, S.A.; Atlas, S.J.; Oo, S.A.; Percac-Lima, S. Use of maternal health services: Comparing refugee, immigrant and US-born populations. *Matern. Child Health J.* **2016**, *20*, 2494–2501. [CrossRef] [PubMed]
14. Hampel, A.; Solbach, P.; Cornberg, M.; Schmidt, R.E.; Behrens, G.M.; Jablonka, A. Current seroprevalence, vaccination and predictive value of liver enzymes for hepatitis B among refugees in Germany. *Bundesgesundheitsblatt Gesundheitsforschung Gesundheitsschutz* **2016**, *59*, 578–583. [CrossRef] [PubMed]
15. Alberer, M.; Malinowski, S.; Sanftenberg, L.; Schelling, J. Notifiable infectious diseases in refugees and asylum seekers: Experience from a major reception center in Munich, Germany. *Infection* **2018**, *46*, 375–383. [CrossRef] [PubMed]
16. Jablonka, A.; Happle, C.; Wetzke, M.; Dopfer, C.; Merkesdal, S.; Schmidt, R.E.; Behrens, G.M.N.; Solbach, P. Measles, Rubella and Varicella IgG Seroprevalence in a Large Refugee Cohort in Germany in 2015: A Cross-Sectional Study. *Infect. Dis. Ther.* **2017**, *6*, 487–496. [CrossRef] [PubMed]
17. Jablonka, A.; Happle, C.; Grote, U.; Schleenvoigt, B.T.; Hampel, A.; Dopfer, C.; Hansen, G.; Schmidt, R.E.; Behrens, G.M. Measles, mumps, rubella, and varicella seroprevalence in refugees in Germany in 2015. *Infection* **2016**, *44*, 781–787. [CrossRef] [PubMed]
18. Grote, U.; Schleenvoigt, B.T.; Happle, C.; Dopfer, C.; Wetzke, M.; Ahrenstorf, G.; Holst, H.; Pletz, M.W.; Schmidt, R.E.; Behrens, G.M. Norovirus outbreaks in German refugee camps in 2015. *Z. Gastroenterol.* **2017**, *55*, 997–1003. [CrossRef] [PubMed]
19. Jablonka, A.; Solbach, P.; Wobse, M.; Manns, M.P.; Schmidt, R.E.; Wedemeyer, H.; Cornberg, M.; Behrens, G.M.N.; Hardtke, S. Seroprevalence of antibodies and antigens against hepatitis A-E viruses in refugees and asylum seekers in Germany in 2015. *Eur. J. Gastroenterol. Hepatol.* **2017**, *29*, 939–945. [CrossRef] [PubMed]

20. Vetter, K.; Goeckenjan, M. Prenatal care in Germany. *Bundesgesundheitsblatt Gesundheitsforschung Gesundheitsschutz* **2013**, *56*, 1679–1685. [CrossRef] [PubMed]
21. Federal Statistical Office of Germany. Available online: https://www.destatis.de/DE/ZahlenFakten/GesellschaftStaat/Bevoelkerung/Geburten/Glossar/GebaerfaehigesAlter.html (accessed on 28 June 2018).
22. Womens Refugee Commission. Available online: https://www.womensrefugeecommission.org/empower/resources/practitioners-forum/facts-and-figures (accessed on 28 June 2018).
23. Abi Nader, H.; Watfa, W. Why be a refugee camp doctor: The challenges, rewards and medical education aspects. *Int. J. Med. Educ.* **2017**, *8*, 307–308. [CrossRef] [PubMed]
24. Efird, J.T.; Bith-Melander, P. Refugee Health: An Ongoing Commitment and Challenge. *Int. J. Environ. Res. Public Health* **2018**, *15*, 131. [CrossRef] [PubMed]
25. Winn, A.; Hetherington, E.; Tough, S. Caring for pregnant refugee women in a turbulent policy landscape: Perspectives of health care professionals in Calgary, Alberta. *Int. J. Equity Health* **2018**, *17*, 91. [CrossRef] [PubMed]
26. Simsek, Z.; Yentur Doni, N.; Gul Hilali, N.; Yildirimkaya, G. A community-based survey on Syrian refugee women's health and its predictors in Sanliurfa, Turkey. *Women Health* **2017**, *21*, 1–15. [CrossRef] [PubMed]
27. Buber-Ennser, I.; Kohlenberger, J.; Rengs, B.; Al Zalak, Z.; Goujon, A.; Striessnig, E.; Potančoková, M.; Gisser, R.; Testa, M.R.; Lutz, W. Human Capital, Values, and Attitudes of Persons Seeking Refuge in Austria in 2015. *PLoS ONE* **2016**, *11*, e0163481. [CrossRef] [PubMed]
28. Jablonka, A.; Behrens, G.M.; Stange, M.; Dopfer, C.; Grote, U.; Hansen, G.; Schmidt, R.E.; Happle, C. Tetanus and diphtheria immunity in refugees in Europe in 2015. *Infection* **2017**, *45*, 157–164. [CrossRef] [PubMed]
29. Jablonka, A.; Dopfer, C.; Happle, C.; Sogkas, G.; Ernst, D.; Atschekzei, F.; Hirsch, S.; Schäll, A.; Jirmo, A.; Solbach, P.; et al. Tuberculosis Specific Interferon-Gamma Production in a Current Refugee Cohort in Western Europe. *Int. J. Environ. Res. Public Health* **2018**, *15*. [CrossRef] [PubMed]
30. Sachs, L. Safe motherhood in refugee settings. *Afr. Health.* **1997**, *19*, 24–25. [PubMed]
31. Pavli, A.; Maltezou, H. Health problems of newly arrived migrants and refugees in Europe. *J. Travel Med.* **2017**, *24*. [CrossRef] [PubMed]
32. Eiset, A.H.; Wejse, C. Review of infectious diseases in refugees and asylum seekers-current status and going forward. *Public Health Rev.* **2017**, *38*, 22. [CrossRef] [PubMed]
33. Bukasa, A.; Campbell, H.; Brown, K.; Bedford, H.; Ramsay, M.; Amirthalingam, G.; Tookey, P. Rubella infection in pregnancy and congenital rubella in United Kingdom, 2003 to 2016. *Euro Surveill.* **2018**, *23*. [CrossRef] [PubMed]
34. McElroy, R.; Laskin, M.; Jiang, D.; Shah, R.; Ray, J.G. Rates of rubella immunity among immigrant and non-immigrant pregnant women. *J. Obstet. Gynaecol. Can.* **2009**, *31*, 409–413. [CrossRef]
35. Plotinsky, R.N.; Talbot, E.A.; Kellenberg, J.E.; Reef, S.E.; Buseman, S.K.; Wright, K.D.; Modlin, J.F. Congenital rubella syndrome in a child born to Liberian refugees: Clinical and public health perspectives. *Clin. Pediatr.* **2007**, *46*, 349–355. [CrossRef] [PubMed]
36. De Maio, F.G. Immigration as pathogenic: A systematic review of the health of immigrants to Canada. *Int. J. Equity Health* **2010**, *9*, 27. [CrossRef] [PubMed]
37. Anderson, F.M.; Hatch, S.L.; Comacchio, C.; Howard, L.M. Prevalence and risk of mental disorders in the perinatal period among migrant women: A systematic review and meta-analysis. *Arch. Womens Ment. Health* **2017**, *20*, 449–462. [CrossRef] [PubMed]
38. Gogol, K.N.; Gotsiridze, E.G.; Guruli, Z.V.; Kintraia, N.P.; Tsaava, F.D. The expectancy-stress factor in pregnant refugee women. *Georgian Med. News* **2006**, 13–16.
39. Urquia, M.L.; Glazier, R.H.; Blondel, B.; Zeitlin, J.; Gissler, M.; Macfarlane, A.; Ng, E.; Heaman, M.; Stray-Pedersen, B.; Gagnon, A.J.; et al. International migration and adverse birth outcomes: Role of ethnicity, region of origin and destination. *J. Epidemiol. Community Health* **2010**, *64*, 243–251. [CrossRef] [PubMed]
40. Alnuaimi, K.; Kassab, M.; Ali, R.; Mohammad, K.; Shattnawi, K. Pregnancy outcomes among Syrian refugee and Jordanian women: A comparative study. *Int. Nurs. Rev.* **2017**, *64*, 584–592. [CrossRef] [PubMed]
41. Gungor, E.S.; Seval, O.; Ilhan, G.; Verit, F.F. Do Syrian refugees have increased risk for worser pregnancy outcomes? Results of a tertiary center in Istanbul. *Turk J. Obstet. Gynecol.* **2018**, *15*, 23–27. [PubMed]

42. Erenel, H.; Aydogan Mathyk, B.; Sal, V.; Ayhan, I.; Karatas, S.; Koc Bebek, A. Clinical characteristics and pregnancy outcomes of Syrian refugees: A case-control study in a tertiary care hospital in Istanbul, Turkey. *Arch. Gynecol. Obstet.* **2017**, *295*, 45–50. [CrossRef] [PubMed]
43. Gornall, J. Healthcare for Syrian refugees. *BMJ* **2015**, *351*, h415. [CrossRef] [PubMed]

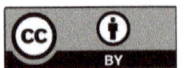

© 2018 by the authors. Licensee MDPI, Basel, Switzerland. This article is an open access article distributed under the terms and conditions of the Creative Commons Attribution (CC BY) license (http://creativecommons.org/licenses/by/4.0/).

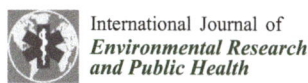

Review

Prevalence of Sexual Violence in Migrants, Applicants for International Protection, and Refugees in Europe: A Critical Interpretive Synthesis of the Evidence

Lotte De Schrijver [1], Tom Vander Beken [2], Barbara Krahé [3] and Ines Keygnaert [1,*]

1. UGent-International Centre for Reproductive Health, 9000 Ghent, Belgium; lotte.deschrijver@ugent.be
2. UGent-Institute for International Research on Criminal Policy, 9000 Ghent, Belgium; tom.vanderbeken@ugent.be
3. Department of Psychology, University of Potsdam, 14476 Potsdam, Germany; krahe@uni-potsdam.de
* Correspondence: ines.keygnaert@ugent.be; Tel.: +32-09-332-35-64

Received: 26 August 2018; Accepted: 7 September 2018; Published: 11 September 2018

Abstract: *(1) Background*: Sexual violence (SV) is a major public health problem, with negative socio-economic, physical, mental, sexual, and reproductive health consequences. Migrants, applicants for international protection, and refugees (MARs) are vulnerable to SV. Since many European countries are seeing high migratory pressure, the development of prevention strategies and care paths focusing on victimised MARs is highly needed. To this end, this study reviews evidence on the prevalence of SV among MAR groups in Europe and the challenges encountered in research on this topic. *(2) Methods*: A critical interpretive synthesis of 25 peer-reviewed academic studies and 22 relevant grey literature documents was conducted based on a socio-ecological model. *(3) Results*: Evidence shows that SV is highly frequent in MARs in Europe, yet comparison with other groups is still difficult. Methodologically and ethically sound representative studies comparing between populations are still lacking. Challenges in researching SV in MARs are located at the intrapersonal, interpersonal, community, societal, and policy levels. *(4) Conclusions*: Future research should start with a clear definition of the concerned population and acts of SV to generate comparable data. Participatory qualitative research approaches could be applied to better grasp the complexity of interplaying determinants of SV in MARs.

Keywords: sexual violence; migrants; refugees; asylum seekers; applicants for international protection; Europe; prevalence

---

1. Introduction

Sexual violence (SV) is a major health, judicial, and societal concern [1,2] and can have numerous serious short- and long-term physical, psychological, and social consequences for victims, but also for family members, peers, and assailants [1,3–5]. It is a global and serious public health and human rights problem [5]. SV occurs all over the world, in all cultures, at every societal level, among people from all genders, and in all age categories [1]. Regardless of the context in which SV occurs (during war and conflict, within an intimate partnership or larger family or community structure), it is considered a deeply violating and painful experience for those affected [5]. SV can be broadly defined as a range of behaviours including sexual harassment, sexual violence without penetration, and attempted and completed rape, and can occur in a myriad of contexts and relationships [6]. It includes victimization, perpetration, and the witnessing of transgressive and violent sexual acts, taking place between strangers or in close and intimate relationships, motivated by individual or political reasons, in the context of conflict, exploitation, or targeting of a specific group [7]. In this paper, we will use the term "SV" to refer to this broad range of behaviours. However, since there is a diversity in the use of terms referring to SV, we will use the terminology of the original papers in the "results" section in order to be clear about the specific types or subcategories of SV addressed in the respective studies.

Both scientific and grey literature identify applicants for international protection and refugees as being especially vulnerable to SV exposure [8,9]. However, the extent to which this vulnerability is reflected in the prevalence of SV is not yet made clear. There is a lack of qualitative and comparable research on this topic. Moreover, the implementation of prevention and response policies based on the evidence is rare.

In the last decade, the world has seen an increase in the number of people forced to flee from their homes. In 2014, the United Nations High Commissioner for Refugees (UNHCR), counted 59.5 million forcibly displaced people worldwide, which was a 16% increase compared to the previous year [10]. The numbers have gone up since then. Today, the UN Agency estimates that 65.6 million men, women, and children have been forced to leave their home countries. This figure includes 22.5 million refugees, of whom over half are minors under the age of 18 [11].

The terms "migrant", "asylum seeker/applicant for international protection", and "refugee" are often considered as synonyms but refer to different populations. In this paper, the definitions proposed by the UNHCR will be used. A migrant is someone who consciously and voluntarily decides to leave his/her country of origin and who could decide to go back without having to fear for their safety. Others who leave their home country do not have that option [12]. Asylum seekers or applicants for international protection flee their home country and are awaiting a decision on their request for international protection [12]. Refugees are those applicants that have received a positive decision regarding their request for international protection. The abbreviation "MARs" will be used here to refer to migrants, applicants for international protection, and refugees. Although the focus of this study is mainly on the latter two, the term "migrant" is also included, because a migrant may have been an applicant or refugee in the past.

Although the number of applications for international protection has recently declined, applicants and refugees still remain a group not to be neglected [13]. Although Europe has a long history as an area for migratory transit and/or as a destination, the high numbers of MARs have provided some challenges. One of them is the responsibility to guard, guarantee, or aid in achieving the health and well-being of MARs.

To take up this responsibility, a clear overview of the specificities regarding the population's experienced threats to health and well-being should be identified in order to develop and provide adequate and appropriate care. Since the harsh conditions in which MARs may find themselves may hamper their access to protection and medical, forensic, and/or psychological care in European countries, it is essential to research the impact of SV on the lives of those belonging to vulnerable groups. This will contribute to a better understanding of the mechanisms involved and to recommendations with an eye to improving the health and wellbeing of all individuals belonging to this group.

A first step in the research chain is to estimate the magnitude of the problem in this population. The objective of our study is to critically review the evidence on the prevalence of SV in MARs in Europe and to discuss the challenges of conducting research on SV in this specific population to inform future prevalence studies. To address the study objectives, this review will look into prevalence studies on SV in MARs in Europe through the method of a critical interpretive synthesis (CIS).

2. Methods

2.1. Critical Interpretive Synthesis

In order to critically discuss the evidence and challenges of research on SV prevalence in MAR, we opted to conduct a critical interpretive synthesis (CIS). This method not only uses the conventional search process of traditional systematic reviews, but focusses on identifying and selecting a diverse sample of documents [14] stemming from both academic and policy as well as legal frameworks. A CIS thus also considers studies that would not meet the criteria for inclusion in a systematic review, in particular grey literature including research reports from non-governmental organisations (NGOs) working directly with the population, for example. This broadens the scope significantly and helps us to better grasp the heterogeneous body of literature on SV in MARs [15].

The strength of a CIS lies in promoting an understanding of phenomena and theory construction through an inductive and interpretive combination of constructs and evidence from different approaches and study fields, resulting in a new coherent whole [16]. This methodology allows us to integrate different kinds of sources, regardless of whether they are peer reviewed or grey literature, and to add a qualitative dimension to the analysis [16].

Different from traditional systematic review methodologies, a CIS does not draw upon an a priori defined research question representing a specific hypothesis, but rather identifies and refines relevant questions during the review process itself [17]. Its process is characterised by a dynamic, interactive, and recursive nature with recognition of the necessity of flexibility and reflexivity during the search, sampling, and analysis of the data [16,18]. Instead of a linear progression, the CIS review strategy is more circular and evolves organically, explicitly acknowledging that some aspects of the process will not be auditable or reproducible as it is grounded in the evidence retrieved by specific research teams with their particular backgrounds and awareness of relevant literature from various fields and sources [16,18]. The non-linear progress of this method also allows for including new sources based on the findings of the interpretive synthesis and to analyse the data in the light of different research areas and specific background knowledge of the research team, which may ultimately contribute to the construction of new theoretical frameworks [16]. New theories and concepts arising as a result of a CIS may serve as a starting point for future studies [16].

To answer the predetermined research objectives, we synthesized and approached the literature through the lens of a socio-ecological model. This approach [19,20] can be used to study SV from a perspective in which four interlinked levels play a key role. It suggests that the interactions between the individuals and their environment shape their development over time [19]. Within a complex system of relationships affected by multiple levels of the surrounding environment [20], research on SV takes place in a social context. These interactions between different social contexts can be categorized in various systems.

At the first level of the socio-ecological model, we find the intrapersonal processes taking place within the individuals themselves. These internal processes are bi-directionally influenced by the immediate surrounding of the individual, the second level. The relationship between the individuals and their direct context is, in turn, affected by the relationships between several different microsystems within a community, representing the third level. At the fourth level, communities are influenced by processes taking place at the societal and public policy levels [19,20].

Starting from this model, we begin by looking at relevant factors in the light of SV prevalence in MARs identified at the individual level, followed by challenges at the interpersonal level, in order to continue with the organisational and community level and finally the societal and public policy level.

The CIS method combined with a socio-ecological approach guides us in considering why little is known about the prevalence of SV in Europe, how the identified research challenges relate to each other [18], and how they may influence recommendations for practice [17] and future research. Although papers on related topics have been published in the past, these mainly concerned systematic reviews and did not include relevant non-academic sources. The approach we used here allows us to add to the knowledge base on this topic by critically evaluating on which socio-ecological levels researchers and policymakers should focus in order to improve research strategies and policies concerning SV in MARs in Europe.

2.2. Sample of Studies

Between 1 May and 31 August 2017, we selected peer-reviewed articles relevant to the research objectives of this study through a database search. During the first phase of the CIS, articles were deemed relevant if they contributed original data, theoretical or methodological information, or policy considerations to the problem of SV in MARs living in Europe, regardless of the specific research question, the study field, or research design. This search was part of a larger study called "UN-MENAMAIS-UNderstanding the MEchanisms, NAture, MAgnitude and Impact of Sexual violence in Belgium" and took place simultaneously with the search action for a CIS on the risk factors and consequences of SV and help-seeking behaviours after SV victimization in MARs. These results will be presented elsewhere.

The following inclusion criteria were used: papers on SV in MARs in Europe had to be published after the year 2000 in English, French, or Dutch. Any author's definition of sexual violence (i.e., rape and any other form of sexual violence) was accepted, but studies that combined sexual and non-sexual violence into one category in the analysis were excluded in order to maximize the comparability of the prevalence numbers. However, we did use these sources in order to obtain a deeper sense of the background concerning the issue of SV in MARs. If different forms of violence were studied in one single study and rates of SV could be separated from the other types of violence, the paper was still included. The Medical Subject Heading (MeSH, which refers to the controlled vocabulary used to index all of the articles in PubMed) terms and key words presented in Table 1 were used in different combinations and databases.

Table 1. Search terms. MeSH: Medical Subject Heading.

MeSH Terms	Keywords	Databases	Alerts
Prevalence; sex offences; child abuse; sexual human trafficking; rape; refugees; transients and migrants; sexual minorities	Sexual violence; rape; sexual assault; sexual abuse; child abuse; human trafficking; sexual exploitation; forced prostitution; sexual harassment; sexual slavery; attempted rape; refugees; asylum seekers; migrants; undocumented migrants; legal status; irregular; illegal; lesbian, gay, bisexual, transgender & intersex (LGBTI); conflict related sexual violence; war; European Union (EU); Europe; high-income countries; Western countries; help-seeking; help-seeking behaviour; disclosure; selective disclosure; health care; access; barriers	PubMed Google Scholar Science Direct	Crimpapers Science Direct

In addition to peer-reviewed articles, we also considered grey literature. With the term "grey literature", we refer to those documents that have not necessarily undergone a peer-review process and/or are not included in academic bibliographical retrieval systems and often remain unpublished and limited in distribution [21,22]. It includes reports of different natures, including dissertations, technical specifications, standards and guidelines, official documentation, and so on [21]. These sources were derived from the reference lists of studies used in the first phase and sources provided by experts and alerts.

Initially, we identified a total of 2380 peer-reviewed articles on the prevalence of SV, its consequences, the associated risk factors, and help-seeking behaviour after SV in MARs in the database search and 93 through other sources. Of those, 138 documents were selected as relevant for the general CIS on SV in MARs in Europe (cf. above). Ninety-one documents were excluded from the CIS because they did not address our research question on SV prevalence in the population of interest as they were of poor quality or were not fully accessible for our research team. We ultimately included 25 peer-reviewed articles and 22 grey literature documents in the CIS on the results and challenges of SV prevalence studies in MARs in Europe. To have an idea of the prevalence of SV in MARs in

Europe, only papers addressing the problem of SV in MARs living in Europe were included in the analyses. The studies retained in the CIS discuss SV prevalence in MARs in the following 12 European countries: Belgium, France, Germany, Greece, Hungary, Ireland, Malta, the Netherlands, Portugal, Spain, Sweden, Switzerland, Turkey and the United Kingdom. One study reported a survey conducted in all EU countries.

3. Results

3.1. Prevalence of SV in Migrants, Applicants for International Protection, and Refugees in Europe

Compared to the attention given to SV in the general population, research on SV in MARs is extremely scarce. In this section, we discuss the prevalence of SV victimization and perpetration in MARs in Europe. The findings regarding both victimization and perpetration will be presented together when they stem from the same studies.

As we will discuss in more detail later, estimating the prevalence of SV in MARs involves several challenges. The combination of these challenges led to the identification of only five studies on the prevalence of SV in MARs in Europe that matched our predetermined inclusion criteria, and may be the primary reason for the scarcity of data on prevalence, consequences, and mediating factors of SV in this population.

One frequently cited paper concerns a community-based participatory study by Keygnaert et al. from 2012 [23] on sexual and gender-based violence (SGBV) in refugees, applicants, and undocumented migrants in Belgium and the Netherlands. This study showed that approximately 57% of the participants indicated that they had been confronted with SV experiences, comprising rape and sexual exploitation among others. Compared to the general population, the nature of the experienced SV included more incidences of multiple and gang rape [23]. A fifth of all respondents in this study reported having been sexually victimised themselves. A total of 332 acts of SGVB were described in 223 interviews, including 188 cases of SV, of which 47 were personal experiences and 141 were experienced by a close peer of the respondent [23]. These results indicate a high risk for MARs of becoming confronted with SV. At a more detailed level, 69% of individuals victimized since their arrival in Europe were women, and 29% were men. In 2% of the cases, the gender of the victim remained unclear or multiple victims of both sexes were involved. The opposite pattern can be found when asking about who the assailants were. In 72.6% of the cases, the assailant was a man, in 1.5% it concerned a transgender assailant, in 19.6%, the gender was not clearly specified, and only in 6% of the cases the assailant was a woman [23]. In line with findings from studies in the general population [4,24], most victims knew their assailants [23]. The assailant was in most cases an intimate partner (31%) and less frequently a professional (23%), a family member (16%), an acquaintance (15%), or a stranger (12%) [23]. In a third of the incidences, the assailant was a European citizen [23].

When looking further into the European situation, another much-cited study by Keygnaert et al. [25] from 2014 in eight European countries (Belgium, Greece, Hungary, Ireland, Malta, the Netherlands, Portugal, and Spain) examined the prevalence of SV in refugees, applicants for International protection, and undocumented migrants in a wider European context. This community-based participatory study showed that in the European asylum reception sector, both sexes as well as both residents and professionals are at risk of being exposed to different forms of violence, including SV, with 58.3% of the 562 respondents reporting having being directly (23.3%) or indirectly (76.6%) confronted with SV [25]. This study also showed that victimization and perpetration of violence seem to be more gender-balanced in comparison with the general population. Both sexes indicated a comparable tendency to have experienced all types of violence perpetration and victimization. However, men were more likely to be involved in SV perpetration and emotional victimization, whereas women tended to be more likely to become the victim of SV and perpetrate emotional violence [25].

It should be noted here that the findings may be an underestimation since many of the respondents in the study indicated that they did not want to disclose or were hesitant to disclose personal SV experiences as long as they remained and/or worked in reception centres. Fear of reprisals by community members and feared impact on their asylum case or stay in the facility may have influenced the number of reported cases [25]. Although these studies give us an idea of the magnitude of the problem in this population, their objective was not to present representative prevalence numbers.

In the same period, the European Union Agency for Fundamental Rights (FRA) [9] published an EU-wide survey about violence against women (VAW), which included a section on the prevalence of violence in migrant populations. They concluded that women who were not a citizen of their current country of residence were more likely than women without a migration history to become victims of physical and/or SV by both partners and non-partners after the age of 15. However, they did not find notable differences from the general population in physical, sexual, or psychological violence before the age of 15, and sexual harassment and stalking after the age of 15 [9]. Unfortunately, these numbers cannot be broken down according to legal status, do not consider SV against men, and are not comparable with the figures by Keygnaert et al. in 2012 and 2014 [23,25].

In 2015, Doctors of the World (*Médicins du Monde*, MdM) [26] disseminated a report on the access to healthcare in 2014 for vulnerable people, such as MARs in 11 countries (Belgium, France, Germany, Greece, the Netherlands, Spain, Sweden, Switzerland, the United Kingdom, Turkey, and Canada). The data were collected by means of social and medical questionnaires administered to patients who attended a MdM consultation in one of the 11 countries [26]. Unfortunately, questions on SV were not asked in every country and strongly depended on the healthcare providers' willingness to address the issue. Even though the numbers could not be generalized, the results indicate that applicants for international protection were disproportionately highly represented among victims of violence [26] and thus may support the hypothesis that MARs are more vulnerable to SV than the general population. Among the patients who were questioned about their experiences with SV, 27.6% (37.6% of women and 7.3% of men) reported sexual assault. Rape was mentioned by 14.9% of those patients (24.1% of the women and 5.4% of the men). Interestingly, male patients reported a quarter of the total number of sexual assaults [26]. The figures cannot be considered representative, but they provide an impression of the current situation.

Another important finding in this study, which continues in the line of the results found by Keygnaert et al. [23,25,27], relates to the experiences of SV throughout the trajectory of MARs from country of origin to country of destination. MARs do not only experience SV before migrating, but also during and after their arrival in Europe [26,27]. In the population studied by MdM, 21.1% of the reported rapes and 17.7% of the sexual assaults took place after the victim's arrival in the host country. This is an important finding since most studies on SV in MARs only consider violence cases in the country of origin, ignoring the experiences en route or after arrival. Keygnaert et al. [27] found in another study published in 2014 on SV among sub-Saharan migrants in Morocco that 45% of them had experienced SV in a direct or indirect manner during their migration or in Morocco itself. These are important findings to consider when asking about SV in this population. Identifying aspects related to SV before leaving the country of origin, during transit, and after arrival in the host country is necessary in order to provide appropriate and adequate policy recommendations and prevention strategies.

In 2009, the Refugee Council's Vulnerable Women's Project (VWP) [28] published some numbers in line with the trends reported here. In a 21-month period (2006–2008), the project supported 153 refugee and asylum-seeking women in the United Kingdom. Of those, 76% indicated that they had been raped either in their home country or in the United Kingdom, had been sexually abused (22%), or had been confronted with threats of being raped or sexually abused while in detention in their country of origin (9%). Men were not included in this study [28].

We will briefly discuss some non-European studies on conflict-related SV (CRSV) to illustrate the specific SV experiences that may have taken place before the migration process started. During the Rwandan genocide for example, up to half a million women were raped. In parts of Liberia, more than

90% of women and girls above the age of three became the victim of CRSV, and in parts of Eastern Congo, it is estimated that about 75% of the women were confronted with SV [28]. CRSV presents itself in specific forms, such as gang rape, depending on the war in which it takes place and the underlying function of the practice [29–32].

Although clear and robust prevalence rates of SV in MARs in Europe are lacking, the evidence we have right now supports the hypothesis that MARs are vulnerable to becoming victims of SV. In addition, it is in line with the wide recognition that in times of conflict everyone is more exposed to violence and more particularity to SGBV [33]. The numbers reported on the situation in Europe also follow the same trend as shown in a systematic review and meta-analysis from 2014 on SV among female refugees in complex humanitarian emergencies. Vu et al. [34] estimate the prevalence of SV in this population as approximately one in five women. Given the multiple barriers associated with disclosing the experiences, the researchers stress that these numbers are most likely an underestimation.

3.2. Challenges in Conducting, Comparing, and Interpreting Research in Migrants, Applicants for International Protection, and Refugees

The challenges in conducting research on MARs were approached and analysed in this study from a socio-ecological perspective [19,20] in which four interlinked levels play a key role. We start by (1) looking at the issues identified on the individual level, and continue with (2) the interpersonal level, followed by (3) challenges at a broader organisational and community level. We will finish this analysis with (4) a discussion of barriers in conducting research at a societal and public policy level.

3.2.1. Research Challenges at the Individual Level

At the individual level, two perspectives need to be taken into account, namely that of the researcher and that of the research participant. Given the experience of the MAR population with violent conflict, displacement, and human rights violations, most researchers struggle with approaching their study population purely as objects of research without trying to make a difference and reduce suffering [35,36]. From the researchers' point of view, remaining neutral can be quite a challenge. In addition, from an ethical perspective, one may question the motives for researching MARs if researchers cannot offer them anything in return.

From the point of view of the research participant, factors related to disclosing sensitive information about themselves can be a perceived or real threat to personal safety (infra). This may result in (dis)trust from migrants of the so-called authorities and may influence their willingness to participate.

3.2.2. Research Challenges at the Interpersonal Level

Many researchers are intrinsically motivated to work with this population because they want to contribute to improving their situation [35]. At the same time, research can only have a substantial impact for a group of people if the results are published. Both ethical considerations and logistic challenges are central to finding the balance between applying high academic standards to the research design and making a difference to the participants. It is not always possible for researchers to reveal the details of how they conducted the study (e.g., identification and selection of participants, handling of local security issues, context of the interviews, access to illegal immigrants, illegal activities performed by MARs, etc.), because of the privacy of research participants and the fact that their safety might be at stake. The political and legal issues related to the situation of applicants for international protection and refugees means that they have fewer rights and are at risk when participating in research [35,36]. Because of the protection of the safety of the participants, some elements of the research design may not always be revealed. The manner of gaining access to undocumented migrants is one example. Participating in research on illegal behaviour may put both respondents and researchers at risk [36]. Withholding concrete and detailed descriptions of the research process and the gatekeepers involved as a way of protecting individual participants and the community as a whole [36] may lead to a lack of reproducibility of the study and threaten the transparency of the results.

Researchers and their respondents often do not speak the same language and might have different cultural backgrounds [35], meaning that interpreters or cultural mediators have to be involved in order to gather data. However, including a third party into qualitative research brings along new challenges, such as erroneous translations, difficulties in establishing a relation of trust between the interviewer and the interviewee, and the risk of interviewees refraining from disclosure in the presence of a third party out of fear of the effects on the community to which they belong.

These challenges could be reduced through the use of a community-based participatory research approach [6,37]. This approach creates bridges between scientists and communities and establishes mutual trust by sharing knowledge and valuable experiences [6]. By participating within the community, researchers gain a deeper understanding of the unique circumstances in which a given community lives. It facilitates open dialogue on sensitive issues and helps to define mutual agreements about the collaborative research process [6].

3.2.3. Research Challenges at the Organisational and Community Level

Another significant challenge relates to the fact that the research population of MARs is mobile and hard to reach. Firstly, when the study population is characterised by being on the move, it is difficult to investigate effects over longer periods of time. This is specifically relevant in the light of the impact of SV on the lives of victims, assailants, and their families/peers. Longitudinal designs are very hard to establish.

Another fundamental problem in conducting representative studies on all kinds of migrant populations lies in the difficulties of getting access to a certain community. To start with, MARs are not equally distributed over Europe, nor within each country. They often live in big cities or near a certain reception centre, and even within these broader areas they tend to live in specific neighbourhoods. This means that achieving nationwide randomized samples is very costly and resource-intensive [38,39]. Furthermore, due to their legal status (or rather the lack thereof), subpopulations of MARs often remain hidden [38,39]. The combination of these factors makes MARs a population that is hard to reach.

3.2.4. Research Challenges at the Societal and Public Policy Level

The societal level in the socio-ecological model looks at the broad societal factors that create a challenging climate to conduct research on a vulnerable population such as MAR. First of all, regulations regarding legal statuses can significantly influence research opportunities. Ethical considerations play an important role here. Is it ethical to ask research questions which may ultimately lead to policies that may negatively impact the living situation of the studied community? Düvell et al. [36] gave the example of documenting *how* undocumented migrants enter a country compared to studying the *why* question with regard to this behaviour. Researchers' findings may be used by policymakers to the disadvantage of the communities that participate [36]. A thorough reflection of the justification of why one wants to conduct a certain study and how the findings may be used afterwards should always be part of the preparatory phase.

Secondly, the extent to which people with different legal statuses are integrated into the larger administrative and demographic organisation of a society can have a strong impact too. A common practice to register migrants in the European Union is missing [38,39]. A related obstacle concerns the difficulty of including MARs in representative studies. MARs are often excluded from large national studies because of language problems [24] and a lack of complete demographic information [38,39]. Undocumented migrants also remain excluded from these studies since they are not represented in national registries [38,39].

3.3. Challenges in Conducting Research on Sexual Violence

In addition to dealing with the specific challenges involved in studying MARs, research on SV itself can equally be a challenging task. Again, several reasons for the lack of an extensive, systematic knowledge base on this topic can be classified according to a socio-ecological framework.

3.3.1. Research Challenges at the Individual Level

The primary reason for the difficulty of establishing the magnitude of the problem lies in the fact that those involved commonly hide the experience (infra) and health care workers do not recognize it. This may be out of fear of being stigmatized or of further violence after disclosure [24,28,40,41]. One cannot count or study what remains hidden.

3.3.2. Research Challenges at the Organisational, Community, and Interpersonal Level

The organisation and structure within the community and institutions create a specific barrier in gaining access to populations. The refusal by community gatekeepers or those in charge of institutions reduces the access to individuals that may be relevant for researchers [6,38,39]. This leads to bias and a lack of generalizable data.

Linked to gaining access to a certain community to talk about SV are interpersonal barriers related to the sensitivity of the researched topic. Disclosure of SV is one of the most important interpersonal challenges identified with regard to investigating SV. Respondents need to be actively motivated to discuss their experiences with SV to provide researchers with the necessary details to arrive at conclusions that correspond with the lived reality of the participants. Therefore, certain criteria should be met. Participants will be more likely to talk about their experiences if they perceive the interviewer as trustworthy, as someone who understands them, as someone who responds in an accepting and not stigmatizing manner, and if they expect disclosure to lead to future benefits [42–44]. These benefits could be personal, but could also be related, for example, to the prevention of future victimization of others. Drawing the bigger picture of a study in that light could be very useful. Informing participants about what will ultimately happen with the findings of the study may be one way to increase the motivation for participation. Another strategy may be to involve them in the dissemination of the results within the community and to policymakers afterwards [2]. The use of a participatory research design could thus be a promising approach to incentivise engagement in SV research.

3.3.3. Research Challenges at the Societal and Public Policy Level

At a broader societal level, it appears that defining SV remains a significant challenge. What falls under the category of SV is not always clear. Publications on the theme use different terms to describe the same concepts and phenomena or describe different types of SV with the same terminology. Further, the societal construction and awareness of SV often seems to be limited to female victims of rape perpetrated by men [6,45,46]. The victimization of males and transgender people is generally neglected [45,46]. Stereotypical thinking about victims and sexual violence is strongly reinforced in ruling rape myths [47]. As we will discuss below, this impacts the policies and funding of studies in specific populations and the focus of research questions.

Definitions of Sexual Violence

Defining SV in a consistent manner is an important issue in researching and reporting SV to avoid confusion and enhance the comparability of findings [48]. In a number of studies for example, data on both sexual and physical violence are collected and/or analysed as one single item. When presented as a single item, the nature of the violence and the underlying dynamics remain unclear. Both physical and sexual violence encompass a multitude of types of violent acts, may emerge in diverse contexts, and result in different consequences. At the same time, physical and SV show some overlap, are often linked to each other, and may be hard to distinguish from one another in certain situations [6,49].

Specifically, in the light of intimate partner violence (IPV), the distinction between the two may be unclear. SV encompasses all sexual acts against someone's will. It may be difficult to judge whether a sexual act in an intimate relationship is against a partner's will. For example, when partners have sex with their partner against their will to avoid physical violence, does this count as SV or not? A clear distinction between the two is often not described, and definitions are lacking.

The lack of a clear and encompassing definition of SV may result in policies and research funding that focus solely on those forms of SV (such as completed rape of women) that meet the lay understanding of the general public rather than corresponding to how the phenomenon is really perceived and experienced by those people affected by it [6].

Violence against Women and Gender-Based Violence (GBV) as Umbrella Terms

The same problem arises in the study of VAW or GBV. SV is often discussed under those broader umbrellas that are often used interchangeably [28]. GBV is generally used to describe and capture all forms of violence that occur as a result of "the normative role expectations associated with each gender, along with the unequal power relationships between men and women within the context of a specific society" [50] (p 14).

VAW could be considered as a subcategory of GBV in which violence is directed at girls and women and goes beyond what we consider as SV alone. It refers to many forms of violence, including IPV and rape/sexual assault and other forms of SV perpetrated by someone other than a partner (non-partner sexual violence), as well as female genital mutilation (FGM), honour killings, and the trafficking of women [4]. Note that while women, girls, men, and boys can all become victims of GBV [23,27,51], the main focus within this research area has traditionally been on women and girls. To illustrate, an estimated 35% of all women worldwide are confronted at least once during their life with physical and/or sexual violence, IPV, or SV by a non-partner [4]. When it comes to lifetime prevalence in men however, these numbers are not available.

From a gender perspective, as a result of a ruling patriarchy, power relations, and hierarchical constructions of masculinity and femininity, women appear to be more vulnerable to structural gender inequality [24,52]. Therefore, the primary focus within GBV lies on VAW [24], which creates a gap in the knowledge about GBV against boys and men [1,51] and undermines the comparison of female and male experiences of victimization.

Defining Human Trafficking and Sexual Exploitation

Other umbrella terms related to SV and often used in the context of MARs are "human trafficking", "sexual exploitation", and "SV as a weapon of war or conflict-related SV" (CRSV). These types of violence could play a role both in the decision to leave the home country or in the specific vulnerabilities of MARs while in transit or after arrival in the host country in Europe.

Trafficking in persons or *human trafficking* are often used as synonyms. Trafficking is characterized by the exploitation of vulnerable people in specific kinds of way. The United Nations Office on Drugs and Crime (UNODC) defines it on their webpage as "recruitment, transportation, transfer, harbouring or receipt of persons, by means of the threat or use of force or other forms of coercion, of abduction, of fraud, of deception, of the abuse of power or of a position of vulnerability or of the giving or receiving of payments or benefits to achieve the consent of a person having control over another person, for the purpose of exploitation" [53]. One way of exploitation is *sexual exploitation*, a form of SV that again covers a range of different forms of sexual violence, such as forced prostitution, sexual slavery, transactional sex, solicitation of transactional sex, and having an exploitative relationship [54,55]. The UN describes it in its glossary as "any actual or attempted abuse of position of vulnerability, differential power or trust, for sexual purposes, including, but not limited to, profiting monetarily, socially or politically from the sexual exploitation of another" [55].

Estimates of trafficking for sexual exploitation are difficult to ascertain for a number of reasons. One of the complexities is the fact that the boundaries of trafficking and exploitation are often hard to define [56,57]. Again, consensus on a clear definition of the practices is lacking. Ascertaining prevalence rates can thus be a challenging task. Nevertheless, there are enough indications of the magnitude of this problem to draw the conclusion that it is a serious issue, especially among MARs. The number of migrant girls and women under sexual exploitation at any given time in the United Kingdom is estimated by the Refugee Council to range between 4000 and 10,000 [28]. A survey from 2012 by the International Labour Organization (ILO) showed that an estimated 22% of people in forced labour were sexually exploited. The organization also estimated that two-thirds of all the revenues from forced labour globally were the result of some form of forced sex work, amounting to around 99 billion US dollars or 85 billion euros a year [58].

As we will discuss later, migrants are especially at risk of ending up in forced labour and experiencing SV in this context. According to the ILO, 44% of the victims had migrated within or across countries prior to being trafficked [58]. The ILO also indicates that the vast majority of victims of sexual exploitation are women and girls [56–58]. Importantly, we should not forget that the focus on females as being the only victims might lead to a biased image. Based on different literature reviews, multiple authors concluded that the existence of male sex workers was not acknowledged in the identified sources [59,60].

In those cases where male sex workers were mentioned, they seemed to be considered as less severely victimized. In contrast to female sex workers, they were assigned much more agency. Further, in studies on male victimization, the focus was more on the danger of HIV infection rather than on the violence component [59], emphasizing the public-health threat rather than the need for care [6] of male victims. Providing health care for MARs appears to be motivated primarily by removing a threat to public health [61,62]. In this regard, focusing on infectious diseases is often more accepted than, for example, investing in mental health care, which is often considered as only benefitting the individual involved.

Keygnaert and Guieu [61] argue that the binary approach in SV research, seeing women as victims and men as perpetrators, ignores the complexity and multiplicity of the experience of violence, women's agency and victimisation of male, lesbian, gay, bisexual and transgender (LGBT) individuals victimization, and the role of reigning social norms leading to acceptance of violence [61]. Interestingly, in studies on male sex workers, sexual orientation seemed to be an important aspect, whereas female victims of sexual exploitation were automatically considered to be heterosexual [59]. SV against men seems to be recognized only when it concerns the rape of male prisoners or sexual torture of homosexual men [41,63].

Conflict-Related Sexual Violence (CRSV)

SV may also occur as a component of war and conflict. Situations during or after conflict are contexts with a high prevalence of SV [1]. CRSV refers to a potential weapon of war, ethnic cleansing, or genocide, and is widely acknowledged as a serious problem of international security [30]. This type of SV may be different from other types in that it is used as a strategical means to attain a goal, namely achieving power and dominance over a group considered as inferior [29]. SV probably occurs in all conflicts, but the prevalence and severity differs widely [30,31,64,65]. The term "CRSV" covers all acts of SV that can be considered as strategical mechanisms deployed to attain military or political goals [66]. However, wartime rape is not necessarily always an intentional war strategy, but is often a tolerated weapon rather than an ordered way of attacking the enemy [29]. It is used as a way of torturing people to exercise control over a specific group of people (e.g., ethnic minorities) or as a way to punish or offend individuals and the group to which they belong [28,32].

It is important to consider all actors in conflict situations as possible victims and assailants. Making the distinction between the two roles in conflict areas can be very difficult [32]. Militias, rebels, state officers, and civilians are at risk of becoming victims, assailants, or both in the context of war, with armed state actors being identified as more frequently perpetrating SV than rebel groups [29]. In the literature concerning CRSV, we can again identify a gender bias given that researchers generally do not ask about the sex of the assailants, but assume they are male [29]. Where testimonies about CRSV against men do exist, they are often minimalised, not classified as SV, or ignored. Although the literature is scarce, forced fellatio and masturbation, genital mutilation, forced rape by civilian men, and forced insertion of objects in the anus of prisoners have been described during conflict [41,51,67]. Given this observation, it becomes clear that better knowledge about SV against boys and men is needed.

In combination with the diversity of SV in conflict areas, making statements about the general prevalence of CRSV is again not possible to date. In addition, apart from problems with defining SV from an relational and societal perspective, the terms "rape", "sexual assault", "sexual abuse", and "sexual violence", which are important to distinguish as they might include or exclude different acts a victim had been subjected to, are often considered to be synonymous and are in many papers used interchangeably [1]. This may result in blurred prevalence numbers.

Due to the lack of clear definitions used in studies, comparable prevalence data on CRSV is difficult to collect.

4. Discussion

By discussing the evidence and challenges of SV prevalence research in MARs in Europe based on a CIS in the light of a socio-ecological model, this paper adds to the limited knowledge base on this topic. It does so by placing the findings from both peer-reviewed studies and grey literature next to each other and by analysing both the specific challenges of conducting SV research and prevalence studies in MAR populations. The findings of this CIS allow us to formulate some recommendations for future research. Firstly, there is a pressing need for high-quality representative prevalence studies on SV in MARs in Europe. Secondly, the identified challenges in conducting research on MARs lead to the conclusion that a clean and ethical design for conducting research within this particular population may be hard to reach and that creative approaches and mixed methods may be necessary. Designing a study with this population would require attention to the specificities of MARs and their situation. This means that we, as researchers, need to look for ways of reaching MARs who could fall out of samples because of their legal status and cultural/language barriers. In addition, we need to guarantee the safety of the participants. This can be done through a thorough analysis of the safety threats on all levels of a socio-ecological approach and through addressing them in an ethical and concrete way before the start of the study. Past researchers have experienced that participants were more willing to talk about the experiences if they were not dependent for care or reception on the facilities in which they were interviewed [23,25]. Considering the dependent situation in which MARs may find themselves is one example of how we can estimate the safety threats for participants in SV research.

By working with interviewers who speak the same language and have the same cultural background as the participants, misinterpretation of the data due to linguistic errors could be avoided. However, researchers should be sensitive to the possible introduction of cultural biases by those interviewers and discuss the interpretations with them. Further, although this might avoid the problem of having to work with interpreters, it might induce a barrier on the side of the respondent as this person might take into consideration the cultural habits of disclosure on such topics and potential harmful community reactions to this disclosure and therefore decide not to disclose certain information because of shared cultural identity. Training the interviewers sufficiently in asking questions about sensitive issues, keeping confidentiality, trusting and bonding, and coping with this information thus becomes key in this approach. Emphasizing the confidentiality of the shared information is crucial in every encounter in order to reassure the interviewee that the disclosed information will not be passed on to other persons in the community. In order to maintain participants' motivation, limiting the data collection to only one interview or questionnaire per person may help to avoid attrition at follow-up.

Aside from elements influencing the feasibility and quality of research with MAR populations, challenges regarding researching the topic of SV should be addressed. First, SV needs to be defined clearly. The definition should be inclusive, that is, applicable to men, women, and transgender people of all ages, regardless of their legal status, sexual orientation, or gender identity. To achieve this objective, the acts falling under SV should be described as concrete and observable behaviours [48]. When inquiring about SV, attention should be given not only to the violent acts themselves, but also to the gender of both the victim and assailant, the context in which the violence took place, and the relation between the victim and assailant [68]. Given the broad range of types of SV MARs may have encountered, both open and closed questions regarding SV are necessary to cover the entire range of possibilities and to avoid interpretation bias [69].

When doing research on sensitive issues such as experiences of SV, it is important to consider the possibility that the study participants may experience unintended negative consequences as a result of their participation. Therefore, it may be useful to provide some follow-up support to ensure that they have not come to harm as a result of the study [70–72].

Developing a clean research design for SV research in MARs is quite a challenge. A balancing exercise between ethical considerations and academic standards will be key.

5. Conclusions

Sexual violence experiences in MARs living in Europe is widespread, yet representative studies providing a solid data base are lacking. Future research should start with a clear definition of the population and acts of SV in order to generate high-quality and comparable data. Given the necessity of acknowledging the specific experiences related to different migratory stages and motivations, mixed-method research using interviewers trained in cultural and linguistic skills should be applied to fully grasp the complex manifestations of SV in MARs.

Ultimately, the goal of prevalence studies is to have a clear view on the magnitude of the problem of SV in MARs in order to inform policymakers in their decision-making process regarding actions to improve preventive measures and the allocation of sufficient resources to care programs for both victims of SV and assailants. Although MARs are considered a specific minority group, they still are a subgroup of the general population and should thus be entitled to any general strategy to eliminate the negative consequences of SV and the victimization experience itself. In order to identify specific vulnerabilities and consequences of SV related to legal status or migratory history, comparison with the general population is necessary. Therefore, SV prevalence studies should be designed in such a way that they are applicable to representative samples from both the general population and specific subpopulations such as MARs, taking the research associated with hard-to-reach subgroups into consideration and allowing for comparisons of the findings between different populations.

Author Contributions: L.D.S. performed the CIS and wrote the paper. I.K. is the initiator and supervisor of the study and actively contributed to the data collection, CIS analysis, and writing of the paper. T.V.B. is co-supervisor of the study and contributed to the reflection process of the CIS and writing of the paper. B.K. contributed relevant literature and feedback on the structure and writing of the paper.

Funding: The research that lead to these results was subsidized by the Belgian Federal Science Policy via contract BR/175/A5/UN-MENAMAIS.

Conflicts of Interest: The authors declare no conflict of interest.

References

1. World Health Organization. *Guidelines for Medico-Legal Care for Victims of Sexual Violence*; WHO Press: Geneva, Switzerland, 2003.
2. Keygnaert, I. Seksueel geweld tegen vluchtelingen, asielzoekers en mensen zonder wettig verblijf in België en Nederland. In *Vrouwen Onder Druk: Schendingen van de Seksuele Gezondheid Bij Kwetsbare Vrouwen*; Lannoo: Tielt, Belgium, 2010; pp. 69–88.
3. World Health Organization. *World Report on Violence and Health*; WHO Press: Geneva, Switzerland, 2002. Available online: http://www.who.int/violence_injury_prevention/violence/world_report/en/ (accessed on 7 July 2017).

4. World Health Organization. *Global and Regional Estimates of Violence Against Women: Prevalence and Health Effects of Intimate Partner Violence and Nonpartner Sexual Violence*; WHO Press: Geneva, Switzerland, 2013.
5. Sexual and Reproductive Health. Sexual Violence. Available online: http://www.who.int/reproductivehealth/topics/violence/sexual_violence/en/ (accessed on 7 July 2017).
6. Keygnaert, I. *Sexual Violence and Sexual Health in Refugees, Asylum Seekers and Undocumented Migrants in Europe and the European Neighbourhood: Determinants and Desirable Prevention*; Ghent University: Gent, Belgium, 2014.
7. Depraetere, J.; De Schrijver, L.; Nobels, A.; Inescu, A.; Keygnaert, I. The myriad of sexual violence definitions. In *UN-MENAMAIS Literature Review: Understanding the Mechanisms, Nature, Magnitude and Impact of Sexual Violence in Belgium—A Critical Interpretative Synthesis*; Keygnaert, I., Ed.; Ghent University: Ghent, Belgium, 2018.
8. Freedman, J. Sexual and gender-based violence against refugee women: A hidden aspect of the refugee "crisis". *Reprod. Health Matters* **2016**, *24*, 18–26. [CrossRef] [PubMed]
9. European Union Agency for Fundamental Rights. *Violence against Women: An Eu-Wide Survey*; Publications Office of the European Union: Luxembourg, 2014.
10. Myria. *De Asielcrisis Van 2015: Cijfers en Feiten*; Myria: Brussels, Belgium, 2015.
11. Figures at a Glance. Available online: http://www.unhcr.org/figures-at-a-glance.html (accessed on 23 August 2017).
12. Bradby, H.; Humphris, R.; Newall, D.; Phillimore, J. Public health aspects of migrant health: A review of the evidence on health status for refugees and asylum seekers in the European Region. In *Health Evidence Network Synthesis Report 44*; WHO Regional Office for Europe: Copenhagen, Denmark, 2015.
13. Myria. *Migratie in Cijfers en in Rechten 2017*; Myria: Brussels, Belgium, 2017.
14. Morrison, L.G.; Yardley, L.; Powell, J.; Michie, S. What design features are used in effective e-health interventions? A review using techniques from critical interpretive synthesis. *Telemed. E-Health* **2012**, *18*, 137–144. [CrossRef] [PubMed]
15. Keygnaert, I.; Depraetere, J. Introduction. In *UN-MENAMAIS Literature Review: Understanding the Mechanisms, Nature, Magnitude and Impact of Sexual Violence in Belgium—A Critical Interpretative Synthesis*; Keygnaert, I., Ed.; Ghent University: Ghent, Belgium, 2018.
16. Dixon-Woods, M.; Cavers, D.; Agarwal, S.; Annandale, E.; Arthur, A.; Harvey, J.; Hsu, R.; Katbamna, S.; Olsen, R.; Smith, L.; et al. Conducting a critical interpretive synthesis of the literature on access to healthcare by vulnerable groups. *BMC Med. Res. Methodol.* **2006**, *6*, 35. [CrossRef] [PubMed]
17. Flemming, K. Synthesis of quantitative and qualitative research: An example using Critical Interpretive Synthesis. *J. Adv. Nurs.* **2010**, *66*, 201–217. [CrossRef] [PubMed]
18. Entwistle, V.; Firnigl, D.; Ryan, M.; Francis, J.; Kinghorn, P. Which experiences of health care delivery matter to service users and why? A critical interpretive synthesis and conceptual map. *J. Health Serv. Res. Policy* **2012**, *17*, 70–78. [CrossRef] [PubMed]
19. Bronfenbrenner, U. *The Ecology of Human Development: Experiments by Nature And Design*; Harvard University Press: Cambridge, MA, USA; London, UK, 1979; Volume 32, pp. 513–531.
20. Berk, L.E. *Child Development*, 7th ed.; Pearson Education: Boston, MA, USA, 2006.
21. Alberani, V.; De Castro Pietrangeli, P.; Mazza, A.M. The use of grey literature in health sciences: A preliminary survey. *Bull. Med. Libr. Assoc.* **1990**, *78*, 358–363. [PubMed]
22. McAuley, L.; Pham, B.; Tugwell, P.; Moher, D. Does the inclusion of grey literature influence estimates of intervention effectiveness reported in meta-analyses? *Lancet* **2000**, *356*, 1228–1231. [CrossRef]
23. Keygnaert, I.; Vettenburg, N.; Temmerman, M. Hidden violence is silent rape: Sexual and gender-based violence in refugees, asylum seekers and undocumented migrants in Belgium and the Netherlands. *Cult. Health Sex.* **2012**, *14*, 505–520. [CrossRef] [PubMed]
24. Watts, C.; Zimmerman, C. Violence against women: Global scope and magnitude. *Lancet* **2002**, *359*, 1232–1237. [CrossRef]
25. Keygnaert, I.; Dias, S.F.; Degomme, O.; Deville, W.; Kennedy, P.; Kovats, A.; De Meyer, S.; Vettenburg, N.; Roelens, K.; Temmerman, M. Sexual and gender-based violence in the European asylum and reception sector: A perpetuum mobile? *Eur. J. Public Health* **2014**, *25*, 90–96. [CrossRef] [PubMed]
26. Chauvin, P.; Simonnot, N.; Vanbiervliet, F.; Vicart, M.; Vuillermoz, C. *Access to Healthcare for People Facing Multiple Vulnerabilities in Health in 26 Cities Across 11 Countries: Report on the Social and Medical Data Gathered in 2014 in Nine European Countries, Turkey and Canada*; Doctors of the World-Médecins du Monde International Network: Paris, France, 2015.

27. Keygnaert, I.; Dialmy, A.; Manco, A.; Keygnaert, J.; Vettenburg, N.; Roelens, K.; Temmerman, M. Sexual violence and sub-Saharan migrants in Morocco: A community-based participatory assessment using respondent driven sampling. *Glob. Health* **2014**, *10*, 32. [CrossRef] [PubMed]
28. Refugee Council. *The Vulnerable Women's Project: Refugee and Asylum Seeking Women Affected by Rape or Sexual Violence. A Literature Review*; Refugee Council: London, UK, 2009; Volume 2, p. 2012.
29. Cohen, D.K.; Green, A.H.; Wood, E.J. *Wartime Sexual Violence*; USIP: Washington, DC, USA, 2013.
30. Cohen, D.K.; Nordås, R. Sexual violence in armed conflict: Introducing the SVAC dataset, 1989–2009. *J. Peace Res.* **2014**, *51*, 418–428. [CrossRef]
31. Wood, E.J. Sexual violence during war: Variation and accountability. In *Collective Crimes and International Criminal Justice: An Interdisciplinary Approach*; Intersentia: Antwerp, Belgium, 2010.
32. Deleu, N. *Naar een Inclusief Referentiecentrum Seksueel Geweld in België: Op Welke Manier Kan er rekEning Gehouden Worden Met Noden van Mensen Uit Door Oorlof Getroffen Gebieden?* Ghent University: Ghent, Belgium, 2016.
33. More than Numbers Regional Overview: Responding to Gender-Based Violence in the Syria Crisis. Available online: http://www.unfpa.org/sites/default/files/pub-pdf/unfpa_gbv_take10-may17-single41.pdf (accessed on 21 November 2017).
34. Vu, A.; Adam, A.; Wirtz, A.; Pham, K.; Rubenstein, L.; Glass, N.; Beyrer, C.; Singh, S. The Prevalence of sexual violence among female refugees in complex humanitarian emergencies: A systematic review and meta-analysis. *PLoS Curr.* **2014**. [CrossRef] [PubMed]
35. Jacobsen, K.; Landau, L.B. The dual imperative in refugee research: Some methodological and ethical considerations in social science research on forced migration. *Disasters* **2003**, *27*, 185–206. [CrossRef] [PubMed]
36. Düvell, F.; Triandafyllidou, A.; Vollmer, B. Ethical issues in irregular migration research in Europe. *Popul. Space Place* **2010**, *16*, 227–239. [CrossRef]
37. Stacciarini, J.M.; Shattell, M.M.; Coady, M.; Wiens, B. Community-based participatory research approach to address mental health in minority populations. *Community Ment. Health J.* **2011**, *47*, 489–497. [CrossRef] [PubMed]
38. Leye, E.; De Schrijver, L.; Van Baelen, L.; Andro, A.; Lesclingand, M.; Ortensi, L.; Farina, P. *Estimating FGM Prevalence in Europe. Findings of a Pilot Study. Research Report*; Ghent University: Ghent, Belgium, 2017.
39. Van Baelen, L.; De Schrijver, L.; Leye, E. Towards a better estimation of prevalence of female genital mutilation in the European Union: Situation analysis. Unpublished report. 2017.
40. Eapen, R.; Falcione, F.; Hersh, M.; Obser, K.; Shaar, A. *Initial Assessment Report: Protection Risks for Women and Girls in the European Refugee and Migrant Crisis*; UNHCR: Geneva, Switzerland, 2016.
41. Oosterhoff, P.; Zwanikken, P.; Ketting, E. Sexual torture of men in Croatia and other conflict situations: An open secret. *Reprod. Health Matters* **2004**, *12*, 68–77. [CrossRef]
42. De Schrijver, L. *Selective Disclosure bij Coming out: Een Exploratief Onderzoek bij Holebi's*; KU Leuven Faculteit Psychologie en Pedagogische Wetenschappen: Leuven, Belgium, 2013.
43. Bottoms, B.L.; Peter-Hagene, L.C.; Epstein, M.A.; Wiley, T.R.A.; Reynolds, C.E.; Rudnicki, A.G. Abuse characteristics and individual differences related to disclosing childhood sexual, physical, and emotional abuse and witnessed domestic violence. *J. Interpers. Violence* **2016**, *31*, 1308–1339. [CrossRef] [PubMed]
44. Vangelisti, A.; Caughlin, J.; Timmerman, L. Criteria for revealing family secrets. *Commun. Monogr.* **2001**, *68*, 1–27. [CrossRef]
45. Krug, E.G.; Mercy, J.A.; Dahlberg, L.L.; Zwi, A.B. The world report on violence and health. *Lancet* **2002**, *360*, 1083–1088. [CrossRef]
46. Peterson, Z.D.; Voller, E.K.; Polusny, M.A.; Murdoch, M. Prevalence and consequences of adult sexual assault of men: Review of empirical findings and state of the literature. *Clin. Psychol. Rev.* **2011**, *31*, 1–24. [CrossRef] [PubMed]
47. Peterson, Z.D.; Muehlenhard, C.L. Was it rape? The function of women's rape myth acceptance and definitions of sex in labeling their own experiences. *Sex Roles* **2004**, *51*, 129–144. [CrossRef]
48. Cook, S.L.; Gidycz, C.A.; Koss, M.P.; Murphy, M. Emerging issues in the measurement of rape victimization. *Violence Women* **2011**, *17*, 201–218. [CrossRef] [PubMed]

49. Black, M.C.; Basile, K.C.; Breiding, M.J.; Smith, S.G.; Walters, M.L.; Merrick, M.T.; Stevens, M.R. *The National Intimate Partner and Sexual Violence Survey: 2010 Summary Report*; National Center for Injury Prevention and Control, Centers for Disease Control and Prevention: Atlanta, GA, USA, 2011; Volume 19, pp. 39–40.
50. Bloom, S.S. *Violence against Women and Girls: A Compendium of Monitoring and Evaluation Indicators*; USAID: Washington, DC, USA, 2008.
51. Carpenter, R.C. Recognizing gender-based violence against civilian men and boys in conflict situations. *Secur. Dialogue* **2006**, *37*, 83–103. [CrossRef]
52. World Health Organization. *Preventing Intimate Partner and Sexual Violence against Women: Taking Action and Generating Evidence*; World Health Organization: Geneva, Switzerland, 2010.
53. Human Trafficking. Available online: https://www.unodc.org/unodc/en/human-trafficking/what-is-human-trafficking.html (accessed on 15 September 2017).
54. Miller, E.; Decker, M.R.; Silverman, J.G.; Raj, A. Migration, sexual exploitation, and women's health: A case report from a community health center. *Violence Women* **2007**, *13*, 486–497. [CrossRef] [PubMed]
55. Task Team on the SEA Glossary for the Special Coordinator on Improving the United Nations Response to Sexual Exploitation and Abuse. *United Nations Glossary on Sexual Exploitation and Abuse. Thematic Glossary of Current Terminology Related to Sexual Exploitation and Abuse (SEA) in the Context of the United Nations*; United Nations: New York, NY, USA, 2016.
56. Hume, D.L.; Sidun, N.M. *Human Trafficking of Women and Girls: Characteristics, Commonalities, and Complexities*; Taylor & Francis: Didcot, UK; Abingdon, UK, 2017.
57. Lopez, D.A.; Minassians, H. The Sexual Trafficking of Juveniles: A Theoretical Model. *Vict. Offenders* **2018**, *13*, 257–276. [CrossRef]
58. International Labour Organization (ILO). *Profits and Poverty: The Economics of Forced Labor*; International Labour Organization: Geneva, Switzerland, 2014.
59. Dennis, J.P. Women are victims, men make choices: The invisibility of men and boys in the global sex trade. *Gend. Issues* **2008**, *25*, 11–25. [CrossRef]
60. Oram, S.; Stöckl, H.; Busza, J.; Howard, L.M.; Zimmerman, C. Prevalence and risk of violence and the physical, mental, and sexual health problems associated with human trafficking: Systematic review. *PLoS Med.* **2012**, *9*, e1001224. [CrossRef] [PubMed]
61. Keygnaert, I.; Guieu, A. What the eye does not see: A critical interpretive synthesis of European Union policies addressing sexual violence in vulnerable migrants. *Reprod. Health Matters* **2015**, *23*, 45–55. [CrossRef] [PubMed]
62. Keygnaert, I.; Guieu, A.; Ooms, G.; Vettenburg, N.; Temmerman, M.; Roelens, K. Sexual and reproductive health of migrants: Does the EU care? *Health Policy* **2014**, *114*, 215–225. [CrossRef] [PubMed]
63. Amnesty International. *Crimes of Hate, Conspiracy of Silence: Torture and Ill-Treatment Based on Sexual Identity*; Amnesty International: London, UK, 2001.
64. Wood, E.J. Variation in sexual violence during war. *Politics Soc.* **2006**, *34*, 307–342. [CrossRef]
65. Wood, E.J. Armed groups and sexual violence: When is wartime rape rare? *Politics Soc.* **2009**, *37*, 131–161. [CrossRef]
66. Bastick, M.; Grimm, K.; Kunz, R. *Sexual Violence in Armed Conflict*; Center for the Democratic Control of Armed Forces: Geneva, Switzerland, 2007.
67. Carlson, E.S. The hidden prevalence of male sexual assault during war: Observations on blunt trauma to the male genitals. *Br. J. Criminol.* **2005**, *46*, 16–25. [CrossRef]
68. Krahé, B.; Vanwesenbeeck, I. Mapping an agenda for the study of youth sexual aggression in Europe: Assessment, principles of good practice, and the multilevel analysis of risk factors. *J. Sex. Aggress.* **2016**, *22*, 161–176. [CrossRef]
69. Krebs, C.P.; Lindquist, C.H.; Warner, T.D.; Fisher, B.S.; Martin, S.L.; Childers, J.M. Comparing sexual assault prevalence estimates obtained with direct and indirect questioning techniques. *Violence Women* **2011**, *17*, 219–235. [CrossRef] [PubMed]
70. Stark, L.; Ager, A. A systematic review of prevalence studies of gender-based violence in complex emergencies. *Trauma Violence Abuse* **2011**, *12*, 127–134. [CrossRef] [PubMed]

71. Kuyper, L.; Wijsen, C.; de Wit, J. Distress, need for help, and positive feelings derived from participation in sex research: Findings of a population study in the Netherlands. *J. Sex Res.* **2014**, *51*, 351–358. [CrossRef] [PubMed]
72. Yeater, E.; Miller, G.; Rinehart, J.; Nason, E. Trauma and sex surveys meet minimal risk standards: Implications for institutional review boards. *Psychol. Sci.* **2012**, *23*, 780–787. [CrossRef] [PubMed]

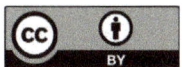

© 2018 by the authors. Licensee MDPI, Basel, Switzerland. This article is an open access article distributed under the terms and conditions of the Creative Commons Attribution (CC BY) license (http://creativecommons.org/licenses/by/4.0/).

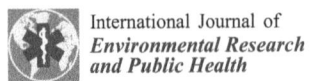

Review

The Effectiveness and Cost-Effectiveness of Hepatitis C Screening for Migrants in the EU/EEA: A Systematic Review

Christina Greenaway [1,2,3,*], Iuliia Makarenko [2], Claire Nour Abou Chakra [4], Balqis Alabdulkarim [2], Robin Christensen [5], Adam Palayew [3], Anh Tran [6], Lukas Staub [6], Manish Pareek [7], Joerg J. Meerpohl [8], Teymur Noori [9], Irene Veldhuijzen [10], Kevin Pottie [11,12], Francesco Castelli [13,†,‡] and Rachael L. Morton [6]

1. Division of Infectious Diseases, Jewish General Hospital, McGill University, Montreal, QC H3T 1E2, Canada
2. Centre for Clinical Epidemiology of the Lady Davis Institute for Medical Research, Jewish General Hospital, Montreal, QC H3T 1E2, Canada; makarenko.j@gmail.com (I.M.); Balqis.alabdulkarim@mail.mcgill.ca (B.A.)
3. Department of Epidemiology, Biostatistics, and Occupational Health, McGill University, Montreal, QC H3A 1A2, Canada; apalayew@gmail.com
4. Department of Microbiology and Infectious Diseases, Université de Sherbrooke, Sherbrooke, QC J1H 5N4, Canada; Claire.Nour.Abou.Chakra@USherbrooke.ca
5. Musculoskeletal Statistics Unit, The Parker Institute, Bispebjerg and Frederiksberg Hospital & Department of Rheumatology, Odense University Hospital, DK2000 Odense, Denmark; Robin.Christensen@regionh.dk
6. NHMRC Clinical Trials Centre, The University of Sydney, Sydney 1450, Australia; anh.tran@ctc.usyd.edu.au (A.T.); lukas.staub@ctc.usyd.edu.au (L.S.); Rachael.morton@ctc.usyd.edu.au (R.L.M.)
7. Department of Infection, Immunity and Inflammation, University of Leicester, Leicester LE1 7RH, UK; manish.pareek@leicester.ac.uk
8. Institute for Evidence in Medicine (for Cochrane Germany Foundation), Medical Center, University of Freiburg, 79110 Freiburg, Germany; meerpohl@ifem.uni-freiburg.de
9. European Centre for Disease Prevention and Control, 169 73 Solna, Sweden; teymur.noori@ecdc.europa.eu
10. Centre for Infectious Disease Control, National Institute for Public Health and the Environment (RIVM), 3720 BA Bilthoven, The Netherlands; irene.veldhuijzen@rivm.nl
11. C.T. Lamont Primary Health Care Research Centre, Bruyère Research Institute, Ottawa, ON K1N 5C8, Canada; kpottie@uottawa.ca
12. Centre for Global Health, University of Ottawa, Ottawa, ON K1N 5C8, Canada
13. Division of Infectious Diseases, University of Brescia, 255123 Brescia, Italy; francesco.castelli@unibs.it
* Correspondence: ca.greenaway@mcgill.ca; Tel.: +1-514-340-8222; Fax: +1-514-340-7546
† UNESCO Chair holder "Training and empowering human resources for health development in resource-limited countries".
‡ The authors are responsible for the choice and presentation of views contained in this article and for opinions expressed therein, which are not necessarily those of UNESCO and do not commit the Organization.

Received: 17 July 2018; Accepted: 10 September 2018; Published: 14 September 2018

Abstract: Chronic hepatitis C (HCV) is a public health priority in the European Union/European Economic Area (EU/EEA) and is a leading cause of chronic liver disease and liver cancer. Migrants account for a disproportionate number of HCV cases in the EU/EEA (mean 14% of cases and >50% of cases in some countries). We conducted two systematic reviews (SR) to estimate the effectiveness and cost-effectiveness of HCV screening for migrants living in the EU/EEA. We found that screening tests for HCV are highly sensitive and specific. Clinical trials report direct acting antiviral (DAA) therapies are well-tolerated in a wide range of populations and cure almost all cases (>95%) and lead to an 85% lower risk of developing hepatocellular carcinoma and an 80% lower risk of all-cause mortality. At 2015 costs, DAA based regimens were only moderately cost-effective and as a result less than 30% of people with HCV had been screened and less 5% of all HCV cases had been treated in the EU/EEA in 2015. Migrants face additional barriers in linkage to care and treatment due to several patient, practitioner, and health system barriers. Although decreasing HCV costs have made treatment more accessible in the EU/EEA, HCV elimination will only be possible in the region if health systems include and treat migrants for HCV.

Keywords: hepatitis C; screening; migrants; viral hepatitis elimination; European Union

1. Introduction

Chronic hepatitis C is an important public health problem in the EU/EEA, with an estimated 3.24 million persons having active hepatitis C virus (HCV) infection [1,2]. It is a leading cause of chronic liver disease and liver cancer in the EU/EEA due to undetected and untreated infections [3–5]. Since 2013, the landscape of HCV treatment has changed rapidly as pan-genotypic DAA HCV treatment regimens that cure most infections (>95% of cases) have become available, making HCV elimination possible [6–9]. In 2015 however, only 34% of HCV infected persons had been diagnosed and less than 5% of all HCV cases had been treated [2]. Identifying and treating all groups at risk for HCV in the EU/EEA will be essential to address the health and economic burden due to HCV in the EU/EEA and to reach WHO elimination goals by 2030 [3,5,9–11].

HCV screening and control programs in the EU/EEA primarily focus on persons who inject drugs (PWID), as they are the largest and highest burden population [1]. Migrants from intermediate and high HCV prevalence countries (anti-HCV $\geq$ 2% and $\geq$5%, respectively) are an additional important and underappreciated group at increased HCV risk in the EU/EEA and often do not have identifiable HCV risk factors [12,13]. They are most likely to have been exposed to HCV in their countries of origin through receipt of contaminated blood products or unsafe injections or procedures, and have a prevalence of HCV that reflects that of their countries of origin [14,15]. The increased flow of migrants from intermediate and high HCV prevalence countries into the EU/EEA over the past few decades has resulted in a disproportionately high number of reported HCV cases (14%) occurring among migrants, who account for up to one half of all cases in some low HCV prevalence EU/EEA countries [12,13]. HCV diagnosis among migrants living in low incidence countries is delayed due to several patient, practitioner, and infrastructural barriers that may result in a higher burden of liver-associated complications compared to host populations [16,17]. We conducted a systematic review (SR) to estimate the effectiveness, resource use, costs, and cost-effectiveness of HCV screening programs for migrants in the EU/EEA.

2. Methods

2.1. Overall Approach and Key Questions

Using the Grading of Recommendations Assessment, Development, and Evaluation (GRADE) approach, the Campbell and Cochrane Collaboration Equity Methods Group and review team including clinicians, public health experts and researchers from across the EU/EEA, we conducted evidence syntheses. "Migrants", a focus of this review, included asylum seekers, refugees, undocumented migrants, and other foreign-born residents. A detailed description of the methods have been published and were registered in PROSPERO (CRD42016045798) [18].

We used the GRADE approach to rate the certainty of evidence starting with a simplified categorization of study types (i.e., meta-analyses, RCTs, and observational studies). The rating scheme allows for factors that may raise or lower the level of certainty. Factors that lower certainty of evidence include, risk of bias, inconsistency across studies, indirectness, and publication bias. Factors that increase certainty of evidence include large effect size and an observed dose-response effect. The final certainty ratings are reflective of the certainty in the estimated effect in the context of bias and limitations. Evidence was graded as high, moderate, low, or very low certainty, based on how likely further research would change the confidence in the estimate of effect. Low certainty and very low certainty do not mean absence of evidence for effectiveness, but rather signal highlights the need for more research to improve the precision of the estimate of effect.

This review followed the Grading of Recommendations Assessment, Development, and Evaluation (GRADE) and Cochrane methodological approach [18]. We used the Preferred Reporting Items for Systematic Reviews and Meta-Analyses (PRISMA) Checklist for reporting the results of the systematic reviews (SR) [18,19]. The review team developed two overarching research questions (PICO: Population, Intervention, Comparison, Outcome) and a logic model (Figure S1). The logic model showed key questions/concepts along the evidence chain along the screening effectiveness pathway [18,20,21]. The two overarching research questions (PICO) we sought to answer were:

- What is the effectiveness of screening migrants arriving and living in the EU/EEA for HCV?
- What is the cost, resource utilization, and cost-effectiveness for screening migrants for HCV?

The following key questions were identified along the screening effectiveness pathway. (1) What is the test accuracy and performance characteristics of screening tests for HCV? (2) What is the efficacy of new direct acting antiviral (DAA) treatments for HCV to decrease HCV associated morbidity and mortality? (3) What is the uptake of HCV of screening and treatment? (4) What is the cost-effectiveness of a screen-treat approach for HCV in the general population and the migrant population when treated with DAAs? [18].

2.2. Search Strategy and Selection Criteria

We conducted two searches, one for SRs and guidelines on the effectiveness and cost-effectiveness of HCV screening programs in migrants and a second search for SRs and primary studies on the resource use, costs, and cost-effectiveness of HCV screening programs in migrants. For the first search, Medline via OVID, EMBASE, CINAHL, Epistemonikos, and Cochrane CENTRAL were searched for publications between 1 January 2010 and 12 May 2016. A combination of key terms was used including "hepatitis C/HCV", "screening", "migrants", "costs", "cost-effectiveness" AND "guidelines", and "reviews". The search terms and the search strategy for Ovid Medline are included in the supplementary material (Table S1). We also searched grey literature websites for published guidelines and reports at CDC, ECDC, EASL (European Association for the Study of the Liver), and WHO. We applied no language restrictions to the search. In the second search, using terms of "hepatitis C/HCV", "screening", "costs", and "cost-effectiveness", Medline via Ovid, EMBASE, the NHS Economic Evaluation Database (NHS EED), Database of Abstracts of Reviews of Effects (DARE), and the Cost Effectiveness Analysis Tufts registry and Google scholar databases were searched for publications between 1 January 2000 and 31 May 2016. Reference lists of relevant reviews were also searched.

2.3. Study Selection and Quality Assessment

Two authors screened the titles and abstracts, assessed selected full-text articles for eligibility, and extracted data from included articles. Disagreements were resolved by consensus or by a third author. For the screening effectiveness search we included systematic reviews on the impact of HCV screening or antiviral therapies on the development of liver related morbidities such as cirrhosis, hepatocellular carcinoma, and the need for liver transplantation and all-cause or attributable mortality. For the cost-effectiveness search we included individual economic studies of screening strategies that included an arm of direct acting antiviral (DAA) therapies or studies of the cost-effectiveness of DAA therapies [8]. We only included studies published in full and in English or French. If more than one version of a SR was identified, the most recent was considered. Studies were excluded if they focused only on nongeneralizable subgroups (such as PWIDs) (Figures 1 and 2).

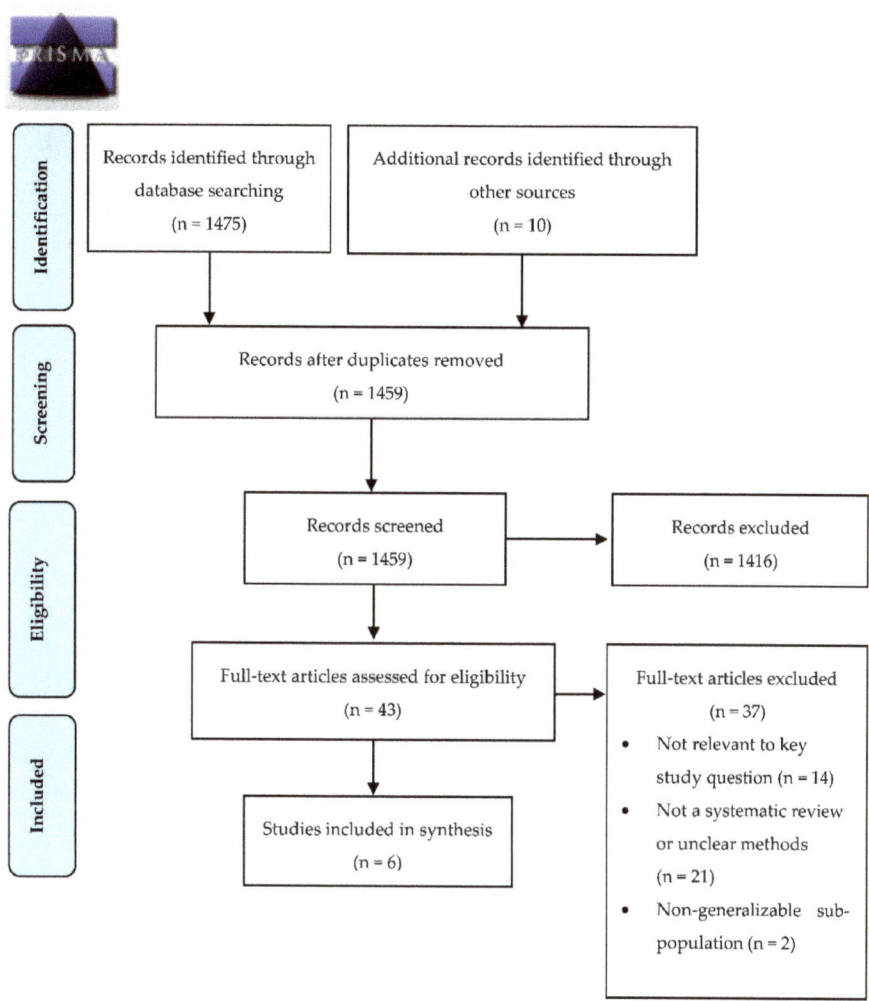

Figure 1. Preferred Reporting Items for Systematic Reviews and Meta-Analyses (PRISMA) diagram for the effectiveness of hepatitis C screening.

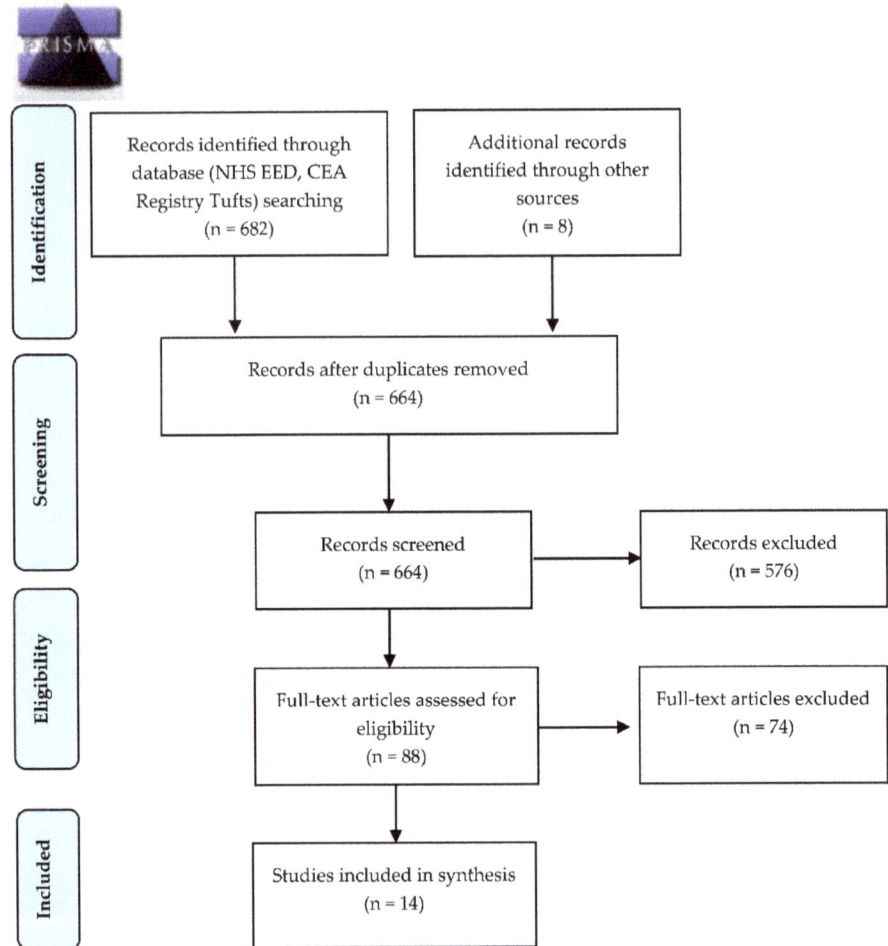

Figure 2. PRISMA diagram for the resource use, costs, and cost-effectiveness for hepatitis C screening.

The methodologic quality of SRs was assessed by two authors using the AMSTAR tool (A Measurement Tool to Assess Systematic Reviews) [22]. The GRADE criteria were applied to assess the certainty of evidence in preselected outcome measures in the SRs (GRADE Tables S2–S5) [23]. For the second search which included individual studies the certainty of economic evidence in each study was assessed using the relevant items from the 1997 Drummond checklist [24].

2.4. Data Extraction and Synthesis

The following information was extracted from each study: study design, objectives, analyses, quality of the individual studies included in the systematic review, population examined, number of included studies, total number of participants included, intervention, outcome, and the results. For the economic studies we extracted the following data; economic methods used (e.g., microcosting study, within-trial cost–utility analysis, Markov model), description of the case base population, the intervention and comparator, absolute size and relative difference in resource use, cost-effectiveness results (e.g., incremental net benefit (INB) or incremental cost-effectiveness ratio (ICER)), and three specific questions for the GRADE Evidence to Decision table: the size of the resource requirements, the certainty of evidence around resource requirements, and whether the cost-effectiveness results favored the intervention or comparison [25]. Key results were converted to 2015 Euros using the Cochrane web-based currency conversion tool: https://eppi.ioe.ac.uk/costconversion/default.aspx.

3. Results

3.1. Search Results

In the search for the effectiveness of HCV screening we retrieved 1475 references and identified 10 additional records through other sources (Figure 1). After duplicates were removed, 1459 references were screened by title and abstract. A total of 43 references were then selected for full text assessment. We did not identify any randomized controlled trials or SRs on the effectiveness of HCV screening in the general or migrant populations. We therefore included five SRs and one guideline that addressed the key questions along the screening evidence chain: the performance of HCV diagnostic tests (n = 2) [6,26], the impact of HCV treatment on preventing HCC and all-cause mortality (n = 3) [27–29], and the HCV care continuum (n = 1) (Table 1) [30]. In the economic search, 682 articles were retrieved and an additional eight records identified through other sources (Figure 2). After duplicate removal, 664 references were screened by title and abstracts. Of these, a total of 88 references underwent full text assessment and 14 individual studies of populations living in low HCV prevalence countries were included (Table 2) [31–44].

3.2. Performance of Diagnostic Tests

The performance of diagnostic testing for HCV has been recently summarized in the 2017 WHO Guidelines on Hepatitis B and C testing [6]. WHO estimates the sensitivity and specificity of 3rd generation HCV enzyme immunoassays (EIA) to be 98% and 99%, respectively [6]. Similarly, the sensitivity of the confirmatory test to detect virus nucleic acid (nucleic acid test; NATs) is estimated to be 96.2% (95% CI, 94.4–97.5) and the specificity to be 98.9% (98.3–99.3) [6]. There was no reported evidence suggesting that migrants or any other group would encounter lower performance rates. The accuracy of point of care testing, a strategy that potentially could increase screening uptake, was reviewed by Khuroo et al. who found that these tests performed well in low, middle, and high income countries [26]. The sensitivity (95.8% (93.9–97.1)) was slightly lower compared to EIAs but demonstrated comparable specificity (99.0% (98.5–99.3)) [26]. The GRADE certainty of the evidence in the Khuroo study was very low (S3 GRADE Table 1).

Table 1. Characteristics of studies on the effectiveness of hepatitis C screening.

Study	Quality of Systematic Review/GRADE Certainty of Evidence	Design	Population	Intervention/Outcomes	Results
Khuroo 2015 [26]	Quality of systematic Review AMSTAR: 8/11 GRADE Certainty of Evidence Very Low	Systematic Review Up to March 2012. N = 30 studies: 25—full-text article 2—WHO reports 1—WHO draft report 2—letters to editor	Adults > 18 years 17,151 participants 16 studies were conducted in low/middle income countries (India n = 4, Brazil n = 2, Cameroon n = 2, China n = 2, Egypt n = 1, Malawi n = 1, South Korea n = 2, Thailand n = 1, and Zimbabwe n = 1) 14 studies conducted in high income countries (United States n = 8, Germany n = 1, Italy n = 1, Spain n = 1) (Report for WHO n = 3)	**Intervention:** Point-of-care test: any commercially available assay at or near the site of patient care with <30 min turn-around time. Reference standard: third generation EIA, microenzyme immunoassay, CIA, RIBA, NAT **Outcome:** Sensitivity, specificity, LR+/−, Diagnostic OR (95% CI)	Pooled sensitivity: 97.4% (95% CI = 95.9–98.4) specificity: 99.5% (99.2–99.7) +LR: 80.17 (55.35–116.14) −LR: 0.03 (0.02–0.04) Diagnostic OR: 3032.85 (1595.86–5763.78) OraQuick test had the highest sensitivity and specificity: sensitivity: 99.5 (98.9–99.8) specificity: 99.8 (99.6–99.9)
Kimer 2012 [27]	Quality of systematic Review AMSTAR: 7/11 GRADE Certainty of Evidence Very Low	Systematic Review Up to 2012 N = eight RCTs, five prospective cohorts	RCTs conducted in France, Italy, Spain, Japan, and USA in patients with HCV-related cirrhosis or fibrosis and treated with antiviral therapy 1156 patients with therapy 1074 controls Prospective cohorts: Patients with HCV-related cirrhosis	**Intervention:** Antiviral therapy (PR, IFN, PEG-IFN) **Outcome:** RR, 95% CI of HCC development; number needed to treat to prevent 1 case of HCC = 1/risk difference overall mortality liver-related mortality liver-related morbidity	Risk of HCC among received antiviral therapy vs. did not receive: Absolute number of HCC: 81/1156 vs. 129/1174 RR (95% CI): 0.53 (0.34–0.81) SVR and non-SVR compared to no therapy—RR (95% CI): SVR: RR = 0.15 (0.05–0.45) Non-SVR: RR = 0.57 (0.37–0.85) Number needed to treat to prevent one case of HCC: eight patients.
Simmons 2015 [28]	Quality of systematic Review AMSTAR: 8/11 GRADE Certainty of Evidence Very low to low	Systematic Review 1990–2014 N = 31 studies: General population: 17 studies; Cirrhotic: nine studies; HIV co-infected: five studies	Adults (>18 years old) chronically infected with HCV of any genotype treated with any antiviral regimen stratified into 3 groups: 1- patients at any disease stage 2- cirrhotic patients 3- HIV/HCV co-infected Total: 33,336 participants General population: 28,398 Cirrhotic: 2604 HIV co-infected: 2358	**Intervention:** PR; IFN; PEG-IFN; IFN-beta **Outcome:** all-cause mortality; pooled adjusted HR (95% CI); pooled estimates for the 5-year mortality	Mortality of achieved SVR vs. non-SVR, aHR (95% CI): General population: 0.50 (0.37–0.67) Cirrhotic group: 0.26 (0.18–0.74) HIV co-infected group: 0.21 (0.10–0.45) Pooled 5-year mortality rates for SVR vs. non-SVR, IR (95% CI): General population: 1.98 (1.00–3.45) vs. 7.75 (5.86–10.98) Cirrhotic group: 4.90 (3.45–7.28) vs. 15.88 (11.44–21.80) Co-infected group: 1.49 (0.50–2.96) vs. 11.44 (6.33–19.3)

Table 1. Cont.

Study	Quality of Systematic Review/CRADE Certainty of Evidence	Design	Population	Intervention/Outcomes	Results
Public Health Agency of Canada, Canadian Task Force on Preventative Health Care 2016 [29]	Quality of Systematic Review AMSTAR: 11/11 GRADE Certainty of Evidence Very low to moderate	Systematic Review Up to November 2015 N = Benefits of treatment: 11 studies; Harms of treatment: 7	Treatment-naïve nonpregnant HIV/HBV negative adults Wide range of fibrosis scores +80% noncirrhotic RCTs (n = 7) 6/7 RCTs all patients were Genotype 1 2431 participants ranged from 121 to 499 participants in a study. Recruitment sites included: United States, Australia, Austria, Belgium, Canada, Denmark, France, Germany, New Zealand, Norway, Poland, Russia, Spain, Japan, Italy, Mexico, Puerto Rico, Romania, Ukraine, United Kingdom, Sweden, the Netherlands, Bulgaria, Portugal, Slovakia, China, and the Republic of Korea.	**Intervention:** DAA-based vs. PR regimens. DDA therapies included those that were approved at the time of the study and those anticipated to be approved by February 2016 for all HCV genotypes. **Outcomes:** All-cause mortality; hepatic mortality; hepatic decompensation; hepatocellular carcinoma; need for liver transplantation.	Hepatic mortality: 60 fewer/1000 (95% CI 59–62) Hepatocellular carcinoma: 18 fewer/1000 (17–19) Decompensated cirrhosis: 46 fewer/1000 (46–47) Need for liver transplantation: 4 fewer/1000 (4–6) In cirrhotic individuals DAA-based regimens compared to PR resulted in 30 fewer/1000 people affected by hepatic mortality.
Yehia 2014 [30]	Quality of systematic Review AMSTAR: 3/1 Data quality not formally assessed	Systematic Review 2003–2013 N = 10 studies	Only studies from the US that collected data after 2000 were included. Studies of the general population excluded those with only a single study site, exclusively focused on specific populations (e.g., only immigrants, injection drug users, those with HIV/HCV co-infection) **Study subjects for each question** Chronic infection: 15,079 Diagnosed/Aware: 203 Access to Care: 101 HCV RNA confirmed: 8810 Liver biopsy: 180,703 Prescribed HCV treatment: 46,452 Achieved SVR: 18,105	Examined data addressing seven key steps along the HCV care and treatment cascade	**Care/Treatment cascade:** 100% Chronic HCV infected (3,500,000) 50% Diagnosed and aware 43% Access to outpatient care 27% HCV RNA confirmed 17% Underwent liver biopsy 16% Prescribed HCV treatment 9% Achieved SVR

AMSTAR: A MeaSurement Tool to Assess systematic Reviews [22]; aHR: adjusted hazard ratio; CI: confidence interval; CIA: chemiluminescence immunoassay; DAA: direct acting antiviral; EIA: enzyme immunoassay; GRADE: the grading of recommendation assessment, development and evaluation; HCC: hepatocellular carcinoma; HCV: hepatitis C virus; HIV: human immunodeficiency virus; HR: hazard ratio; IFN: interferon; IR: incidence rate; LR: likelihood ratio; NAT: nucleic acid test; OR: odds ratio; PEG-IFN: pegylated interferon; PR: pegylated-interferon-ribavirin; RBV: ribavirin; RCT: randomized controlled trial; RIBA: recombinant immunoblot assay; RNA: ribonucleic acid; RR: risk ratio; SVR: sustained virological response; US: United States; WHO: World Health Organization.

3.3. Impact of Therapy on Long-Term Outcomes

Interferon free DAAs are the recommended therapy for all HCV genotypes in the EU/EEA [8]. These regimens are well tolerated and cure > 95% of cases based on achieving sustained virologic response (SVR0, which is considered to be a reliable surrogate outcome for HCV cure) [7,8]. Within the search dates we did not identify any studies that examined the impact of DAA therapies on long-term HCV liver related outcomes or mortality, as these agents only became available in 2013. Three SRs that assessed the impact of older interferon (IFN) based HCV treatment on preventing liver related sequelae and all-cause mortality were included [27–29]. These three SRs included studies from Europe, North America, Australia, and Asia, and found that IFN-based HCV therapy significantly decreased rates of hepatocellular carcinoma (HCC), hepatic decompensation, and all-cause mortality in those on HCV treatment, and particularly in those who achieved SVR [27–29]. In a meta-analysis by Kimer et al., the risk of HCC was lower in those on antiviral HCV therapy (IFN or PEG-IFN alone or with ribavirin) compared to placebo or no intervention (RR = 0.53, 95% CI 0.34–0.81). This effect was much more pronounced among virological responders compared to nonresponders [27]. In the SR by Simmons et al., the adjusted hazard ratio (aHR) of all-cause mortality rate was lower in patients on treatment for chronic HCV after a median follow-up time of 5.4 years [28]. In those achieving SVR, compared with non-SVR, the aHR was 0.50 (95% CI: 0.37–0.67) in the general population, and 0.26 (95% CI: 0.18–0.37) in the cirrhotic group [28]. Finally, in the SR conducted by the Public Health Agency of Canada (PHAC), a reduction in hepatic mortality (60 fewer/1000, 95% CI: 59–62), HCC (18 fewer/1000, 95% CI: 17–19), hepatic decompensation or decompensated cirrhosis (46 fewer/1000, 95% CI: 46–47), and need for liver transplantation (4 fewer/1000, 95% CI: 4–5) among those treated with DAA to PEG-IFN was found [29]. The GRADE certainty of the evidence of the data in these three systematic reviews was very low to moderate (GRADE Tables S3–S5).

3.4. The HCV Care Continuum and Pathway

In a SR of studies of the HCV care continuum in the pre-DAA period among in the general population in the US from 2003–2013, only 50% of HCV cases were diagnosed and aware of their infection, 27% had HCV RNA confirmatory testing, 16% were prescribed HCV therapy, and 9% achieved SVR [30]. The results of this study were not stratified by risk group nor did they report on the barriers to uptake of the steps along the care cascade. A modeling study in Europe published after the search timeframe also demonstrated a weak HCV care continuum in 2015, consistent with the US SR by Yehia [2]. They found that in Europe in 2015, only 36% of HCV infected persons have been screened and, of those diagnosed, only 12.7% and 11.3% had been treated and cured, respectively [2]. They found that, to achieve WHO elimination targets, expansion of screening programs in the EU/EAA would be needed along with unrestricted access to treatment for all found to be infected.

3.5. Resource Use, Costs and Cost-Effectiveness

Screening for HCV in those treated with DAAs is cost-effective even at higher 2015 costs. A UK study evaluated the cost-effectiveness of screening and treating pregnant women attending antenatal clinics [44]. The incremental cost effectiveness ratio (ICER) for screening and treatment (PR) compared with no screening and no treatment was £2400 (€2745) per QALY gained. For screening and treating with DAAs compared with no screening and no treatment, the ICER was still cost-effective at £9139 (€10,455)/QALY gained. A Canadian study evaluated the cost-effectiveness of screening for HCV in different age groups and then treating with DAAs in the Canadian population where the HCV seroprevalence ranged from 0.3 to 0.8% [32]. The ICER for IFN-free DAAs vs. older therapies ranged from CAN$34,359 (€21,977) to CAN$44,034 (€28,166) per QALY gained [32]. In the US, Rein et al. found that screening followed by DAA therapy was moderately cost-effective with ICERs ranging from US$47,237 (€40,665) to US$72,169 (€62,128) per QALY gained [36].

The Drummond Criteria [24]: (i) Was a well-defined question posed in answerable form? (ii) Was a comprehensive description of the competing alternatives given (i.e., can you tell who did what to whom, where, and how often)? (iii) Was the effectiveness of the program or services established? (iv) Were all the important and relevant costs and consequences for each alternative identified? (v) Were costs and consequences measured accurately in appropriate physical units (e.g., hours of nursing time, number of physician visits, lost working days, and gained life years)? (vi) Were the cost and consequences valued credibly? (vii) Were costs and consequences adjusted for differential timing? (viii) Was an incremental analysis of costs and consequences of alternatives performed? (ix) Was allowance made for uncertainty in the estimates of costs and consequences? (x) Did the presentation and discussion of study results include all issues of concern to users?

Non-pan-genotypic DAA therapies have also been found to be moderately cost-effective, however they had a large budget impact at the 2015 cost of treatment [31]. Deuffic-Burban found that DAAs were moderately cost-effective for genotypes 1 and 4 regardless of fibrosis stage, ranging from €40,000 to €88,000 per quality-adjusted life year (QALY) gained (Table 2). IFN-based regimens were estimated to be more cost-effective for genotypes 2 or 3 at €21,300 to €19,400 per QALY gained regardless of fibrosis stage [31]. DAAs were found to be moderately cost-effective for genotype 1 & 4 at a median threshold of €24,000/QALY gained and maximum upper limit of €80,000/QALY gained however, introducing these regimens on a wide scale would have a substantial budget impact of €3.5–7.2 billion on the French health care system [31,45]. Several US studies have evaluated the cost-effectiveness of DAA therapies compared to older PEG-INF-RBV therapies and found that DAA therapies were moderately cost-effective at a willingness-to-pay threshold of $50,000 US (€39,210), but varied significantly by HCV genotype, presence of liver fibrosis, and treatment history [33–38]. In the US, DAAs were moderately cost-effective for genotypes 1 & 4 whereas IFN-RBV was more cost-effective for genotypes 2 & 3. DAAs were more cost-effective in the presence of cirrhosis and treatment naïve patients. Providing DAAs to all eligible HCV patients would also have a huge budget impact, costing an additional US$65 (€56) billion over a 5-year period, whereas the resulting cost-offsets were estimated at only US$16 (€14) billion [34].

Table 2. Included studies on the cost, resource use, and cost-effectiveness of HCV screening and direct acting antiviral therapies.

Study	Quality/Certainty of Economic Evidence	Design/Population	Intervention(s)	Cost-Effectiveness (ICER or INB)	Resource Requirements
Cost-effectiveness of HCV Screening and DAA therapy					
Brett-Major 2016 [41]	Certainty of evidence: moderate Allowance was made for uncertainty in the estimates of costs, HCV rates, and ranges were provided. Threshold sensitivity analysis undertaken. PSA not performed. Justification for choice of ranges was provided for all parameters. Cost offsets (and net savings) rather than cost-effectiveness was reported	**Design:** Decision-analytic costing model; results reported in US dollars **Population:** Applicants to US military service HCV prevalence 0.48–0.98/1000	**Three strategies:** 1- Enzyme immunoassay (EIA) screening 2- EIA + nucleic acid testing (NAT) screening 3- no screening Treatment with SOF based regimens	Not applicable (Costing study)	High costs. With no screening, the cost to the Department of Defence of treating the estimated 93 cases of chronic HCV cases from a single year's accession cohort was $9.3 million [€7,293,134]. Screening with the HCV antibody test followed by the nucleic acid test for confirmation yielded a net annual savings and a $3.1 million dollar [€2,431,04] advantage over not screening.
He 2016 [42]	Certainty of evidence: moderate Allowance was made for uncertainty in the estimates of costs and consequences, and ranges were provided. PSA not performed. Justification for choice of ranges was not provided for all parameters. Cost-effectiveness results were sensitive to the time horizon.	**Design:** Dynamic microsimulation model of transmission/progression of HCV, and cost-effectiveness and budget impact analysis; results reported in US dollars **Population:** Population in US prisons HCV prevalence 25% and 50% undiagnosed	**Three strategies:** 1- risk-based screening 2- universal opt-out screening 3- no screening Treatment with SOF based regimens	ICER ($/QALY gained): **1 year risk-based vs. no screening:** $19,635 [€15,552] **1 year universal vs. no screening:** $20,571 [€16,293] **5 year universal vs. no screening:** $24,046 [€19,046] **10 year universal vs. no screening:** $29,234 [€23,155]	Low to moderate costs. **Screening cost per 2 million prisoners:** 1year risk-based vs. no screening: +$37M [€29M] 1year universal vs. no screening: +$107M [€84M] 5year universal vs. no screening: +$178M [€140M] 10year universal vs. no screening: +$249M [€197M] **Treatment cost per 2 million prisoners:** No Screening: $59,035M [€46,759M] 1year risk-based vs. no screening: +$816M [€646M] 1year universal vs. no screening: +$1480M [€1172M] 5year universal vs. no screening: +$1951M [€1545M] 10year universal vs. no screening: +$2190M [€1734M]

Table 2. Cont.

Study	Quality/Certainty of Economic Evidence	Design/Population	Intervention(s)	Cost-Effectiveness (ICER or INB)	Resource Requirements
Cost-effectiveness of HCV Screening and DAA therapy					
Orkin 2016 [43]	Certainty of evidence: low. Allowance was not made for uncertainty in the estimates of costs and consequences. No source for unit prices (costs) was given. PSA not performed. Justification for choice of ranges was not provided for all parameters. Cost-effectiveness results were not reported.	**Design:** Prospective 1 week-long snapshot observational study with assumed costs for testing and treating; results reported in British pounds. **Population:** People visiting emergency departments in the UK. HCV prevalence 1.84%	**One strategy:** Routine combined HIV, HCV, and HBV testing	Not applicable	Low to moderate costs. Assuming the cost per diagnosis is £7 [€8], the cost per new case detected would be £988 [€1109] for HCV, £1351 [€1517] for HBV, and £2478 [€2783] for HIV.
Rein 2015 [36]	Certainty of evidence: high. Allowance was made for uncertainty in the estimates of costs and consequences, and ranges were provided. PSA was performed. Justification for choice of ranges was provided for all parameters. Cost-effectiveness results were sensitive to treatment cost, SVR probability, QALY post SVR, fibrosis rate	**Design:** Monte Carlo simulation model; results presented in US dollars. **Population:** General population aged ≥20, and patients with chronic HCV genotype 1, 2, 3, and 4 in US. HCV prevalence rate: varies by birth decade, race, and sex. Heavy alcoholics 0.089 HIV+ 0.02	Screening followed by treatment **Five strategies:** 1- PR 2- PI+PR 3- SOF+PR 4- SOF+SIM 5- SOF+RBV	**Genotype 1/4—ICER ($/QALY):** PR vs. no treatment: $59,792 [€47,359] PR extensively dominated by PI+PR PI + PR vs. no treatment:$43,530 [€34,478] SOF+PR vs. PI+PR: $47,237 [€37,414] SOF+SIM vs. SOF+PR: $72,169 [€57,162]	Treatment costs: **Genotype 1&4:** PR: $61,224 [€48,493] PI+PR: $78,812 [€62,424] SOF+PR: $99,306 [€78,656] SOF+SIM: $150,360 [€119,094] **Genotype 2:** PR: $30,612 [€24,246] SOF+RBV: $88,158 [€69,826] **Genotype 3:** PR: $30,612 [€24,246] SOF+RBV: $176,316 [€139,653] Other costs: Testing: antibody: $25 [€19] RNA: $59 [€45] Post-diagnostic evaluation: if coordinated with treatment: $832 [€658] if not treated: $869 [€688]

Table 2. Cont.

Study	Quality/Certainty of Economic Evidence	Design/Population	Intervention(s)	Cost-Effectiveness (ICER or INB)	Resource Requirements
Cost-effectiveness of HCV Screening and DAA therapy					
Selva-patt 2015[+]	Certainty of evidence: moderate. Allowance was made for uncertainty in the estimates of costs and consequences, and ranges were provided. PSA not performed. Justification for choice of ranges was not provided for all parameters. Cost-effectiveness results were sensitive to the prevalence of HCV infection among the screened women and the proportion of identified women treated.	**Design:** Markov cohort simulation model; results reported in British pounds **Population:** Pregnant women attending antenatal clinics in the UK HCV prevalence 0.38%	**Two strategies:** 1- screening and treatment (PR) 2- no screening and no treatment Base-case: Treatment with PR based regimen (IFN/RBV) Additional scenarios: 1- IFN/RBV+SOF 2- IFN/RBV → Ø SVR → IFN/RBV+SOF	ICER (£/QALY): Screening + PR vs. no screening + no treatment: £2400 [€2745] (screening + newer direct-acting antiviral regimens vs. no screening + no treatment) £9139 [€10,455])	Moderate costs. Total costs of screening and confirmation of 44 new diagnoses: £240,641 [€275,299] Cost per newly diagnosed individual: £5469 [€6256]
Wong 2015[32]	Certainty of evidence: moderate. Allowance was made for uncertainty in the estimates of costs and consequences, and ranges were provided. PSA was performed. Justification for choice of ranges was provided for all parameters. Cost-effectiveness results were sensitive to rates of chronic HCV infection, seroprevalence, costs (excluding the cost of antiviral therapy), treatment uptake and quality of life (utilities).	**Design:** Decision-analytic Markov model; results reported in Canadian dollars **Population:** General Canadian population, 2 age groups: 25–64 and 45–64 years old HCV prevalence assumed is 0.5%	**Four strategies:** 1- No screening 2- Screen and treat with PR 3- Screen and treat with: a G1: Interferon free DAA b G2/3: SOF+RBV c G4/5/6: PR 4- Screen and treat with: a G1: SIM+PR b G2/3: SOF+RBV c G4/5/6: PR	ICER (CAN $/QALY) of screening and treatment vs. no screening: **Age 25–64 years:** PR: $38,117 [€25,502] IFN-free DAA (genotype 1), SOF+RBV (genotype 2/3),or PR (genotype 4/5/6): $34,783 [€23,271] PR+RBV (genotype 1), SOF+RBV (genotype 2/3), or PR (genotype 4/5/6): $42,398 [€28,366] **Age 45–64 years:** PR: $34,359 [€22,988] SIM+PR (G1), SOF+RBV (G2/3), or PR (G4/5/6): $44,034 [€29,461] IFN-free DAA (G1), SOF+RBV (G2/3), or PR (G4/5/6): $35,562 [€23,793]	Moderate to high costs: CAN$70,000 [€46,834] $84,000 [€56,201]/person. Costs of antiviral therapies (CAN $): SIM-based: 24 weeks: $46,157 [€30,881]; 48 wk: $55,811 [€37,340] SOF-based: 12 wk: $55,000 [€36,798] ABT-based: 48 wk: $19,948 [€13,346]; 24 wk: $59974 [€6673] Costs of adverse events (weekly): anemia: $107 [€71], depression: $73 [€48], pruritus: $12 [€8], rash: $12 [€8] HCV-tests: anti-HCV: $14 [€9], HCV RNA: $100 [€66] **For age 25–64 years,** No screening: $71,327 [€47,722]; Screen and treat: PR: $71,450 [€47,804] IFN-free DAA (G1), SOF+RBV (G2/3) or PR (G4/5/6): $71,593 [€47,900] SIM+PR (G1), SOF+RBV (G2/3) or PR (G4/5/6): $71,593 [€47,900] **For age 45–64:** No screening: $83,335 [€55,756] Screen and treat: PR: $83,476 [€55,850] IFN-free DAA (G1), SOF+RBV (G2/3) or PR (G4/5/6): $83,672 [€55,981] SIM+PR (G1), SOF+RBV (G2/3) or PR (G4/5/6): $83,673 [€55,982]

Table 2. Cont.

Study	Quality/Certainty of Economic Evidence	Design/Population	Intervention(s)	Cost-Effectiveness (ICER or INB)	Resource Requirements
Cost-effectiveness of HCV Screening and DAA therapy					
Chhatwal 2015 [34]	Certainty of evidence: high. Allowance was made for uncertainty in the estimates of costs and consequences, and ranges were provided. PSA was performed. Justification for choice of ranges was provided for all parameters. Cost-effectiveness results were most sensitive to quality of life after successful treatment, cost of SOF, drug efficacy	**Design:** Decision-analytic Markov model; results reported in US dollars. **Population:** Treatment naïve and treatment-experienced HCV population in US	**Two strategies:** 1- SOF-LDV 2- IFN-based therapy	SOF-LDV vs. IFN-based therapy—ICER ($/QALY): **Treatment naïve patients:** No cirrhosis: $61,517 [€48,725.] Cirrhosis: $20,673 [€16,374.] **Treatment experienced patients:** No cirrhosis: $69,707 [€55,212] Cirrhosis: $92,302 [€73,109]	Treating eligible HCV patient would cost an additional $65 billion [€51.5 billion] over a 5 year period **The weekly costs by third-party payer** SOF: $7000 [€5544] LDV: $875 [€693] PEG-IFN: $587 [€464] RBV: $309 [€244] BOC: $1100 [€871] TEL: $4100 [€3247]
Deuffic-Burban 2016 [3] *	Certainty of evidence: moderate. Allowance was made for uncertainty in the estimates of costs and consequences, and ranges were provided. PSA not performed. Limited justification for choice of ranges. Cost-effectiveness results were sensitive to the price of new DAAs particularly for treating genotype 1	**Design:** Decision-analytic Markov model; results reported in Euros. **Population:** Patients with chronic HCV aged ≥18, aware of their infection, in fibrosis stage F1-F4 or decompensated cirrhosis, treated in France. HCV prevalence	**Three strategies:** 1- TVR/BOC-based triple therapy for genotype 1 and dual therapy with PR for genotypes other than 1 (at F2) 2- SOF/SIM+PR 3- IFN-free DAAs with or without RBV Strategies 2 & 3 evaluated starting treatment at ≥F3, ≥F2 or regardless of fibrosis	**Genotype 1:** IFN-free was a cost-effective vs. IFN-based: ICER: €40,400 to €88,300/QALY QALY/person: 12.59 vs. 12.11 for IFN-based therapy **Genotypes 2 or 3:** IFN-based was the most cost-effective: ICER: €21,300/QALY for genotype 2 ICER: €19,400/QALY for genotype 3 **Genotype 4:** IFN-free regimens was cost-effective: ICER: €23,000 to €58,200/QALY	Moderate to high resource Treating all CHC-screened patients over 5 years would cost: €3.5–7.2 billion **Cost of treatment/week:** SOF: €3417 OBV/PTV-r: €3259 DCV: €2125 SIM: €1750 TEL: €1042 LDV: €417 BOC: €378 DAV: €284 PEG-IFN: €158 RBV: €55 Costs related to adverse events (cost per event): Severe anaemia: €2564 Severe depression: €1619 Severe rash: €2942 Moderate anaemia: €4200

Table 2. Cont.

Study	Quality/Certainty of Economic Evidence	Design/Population	Intervention(s)	Cost-Effectiveness (ICER or INB)	Resource Requirements
Cost-effectiveness of HCV Screening and DAA therapy					
Hagan 2014 [37]	Certainty of evidence: moderate. Allowance was made for uncertainty in the estimates of costs and consequences, and ranges were provided. PSA not performed. Justification for choice of ranges was provided for all parameters. Cost-effectiveness results were sensitive to SVR rates	**Design:** Decision-analytic Markov model; results reported in US dollars **Population:** Chronic HCV genotype 1, in 50 years old in US HCV prevalence 1.6%	**Two strategies:** 1- SOF/RBV 2- SOF/SIM	SOF-SIM dominated SOF-RBV: yielded lower costs and more QALYs SOF-SIM: $165,336 [€133,108] and 14.69 QALYs SOF-RBV: $243,586 [€196,106] and 14.45 QALYs	Costs of drugs per course: 24-weeks SOF/RBV: $169,000 12-weeks SOF/SIM: $150,000 Treatment-associated medical care: SOF/RBV: $2100 (1890–2310) [€1690 (€1521–€1859)] SOF/SIM: $1160 (1044–1276) [€933 (€840–€1027)]
Leidner 2015 [40]	Certainty of evidence: moderate. Allowance was made for uncertainty in the estimates of costs and consequences, and ranges were provided. PSA not performed. Justification for choice of ranges was provided for all parameters. Cost-effectiveness results were sensitive to post-treatment quality of life (utilities) and treatment costs.	**Design:** Decision-analytic Markov model; results reported in US dollars **Population:** 55-year old patient in US with genotype 1 HCV infection	**Two strategies:** 1- treatment at fibrosis stages F3 and F4 2- treatment strategies at earlier stages of liver disease (fibrosis stages F2, F1, or F0).	ICER ($/QALY): **Patients diagnosed at F0:** treatment at F2 vs. F3: $97,900 [€80,102] treatment at F0 vs. F2: $242,900 [€198,741] **Patients diagnosed at F1:** treatment at F2 vs. F3: $59,500 [€48,683] treatment at F1 vs. F2: $174,100 [€142,449] **Patients diagnosed at F2:** treatment at F2 vs. F3: $37,300 [€30,518] The threshold of treatment costs: for ICER $50,000/QALY: $20,200 [€16,527] for ICER $100,000/QALY: $42,400 [€34,691]	Moderate to high costs. Larger costs for patients with advanced or end stage liver disease, compared to early stage liver disease. Nontreatment and treatment costs: **Patients starting at F0:** treatment at F3: $33,600 [€27,491] treatment at F2: $45,000 [€36,819] treatment at F1: $70,800 [€57,928] treatment at F0: $11,100 [€9082] **Patients starting at F1:** treatment at F3: $59,200 [€48,437] treatment at F2: $77,400 [€63,328] treatment at F1: $113,200 [€92,620] **Patients starting at F2:** treatment at F3: $91,000 [€74,456] treatment at F2: $113,600 [€92,947]

Table 2. Cont.

Study	Quality/Certainty of Economic Evidence	Design/Population	Intervention(s)	Cost-Effectiveness (ICER or INB)	Resource Requirements
Cost-effectiveness of HCV Screening and DAA herapy					
Linas 2015 [39]	Certainty of evidence: high Allowance was made for uncertainty in the estimates of costs and consequences, and ranges were provided. PSA was performed. Justification for choice of ranges was provided for all parameters. Cost-effectiveness results were sensitive to cost of SOF	**Design:** Monte Carlo simulation. Results reported in US dollars **Population:** Chronic HCV genotype 2 or 3 in the US	**Three strategies:** 1- SOF 2- PR 3- No therapy	ICER ($/QALY) **Genotype 2** **No cirrhosis (naïve):** 24 wk PR vs. no therapy: $3000 [€2415] 12 wk SOF-RBV vs. 24 wk PR: $238,000 [€191,609] **No cirrhosis (treatment experienced):** 12 wk SOF-RBV vs. no therapy: $63,700 [€51,283] 16 wk SOF-RBV vs. 12 wk SOF-RBV: $468,000 [€376,777] **Cirrhosis (treatment naïve):** 24 wk PR vs. no therapy: $8700 [€7004] 12 wk SOF-RBV vs. 24 wk PR: $35,500 [€28,580] **Cirrhosis (treatment experienced):** 12 wk SOF-RBV dominated by no therapy SOF-RBV 16 wk vs. 12 wk: $27,300 [€21,978] **Genotype 3** **No cirrhosis (treatment-naïve):** 24 wk PR vs. no treatment: $4800 [€3864] 12 wk SOF-RBV dominated by 24 wk PR 12 wk PR-SOF vs. 24 wk PR: $263,000 [€211,736] 24 wk SOF-RBV vs. 12 wk PR-SOF: $266,000 [€214,151] **No cirrhosis (treatment-experienced):** 12 wk PR-SOF vs. no treatment: $82,000 [€66,016] 12 wk SOF-RBV and 16 wk SOF-RBV both dominated by 12 wk PR-SOF SOF-RBV 24 wk vs. 16 wk: $1,100,000 [€805,080] **Cirrhosis (treatment-naïve):** 24 wk PR vs. no treatment: $13,600 [€10,949] 12 wk SOF-RBV dominated by 12 wk PR 12 wk PR-SOF vs. 24 wk PR: $22,600 [€18,194] 24 wk SOF-RBV vs. 12 wk PR-SOF: $107,000 [€96,143] **Cirrhosis (treatment-experienced):** 12 wk PR-SOF vs. no treatment: $22,300 [€17,953] 12 wk, 16 wk and 24 wk SOF-RBV all dominated by 12 wk PR-SO	Total HCV therapy costs per number of weeks (base case value and range from sensitivity analysis): 24 wk PR: $25,300 (12,800–37,800) [€20,368 (10,305–30,432)] 12 wk SOF-RBV: $91,500 (2000–97,500) [€73,664 (1610–78,495)] 16 wk SOF-RBV: $121,900 (30,000–129,900) [€98,139 (24,152–104,579)] 24 wk SOF-RBV: $182,900 (4900–194,900) [€147,249 (3944–156,910)] 12 wk PR-SOF: $9000 (3000–$105,000) [€7245 (2415–84,533)]

Table 2. Cont.

Study	Quality/Certainty of Economic Evidence	Design/Population	Intervention(s)	Cost-Effectiveness (ICER or INB)	Resource Requirements
Cost-effectiveness of HCV Screening and DAA therapy					
Najafzadeh 2015 [33]	Certainty of evidence: high. Allowance was made for uncertainty in the estimates of costs and consequences, and ranges were provided. PSA was performed. Justification for choice of ranges was provided for all parameters. Cost-effectiveness results were sensitive to treatment cost	**Design:** Discrete event simulation **Population:** Treatment-naïve patients infected with chronic HCV genotype 1, 2, or 3 in the US.	Five strategies (genotype 1): 1- BOC+PR 2- SOF+PR 3- SOF+SIM 4- SOF+DCV 5- SOF+LDV 4 strategies (genotype 2/3): 1- PR 2- SOF+RBV 3- SOF+DCV 4- SOF+LDV+ RBV (genotype 3 only)	ICER ($/QALY): **Genotype 1** BOC+PR: reference SOF+PR: $21,528 [€17,051] SOF+SIM: $71,445 [€56,589] SOF+DCV: $63,355 [€50,181] SOF+LDV: $12,825 [€10,158] **Genotype 2:** PR: reference SOF+RBV: $110,168 [€87,260] SOF+DCV: $691,574 [€48,770] **Genotype 3:** PR: reference SOF+RBV: dominated by PR SOF+DCV: $396,229 [€313,839] SOF+LDV+RBV: $73,236 [€58,007]	Drug costs: **Genotype 1:** BOC+PR: $100,926 [€79,940] SOF+PR: $120,648 [€95,561] SOF+SIM: $171,023 [€135,461] SOF+DCV: $169,747 [€134,450] SOF+LDV: $115,358 [€91,371] **Genotype 2:** PR: $54,005 [€42,775] SOF+RBV: $109,958 [€87,093] SOF+DCV: $316,845 [€250,962] **Genotype 3:** PR: $58,323 [€46,195] SOF+RBV: $207,872 [€164,648] SOF+DCV: $317,830 [€251,742] SOF+LDV+RBV: $120,464 [€95,415]
Saab 2014 [38]	Certainty of evidence: moderate. Allowance was made for uncertainty in the estimates of costs and consequences, and ranges were provided. PSA was performed. Justification for choice of ranges was not provided for all parameters. Cost-effectiveness results were most sensitive to cirrhosis prevalence and fibrosis rate, recurrence rates in patients achieving SVR.	**Design:** Decision-analytic Markov model; results reported in US dollars **Population:** Patients with chronic HCV genotype 1 in US	Five Strategies: 1- SOF+PR 2- PR 3- BOC+PR 4- TEL+PR 5- SIM+PR	ICER ($/QALY): **Treatment naïve (without cirrhosis)** SOF+PR compared with PR: ≤$29,271 [€23,565] No treatment: $2071 [€1667] SOF+PR dominated BOC+PR, TEL+PR and SIM+PR **Treatment naïve (with cirrhosis)** SOF+PR compared with PR: ≤$16,939 [€13,637] BOC+PR: $8450 [€6802] SIM+PR: $1899 [€1528] No treatment: $17,299 [€13,927] SOF+PR dominated TEL+PR **Treatment experienced (all patients)** SOF+PR compared with PR: ≤$4290 [€3453] No treatment: $16,617 [€13,378] SOF+PR dominated BOC+PR, TEL+PR and SIM+PR	Total lifetime costs: **Treatment-naïve without cirrhosis:** SOF+PR: $116,715 [€93,964] PR: ≤$95,333 [€76,750] BOC+PR: $124,229 [€100,014] TEL+PR: $128,879 [€103,757] SIM+PR: $120,318 [€96,865] No treatment: $112,093 [€90,243] **Treatment-naïve with cirrhosis** SOF+PR: $209,923 [€169,004] PR: ≤$172,814 [€139,129] BOC+PR: $199,192 [€160,365] TEL+PR: $211,996 [€170,673] SIM+PR: $207,758 [€167,261] No treatment: $140,210 [€112,880] **Treatment-experienced all patients:** SOF+PR: $148,812 [€119,805] PR: ≤$145,009 [€116,743] BOC+PR: $165,983 [€133,629] TEL+PR: $165,428 [€133,182] SIM+PR: $168,251 [€135,455] No treatment: $115,911 [€93,317]

Table 2. Cont.

Study	Quality/Certainty of Economic Evidence	Design/Population	Intervention(s)	Cost-Effectiveness (ICER or INB)	Resource Requirements
Cost-effectiveness of HCV Screening and DAA therapy					
Younossi 2015 [35]	Certainty of evidence: moderate. Allowance was made for uncertainty in the estimates of costs and consequences, and ranges were provided. PSA was performed. Justification for choice of ranges was not provided for patient distribution, regimen efficacy, costs, or utilities. Cost-effectiveness results were robust across the limited ranges tested.	**Design:** Decision-analytic Markov model; results reported in US dollars. **Population:** Patients with chronic HCV genotype 1 in US.	**Six strategies:** 1- LDV/SOF 2- SOF+PR 3- SIM+PR 4- SOF+SIM 5- SOF+RBV 6- BOC+PR	**LDV/SOF (ICER):** **Treatment-naïve patients:** dominant over no treatment dominant over SOF+PR (12/24 weeks) less expensive and less effective than SOF+SIM dominant over SOF+RBV dominant over BOC+PR Results similar for patients with and without cirrhosis; and for treatment experienced patients with PR or Protease inhibitor (PI) + RBV	Drug costs/pack: BOC: $6687 [€5296] LDV/SOF: $31,500 [€24,950] PEG-IFN: $3310 [€2621] SIM: $22,120 [€17,520] SOF: $28,000 [€22,177] RBV: $1153 [€913]; Generic: $238 [€188] **Total lifetime costs by strategy (treatment naïve):** No treatment: $141,856 [€112,359] LDV/SOF: $90,127 [€71,386] SOF+PR: $119,846 [€94,925] SIM+PR: $128,793 [€102,012] SOF+SIM: $191,631 [€151,784] SOF+RBV: $229,200 [€181,541] BOC+PR: $127,759 [€101,193]

ABT: a protease inhibitor; BOC: boceprevir; CAD: Canadian dollar; DAA: direct acting antiviral; DAV: dasabuvir; DCV: daclatasvir; F: fibrosis stage; G: genotype; HBV: hepatitis B virus; HCV: hepatitis C virus; HIV: human immunodeficiency virus; ICER: incremental cost-effectiveness ratio; IFN: interferon; INB: incremental net benefit LDV: ledipasvir; OBV: ombitasvir; PI: protease inhibitor; PEG-IFN: pegylated interferon; PR: pegylated-interferon-ribavirin; PSA: probabilistic sensitivity analysis; PTV-r: paritaprevir-ritonavir; QALY: quality-adjusted life years; RBV: ribavirin; RNA: ribonucleic acid; SIM: simeprevir; SOF: sofosbuvir; SVR: sustained virological response; TEL/TVR: telaprevir; US: United States. * Costs were expressed in 2015 Euro in the original publication.

4. Discussion

The data in this review supports the effectiveness and cost-effectiveness of HCV screening in populations at risk for HCV infection, including migrants from intermediate and high HCV prevalence countries (anti-HCV $\geq$ 2% and $\geq$5%, respectively). Screening tests to detect the presence of HCV antibodies performed equally well in all populations. In the laboratory setting or at the point-of-care both are highly sensitive and specific [6,26]. DAA therapies are highly efficacious and well tolerated with >95% cure rates in a range of populations in different countries [7]. Achieving SVR with HCV therapy is associated with decreased risk and rate of liver disease progression, lower rates of HCC development, and improved survival [27–29,46]. At 2015 costs, DAA based regimens were only moderately cost-effective and as a result less than 30% of those with HCV had been screened and less than 5% of all HCV cases had been treated in the EU/EEA in 2015 [2,31]. Migrant populations in the EU/EEA face difficulties accessing care and treatment as a result of numerous barriers at the patient, provider, and health system level [16,47]. To reach HCV elimination goals in the EU/EEA dramatic scale up of HCV testing with diagnosis of all groups at HCV risk, including migrants, and linking those found to be positive to care and treatment will be required.

Migrants living in the EU/EEA bear a disproportionate burden of HCV [1,13]. They are older and more likely to have advanced liver disease and hepatocellular carcinoma compared to non-migrants at the time of HCV diagnosis [17,48,49]. This is likely due to missed or delayed diagnoses. In a survey in Finland, 63% of migrants found to be HCV positive had not been previously diagnosed [50]. Seventy percent of these HCV positive migrants had been living in Finland for more than five years. Similarly, in a population based study in Canada, it took a mean of 10 years after arrival for migrants to be diagnosed with HCV [48]. Another Canadian study found that it was cost-effective to screen immigrants for HCV followed by DAA treatment at an anti-HCV prevalence of 1.9%, which is the mean HCV seroprevalence of migrants living in the EU/EEA [12,13,51]. These data taken together suggest that early screening of migrants based on the HCV prevalence in the country of origin with linkage to care and treatment could prevent liver related sequelae in the migrant population and would be cost-effective. In an ECDC survey, 18 of 21 responding countries had national guidance on HCV testing; however, only six countries (29%) had guidance on testing migrants for HCV [52]. This highlights an important gap and an opportunity for health promotion among the migrant population.

Migrants face multiple barriers in accessing healthcare services resulting in gaps along all steps of the HCV care continuum [16,53]. Many groups of newly arriving migrants, including asylum seekers and undocumented migrants, lack entitlement to health care in the EU/EEA, thus preventing them from being diagnosed or receiving treatment [54]. Individual barriers include lack of knowledge and awareness of risk factors, fear, and stigma of blood-borne diseases, and socioeconomic, linguistic, and cultural barriers [47,55–57]. Providers are frequently unaware that birth in an HCV endemic country is an important risk factor for HCV. Language and cultural discordance between patients and providers may lead to poor communication and low quality of care [16,53,58]. Lack of screening guidelines and programs and the lack of access to interpreters are important health system barriers. Barriers to effective screening and treatment programs may also include lack of political will to address migrant health issues or negative national attitudes toward migrants. Resulting policies may deny migrants the entitlement to health care or prevent the development of migrant-friendly heath care systems [58].

Evidence from primary studies of migrant populations suggests that HCV screening uptake and linkage to care could be improved by implementing decentralized community-based screening strategies, and cooperation with community-based organizations to overcome cultural and language barriers [59–64]. Furthermore, integrated point-of-care testing for HCV, HBV, and HIV increased testing uptake [59,65]. HCV screening and treatment programs for migrants in the EU/EEA will need to be tailored to their specific needs. In addition, it will be necessary to ensure universal access to health care in order to enhance uptake along the entire HCV care continuum.

The greatest barrier to scaling up HCV treatment in the EU/EEA has been the high cost of therapy, which has decreased dramatically in the past two years [66]. As a result, many countries in the EU/EEA have lifted restrictions and provide more widespread availability of HCV therapy in the region [67]. Dropping prices and simpler short treatment regimens have helped create an opportunity to eliminate HCV in the EU/EEA. Recent guidance from the WHO has highlighted the need to increase HCV case detection and linkage to HCV care [6]. This includes screening persons originating from countries with an intermediate ($\geq$2%) and high ($\geq$5%) HCV prevalence, which includes many of the migrants living in the EU/EEA. Consideration of existing prevention and control efforts and the capacity of existing systems must also be taken into account [68]. Knowledge of the HCV epidemiology in each EU/EEA Member State will be needed to identify those migrant groups at highest HCV risk, given that the top countries of origin of HCV infected migrants in each country varies (Table S6) [13]. Each country will need to assess their own capacity to increase HCV testing in at risk populations and to ensure that programs are in place that effectively link those with active HCV to care and provide HCV treatment.

Strengths and Limitations

The major strength of our study is that we used a systematic review process to identify relevant studies and the GRADE methodology to evaluate the certainty of the evidence. Our study had the following limitations. The findings were limited by the low to moderate certainty of the evidence of the included studies. Our study was also limited by the low number of studies reporting on linkage to care for migrants to EU/EEA. Finally, the included cost-effective studies modeled the 2015 cost of DDA therapies. We anticipate however, that HCV screening and treatment will be even more cost-effective given the dramatic decrease in cost of DAA therapy in the EU/EEA since 2015 [66,67].

5. Conclusions

In many EU/EEA countries migrants originating from intermediate and high HCV prevalence countries make up a large proportion of all HCV cases and have poorer liver related outcomes due to delayed diagnosis and treatment. This health disparity is due to the numerous barriers migrants face accessing HCV diagnosis, care, and treatment. Migrant focused programs will need to ensure entitlement to health services and will be most effective if they address linguistic and cultural barriers, are community-based, and integrated with screening for other diseases such as HIV and HBV. Although decreasing HCV costs have made treatment more accessible in the EU/EEA, HCV elimination will only be possible in the region if health systems include and treat migrants for HCV [66].

Supplementary Materials: The following are available online at http://www.mdpi.com/1660-4601/15/9/2013/s1, Figure S1: Analytic Framework for HCV Screening in Migrants; Table S1. Effectiveness and Cost-effectiveness Search Strategy; Tables S2–S5. Study profile GRADE; Table S6. Chronic HCV burden in migrants: the 10 migrant groups from intermediate/high HCV prevalence countries with the highest number of HCV cases in host EU/EEA countries.

Author Contributions: Conceptualization: C.G., I.V., F.C., R.L.M., and K.P. Methodology: K.P., J.J.M., and R.C. Resources: I.V., F.C., R.L.M., M.P., and T.N., Writing—original draft: C.G., I.M., and B.A. Data curation: C.N.A.C., I.M., A.P., R.L.M., A.T., L.S., and J.J.M. Writing—review & editing: All authors.

Funding: This work is supported by the European Centre for Disease Prevention and Control (ECDC); FWC No ECDC/2015/016; Specific Contract No 1 ECD.5748. Manish Pareek is supported by the National Institute for Health Research (NIHR Post-Doctoral Fellowship, Manish Pareek, PDF-2015-08-102). The views expressed in this publication are those of the author(s) and not necessarily those of the NHS, the National Institute for Health Research, or the Department of Health. A/Prof Rachael Morton is supported by an Australian NHMRC Sidney Sax Overseas Fellowship #1054216. The Parker Institute, Bispebjerg, and Frederiksberg Hospital (Christensen) is supported by a core grant from the Oak Foundation (OCAY-13-309).

Conflicts of Interest: C.G. was the first author on five of the infectious disease conditions including hepatitis C in the Canadian Migrant Health Guidelines; K.P. led the overall guidelines. M.P. reports an institutional grant (unrestricted) for project related to blood-borne virus testing from Gilead Sciences outside the submitted work. I.M., C.N.A.C., B.A., A.P., I.V., F.C., R.M., A.T., L.S., J.J.M., R.C., and T.N. declare no conflicts of interest. The funding sponsors had no role in the design of the study; in the collection, analyses, or interpretation of data; in the writing of the manuscript, and in the decision to publish the results.

References

1. European Centre for Disease Prevention and Control. *Systematic Review on Hepatitis B and C Prevalence in the EU/EEA*; ECDC: Stockholm, Sweden, 2016.
2. Razavi, H.; Robbins, S.; Zeuzem, S.; Negro, F.; Buti, M.; Duberg, A.S.; Roudot-Thoraval, F.; Craxi, A.; Manns, M.; Marinho, R.T.; et al. Hepatitis C virus prevalence and level of intervention required to achieve the WHO targets for elimination in the European Union by 2030: A modelling study. *Lancet Gastroenterol. Hepatol.* **2017**, *2*, 325–336. [CrossRef]
3. Mühlberger, N.; Schwarzer, R.; Lettmeier, B.; Sroczynski, G.; Zeuzem, S.; Siebert, U. HCV-related burden of disease in Europe: A systematic assessment of incidence, prevalence, morbidity, and mortality. *BMC Public Health* **2009**, *9*, 34. [CrossRef] [PubMed]
4. Mathurin, P. HCV burden in Europe and the possible impact of current treatment. *Dig. Liver Dis.* **2013**, *45* (Suppl. 5), S314–S317. [CrossRef] [PubMed]
5. El Khoury, A.C.; Wallace, C.; Klimack, W.K.; Razavi, H. Economic burden of hepatitis C-associated diseases: Europe, Asia Pacific, and the Americas. *J. Med. Econ.* **2012**, *15*, 887–896. [CrossRef] [PubMed]
6. WHO. *Guidelines on Hepatitis B and C Testing*; World Health Organization: Geneva, Switzerland, 2017.
7. Falade-Nwulia, O.; Suarez-Cuervo, C.; Nelson, D.R.; Fried, M.W.; Segal, J.B.; Sulkowski, M.S. Oral direct-acting agent therapy for hepatitis c virus infection: A systematic review. *Ann. Intern. Med.* **2017**, *166*, 637–648. [CrossRef] [PubMed]
8. European Association for the Study of the Liver. EASL Recommendations on Treatment of Hepatitis C 2018. *J. Hepatol.* **2018**, *69*, 461–511. [CrossRef] [PubMed]
9. World Health Organisation. *Combating Hepatitis B and C to Reach Elimination by 2030*; WHO: Geneva, Switzerland, 2016.
10. World Health Organization Regional Office for Europe. *Action Plan for the Health Sector Response to Viral Hepatitis in the WHO European Region*; WHO/Europe: Copenhagen, Denmark, 2016.
11. World Health Organisation. *Global Health Sector Strategy on Viral Hepatitis 2016–2021. Towards Ending Viral Hepatitis*; WHO: Geneva, Switzerland, 2016.
12. Falla, A.M.; Ahmad, A.A.; Duffell, E.; Noori, T.; Veldhuijzen, I.K. Estimating the scale of chronic hepatitis C virus infection in the EU/EEA: A focus on migrants from anti-HCV endemic countries. *BMC Infect. Dis.* **2018**, *18*, 42. [CrossRef] [PubMed]
13. European Centre for Disease Prevention and Control. *Epidemiological Assessment of Hepatitis B and C among Migrants in the EU/EEA*; ECDC: Stockhlom, Sweden, 2016.
14. Pepin, J.; Abou Chakra, C.; Pepin, E.; Nault, V.; Valiquette, L. Evolution of the global burden of viral infections from unsafe medical injections, 2000–2010. *PLoS ONE* **2014**, *9*, e99677. [CrossRef] [PubMed]
15. Greenaway, C.; Thu Ma, A.; Kloda, L.A.; Klein, M.; Cnossen, S.; Schwarzer, G.; Shrier, I. The Seroprevalence of Hepatitis C Antibodies in Immigrants and Refugees from Intermediate and High Endemic Countries: A Systematic Review and Meta-Analysis. *PLoS ONE* **2015**, *10*, e0141715.
16. Seedat, F.; Hargreaves, S.; Nellums, L.B.; Ouyang, J.; Brown, M.; Friedland, J.S. How effective are approaches to migrant screening for infectious diseases in Europe? A systematic review. *Lancet Infect. Dis.* **2018**. [CrossRef]
17. Chen, W.; Tomlinson, G.; Krahn, M.; Heathcote, J. Immigrant patients with chronic hepatitis C and advanced fibrosis have a higher risk of hepatocellular carcinoma. *J. Viral. Hepat.* **2012**, *19*, 574–580. [CrossRef] [PubMed]
18. Pottie, K.; Mayhew, A.; Morton, R.; Greenaway, C.; Akl, E.A.; Rahman, P.; Zenner, D.; Pareek, M.; Tugwell, P.; Welch, V.; et al. Prevention and assessment of infectious diseases among children and adult migrants arriving to the European Union/European Economic Association: A protocol for a suite of systematic reviews for public health and health systems. *BMJ Open* **2017**, *7*, e014608. [CrossRef] [PubMed]
19. Moher, D.; Liberati, A.; Tetzlaff, J.; Altman, D.G. Preferred reporting items for systematic reviews and meta-analyses: The PRISMA statement. *Ann. Intern. Med.* **2009**, *151*, 264–269. [CrossRef] [PubMed]
20. Woolf, S.; Schunemann, H.J.; Eccles, M.P.; Grimshaw, J.M.; Shekelle, P. Developing clinical practice guidelines: Types of evidence and outcomes; values and economics, synthesis, grading, and presentation and deriving recommendations. *Implement. Sci.* **2012**, *7*, 61. [CrossRef] [PubMed]

21. Owens, D.K.; Whitlock, E.P.; Henderson, J.; Pignone, M.P.; Krist, A.H.; Bibbins-Domingo, K.; Curry, S.J.; Davidson, K.W.; Ebell, M.; Gillman, M.W.; et al. Use of Decision Models in the Development of Evidence-Based Clinical Preventive Services Recommendations: Methods of the U.S. Preventive Services Task Force. *Ann. Intern. Med.* **2016**, *165*, 501–508. [CrossRef] [PubMed]
22. Shea, B.J.; Hamel, C.; Wells, G.A.; Bouter, L.M.; Kristjansson, E.; Grimshaw, J.; Henry, D.A.; Boers, M. AMSTAR is a reliable and valid measurement tool to assess the methodological quality of systematic reviews. *J. Clin. Epidemiol.* **2009**, *62*, 1013–1020. [CrossRef] [PubMed]
23. Guyatt, G.; Oxman, A.D.; Akl, E.A.; Kunz, R.; Vist, G.; Brozek, J.; Norris, S.; Falck-Ytter, Y.; Glasziou, P.; Jaeschke, R. GRADE guidelines: 1. Introduction—GRADE evidence profiles and summary of findings tables. *J. Clin. Epidemiol.* **2011**, *64*, 383–394. [CrossRef] [PubMed]
24. Drummond, M.F.; Sculpher, M.J.; Claxton, K.; Stoddart, G.L.; Torrance, G.W. *Methods for the Economic Evaluation of Health Care Programmes*, 2nd ed.; Oxford University Press: New York, NY, USA, 1997; p. 396.
25. Alonso-Coello, P.; Oxman, A.D.; Moberg, J.; Brignardello-Petersen, R.; Akl, E.A.; Davoli, A.; Treweek, S.; Mustafa, R.; Vandvik, P.; Meerpohl, J.; et al. GRADE Evidence to Decision (EtD) frameworks: A systematic and transparent approach to making well informed healthcare choices. 2: Clinical practice guidelines. *Br. Med. J.* **2016**, *353*, i2089. [CrossRef] [PubMed]
26. Khuroo, M.S.; Khuroo, N.S.; Khuroo, M.S. Diagnostic accuracy of point-of-care tests for hepatitis C virus infection: A systematic review and meta-analysis. *PLoS ONE* **2015**, *10*, e0121450. [CrossRef] [PubMed]
27. Kimer, N.; Dahl, E.K.; Gluud, L.L.; Krag, A. Antiviral therapy for prevention of hepatocellular carcinoma in chronic hepatitis C: Systematic review and meta-analysis of randomised controlled trials. *BMJ Open* **2012**, *2*, e001313. [CrossRef] [PubMed]
28. Simmons, B.; Saleem, J.; Heath, K.; Cooke, G.S.; Hill, A. Long-Term Treatment Outcomes of Patients Infected With Hepatitis C Virus: A Systematic Review and Meta-analysis of the Survival Benefit of Achieving a Sustained Virological Response. *Clin. Infect. Dis.* **2015**, *61*, 730–740. [CrossRef] [PubMed]
29. Public Health Agency of Canada. *Treatment for Hepatitis C Virus: A Systematic Review and Meta-Analysis*; Canadian Preventative Task Force: Ottawa, ON, Canada, 2016.
30. Yehia, B.R.; Schranz, A.J.; Umscheid, C.A.; Lo Re, V., III. The treatment cascade for chronic hepatitis C virus infection in the United States: A systematic review and meta-analysis. *PLoS ONE* **2014**, *9*, e101554. [CrossRef] [PubMed]
31. Deuffic-Burban, S.; Obach, D.; Canva, V.; Pol, S.; Roudot-Thoraval, F.; Dhumeaux, D.; Mathurin, P.; Yazdanpanah, Y. Cost-effectiveness and budget impact of interferon-free direct-acting antiviral-based regimens for hepatitis C treatment: The French case. *J. Viral Hepat.* **2016**, *23*, 767–779. [CrossRef] [PubMed]
32. Wong, W.W.; Tu, H.-A.; Feld, J.J.; Wong, T.; Krahn, M. Cost-effectiveness of screening for hepatitis C in Canada. *CMAJ* **2015**, *187*, E110–E121. [CrossRef] [PubMed]
33. Najafzadeh, M.; Andersson, K.; Shrank, W.H.; Krumme, A.A.; Matlin, O.S.; Brennan, T.; Avorn, J.; Choudhry, N.K. Cost-effectiveness of novel regimens for the treatment of hepatitis C virus. *Ann. Intern. Med.* **2015**, *162*, 407–419. [CrossRef] [PubMed]
34. Chhatwal, J.; Kanwal, F.; Roberts, M.S.; Dunn, M.A. Cost-effectiveness and budget impact of hepatitis C virus treatment with sofosbuvir and ledipasvir in the United States. *Ann. Intern. Med.* **2015**, *162*, 397–406. [CrossRef] [PubMed]
35. Younossi, Z.M.; Park, H.; Saab, S.; Ahmed, A.; Dieterich, D.; Gordon, S.C. Cost-effectiveness of all-oral ledipasvir/sofosbuvir regimens in patients with chronic hepatitis C virus genotype 1 infection. *Aliment. Pharmacol. Ther.* **2015**, *41*, 544–563. [CrossRef] [PubMed]
36. Rein, D.B.; Wittenborn, J.S.; Smith, B.D.; Liffmann, D.K.; Ward, J.W. The cost-effectiveness, health benefits, and financial costs of new antiviral treatments for hepatitis C virus. *Clin. Infect. Dis.* **2015**, *61*, 157–168. [CrossRef] [PubMed]
37. Hagan, L.M.; Sulkowski, M.S.; Schinazi, R.F. Cost analysis of sofosbuvir/ribavirin versus sofosbuvir/simeprevir for genotype 1 hepatitis C virus in interferon-ineligible/intolerant individuals. *Hepatology* **2014**, *60*, 37–45. [CrossRef] [PubMed]
38. Saab, S.; Gordon, S.C.; Park, H.; Sulkowski, M.; Ahmed, A.; Younossi, Z. Cost-effectiveness analysis of sofosbuvir plus peginterferon/ribavirin in the treatment of chronic hepatitis C virus genotype 1 infection. *Aliment. Pharmacol. Ther.* **2014**, *40*, 657–675. [CrossRef] [PubMed]

39. Linas, B.P.; Barter, D.M.; Morgan, J.R.; Pho, M.T.; Leff, J.A.; Schackman, B.R.; Horsburgh, C.R.; Assoumou, S.A.; Salomon, J.A.; Weinstein, M.C.; et al. The cost-effectiveness of sofosbuvir-based regimens for treatment of hepatitis c virus genotype 2 or 3 infection. *Ann. Intern. Med.* **2015**, *162*, 619–629. [CrossRef] [PubMed]
40. Leidner, A.J.; Chesson, H.W.; Xu, F.; Ward, J.W.; Spradling, P.R.; Holmberg, S.D. Cost-effectiveness of hepatitis C treatment for patients in early stages of liver disease. *Hepatology* **2015**, *61*, 1860–1869. [CrossRef] [PubMed]
41. Brett-Major, D.M.; Frick, K.D.; Malia, J.A.; Hakre, S.; Okulicz, J.F.; Beckett, C.G.; Jagodinski, L.L.; Forgione, M.A.; Gould, P.L.; Harrison, S.A.; et al. Costs and consequences: Hepatitis C seroprevalence in the military and its impact on potential screening strategies. *Hepatology* **2016**, *63*, 398–407. [CrossRef] [PubMed]
42. He, T.; Li, K.; Roberts, M.S.; Spaulding, A.C.; Ayer, T.; Grefenstette, J.J.; Chhatwal, J. Prevention of Hepatitis C by Screening and Treatment in U.S. Prisons. *Ann. Intern. Med.* **2016**, *164*, 84–92. [CrossRef] [PubMed]
43. Orkin, C.; Flanagan, S.; Wallis, E.; Ireland, G.; Dhairyawan, R.; Fox, J.; Nandwani, R.; O'Connell, R.; Lascar, M.; Bulman, J.; et al. Incorporating HIV/hepatitis B virus/hepatitis C virus combined testing into routine blood tests in nine UK Emergency Departments: The "Going Viral" campaign. *HIV Med.* **2016**, *17*, 222–230. [CrossRef] [PubMed]
44. Selvapatt, N.; Ward, T.; Bailey, H.; Bennett, H.; Thorne, C.; See, L.M.; Tudor-Williams, G.; Thursz, M.; McEwan, P.; Brown, A. Is antenatal screening for hepatitis C virus cost-effective? A decade's experience at a London centre. *J. Hepatol.* **2015**, *63*, 797–804. [CrossRef] [PubMed]
45. Ryen, L.; Svensson, M. The Willingness to Pay for a Quality Adjusted Life Year: A Review of the Empirical Literature. *Health Econ.* **2015**, *24*, 1289–1301. [CrossRef] [PubMed]
46. Backus, L.I.; Belperio, P.S.; Shahoumian, T.A.; Mole, L.A. Direct-acting antiviral sustained virologic response: Impact on mortality in patients without advanced liver disease. *Hepatology* **2018**. [CrossRef] [PubMed]
47. Owiti, J.A.; Greenhalgh, T.; Sweeney, L.; Foster, G.R.; Bhui, K.S. Illness perceptions and explanatory models of viral hepatitis B & C among immigrants and refugees: A narrative systematic review. *BMC Public Health* **2015**, *15*, 151.
48. Greenaway, C.; Azoulay, L.; Allard, R.; Cox, J.; Tran, V.A.; Abou Chakra, C.N.; Steele, R.; Klein, M. A population-based study of chronic hepatitis C in immigrants and non-immigrants in Quebec, Canada. *BMC Infect. Dis.* **2017**, *17*, 140. [CrossRef] [PubMed]
49. Nguyen, L.; Nguyen, M. Systematic review: Asian patients with chronic hepatitis C infection. *Aliment. Pharmacol. Ther.* **2013**, *37*, 921–936. [CrossRef] [PubMed]
50. Tiittala, P.; Ristola, M.; Liitsola, K.; Ollgren, J.; Koponen, P.; Surcel, H.M.; Hiltunen-Back, E.; Davidkin, I.; Kivela, P. Missed hepatitis b/c or syphilis diagnosis among Kurdish, Russian, and Somali origin migrants in Finland: Linking a population-based survey to the national infectious disease register. *BMC Infect. Dis.* **2018**, *18*, 137. [CrossRef] [PubMed]
51. Wong, W.W.L.; Erman, A.; Feld, J.J.; Krahn, M. Model-based projection of health and economic effects of screening for hepatitis C in Canada. *CMAJ Open* **2017**, *5*, E662–E672. [CrossRef] [PubMed]
52. European Centre for Disease Prevention and Control. *Hepatitis B and C Testing Activities, Needs, and Priorities in the EU/EEA*; ECDC: Stockholm, Sweden, 2017.
53. Greenaway, C.; Makarenko, I.; Tanveer, F.; Janjua, N. Addressing Hepatitis C in the Foreign-Born Population: A key to HCV Elimination in Canada. *Can. Liver J.* **2018**, *1*, 34–50. [CrossRef]
54. Noret, I.; Frydryszak, D.; Macherey, A.; Simonnot, N. European Network to Reduce Vulnerabilities in Health. Available online: https://mdmeuroblog.wordpress.com/about/ (accessed on 14 September 2018).
55. Institute of Medicine Committee on the Prevention Control of Viral Hepatitis Infection. *Hepatitis and Liver Cancer: A National Strategy for Prevention and Control of Hepatitis B and C*; Colvin, H.M., Mitchell, A.E., Eds.; National Academies Press (US), National Academy of Sciences: Washington, DC, USA, 2010.
56. Ferrante, J.M.; Winston, D.G.; Chen, P.H.; de la Torre, A.N. Family physicians' knowledge and screening of chronic hepatitis and liver cancer. *Fam. Med.* **2008**, *40*, 345–351. [PubMed]
57. Blondell, S.J.; Kitter, B.; Griffin, M.P.; Durham, J. Barriers and Facilitators to HIV Testing in Migrants in High-Income Countries: A Systematic Review. *AIDS Behav.* **2015**, *19*, 2012–2024. [CrossRef] [PubMed]
58. Pareek, M.; Noori, T.; Hargreaves, S.; van den Muijsenbergh, M. Linkage to Care Is Important and Necessary When Identifying Infections in Migrants. *Int. J. Environ. Res. Public Health* **2018**, *15*, 1550. [CrossRef] [PubMed]

59. Fernandez, M.; Manzanares, S.; Jacques, C.; Caylá, J.; Kunkel, J.; Foster, G. Screening for Chronic viral Hepatitis in Migrant Populations—Report on Four HEPscreen Pilot Studies. Available online: http://hepscreen.eu/wp-content/uploads/2014/12/HEPscreen_Final-WP6-report_Pilot-studies.pdf (accessed on 14 September 2018).
60. Jafferbhoy, H.; Miller, M.H.; McIntyre, P.; Dillon, J.F. The effectiveness of outreach testing for hepatitis C in an immigrant Pakistani population. *Epidemiol. Infect.* **2012**, *140*, 1048–1053. [CrossRef] [PubMed]
61. Perumalswami, P.; DiClemente, F.M.; Kapelusznik, L.; Pan, C.; Chang, C.; Friedman, S.L.; Vachon, M.-L.C.; Standen, M.; Khaitova, V.; Factor, S.H.; et al. Hepatitis outreach network (HONE): HBV and HCV screening of ethnic urban populations of New York city with linkage to care. In *Hepatology (Baltimore, Md.)*; John Wiley and Sons Inc.: New York, NY, USA, 2011; Volume 54, pp. 594A–595A.
62. Perumalswami, P.V.; DeWolfe Miller, F.; Orabee, H.; Regab, A.; Adams, M.; Kapelusznik, L.; Aljibawi, F.; Pagano, W.; Tong, V.; Dieterich, D.T.; et al. Hepatitis C screening beyond CDC guidelines in an Egyptian immigrant community. *Liver Int. Off. J. Int. Assoc. Stud. Liver* **2014**, *34*, 253–258. [CrossRef] [PubMed]
63. Perumalswami, P.V.; Factor, S.H.; Kapelusznik, L.; Friedman, S.L.; Pan, C.Q.; Chang, C.; Di Clemente, F.; Dieterich, D.T. Hepatitis Outreach Network: A practical strategy for hepatitis screening with linkage to care in foreign-born communities. *J. Hepatol.* **2013**, *58*, 890–897. [CrossRef] [PubMed]
64. Zuure, F.R.; Bouman, J.; Martens, M.; Vanhommerig, J.W.; Urbanus, A.T.; Davidovich, U.; van Houdt, R.; Speksnijder, A.G.C.L.; Weegink, C.J.; van den Hoek, A.; et al. Screening for hepatitis B and C in first-generation Egyptian migrants living in the Netherlands. *Liver Int.* **2013**, *33*, 727–738. [CrossRef] [PubMed]
65. Bottero, J.; Boyd, A.; Gozlan, J.; Carrat, F.; Nau, J.; Pauti, M.-D.; Rougier, H.; Girard, P.-M.; Lacombe, K. Simultaneous Human Immunodeficiency Virus-Hepatitis B-Hepatitis C Point-of-Care Tests Improve Outcomes in Linkage-to-Care: Results of a Randomized Control Trial in Persons Without Healthcare Coverage. *Open Forum Infect. Dis.* **2015**, *2*, ofv162. [CrossRef] [PubMed]
66. Marshall, A.D.; Cunningham, E.B.; Nielsen, S.; Aghemo, A.; Alho, H.; Backmund, M.; Bruggmann, P.; Dalgard, O.; Seguin-Devaux, C.; Flisiak, R.; et al. Restrictions for reimbursement of interferon-free direct-acting antiviral drugs for HCV infection in Europe. *Lancet Gastroenterol. Hepatol.* **2018**, *3*, 125–133. [CrossRef]
67. Marshall, A.D.; Pawlotsky, J.M.; Lazarus, J.V.; Aghemo, A.; Dore, G.J.; Grebely, J. The removal of DAA restrictions in Europe—One step closer to eliminating HCV as a major public health threat. *J. Hepatol.* **2018**, in press. [CrossRef] [PubMed]
68. Duffell, E.; Hedrich, D.; Mardh, O.; Mozalevskis, A. Towards Elimination of hepatitsi B and C in European Union and European Economic Area Countries: Monitiroing the World Health Organization's global health sector strategy core indicators and scaling up key interventions. *Eurosurveillance* **2017**, *22*, 30476. [CrossRef] [PubMed]

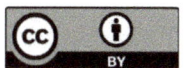

© 2018 by the authors. Licensee MDPI, Basel, Switzerland. This article is an open access article distributed under the terms and conditions of the Creative Commons Attribution (CC BY) license (http://creativecommons.org/licenses/by/4.0/).

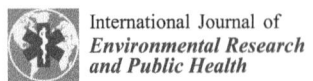

Article

Emergency Department Discharge Outcome and Psychiatric Consultation in North African Patients

Osnat Keidar [1,*,†], Sabrina N. Jegerlehner [1,†], Stephan Ziegenhorn [1], Adam D. Brown [2,3], Martin Müller [1,4], Aristomenis K. Exadaktylos [1] and David S. Srivastava [1]

1. Department of Emergency Medicine, Inselspital, Bern University Hospital, University of Bern, 3010 Bern, Switzerland; sabrina.jegerlehner@insel.ch (S.N.J.); stephan.ziegenhorn@insel.ch (S.Z.); martin.mueller2@insel.ch (M.M.); aristomenis.exadaktylos@insel.ch (A.K.E.); davidshiva.srivastava@insel.ch (D.S.S.)
2. Department of Psychology, New School for Social Research, New York, NY 10011, USA; brownad@newschool.edu
3. Department of Psychiatry, New York University School of Medicine, New York, NY 10016, USA
4. Institute of Health Economics and Clinical Epidemiology, University Hospital of Cologne, 50935 Cologne, Germany
* Correspondence: osnat.keidar@insel.ch
† Both authors contributed equally to the manuscript.

Received: 30 July 2018; Accepted: 12 September 2018; Published: 17 September 2018

Abstract: Studies in Europe have found that immigrants, compared to the local population, are more likely to seek out medical care in Emergency Departments (EDs). In addition, studies show that immigrants utilize medical services provided by EDs for less acute issues. Despite these observed differences, little is known about the characteristics of ED use by North African (NA) immigrants. The main objective of this study was to examine whether there were differences in ED discharge outcomes and psychiatric referrals between NA immigrants and Swiss nationals. A retrospective analysis was conducted using patient records from NA and Swiss adults who were admitted to the ED of the University Hospital in Bern (Switzerland) from 2013–2016. Measures included demographic information as well as data on types of admission. Outcome variables included discharge type and psychiatric referral. A total of 77,619 patients generated 116,859 consultations to the ED, of which 1.1 per cent (n = 1338) were consultations by NA patients. Compared to Swiss national patients, NA patients were younger, with a median age of 38.0 (IQR 28–51 years vs. 52.0 (IQR 32–52) for Swiss and predominantly male (74.4% vs. 55.6% in the Swiss). NA patient admission type was more likely to be "walk-in" or legal admission (7.5% vs 0.8 in Swiss,). Logistic regressions indicated that NA patients had 1.2 times higher odds (95% CI 1.07–1.40, p < 0.003) of receiving ambulatory care. An effect modification by age group and sex was observed for the primary outcome "seen by a psychiatrist", especially for men in the 16–25 years age group, whereby male NA patients had 3.45 times higher odds (95% CI: 2.22–5.38) of having being seen by a psychiatrist. In conclusion differences were observed between NA and Swiss national patients in ED consultations referrals and outcomes, in which NA had more ambulatory discharges and NA males, especially young, were more likely to have been seen by psychiatrist. Future studies would benefit from identifying those factors underlying these differences in ED utilization.

Keywords: North African; immigration; health care; emergency department; disparities

1. Introduction

According to the International Organization for Migration (IOM) a migrant refers to any individual that moves across international borders away from her or his country of origin, regardless of legal status or cause [1]. Current socio-economic, environmental, and political forces in recent years has led to an unprecedented number of people migrating from low and middle-income nations to high-income countries, such as Switzerland [2,3]. Although people are immigrating to Switzerland from a number of geographical regions, a high proportion of individuals are coming from Africa [4]. Recent estimates suggest that approximately 6.7% of all foreign residents come from African countries [5]. More specifically, among those individuals migrating from Africa, a majority are from North African (NA) countries such as Morocco, Egypt, and Tunisia [6]. Supplementary Figures S1 and S2 present the population structure by age groups in male and female for NA and Swiss populations.

Although people from NA represent a small proportion of all individuals migrating to Switzerland, Switzerland has recently seen a rapid rise in migration from NA countries, which has, in part, led to Swiss policy makers pursuing cooperation programs between Switzerland and NA countries on issues of migration and protection [7]. Despite the focus on immigration policy and security issues, not much research, to date, in Switzerland has begun to examine potential health care needs among this population.

Despite the lack of data on the health care needs of individuals from NA in Switzerland, migrants, including those from NA, that arrive to Europe, are at risk for various infection and non-communicable diseases (NCSs). For example, migrants have an increased risk for cardiovascular diseases than the population of the host country [8,9], and in NA migrants in particular a higher risk for Hepatitis B and C, as well as HIV, among other infectious diseases, is reported [10]. Studies also suggest that migration from various countries, including NA, is associated with trauma and greater likelihood of mental health issues [11,12].

One area that might be of particular importance to NA patients, as one station in addressing their health needs, is the utilization of care in Emergency Departments (EDs). In general, European countries, including Switzerland, have reported an increased utilization of EDs among patients with asylum-seeking status [13]. Furthermore, studies have identified a number of important differences in the ways in which immigrants in Europe seek care in EDs [14]. For example, immigrants were more likely to go to the ED for non-acute issues [14,15] and during less "social hours" (e.g., evenings and weekends) [14]. Other studies have reported that the high use of emergency services may be related to inadequate levels of health literacy, a lack of health care system knowledge, lack of access to a general practitioner, undocumented immigration status and language barriers [16–20].

Although migration in and of itself has not been always associated with poor health, the physical, psychological, economic, and social challenges associated with migration have been associated with the presence of psychiatric symptoms. Given the documented challenges that NA migrants face in their country of origin as well as known stressors associated with migration, individuals from NA may be more likely to be in need of psychiatric care in the ED. However, mental health problems in the ED among migrants in general is sparse, and even less is known about NA migrants in particular. Therefore, given the well-documented stressors and exposure to potentially traumatic events associated with migration [21], there is an urgent need to identify whether there are differences between immigrant and non-immigrant utilization of ED resources. If found, such data would point to an important point in the detection and intervention of mental health care services.

To that end, the aim of this study was therefore: (1) to compare the types of admissions to the ED among NA and Swiss-national patients, (2) to examine potential differences in referrals to ambulatory care and psychiatry between NA and Swiss national patients and (3) to identify factors associated with referrals and to ambulatory care and psychiatry. As migration from NA countries is challenging European countries, understanding these aspects should not be a local need, but rather can contribute to the better utilization of healthcare services across the continent, with an aim of improving their health through the implementation of such findings into interventions to improve access and care.

2. Methods

2.1. Design

2.1.1. Setting

The data for the current study was obtained through a retrospective analysis of patient records that had been admitted to the ED of the University Hospital of Bern, Switzerland. It is a level 1 adult ED caring for about 2 million people and in which approximately 46,000 people were treated in 2016 [22]. All adult patients (age ≥ 16 years) admitted to the ED between the 1 January 2013 and the 31 December 2016 were included.

2.1.2. Participants

Patients were identified through the ED electronic patient database and were separated into two groups: (1) patients of NA origin and (2) Swiss nationals. All patients 16 years of age and older were included. According to the Swiss law, the cutoff for treatment in general adult ED is 16. Patients younger than sixteen are referred to the pediatric ED. Exclusion criteria included patients aged less than 16 years, treated in the pediatric ED and with missing documentation of country of origin, triage or leading referred discipline.

2.2. Data Collection

Patients were identified through the ED electronic patient database (E-Care, ED 2.1.3.0, Turnhout, Belgium) and exported into Microsoft Excel (Microsoft Corporation, Redmond, WA, USA) after anonymizing the data.

Variables

Socio-demographic variables included country of origin, determined through the resident card presented at admission. Patients were considered to be from NA if their country of origin was Algeria, Egypt, Libya, Morocco, Sudan or Tunisia. Other variables included type of ED admission (ambulance, walk-in, legal admission [police custody or presence], previous medical contact, and not specified), discipline seen in ED (internal, surgical, psychiatric, other), discharge outcome (ambulatory, hospitalized, death, other), triage level (Swiss triage scale) (1 = life threatening problem that requires an immediate start of treatment to 5 = not urgent condition). The Swiss triage scale is based on the Manchester triage scale which is a five- level scale that was tested for its reliability and validity [23], patient receives an appointment), time of admission (weekday or weekend, where a weekend visit was determined as arrival to ED between Friday 18:00 to Monday 07:00), length of stay in ED (number of hours), and number of ED visits per patient. Ambulatory discharge was determined as being discharged home after the consultation. Seeing a psychiatrist included all ED consultations in which a psychiatrist was the prime or a secondary consultant.

2.3. Statistical Analysis

Statistical analysis was conducted using SPSS Version 22 (BM SPSS Statistics for Windows, IBM Corp., Armonk, NY, USA) and Stata 13.1 (StataCorp, College Station, TX, USA). Descriptive calculation included frequency and percentage of categorical data as well as median and IQR for all continuous variables, as all (age, time in ED and number of visits) had non-normal distribution. Statistical significance was defined as p value < 0.05. For the determination of predicting factors for the two outcome variables (ambulatory discharge and psychiatric consultations), an adjusted logistic regression was conducted. These results ware compared to a model that looked at effect modification for the primary outcomes (ambulatory discharge and psychiatric consultation) by age and sex through an interaction model with presentation of the stratified odds ratios. Age groups were defined as 16–24 [24] (youth promotion measures in Switzerland being aimed at youth aged 16–25 years), 25–39 (young adulthood), 40–64 (later adulthood) and ≥65 (retiring age in Switzerland). As effect modification was identified, only the results of the interaction models were presented for both outcome variables.

3. Results

During the study period, a total of 77,619 Swiss national and NA patients (76,889 Swiss, 98.9%) cumulatively generated 116,859 visits to our ED, with 1338 (1.1%) originated from NA and the others with Swiss nationality. The most common country of origin was Tunisia (405 patients, 30.3%), followed by Morocco (370 patients, 27.7%), Algeria (295 patients, 22.0%), Egypt (142 patients, 10.2%), Sudan (62 patients, 4.6%), and Libya (70 patients, 5.2%) (Figure 1).

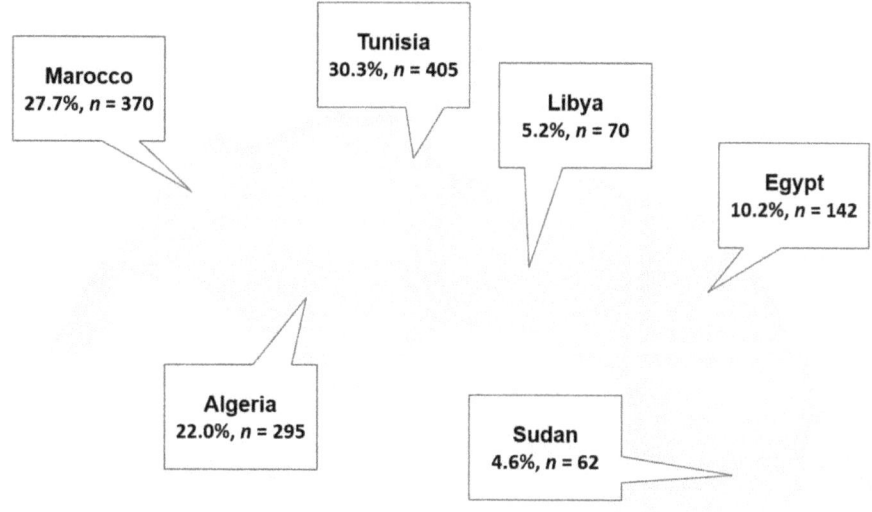

Figure 1. Frequencies of countries of origin of the North African migrant ED population.

3.1. Comparison between NA and Swiss Origin ED Patients' Consultations Characteristics

There were some observed demographic differences between patients from NA and the Swiss population (Table 1). Specifically, patients originating from NA countries were predominantly male (74.4% vs. 55.6% in the Swiss) and younger (median of 38.0 (IQR 28–51 years vs. 52.0 (IQR 32–52) for 154 Swiss). The differences in patient population at discharge reflect the starkly different demographic characteristics of the two populations in our study region (see Figures S1 and S2).

More than half of the visits were walk-in emergencies with the NA patients having significantly more walk-in presentations than the Swiss (55.5% vs. 42.2%). NA patients were assessed in a less acute triage level than the Swiss patients with 79.6% in triage 3 or higher compared to 65.9% in Swiss nationals patients. Additionally, NA patients were more likely to receive an ambulatory care discharge compared to patients from Switzerland (64.2% and 47.4% respectively,) and had shorter length of stay in the ED (median 3.4 h (RQI 2.0–5.4 years) for NA vs 3.6 for Swiss (IQR 3.2 and 3.6 respectively,). However, the median of total visits number was 2.0 for both groups, IQR 1–4 visits for NA and 1–3 for Swiss), with more NA patients having multiple visits (45.4% for NA vs. 33.4% for Swiss). When looking at reasons for admission, the NA patients had higher proportion of admission for general surgical, medical, and psychiatric reasons. In contrast, Swiss patients had higher proportions of admission to specialists (Table 1).

Table 1. Characteristics of ED consultations—comparison between Swiss and NA nationals consultations (*n* = 116,859).

	NA Nationals		Swiss National	
Total, *n* (%)	1338	1.1	115,521	98.9
Gender				
Male	996	74.4	64,250	55.6
Female	342	25.6	51,271	44.4
Reason for admission, *n* (%)				
Surgical	425	31.8	24,756	21.4
Medical	412	30.8	30,637	26.5
Psychiatric	102	7.6	5258	4.6
other discipline	399	29.8	54,870	47.5
Way of admission, *n* (%)				
Ambulance	155	11.6	19,305	16.7
previous medical contact	55	4.1	18,104	15.7
legal admission	101	7.5	946	0.8
walk-in	743	55.5	48,772	42.2
Other	48	3.6	4609	4.0
Triage, *n* (%)				
1 (life threatening)	42	3.6	10,386	9.0
2 (urgent conditions)	232	17.3	28,942	25.1
3 (semi-urgent conditions)	909	67.9	66,308	57.4
4 (low urgent conditions)	113	8.6	7531	6.5
5 (not urgent conditions)	42	3.1	2354	2.0
ED outcome, *n* (%)				
discharge at home	859	64.2	54,989	47.6
hospital admission	268	20.0	41,508	35.9
Death	0	0.0	222	0.2
Not specific	170	12.7	17,510	15.2
Other	41	3.1	1292	1.1
Weekend admission, *n* (%)	437	32.7	39,137	33.9
Multiple visit, *n* (%)	306	45.4	38,632	33.4
Seen by psychiatrist, *n* (%)	193	14.4	8417	7.3
Age, med (IQR)	38.0	28–51	52.0	32–52
Duration in ED (hours), med (IQR)	3.4	2.0–5.4	3.6	2.2–6.2
Number of visits, med (IQR)	2.0	1.0–4.0	2.0	1.0–3.0

3.2. Predictors of Ambulatory Discharge

A logistic regression was performed to determine the effects of possible predicting variables on the odds of being discharged to ambulatory care. NA patients had 1.2 times higher odds (95% CI 1.07–1.40, $p < 0.003$) of being treated as an out-patient in comparison to Swiss national patients, adjusted for age, sex, triage, weekend admission, discipline, weekend consultation and type of admission. To examine effect modification in age groups and sex, an interaction model was conducted. Results are presented in Table 2.

Table 2. Sex and Age group stratified odds ratios * (95% CI) for the outcome ambulant discharge for the comparison NA vs. Swiss (*n* = 116,859). (significant associations in italic and bold).

Sex	Age Group			
	16–24	25–39	40–64	65–Max
Female	0.89 (95% CI: 0.38–2.06)	1.45 (95% CI: 0.96–2.19)	*1.56 (95% CI: 1.01–2.39)*	3.31 (95% CI: 0.93–11.76)
Male	0.94 (95% CI: 0.61–1.46)	1.02 (95% CI: 0.81–1.27)	*1.28 (95% CI: 1.01–1.63)*	1.78 (95% CI: 0.76–4.14)

* adjusted for type of admission, triage category, discipline category, multiple consultation, weekend consultation.

The CI of the odds ratios differed in some of the different age-sex-strata, e.g., in the 40–64 group NA patients were associated with greater odds of ambulatory discharge, but not in the 25–39 age group. Thus, the studied effect is modified by age and sex respectively and their interaction and stratified odds ratios have to be used (Table 2).

3.3. Predictors of Psychiatry Referral

To further understand resource utilization in the ED, a second model was run examining the predictors of psychiatric consultation between NA and Swiss national patients. A logistic regression was conducted. Consultations by NA patients had a 1.75 (95% CI: 1.5–2.0, $p < 0.0001$) times higher odd of being seen by a psychiatrist adjusted for age, sex, triage, weekend visits, and multiple ED visits than consultations by Swiss patients. Again, to examine effect modification of age groups and sex, an interaction model was applied. Results are presented in Table 3.

Table 3. Sex and Age group stratified odds ratios * (95% CI) for the outcome seen by psychiatrist for the comparison NA vs. Swiss (*n* = 116,859) (significant associations in italic and bold).

Sex	Age Group			
	16–24	25–39	40–64	65–Max
Female	1.25 (95% CI: 0.48–3.24)	*0.51 (95% CI: 0.27–0.94)*	0.68 (95% CI: 0.36–1.3)	2.81 (95% CI: 0.37–21.64)
Male	*3.45 (95% CI: 2.22–5.38)*	*1.95 (95% CI: 1.53–2.49)*	*1.94 (95% CI: 1.44–2.61)*	2.98 (95% CI: 0.7–12.68)

* adjusted for triage, multiple consultation, weekend consultation.

There are noted differences in some of the strata between males and females. The odds ratio for seen by psychiatrist in females aged 25–39 years (OR 0.51, 95% CI 0.27–0.94), suggested evidence for a "protective" effect of being NA in adult females regarding being seen by a psychiatrist. In contrast, among males, being NA increased the odds of being seen by a psychiatrist about the factor 2 (OR 1.95, 95% CI 1.53–2.49). Thus, the effect of the association between the exposure (NA vs. Swiss) and the studied outcome (seen by a psychiatrist) is strongly modified by sex, and in the interaction of sex and age. Especially, sex is a strong effect modifier. For age, there seems to be a slight effect modification too. The odds ratio for seen by a psychiatrist in the very young (age 16–24) NA male group is about 3.5 times higher (OR 3.45, 95% CI 2.22–5.38) in comparison with the Swiss national males of the same age, whereas in the young adults (age 25–39) male group the odds ratio point of higher risk was almost twice (OR 1.95, 95% CI 1.53–2.49) in comparison to Swiss national males in the same age (Table 3).

4. Discussion

This is the first study, to our knowledge, comparing the utilization of ED services and referrals in NA immigrants and non-immigrants in a high-income country. Specifically, this study sought to examine whether NA immigrants and non-immigrants would differ in their frequency of ED use and referral type during their ED visit and upon hospital discharge. Converging with a growing body of research showing that immigrants and non-immigrants differ in their utilization of ED services, these data found that NA patients differed from Swiss national patients in a number of important ways. First, the demographic characteristics differed between NA and Swiss-national patients. That is,

NA ED patients were more likely to be male and younger. Second, compared to Swiss national patients, NA patients were more likely to seek care for less acute issues, had greater number of total visits and re-visits, and spent fewer hours in the ED [15,25].

Additionally, a greater proportion of NA patients arrived at the ED through self-referral or through a legal context, whereas Swiss national patients were more likely to have been referred to the ED through another healthcare provider. Third, the two groups differed in terms of referrals and discharge type: NA patients were more likely to see a psychiatrist in the ED and were more likely to be discharged to ambulatory care.

Taken together, these findings begin to shed light on the importance of examining immigrant communities use of healthcare resources within the ED, as it reveals the changes in how patients are using the ED and possibly the healthcare needs. Importantly, these data underscore the importance of studying how immigrants are using the ED, as immigrants appear to be seeking care for non-urgent issues in this setting, rather than through a primary care provider and consecutively generate more visits and lower hospitalization rates than non-immigrant patients.

It is unclear from these data why NA patients are using the ED more often and for less urgent matters. Findings from other studies, however, suggest that immigrants may be more likely to seek care in EDs, compared to seeing other medical specialties, for a variety of legal, cultural, and social factors [26]. In addition, some studies have found that lower levels of healthcare literacy in immigrant communities may impact medical decisions [20,27,28]. Third, although not necessarily the case in Switzerland, immigrants often receive minimal coverage through their insurance, and in some cases, may only receive insurance for emergencies [15]. Therefore, it may be perceived in some immigrant communities that they may not be eligible for care outside the ED. Given this growing number of studies showing a disproportionally greater use of the ED among immigrants, further research is needed to better understand the motivations underlying ED use and barriers to care among other medical specializations.

The greater utilization of the ED among NA patients, both in terms of total and multiple visits, for non-acute medical issues suggests that there is an important need for healthcare systems to consider ways to reduce patient visits. These findings point to the need to develop healthcare literacy programs targeting ED use. A number of community-based strategies for increasing health literacy have proven effective [29,30]. A possible approach for a comprehensive intervention that are hoped to increase patient engagement is the use of the social-ecological model [31]. Future work would benefit from examining whether similar programs may aid in the reduction of ED visits and re-visits for non-acute issues.

Importantly, NA patients in this study were more likely to receive a referral for psychiatric care. Unfortunately, specific mental health disorders were not assessed in this study so the exact cause for the referral is not known. These findings, however, are directly in line with considerable research showing the immigrants are exposed to considerable stress and trauma throughout the migration process, which has been associated with high levels of mental health issues such as depression and PTSD [32,33]. Future work would also benefit from examining the extent to which the patients received the follow-up psychiatric care. Although speculation, one potential reason for the multiple visits, is that the NA patients, for a variety of reasons (e.g., language barriers, lack of trust, cultural beliefs), may not have been enrolled into on-going psychiatric care, and instead continued to seek help from the ED.

These data also point to the potential importance of incorporating brief mental health interventions for immigrants into ED. Given the high rates of psychiatric referrals, offering brief psycho-social interventions within the ED may aid in the reduction of distress and may help to motivate patients to seek additional care. Studies indicate that culturally adapted mental health interventions have a higher potential of being effective, with a focus on groups of same background and in patients' language [34]. An example for such intervention is the International Psychosocial Organization (IPSO) psychos-social counselling program targeted to refugees. The program trains counsellors within the community, to enable a linguistic and culturally sensitive service [35,36]. Future work needs to examine whether similar programs can be integrated into an ED context, for patients identified with mental health problems. Along those lines, these findings indicate that medical staff in the ED might benefit from training in this area as many immigrants may present with complaints that include mental health symptoms. Such training would benefit from the inclusion of culture competence capacity building for physicians and nurses, with existing evidence on the effectiveness among trained professionals in a hospital setting in Switzerland [37]. Similar training was conducted in our ED by the Swiss Red Cross.

It is unclear why NA patients were more likely to arrive in the ED from legal contexts. It may be related to co-occurring and improperly managed mental health concerns, stressors associated with post-migration (e.g., low socio-economic status), and/or potential selection biases in which the police may be more likely to bring an NA patient to the ED in unclear situations. This has the potential to create a vicious circle that leads to lower quality of care and again to readmissions.

Despite the novel contributions of these data to the understanding of how immigrants in the ED, several limitations warrant discussion. First, it is a retrospective study. Follow-up research would benefit from clinical interviews and the employment of prospective methodologies. Second, as previously, mentioned, these data indicate the type of referral but not the specific diagnosis. Also, data on morbidity is not available. Therefore, greater work is needed to better characterize the issues being presented in the ED. Moreover, we cannot provide information on medical condition of pregnant women and children, as they are usually treated at different EDs within our hospital. Lastly, it would be beneficial to stratify in our analysis the Swiss patients into socioeconomic groups, in order to assess if NA population is more closely matched to a particular socioeconomic Swiss group. Unfortunately, this data was not available in our ED records and such analysis could not be conducted.

Notwithstanding these limitations, these data emphasize the importance of the ED in the care of recent immigrants. In particular, they point to an evolving use of the ED in which patients are seeking care more regularly for less acute issues. As studies provide more information on the underlying factors contributing to these patterns, health care providers will need to consider ways to target healthcare literacy more effectively and leverage the types of care provided by ED for immigrants. These findings may be applicable also outside of Switzerland, as the immigration from NA is a continuous phenomenon across Europe, and the culturally sensitive interventions that address these challenges, can serve as a major contribution to a better utilization of ED resources and assist in improving the health of NA migrants. One framework that might be good for integration of such programs across Europe is the Health Promoting Hospitals and Health Services network, that uses the healthy settings approach in an aim to integrate health promotion concepts, values, standards and indicators into the organizational structure and culture of the hospital of the health service, to gain better health to patients, staff and communities. The initiative includes a focus on Migrant friendly and culturally competent health care [38]. In Switzerland, in particular, the "Swiss Hospitals for Equity" network, where our ED is partnering in the activities, aims to improve health and health services to migrants in the hospital setting [39].

5. Conclusions

The study identified differences between the ED patients from Switzerland and NA. NA patients were less likely to be admitted to the hospital and NA males were more likely to be referred to a physiatrist. NA male patients are more likely to be seen by psychiatrist when they seek consultation at the ED, especially in very young adults (16–24) suggesting that those are of special need for special attention and further follow-ups as needed. The different patterns of ED care use between Swiss nationals and NA migrants, were associated with significantly more ambulatory discharges stress the need to focus on ways to ensure access to primary health services to migrant population. Measures that promote equity are paramount in the different population presented to the ED. On the patient level, interventions that focus on case management for patients with re-visits [40] are also recommended, with a hope that using multiple-dimensions approaches could support in slowly closing the health gaps between the two populations.

Supplementary Materials: The following are available online at http://www.mdpi.com/1660-4601/15/9/2033/s1, Figure S1: NA population in Canton Bern by age groups and gender (%), Figure S2: Swiss population in Canton Bern by age groups and gender (%).

Author Contributions: Conceptualization, O.K., S.N.J., M.M., A.K.E. and D.S.S.; Data curation, S.N.J., S.Z. and D.S.S.; Formal analysis, O.K., S.Z. and M.M.; Funding acquisition, A.D.B.; Methodology, O.K. and S.N.J.; Software, M.M.; Validation, S.Z. and D.S.S.; Visualization, A.D.B.; Writing—original draft, O.K., S.N.J. and A.D.B.; Writing—review & editing, O.K., S.N.J., M.M., A.K.E. and D.S.S.

Funding: M.M. was funded by the Bangerter Foundation and the Swiss Academy of Medical Sciences through the "Young Talents in Clinical research" grant (TCR 14/17). This research was also supported by the Fulbright Grant awarded to the Inselspital and to Adam Brown.

Acknowledgments: We thank Sabina Utiger, Meret Ricklin and Jolanta Kluksowa-Rösler from our Emergency Department at Inselspital Bern for data preparation and support. We thank Michael Moses for English Language editing. We also thank Wolf E. Hautz for the research support.

Conflicts of Interest: The authors declare no conflict of interest.

Ethics Approval: The study was granted a waiver from ethical review by the Ethics committee of the Canton Berne under number Ref.-Nr. KEK BE: 010/2016.

Availability of Data and Material: The datasets used and/or analysed during the current study are available from the corresponding author on reasonable request.

Abbreviations

ED	Emergency Department
HPC	Health care providers
NA	North Africa
CDC	Non Communicable Disease
IPSO	International Psychosocial Organization

References

1. International Organization for Migration (IOM). Who Is a Migrant? Available online: https://www.iom.int/who-is-a-migrant (accessed on 26 July 2018).
2. United Nations, Department of Economic and Social Affairs. International Migration Report 2015: Highlights. Available online: https://www.google.com/url?sa=t&rct=j&q=&esrc=s&source=web&cd=1&ved=2ahUKEwj2xaTdwLTdAhUSdt4KHRy6ALEQFjAAegQIAhAC&url=http%3A%2F%2Fwww.un.org%2Fen%2Fdevelopment%2Fdesa%2Fpopulation%2Fmigration%2Fpublications%2Fmigrationreport%2Fdocs%2FMigrationReport2015_Highlights.pdf&usg=AOvVaw1CdU51k4MwZnMzi0--XT74 (accessed on 26 July 2018).
3. International Organization for Migration (IOM). World Migration Report 2015. Migrants and Cities: New Partnerships to Manage Mobility. Available online: publications.iom.int/system/files/wmr2015_en.pdf (accessed on 26 July 2018).
4. Hatton, T.J. Seeking asylum in Europe. *Econ.Policy* **2004**, *19*, 6–62. [CrossRef]
5. Swiss Confederation, Federal Department of Home Affairs. Switzerland Population. Facts and Figures 2016. Available online: www.statistics.admin.ch (accessed on 26 July 2018).
6. Swiss Confedaration, Department of Justice. Migration Report 2015. Available online: https://www.sem.admin.ch/dam/data/sem/publiservice/berichte/migration/migrationsbericht-2015-e.pdf (accessed on 26 July 2018).
7. Swiss Confedaration, Department of Justice. Migration Report 2016. Available online: https://www.sem.admin.ch/dam/.../migration/migrationsbericht-2016-e.pdf (accessed on 1 September 2018).
8. Gadd, M.; Johansson, S.-E.; Sundquist, J.; Wändell, P. Morbidity in cardiovascular diseases in immigrants in Sweden. *J. Int. Med.* **2003**, *254*, 236–243. [CrossRef]
9. Hedlund, E.; Lange, A.; Hammar, N. Acute myocardial infarction incidence in immigrants to Sweden. Country of birth, time since immigration, and time trends over 20 years. *Eur. J. Epidemiol.* **2007**, *22*, 493–503. [CrossRef] [PubMed]

10. Khyatti, M.; Trimbitas, R.-D.; Zouheir, Y.; Benani, A.; Messaoudi, M.-D.E.; Hemminki, K. Infectious diseases in North Africa and North African immigrants to Europe. *Eur. J. Public Health* **2014**, *24*, 47–56. [CrossRef] [PubMed]
11. Abebe, D.S.; Lien, L.; Hjelde, K.H. What we know and don't know about mental health problems among immigrants in Norway. *J. Immigr. Minor Health* **2014**, *16*, 60–67. [CrossRef] [PubMed]
12. Markkula, N.; Lehti, V.; Gissler, M.; Suvisaari, J. Incidence and prevalence of mental disorders among immigrants and native Finns: A register-based study. *Soc. Psychiatry Psychiatr. Epidemiol.* **2017**, *52*, 523–1540. [CrossRef] [PubMed]
13. Muller, M.; Klingberg, K.; Srivastava, D.; Exadaktylos, A.K. Consultations by Asylum Seekers: Recent Trends in the Emergency Department of a Swiss University Hospital. *PLoS ONE* **2016**, *11*, e0155423. [CrossRef] [PubMed]
14. Crede, S.H.; Such, E.; Mason, S. International migrants' use of emergency departments in Europe compared with non-migrants' use: A systematic review. *Eur. J. Public Health* **2018**, *28*, 61–73. [CrossRef] [PubMed]
15. Mahmoud, I.; Hou, X.Y. Immigrants and the utilization of hospital emergency departments. *World J. Emerg. Med.* **2012**, *3*, 245–250. [CrossRef] [PubMed]
16. Norredam, M.; Mygind, A.; Nielsen, A.S.; Bagger, J.; Krasnik, A. Motivation and relevance of emergency room visits among immigrants and patients of Danish origin. *Eur. J. Public Health* **2007**, *17*, 497–502. [CrossRef] [PubMed]
17. Rue, M.; Cabré, X.; Soler-Gonzále, J.; Bosch, A.; Almirall, M.; Serna, M.C. Emergency hospital services utilization in Lleida (Spain): A cross-sectional study of immigrant and Spanish-born populations. *BMC Health Serv. Res.* **2008**, *8*, 81. [CrossRef] [PubMed]
18. Smaland Goth, U.G.; Berg, J.E. Migrant participation in Norwegian health care. A qualitative study using key informants. *Eur. J. Gen. Pract.* **2011**, *17*, 28–33. [CrossRef]
19. Petersen, L.A.; Burstin, H.R.; O'Neil, A.C.; Orav, E.J.; Brennan, T.A. Nonurgent emergency department visits: The effect of having a regular doctor. *Med. Care* **1998**, *36*, 1249–1255. [CrossRef] [PubMed]
20. Gele, A.A.; Pettersen, K.S.; Torheim, L.E.; Kumar, B. Health literacy: The missing link in improving the health of Somali immigrant women in Oslo. *BMC Public Health* **2016**, *16*, 1134. [CrossRef] [PubMed]
21. Bhugra, D. Migration and mental health. *Acta Psychiatrca Scand.* **2004**, *109*, 243–258. [CrossRef]
22. Exadaktylos A, H.W. Emergency medicine in Switzerland. *ICU Manag.* **2015**, *15*, 160–162.
23. Christ, M.; Grossmann, F.; Winter, D.; Bingisser, R.; Platz, E. Modern Triage in the Emergency Department. *Dtsch. Arzteblatt Int.* **2010**, *107*, 892–898. [CrossRef] [PubMed]
24. Swiss Confederation, Federal Department of Home Affairs, Families, Generations and Society Department. Child and Youth Promotion Act. 2008. Available online: http://www.youthpolicy.org/national/Switzerland_2008_Youth_Policy_Strategy.pdf (accessed on 1 September 2018). (In German)
25. Tarraf, W.; Vega, W.; Gonzalez, H.M. Emergency department services use among immigrant and non-immigrant groups in the United States. *J. Immigr. Minor Health* **2014**, *16*, 595–606. [CrossRef] [PubMed]
26. Hacker, K.; Anies, M.; Folb, B.L.; Zallman, L. Barriers to health care for undocumented immigrants: A literature review. *Risk Manag. Healthc Policy* **2015**, *8*, 175–183. [CrossRef] [PubMed]
27. Mantwill, S.; Schulz, P.J. Low health literacy and healthcare utilization among immigrants and non-immigrants in Switzerland. *Patient Educ. Couns.* **2017**, *100*, 2020–2027. [CrossRef] [PubMed]
28. Kreps, G.L.; Sparks, L. Meeting the health literacy needs of immigrant populations. *Patient Educ. Couns.* **2008**, *71*, 328–332. [CrossRef] [PubMed]
29. Ishikawa, H.; Yamaguchi, I.; Nutbeam, D.; Kato, M.; Okuhara, T.; Okada, M.; Kiuchi, T. Improving health literacy in a Japanese community population—A pilot study to develop an educational programme. *Health Expect* **2018**. [CrossRef] [PubMed]
30. Nutbeam, D.; McGill, B.; Premkumar, P. Improving health literacy in community populations: A review of progress. *Health Promot. Int.* **2017**. [CrossRef] [PubMed]
31. McCormack, L.; Thomas, V.; Lewis, M.A.; Rudd, R. Improving low health literacy and patient engagement: A social ecological approach. *Patient Educ. Couns.* **2017**, *100*, 8–13. [CrossRef] [PubMed]
32. Silove, D.; Ventevogel, P.; Rees, S. The contemporary refugee crisis: An overview of mental health challenges. *World Psychiatry* **2017**, *16*, 130–139. [CrossRef] [PubMed]

33. Turrini, G.; Purgato, M.; Ballette, F.; Nosè, M.; Ostuzzi, G.; Barbui, C. Common mental disorders in asylum seekers and refugees: Umbrella review of prevalence and intervention studies. *Int. J. Ment. Health Syst.* **2017**, *11*, 51. [CrossRef] [PubMed]
34. Griner, D.; Smith, T.B. Culturally adapted mental health intervention: A meta-analytic review. *Psychotherapy* **2006**, *43*, 531–548. [CrossRef] [PubMed]
35. International Psychosocial Organization (IPSO). Helping People Help Themselves—Refugees for Refugees. Available online: https://ipsocontext.org/ (accessed on 1 September 2018).
36. Ayoughi, S.; Missmahl, I.; Weierstall, R.; Elbert, T. Provision of mental health services in resource-poor settings: A randomised trial comparing counselling with routine medical treatment in North Afghanistan (Mazar-e-Sharif). *BMC Psychiatry* **2012**, *12*, 14. [CrossRef] [PubMed]
37. Casillas, A.; Paroz, S.; Green, A.R.; Wolff, H.; Weber, O.; Faucherre, F.; Ninane, F.; Bodenmann, P. Cultural competency of health-care providers in a Swiss University Hospital: Self-assessed cross-cultural skillfulness in a cross-sectional study. *BMC Med. Educ.* **2014**, *14*, 19. [CrossRef] [PubMed]
38. Pelikan, J.M. Health promoting hospitals–Assessing developments in the network. *Ital. J. Public Health* **2012**. [CrossRef]
39. Swiss Confedaration, Federal Department of Home Affairs. Swiss Hospitals for Equity. Available online: http://www.hospitals4equity.ch/index.php/en/ (accessed on 1 September 2018).
40. Bodenmann, P.; Velonaki, V.-S.; Griffin, J.L.; Baggio, S.; Iglesias, K.; Moschetti, K.; Ruggeri, O.; Burnand, B.; Wasserfallen, J.-B.; Vu, F.; et al. Case Management may Reduce Emergency Department Frequent use in a Universal Health Coverage System: A Randomized Controlled Trial. *J. Gen. Int. Med.* **2017**, *32*, 508–515. [CrossRef] [PubMed]

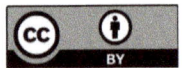

© 2018 by the authors. Licensee MDPI, Basel, Switzerland. This article is an open access article distributed under the terms and conditions of the Creative Commons Attribution (CC BY) license (http://creativecommons.org/licenses/by/4.0/).

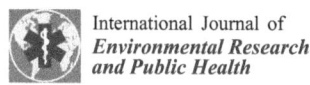

Review

Interventions to Improve Vaccination Uptake and Cost Effectiveness of Vaccination Strategies in Newly Arrived Migrants in the EU/EEA: A Systematic Review

Charles Hui [1,*], Jessica Dunn [1], Rachael Morton [2], Lukas P. Staub [2], Anh Tran [2], Sally Hargreaves [3,4], Christina Greenaway [5], Beverly Ann Biggs [6,7], Robin Christensen [8] and Kevin Pottie [9,10]

1. Division of Infectious Diseases, Children's Hospital of Eastern Ontario, University of Ottawa, Ottawa, ON K1H 8L1, Canada; jdunn@cheo.on.ca
2. NHMRC Clinical Trials Centre, Sydney Medical School, University of Sydney, Camperdown 1450, Australia; rachael.morton@ctc.usyd.edu.au (R.M.); lukas.staub@ctc.usyd.edu.au (L.P.S.); anh.tran@ctc.usyd.edu.au (A.T.)
3. International Health Unit, Section of Infectious Diseases and Immunity, Imperial College London; London W12 0NN, UK; s.hargreaves@imperial.ac.uk
4. The Institute for Infection and Immunity, St George's, University of London, London SW17 0RE, UK
5. Division of Infectious Diseases and Clinical Epidemiology, SMBD-Jewish General Hospital, McGill University, Montreal, QC H3T 1E2, Canada; ca.greenaway@mcgill.ca
6. Department of Medicine/RMH at the Doherty Institute, University of Melbourne, Melbourne 3000, Australia; babiggs@unimelb.edu.au
7. The Victorian Infectious Diseases Service, Royal Melbourne Hospital, Parkville 3050, Australia
8. Musculoskeletal Statistics Unit, The Parker Institute, Bispebjerg and Frederiksberg Hospital, 2000 Frederiksberg, Denmark; robin.christensen@regionh.dk
9. Bruyere Research Institute, Ottawa, ON K1N 5C8, Canada; kpottie@uottawa.ca
10. Departments of Family Medicine and Epidemiology and Community Medicine, University of Ottawa, Ottawa, ON K1G 5Z3, Canada
* Correspondence: chui@cheo.on.ca; Tel.: +1-613-737-7600

Received: 31 July 2018; Accepted: 7 September 2018; Published: 20 September 2018

Abstract: Newly arrived migrants to the EU/EEA (arrival within the past five years), as well as other migrant groups in the region, might be under-immunised and lack documentation of previous vaccinations, putting them at increased risk of vaccine-preventable diseases circulating in Europe. We therefore performed a systematic review conforming to PRISMA guidelines (PROSPERO CRD42016045798) to explore: (i) interventions that improve vaccine uptake among migrants; and (ii) cost-effectiveness of vaccination strategies among this population. We searched MEDLINE, Embase, CINAHL, and Cochrane Database of Systematic Reviews (CDSR) between 1 January 2006 to 18 June 2018. We included three primary intervention studies performed in the EU/EEA or high-income countries and one cost effectiveness study relevant to vaccinations in migrants. Intervention studies showed small but promising impact only on vaccine uptake with social mobilization/community outreach, planned vaccination programs and education campaigns. Targeting migrants for catch-up vaccination is cost effective for presumptive vaccination for diphtheria, tetanus, and polio, and there was no evidence of benefit of carrying out pre-vaccination serological testing. The cost-effectiveness is sensitive to the seroprevalence and adherence to vaccinations of the migrant. We conclude that scarce but direct EU/EEA data suggest social mobilization, vaccine programs, and education campaigns are promising strategies for migrants, but more research is needed. Research should also study cost effectiveness of strategies. Vaccination of migrants should continue to be a public heath priority in EU/EEA.

Keywords: VPD; immunisation strategies; health systems; refugees; migrants; cost effectiveness

1. Introduction

Globally, there are over 258 million people who migrate across international borders, including labour migrants, students, refugees, asylum seekers, undocumented migrants, and other migrant groups [1]. Another 763 million people migrate internally [2]. In the European Union/European Economic Area (EU/EEA) in particular, there has been an unprecedented number of refugees and other migrants between 2014 and 2016 linked to the Syrian war [3], other armed conflicts, climate change and economic crises. In addition, there are around 40 million EU migrants who have moved internally from one European country to another [4].

Control of vaccine preventable diseases (VPDs) is a priority in the EU/EEA [5]. Very little information is available on the occurrence of vaccine preventable diseases specifically among newly arrived migrant populations in the EU/EEA. Although national surveillance systems for VPDs are in place and regular reporting occurs, surveillance is incomplete for migrant health data such as country of birth and time since arrival. There have been EU/EEA measles and polio outbreaks that have been related to under-immunised migrant populations [6–10], but outbreaks have also occurred in non-migrant populations [11–14]. The 2017/2018 pan-European measles epidemic involved internal EU/EEA migrants moving between countries, so it is important also to consider this group alongside migrants arriving from outside of the EU/EEA [15].

Seroprevalence studies have demonstrated sub-optimal immunity to VPD among adult and child migrants [16–24]. Further, the WHO's global data on immunisation coverage report sub-optimal immunisation among the general population worldwide, with global coverage ranging 47–85% depending on the vaccine and even greater variation between geographical region [25]. This includes the EU/EEA, where some countries have not achieved target vaccine coverage with regards to, for example, first dose measles. Among all types of migrants from the top ten countries of birth arriving to the EU/EEA, the range of age-appropriate (i.e., two-dose) measles vaccination coverage ranges 31–99% [26]. Sub-optimal immunity has implications for maintaining herd immunity to minimize outbreaks where seropositivity thresholds within 80–94% are required [25,27]. Collective immunity below these thresholds, whether it is the native-born population, newly-arrived migrants, or a combination, carries the inherent risk of disease transmission and outbreak.

A recent cross-sectional survey study of EU/EEA countries "immigrant" measles vaccination policy demonstrated a significant diversity in strategies with 9 of 31 states having no policy. The remaining 22 states' policies differed widely in utilizing age, immunisation status, method for assessing immunisation status and immigrant type [28]. Furthermore, vaccination policies tailored to migrants and refugees are heterogenous across WHO European region member states [29]. Vaccinations are effective, but there are no specific data on effective implementation strategies for immunization in migrants to EU/EEA. We therefore performed a systematic review to address: (i) what interventions increase uptake of vaccinations in migrants; and (ii) cost-effectiveness of vaccination strategies among migrants.

2. Methods

Using the Grading of Recommendations Assessment, Development and Evaluation (GRADE) approach, the Campbell and Cochrane Collaboration Equity Methods Group and review team, including clinicians, public health experts and researchers from across the EU/EEA, conducted evidence syntheses. A detailed description of the methods can be found in the registered systematic review protocol [30].

The review group followed the PRISMA Reporting guideline [31] for the reporting of this systematic review (PROSPERO CRD42016045798). In summary, the review team developed key research questions and a logic model showing an evidence chain to identify key concepts, to consider the potential role of indirect evidence related to populations and interventions and to support the formulation of search strategies (Supplementary Materials). We aimed to answer the following questions:

What interventions increase the uptake of vaccinations in migrants?
What are cost-effective strategies for vaccinating migrants?

We developed our inclusion and exclusion criteria based on the PICO model (population, intervention, comparator and outcome). "Migrants," a focus for the eligible evidence, included asylum seekers, refugees, undocumented migrants, and other foreign-born residents, with a focus on newly arrived migrants as defined in the protocol as within five years of arrival to the destination country [30]. Internal EU migrants were also included to reflect the large movement of migrants within the EU who were new to the EU/EEA. Only papers addressing migrants to the EU/EEA or other high-income countries were included in the final synthesis. The intervention included any strategy to increase vaccination. The comparators were migrants not exposed to the intervention. We considered the following outcomes: uptake of vaccination and completion of vaccination; disease incidence rates for measles, congenital rubella, diphtheria pertussis, tetanus, Hib, and polio among migrant populations; and cost effectiveness.

Using relevant search terms and strategies, we searched published literature from 1 January 2006 to 18 June 2018 in MEDLINE, Embase, CINAHL, and Cochrane Database of Systematic Reviews (CDSR) for interventions to improve vaccine uptake (File Supplementary A). Searches were designed and conducted by librarian experienced in systematic reviews using a method designed to optimize term selection [32]. The MEDLINE search was validated by testing its ability to retrieve the eligible studies found from the initial search. All were indexed in MEDLINE and the search retrieval was 95%, thus the search was not modified before the final update was run [33]. For economic studies, we searched MEDLINE, Database of Abstracts of Reviews of Effects (DARE), (CDSR) and EMBASE from 1 January 2006 to 26 May 2016, and in addition, NHS EED, CEA Registry (Tufts University) and Google Scholar from 1995 to 2016 (File Supplementary B). No language restrictions were applied to both searches.

For the intervention studies, at least two reviewers (JD, CH, JB, and NN) independently reviewed the titles and abstracts of the papers identified from the search, identifying them as "included" or "not included" based on previously described inclusion/exclusion criteria. Any conflicts were then resolved through discussion by the two review leads (CH and JD). At the second level screening, two independent reviewers performed a full text review per paper (JD, CH, JB, and NN). Conflicts were again resolved via discussion by review leads (CH and JD). The quality of nonrandomized studies was assessed using the Newcastle–Ottawa Scale (NOS) [34]. No studies were excluded based on the NOS.

For the cost effectiveness studies, two reviewers independently reviewed all full text articles (LS and AT) and extracted relevant data from the primary studies that met our inclusion criteria including the economic study design (e.g., micro-costing study, within-trial cost-utility analysis, and decision-analytic model); the intervention and comparator; the difference in resource use; cost-effectiveness results (e.g., incremental net benefit or incremental cost-effectiveness ratio); the certainty of evidence around resource requirements; and whether the cost-effectiveness results favoured the intervention or comparator. Finally, we assessed the certainty of economic evidence in each study using the relevant items from the 1997 Drummond checklist [35].

3. Results

3.1. What Interventions Increase Uptake of Vaccinations in Migrants?

The search for interventions that increase uptake of vaccinations identified 2970 studies. Three studies were included in the final analysis [36–38] (PRISMA Flow Diagram Figure 1). After assessment with the Newcastle–Ottawa Scale (NOS; Table 1), two were determined to be of medium quality [36,38] (NOS 4–6), and one was a low quality study [37] (NOS < 4).

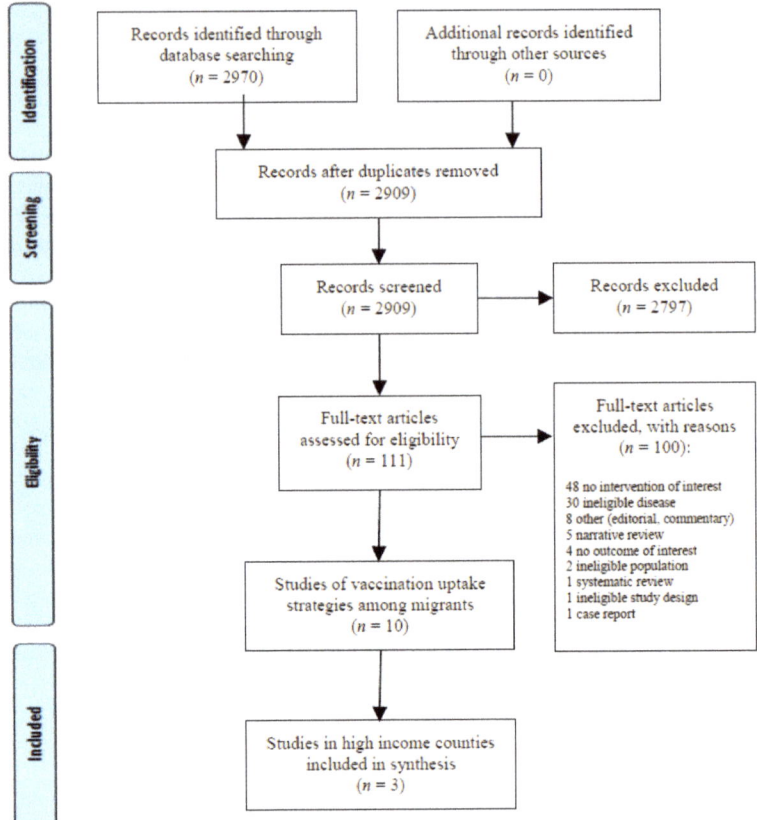

Figure 1. PRISMA Flow Diagram–Interventions to Increase Vaccination Uptake among Migrants.

Two studies were in international migrants to Germany [38] and Australia [36] and one was in internal migrants in Italy [37]. The study characteristics are described in Table 1. Interventions included social mobilization/community outreach [38], planned vaccination programs [36,37], and education campaigns [38]. All the published interventions were associated with positive outcomes of receipt of vaccination. The only outcome reported was vaccine uptake. No disease rates, enrolment in health services or migrant acceptance of vaccination were reported.

Table 1. Characteristics of included studies in high income countries—strategies to increase vaccination uptake.

Study	Quality [1]	Type of study	Setting (Country)	Population	Intervention	Results/Outcomes
Brockmann, 2016 [38]	4/10	Cohort study	Housing units (Germany)	Children, adolescent, adult asylum seekers	Vaccination "concept" facilitated by local public health office: (1) Written letters and posters informing about VPDs (2) In person communication about VPDs (3) Invitations to onsite vaccination campaigns (4) Informational vaccine material in various languages and via interpreters	58% of refugees exposed to concept were vaccinated compared to 6% of refugees vaccinated in facilities without the intervention
Milne, 2006 [36]	4/10	Cross-sectional: assessing uptake of MMR, HepB	School (Australia)	Refugee adolescents, young adults	(1) Self-report survey on immunisation status and primary health care use, with provision of 1 dose MMR. (2) Letter given to student with due date f and written referral to GP; list of GPs and spoken languages available	74% students received MMR vaccine 30% historical vaccination rate
Spadea, 2014 [37]	2/10	Cross-sectional: assessing uptake of MMR and hexavalent (DPT-Hib-IPV-HepB)	Nomadic camp (Italy)	Roma children and women of childbearing age	Vaccination day held on monthly basis	56.4% coverage of hexavalent vaccine (range 44–91%) at three camps 58.4% coverage of MMR vaccine (range 53–83%) at three camps 30% increase in vaccinations compared with previous year

[1] The quality of evidence was assessed using the Newcastle–Ottawa Scale (NOS); rated out of 10 for cross-sectional studies, and out of 9 for case-control or cohort studies.

Of the two studies that were performed in Europe, one was cohort study of asylum seekers living in housing units in Germany employed a vaccination strategy using multiple different interventions [38]. The local public health office informed asylees about relevant VPDs in written letters and posters, as well as in person, and invited them to on-site vaccination campaigns. General practitioners carried out the actual vaccination. Information material regarding vaccination was provided in various languages and via interpreters. Vaccination "certificates" were also provided. In areas utilizing this vaccination strategy, 58% of refugees were vaccinated compared to 6% of refugees vaccinated in facilities without the intervention. Of the total 642 asylees who were vaccinated, 86% received their immunization within the vaccine intervention program. There was a particular focus on male adult asylees who had an eight-fold increase in vaccinations through the strategy. Of note, the program purchased vaccines directly from the manufacturer, saving 50% of the cost compared to buying from a pharmacy. A second European study involved Roma children and women of childbearing age in a nomadic camp in Rome. As part of a tuberculosis outbreak assessment, a monthly vaccination day led to a 56% coverage of hexavalent vaccines and a 58% coverage of MMR vaccines which was a 30% increase in vaccinated subjects compared with the previous year [37]. The third study that was performed in a high income country was a study of refugee adolescents and young adults in an Intensive English Centre high school in Australia employed a survey of immunisation status [36]. The intervention involved the school-based provision of MMR and the first and second dose of a three-dose hepatitis B schedule following an immunisation survey. Of the 165 students who completed the survey (85%), 74% received measles, mumps and rubella (MMR) vaccine in the school as compared with historic levels of 30%. Of the students who received a second dose of hepatitis B vaccine in the school-based program, less than 24% finished the series with a primary care clinician.

3.2. What are Cost-Effective Approaches to Vaccinating Newly Arrived Migrants?

We identified 810 articles for screening. One article conducted among migrants was included in the final analysis [39] (PRISMA flow diagram Figure 2). This cost-effectiveness study was assessed to be of moderate quality using the Drummond checklist. One-way and two-way sensitivity analyses were undertaken, and the cost-effectiveness results were tested for changes across plausible ranges of estimates for costs of serotesting, compliance rates and seroprevalence. Probabilistic sensitivity analyses were not reported.

Results of the economic study are presented in Table 2. This study among migrants compared pre-vaccination serotesting with presumptive vaccination for polio, diphtheria, and tetanus in internationally adopted and immigrant infants to the US [39]. It showed that compared with presumptive vaccination, pre-vaccination serotesting for polio increased the cost per patient from $57 USD to $62 USD (in 2004 dollars) and decreased the percentage of patients protected against polio from 95.3% to 94.0%. Presumptive vaccination was more effective and less expensive than pre-vaccination serotesting when the seroprevalence was <69%. Presumptive vaccination was the preferred method unless the vaccination compliance was extremely high (>96% completion rate). In the same study, the results for diphtheria, tetanus, and acellular pertussis (DTaP) were less definitive. Pre-vaccination serotesting for diphtheria and tetanus increased the cost per patient from $62 USD to $119 USD and increased the percentage of patients protected against both diphtheria and tetanus from 91.5% to 92.3%. Presumptive vaccination was the preferred strategy (with an incremental cost-effectiveness ratio (ICER) of $7148 USD per infant protected) in populations with poor vaccine compliance (where >80% of patients did not complete the full catch-up vaccine series), or populations with low seroprevalence (<51%) of antibodies to diphtheria and tetanus.

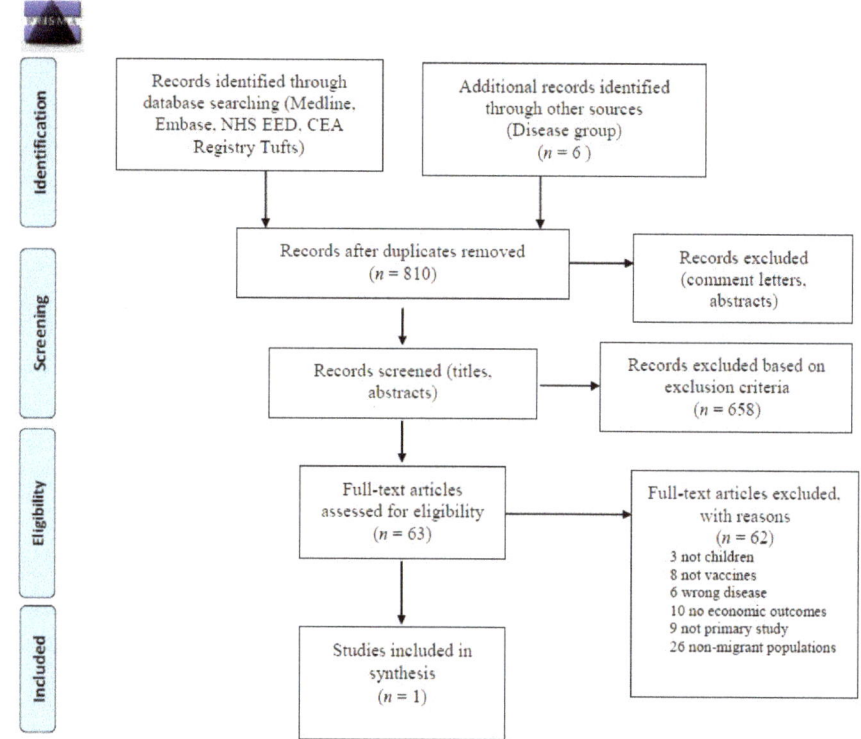

Figure 2. PRISMA 2009 Flow Diagram for Cost-Effectiveness of Vaccination Strategies.

Table 2. Characteristics of Studies—Cost-Effectiveness of Vaccination Strategies.

Study	Certainty of Economic Evidence (Quality)	Design	Population	Intervention	Cost-Effectiveness	Resource Requirements
Cohen et al. 2006 [39]	Some allowance made for uncertainty in the estimates of costs and consequences. The costs are provided as base case, and 25% upper and lower range No probabilistic sensitivity analyses performed. Sensitivity analysis was undertaken for costs of serotesting, compliance rate and seroprevalence. Cost-effectiveness results were sensitive to changes in seroprevalence, cost of serotesting.	Decision-analytic model; results presented in 2004 US dollars	US	1. presumptive vaccination with IPV 2. serotesting for poliovirus type 1, 2, and 3 antibodies followed by vaccination in unprotected patients	For IPV, presumptive vaccination is less costly and more effective, For Dtap, ICER is $7148 USD per person protected.	Difference in costs between 2 interventions are small. For IPV, difference in cost is very minimal: Serotesting is slightly more expensive ($5 USD) than presumptive vaccination. For Dtap, serotesting is more expensive than presumptive vaccine ($57 USD)

4. Discussion

This systematic review identified few data on interventions to increase vaccinations and cost-effectiveness of vaccinations in migrant populations. Several interventions were identified as potentially helpful to increase vaccination rates in migrant populations. The interventions focused on social mobilization and outreach programs, planned vaccinations, and educational campaigns similar to strategies used to improve vaccination rates in low to middle income countries in migrant populations [40–44]. Overall, the interventions in this study described did not address all the vaccination barriers in migrants such as: use of traditional health care [45], socioeconomic status [45], language [46], distance to vaccination service [46,47], continued migration [47], fear of arrest [47], necessity of work [47], lack of vaccination knowledge [46,48,49], cost [49], and lack of health care provider recommendation [50]. None of the interventions focused on health care providers. The interventions were not targeted, having the same strategy for different migrant age groups and all of the interventions were focused on groups of migrants, not at the level of the individual patient-healthcare interaction. Additionally, none of the studies identified that they had engaged migrant populations in the planning or execution of the intervention.

Vaccinations should not be provided in isolation, but the interaction should be viewed as an opportunity to address many important diseases of public health significance [51]. Engaging refugees and other migrant populations in preventive health services remains a challenge in light of the barriers to healthcare [52,53]. A recent consensus statement on access to health services in the EU/EEA by IOM's EQUI HEALTH project [54] highlights the discrepancies in entitlements to statutory health services for migrants; irregular migrants often have highly restrictive access.

The number of studies on the economic analysis for vaccinations in migrant populations is even more limited. Only one study was applicable, suggesting that presumptive polio and DTaP vaccination appear to be more cost effective and less expensive than pre-vaccination serotesting [39]. This modelling was done utilizing data from a very small and unique population of international migrants, international adoptees. Although the economic analysis demonstrated cost effectiveness of vaccination without serological testing, this group has significant resources and understanding of the health systems and entitlements of the country of destination and engages with the health care system on an individual basis. The cost effectiveness differed depending on the serological prevalence of the VPDs and the compliance with vaccinations. Seroprevalence can vary depending on country of origin, type of migrant and age of migrant making it difficult to extrapolate these data.

Two studies published after the economic analysis systematic review was performed examined different costs associated with pre-departure vaccinations, one in the context of a response to an outbreak [55] and the second evaluating the US Vaccination Program for US-bound Refugees (VPR) [56]. The first study showed that pre-departure vaccination of all US bound refugees would not only improve health, reduce importations of VPD, but be cost saving when considering all the resources required for response to outbreak activities. The second US study demonstrated that compared with post-arrival vaccinations, the initiation of the pre-departure VPR where the refugees received one or two doses of selected vaccines before departure and completed the series after arrival demonstrated a net savings per person of $225.93 USD (29% decrease in vaccination costs). The cost savings were sensitive to different variables but demonstrated cost savings across all the estimates. Although the European context is not the same as the orderly US Refugee program, these data could be used to support the vaccination in reception centres before the onward migration in the EU/EEA. Not only is it cost-saving, but there is the potential to prevent unwanted and costly outbreaks of VPDs.

5. Strengths and Limitations

Our study is the first to our knowledge that is a systematic review on interventions that increase vaccinations in migrant populations and cost effectiveness of vaccination strategies in migrant populations. The studies that we found reflect the overall migration health literature of low quality with many being cohort or pre-post studies and no negative studies or long term follow up studies. Other limitations of our study are the lack of comparator data and the fact that the only reported outcome was vaccine uptake. Given the complexities of immunisations in this vulnerable population, a short-term increase in vaccine uptake does not directly translate into decreased VPD incidence or decrease in outbreaks. Finally, there is difficulty in extrapolating this evidence across the very heterogeneous group of migrants (undocumented migrant, refugee, asylum seeker, labour migrant, unaccompanied children, etc.) with different pre-migration immunisation coverage, immunity, and age.

6. Implementation Considerations and Evidence Gaps

The lack of data on migrant specific variables (i.e., country of birth) related to VPDs [7,57–59] makes estimation of the scope of vaccine delivery challenging. Small studies done in special circumstances have shown some sub-optimal vaccine coverage and immunity, but there is a limit to how these data can be extrapolated to all migrants [16,18–20,22–24]. Robust surveillance data on vaccine preventable diseases and vaccine coverage in migrant populations by age group, migration type, source country, and duration of presence in the EU/EEA will be required to design effective immunisation programmes [57,58]. This will require a standardisation of migrant definitions and parameters. Further research on vaccination uptake, immunisation coverage, and cost-effectiveness of different strategies in adults versus children is required to inform potential different migrant guidelines [60]. The optimal method to document immunisations and share immunisation data across jurisdictions in mobile populations to ensure that the migrant receives the correct immunisations at the appropriate time is an understudied area [61]. Documentation could be done via a standardised health record or mobile immunisation record [62,63]. However, they need to be secure, private, and ensure that the information does not disadvantage or be reason for persecution of the migrant. Engaging migrants in the development of interventions is important to the development of effective interventions. Finally, evidence on the comparative effective implementation strategies and cost-effectiveness of different vaccination strategies for migrants will be required to prioritize the VPDs prevention efforts for the EU/EEA.

7. Conclusions

High quality studies assessing interventions to increase vaccinations and the cost effectiveness of vaccinations in migrant populations are scarce. Data on migrant populations, vaccine preventable diseases and vaccinations are required to estimate the scale of the problem and to understand the benefit of interventions on a population scale. Large scale studies on interventions to improve vaccination uptake among different typologies of migrants, and across their migration journey, are required to inform the best and most equitable care of migrants. The economic analyses of these interventions are crucial to inform their implementation.

Supplementary Materials: The following are available online at http://www.mdpi.com/1660-4601/15/9/2065/s1. Table S1. PRISMA 2009 Checklist. File A: Electronic search strategies—interventions to increase vaccination strategies. File B: Electronic search strategies—economic studies.

Author Contributions: Conception and design: C.H., J.D., K.P., A.T., L.S., and R.M. Data acquisition: C.H., J.D., A.T., L.S., and R.M. Data analysis: C.H., J.D., K.P., A.T., L.S., and R.M. Interpretation of results: C.H., J.D., K.P., A.T., L.S., and R.M. Manuscript drafting: C.H., J.D., K.P., A.T., L.S., R.M., S.H., C.G., B.A.B., and R.C. All authors critically revised and approved the final version of the manuscript.

Funding: Rachael Morton is supported by a National Health and Medical Research Council (NHMRC) Fellowship #1054216. Robin Christensen of the Musculoskeletal Statistics Unit, the Parker Institute is supported by grants from the Oak Foundation. Sally Hargreaves is funded by the Imperial NIHR Biomedical Research Centre, the Wellcome Trust (Grant number 209993/Z/17/Z), and the European Society for Clinical Microbiology and Infectious Diseases (ESCMID) through an ESCMID Study Group for Infections in Travellers and Migrants (ESGITM) research grant.

Acknowledgments: We thank Jenna Pepper, MA and Katie O'Hearn, Msc (Children's Hospital of Eastern Ontario Research Institute) for methodological assistance and Margaret Sampson, MLIS, PhD, AHIP (Children's Hospital of Eastern Ontario) for developing the electronic search strategies.

Conflicts of Interest: The authors declare no conflict of interest

References

1. *International Migration Report 2017: Highlights*; United Nations, Department of Economic and Social Affairs, Population Division: New York, NY, USA, 2017.
2. *Cross-National Comparisons of Internal Migration: An Update on Global Patterns and Trends*; United Nations, Department of Economic and Social Affairs, Population Division: New York, NY, USA, 2013.
3. The EU and the Crisis in Syria, Factsheet—EEAS—European External Action Service—European Commission. Available online: https://eeas.europa.eu/headquarters/headquarters-homepage_en/22664/ (accessed on 17 September 2018).
4. *World Migration Report 2018*; International Organization for Migration: Geneva, Switzerland, 2017.

5. European Vaccine Action Plan 2015–2020 (2014). 2017. Available online: http://www.euro.who.int/en/health-topics/disease-prevention/vaccines-and-immunization/publications/2014/european-vaccine-action-plan-20152020-2014 (accessed on 18 March 2017).
6. Filia, A.; Amendola, A.; Faccini, M.; Del Manso, M.; Senatore, S.; Bianchi, S.; Borrini, B.M.; Ciampelli, A.; Tanzi, E.; Filipponi, M.T.; et al. Outbreak of a new measles B3 variant in the Roma/Sinti population with transmission in the nosocomial setting, Italy, November 2015 to April 2016. *Eurosurveillance* **2016**, *21*, 2–6. [CrossRef] [PubMed]
7. Williams, G.A.; Bacci, S.; Shadwick, R.; Tillmann, T.; Rechel, B.; Noori, T.; Suk, J.E.; Odone, A.; Ingleby, J.D.; Mladovsky, P.; et al. Measles among migrants in the European Union and the European Economic Area. *Scand. J. Public Health* **2016**, *44*, 6–13. [CrossRef] [PubMed]
8. Jones, G.; Haeghebaert, S.; Merlin, B.; Antona, D.; Simon, N.; Elmouden, M.; Battist, F.; Janssens, M.; Wyndels, K.; Chaud, P. Measles outbreak in a refugee settlement in Calais, France: January to February 2016. *Eurosurveillance* **2016**, *21*, 30167. [CrossRef] [PubMed]
9. Khetsuriani, N.; Perehinets, I.; Nitzan, D.; Popovic, D.; Moran, T.; Allahverdiyeva, V.; Huseynov, S.; Gavrilin, E.; Slobodianyk, L.; Izhyk, O.; et al. Responding to a cVDPV1 outbreak in Ukraine: Implications, challenges and opportunities. *Vaccine* **2017**, *35*, 4769–4776. [CrossRef] [PubMed]
10. Werber, D.; Hoffmann, A.; Santibanez, S.; Mankertz, A.; Sagebiel, D. Large measles outbreak introduced by asylum seekers and spread among the insufficiently vaccinated resident population, Berlin, October 2014 to August 2015. *Eurosurveillance* **2017**, *22*, 30599. [CrossRef] [PubMed]
11. Derrough, T.; Salekeen, A. Lessons learnt to keep Europe polio-free: A review of outbreaks in the European Union, European Economic Area, and candidate countries, 1973 to 2013. *Eurosurveillance* **2016**, *21*, 30210. [CrossRef] [PubMed]
12. Grammens, T.; Maes, V.; Hutse, V.; Laisnez, V.; Schirvel, C.; Trémérie, J.M.; Sabbe, M. Different measles outbreaks in Belgium, January to June 2016—A challenge for public health. *Eurosurveillance* **2016**, *21*, 30313. [CrossRef] [PubMed]
13. Woudenberg, T.; van Binnendijk, R.S.; Sanders, E.A.M.; Wallinga, J.; de Melker, H.E.; Ruijs, W.L.M.; Hahné, S.J.M. Large measles epidemic in the Netherlands, May 2013 to March 2014: Changing epidemiology. *Eurosurveillance* **2017**, *22*, 30443. [CrossRef] [PubMed]
14. Antona, D.; Lévy-Bruhl, D.; Baudon, C.; Freymuth, F.; Lamy, M.; Maine, C.; Floret, D.; Parent du Chatelet, I. Measles Elimination Efforts and 2008–2011 Outbreak, France. *Emerg. Infect. Dis.* **2013**, *19*, 357–364. [CrossRef] [PubMed]
15. Hargreaves, S.; Nellums, L.B.; Ramsay, M.; Saliba, V.; Majeed, A.; Mounier-Jack, S.; Friedland, J.S. Who is responsible for the vaccination of migrants in Europe? *Lancet* **2018**, *391*, 1752–1754. [CrossRef]
16. Barnett, E.D.; Christiansen, D.; Figueira, M. Seroprevalence of measles, rubella, and varicella in refugees. *Clin. Infect. Dis.* **2002**, *35*, 403–408. [CrossRef] [PubMed]
17. Greenaway, C.; Dongier, P.; Boivin, J.F.; Tapiero, B.; Miller, M.; Schwartzman, K. Susceptibility to measles, mumps, and rubella in newly arrived adult immigrants and refugees. *Ann. Intern. Med.* **2007**, *146*, 20–24. [CrossRef] [PubMed]
18. Mipatrini, D.; Stefanelli, P.; Severoni, S.; Rezza, G. Vaccinations in migrants and refugees: A challenge for European health systems. A systematic review of current scientific evidence. *Pathog. Glob. Health* **2017**, *111*, 59–68. [CrossRef] [PubMed]
19. Toikkanen, S.E.; Baillot, A.; Dreesman, J.; Mertens, E. Seroprevalence of Antibodies against Measles, Rubella and Varicella among Asylum Seekers Arriving in Lower Saxony, Germany, November 2014–October 2015. *Int. J. Environ. Res. Public Health* **2016**, *13*, E650. [CrossRef] [PubMed]
20. Freidl, G.S.; Tostmann, A.; Curvers, M.; Ruijs, W.L.M.; Smits, G.; Schepp, R.; Duizer, E.; Boland, G.; de Melker, H.; van der Klis, F.R.M.; et al. Immunity against measles, mumps, rubella, varicella, diphtheria, tetanus, polio, hepatitis A and hepatitis B among adult asylum seekers in The Netherlands, 2016. *Vaccine* **2018**, *36*, 1664–1672. [CrossRef] [PubMed]
21. Ceccarelli, G.; Vita, S.; Riva, E.; Cella, E.; Lopalco, M.; Antonelli, F.; De Cesaris, M.; Fogolari, M.; Dicuonzo, G.; Ciccozzi, M.; et al. Susceptibility to measles in migrant population: Implication for policy makers. *J. Travel Med.* **2018**, *25*, tax080. [CrossRef] [PubMed]

22. Nakken, C.S.; Skovdal, M.; Nellums, L.B.; Friedland, J.S.; Hargreaves, S.; Norredam, M. Vaccination status and needs of asylum-seeking children in Denmark: A retrospective data analysis. *Public Health* **2018**, *158*, 110–116. [CrossRef] [PubMed]
23. Hubschen, J.M.; Charpentier, E.; Weicherding, P.; Muller, C.P. IgG antibody prevalence suggests high immunization needs in newcomers to Luxembourg, 2012. *Vaccine* **2018**, *36*, 899–905. [CrossRef] [PubMed]
24. Roberton, T.; Weiss, W.; Doocy, S. Challenges in Estimating Vaccine Coverage in Refugee and Displaced Populations: Results From Household Surveys in Jordan and Lebanon. *Vaccines* **2017**, *5*, 22. [CrossRef] [PubMed]
25. Plotkin, S.; Orenstein, W.; Offit, P.; Edwards, K.M. *Plotkin's Vaccines*, 7th ed.; Elsevier: Philadelphia, PA, USA, 2018; pp. 1645–1691.
26. GHO | By Category | Measles, 2nd Dose (MCV2)—Immunization Coverage Estimates by WHO Region. Who Minerva Publish Date Minerva Publish Date. Available online: http://apps.who.int/gho/data/view.main.MCV2vREG?lang=en (accessed on 17 September 2018).
27. Anderson, R.M. The concept of herd immunity and the design of community-based immunization programmes. *Vaccine* **1992**, *10*, 928–935. [CrossRef]
28. Bica, M.A.; Clemens, R. Vaccination policies of immigrants in the EU/EEA Member States-the measles immunization example. *Eur. J. Public Health* **2018**, *28*, 439–444. [CrossRef] [PubMed]
29. Vito, E.D.; Parente, P.; Waure, C.D.; Poscia, A.; Ricciardi, W. *A Review of Evidence on Equitable Delivery, Access and Utilization of Immunization Services for Migrants and Refugees in the WHO European Region*; WHO Regional Office for Europe: Copenhagen, Denmark, 2017.
30. Pottie, K.; Mayhew, A.; Morton, R.; Greenaway, C.; Akl, E.; Rahman, P. Prevention and assessment of infectious diseases among children and adult migrants arriving to the European Union/European Economic Association: A protocol for a suite of systematic reviews for public health and health systems. *BMJ Open* **2017**, *7*, e014608. [CrossRef] [PubMed]
31. Moher, D.; Shamseer, L.; Clarke, M.; Ghersi, D.; Liberati, A.; Petticrew, M.; Shekelle, P.; Stewart, L.A. Preferred reporting items for systematic review and meta-analysis protocols (PRISMA-P) 2015 statement. *Syst. Rev.* **2015**, *4*, 1. [CrossRef] [PubMed]
32. Wm, B. Improving efficiency and confidence in systematic literature searching. In Proceedings of the EAHIL+ICAHIS + ICLC, Edinburgh, UK, 10–12 June 2015.
33. Sampson, M.; McGowan, J. Inquisitio validus Index Medicus: A simple method of validating MEDLINE systematic review searches. *Res. Synth. Methods* **2011**, *16*, 103–109. [CrossRef] [PubMed]
34. Wells, G.; Shea, B.; O'Connell, D.; Peterson, J.; Welch, V.; Losos, M.; Tugwell, P. The Newcastle-Ottawa Scale (NOS) for Assessing the Quality of Nonrandomised Studies in Meta-Analyses. Available online: http://www.ohri.ca/programs/clinical_epidemiology/oxford.asp (accessed on 17 September 2018).
35. Drummond, M.F.; Sculpher, M.J.; Torrance, G.W.; O'brien, B.J.; Stoddart, G.L. *Methods for the Economic Evaluation of Health Care Programmes*, 2nd ed.; Oxford University Press: Oxford, UK, 1997.
36. Milne, B.; Raman, S.; Thomas, P.; Shah, S. Immunisation of refugee and migrant young people: Can schools do the job? *Aust. N. Z. J. Public Health* **2006**, *30*, 526–528. [CrossRef] [PubMed]
37. Spadea, A.; Semyonov, L.; Unim, B.; Giraldi, G.; Corda, B.; D'Amici, A.M.; Ercole, A.; Boccia, A.; La Torre, G. Action against vaccine-preventable infectious diseases and tuberculosis in Nomad Camps: The experience of a Local Health Unit in Rome. *Annali di Igiene Medicina Preventiva e di Comunita* **2014**, *26*, 176–180. [PubMed]
38. Brockmann, S.O.; Wjst, S.; Zelmer, U.; Carollo, S.; Schmid, M.; Roller, G.; Eichner, M. Public Health initiative for improved vaccination for asylum seekers. *Bundesgesundheitsblatt Gesundheitsforschung Gesundheitsschutz* **2016**, *59*, 592–598. [CrossRef] [PubMed]
39. Cohen, A.L.; Veenstra, D. Economic analysis of prevaccination serotesting compared with presumptive immunization for polio, diphtheria, and tetanus in internationally adopted and immigrant infants. *Pediatrics* **2006**, *117*, 1650–1655. [CrossRef] [PubMed]
40. Hu, Y.; Luo, S.; Tang, X.; Lou, L.; Chen, Y.; Guo, J.; Zhang, B. Does introducing an immunization package of services for migrant children improve the coverage, service quality and understanding? An evidence from an intervention study among 1548 migrant children in eastern China. *BMC Public Health* **2015**, *15*, 664. [CrossRef] [PubMed]

41. Ndiaye, S.M.; Ahmed, M.A.; Denson, M.; Craig, A.S.; Kretsinger, K.; Cherif, B.; Kandolo, P.; Moto, D.D.; Richelot, A.; Tuma, J. Polio outbreak among nomads in Chad: Outbreak response and lessons learned. *J. Infect. Dis.* **2014**, *210* (Suppl. 1), S74–S84. [CrossRef] [PubMed]
42. Sengupta, P.; Benjamin, A.I.; Myles, P.R.; Babu, B.V. Evaluation of a community-based intervention to improve routine childhood vaccination uptake among migrants in urban slums of Ludhiana, India. *J. Public Health Oxf. Engl.* **2017**, *39*, 805–812. [CrossRef] [PubMed]
43. Sheikh, M.A.; Makokha, F.; Hussein, A.M.; Mohamed, G.; Mach, O.; Humayun, K.; Okiror, S.; Abrar, L.; Nasibov, O.; Burton, J.; et al. Combined use of inactivated and oral poliovirus vaccines in refugee camps and surrounding communities—Kenya, December 2013. *MMWR—Morb. Mortal. Wkly. Rep.* **2014**, *63*, 237–241. [PubMed]
44. Adam, I.F.; Nakamura, K.; Kizuki, M.; Al Rifai, R.; Vanching, U. Relationship between implementing interpersonal communication and mass education campaigns in emergency settings and use of reproductive healthcare services: Evidence from Darfur, Sudan. *BMJ Open* **2015**, *5*, e008285. [CrossRef] [PubMed]
45. Baker, D.L.; Dang, M.T.; Ly, M.Y.; Diaz, R. Perception of barriers to immunization among parents of Hmong origin in California. *Am. J. Public Health* **2010**, *100*, 839–845. [CrossRef] [PubMed]
46. Harmsen, I.A.; Bos, H.; Ruiter, R.A.C.; Paulussen, T.G.W.; Kok, G.; de Melker, H.E.; Mollema, L. Vaccination decision-making of immigrant parents in the Netherlands; a focus group study. *BMC Public Health* **2015**, *15*, 1229. [CrossRef] [PubMed]
47. Canavati, S.; Plugge, E.; Suwanjatuporn, S.; Sombatrungjaroen, S.; Nosten, F. Barriers to immunization among children of migrant workers from Myanmar living in Tak province, Thailand. *Bull. World Health Organ.* **2011**, *89*, 528–531. [CrossRef] [PubMed]
48. Kowal, S.P.; Jardine, C.G.; Bubela, T.M. "If they tell me to get it, I'll get it. If they don't...": Immunization decision-making processes of immigrant mothers. *Can. J. Public Health* **2015**, *106*, e230–e235. [CrossRef] [PubMed]
49. Wang, L.D.L.; Lam, W.W.T.; Wu, J.T.; Liao, Q. Chinese immigrant parents' vaccination decision making for children: A qualitative analysis. *BMC Public Health* **2014**, *14*, 133. [CrossRef] [PubMed]
50. Devroey, D.; Riffi, A.; Balemans, R.; Van De Vijver, E.; Chovanova, H.; Vandevoorde, J. Comparison of knowledge and attitudes about vaccination between Belgian and immigrant adolescents. *J. Infect. Public Health* **2013**, *6*, 1–9. [CrossRef] [PubMed]
51. European Centre for Disease Prevention and Control. *Infectious Diseases of Specific Relevance to Newly-Arrived Migrants in the EU/EEA—19 November 2015*; ECDC: Stockholm, Sweden, 2015.
52. Blondell, S.J.; Kitter, B.; Griffin, M.P.; Durham, J. Barriers and Facilitators to HIV Testing in Migrants in High-Income Countries: A Systematic Review. *AIDS Behav.* **2015**, *19*, 2012–2024. [CrossRef] [PubMed]
53. Agudelo-Suárez, A.A.; Gil-González, D.; Vives-Cases, C.; Love, J.G.; Wimpenny, P.; Ronda-Pérez, E. A metasynthesis of qualitative studies regarding opinions and perceptions about barriers and determinants of health services' accessibility in economic migrants. *BMC Health Serv. Res.* **2012**, *12*, 461. [CrossRef] [PubMed]
54. Ingleby, D.; Petrova-Benedict, R. Recommendations on Access to Health Services for Migrants in an Irregular Situation: An Expert Consensus. 2016. Available online: http://equi-health.eea.iom.int/images/Expert_consensus_Recommendations.pdf (accessed on 17 September 2018).
55. Coleman, M.S.; Burke, H.M.; Welstead, B.L.; Mitchell, T.; Taylor, E.M.; Shapovalov, D.; Maskery, B.A.; Joo, H.; Weinberg, M. Cost analysis of measles in refugees arriving at Los Angeles International Airport from Malaysia. *Hum. Vaccines Immunother.* **2017**, *13*, 1084–1090. [CrossRef] [PubMed]
56. Joo, H.; Maskery, B.; Mitchell, T.; Leidner, A.; Klosovsky, A.; Weinberg, M. A comparative cost analysis of the Vaccination Program for US-bound Refugees. *Vaccine* **2018**, *36*, 2896–2901. [CrossRef] [PubMed]
57. Catchpole, M.; Coulombier, D. Refugee crisis demands European Union-wide surveillance! *Eurosurveillance* **2015**, *20*, 30063. [CrossRef] [PubMed]
58. Riccardo, F.; Dente, M.G.; Kärki, T.; Fabiani, M.; Napoli, C.; Chiarenza, A.; Giorgi Rossi, P.; Velasco Munoz, C.; Noori, T.; Declich, S. Towards a European Framework to Monitor Infectious Diseases among Migrant Populations: Design and Applicability. *Int. J. Environ. Res. Public Health* **2015**, *12*, 11640–11661. [CrossRef] [PubMed]
59. European Centre for Disease Prevention and Control. *Assessing the Burden of Key Infectious Diseases Affecting Migrant Populations in the EU*; European Centre for Disease Prevention and Control: Stolkholm, Sweden, 2014.

60. Dalla Zuanna, T.; Del Manso, M.; Giambi, C.; Riccardo, F.; Bella, A.; Caporali, M.G.; Dente, M.G.; Declich, S. Immunization Offer Targeting Migrants: Policies and Practices in Italy. *Int. J. Environ. Res. Public Health* **2018**, *15*, E968. [CrossRef] [PubMed]
61. Giambi, C.; Del Manso, M.; Dalla Zuanna, T.; Riccardo, F.; Bella, A.; Caporali, M.G.; Baka, A.; Caks-Jager, N.; Melillo, T.; Mexia, R.; et al. National immunization strategies targeting migrants in six European countries. *Vaccine* **2018**. [CrossRef] [PubMed]
62. Bell, C.; Atkinson, K.M.; Wilson, K. Modernizing Immunization Practice Through the Use of Cloud Based Platforms. *J. Med. Syst.* **2017**, *41*, 57. [CrossRef] [PubMed]
63. Monitoring of Migrant's & Refugee's Health Status—CARE: Common Approach for REfugees and Other Migrants' Health. Available online: http://careformigrants.eu/monitor-of-migrants-refugees-health-status/ (accessed on 17 September 2018).

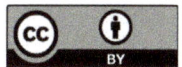

© 2018 by the authors. Licensee MDPI, Basel, Switzerland. This article is an open access article distributed under the terms and conditions of the Creative Commons Attribution (CC BY) license (http://creativecommons.org/licenses/by/4.0/).

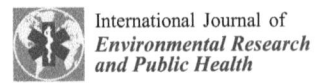

Article

Healthcare Utilization in a Large Cohort of Asylum Seekers Entering Western Europe in 2015

Martin Wetzke [1,2], Christine Happle [1,3], Annabelle Vakilzadeh [4], Diana Ernst [5], Georgios Sogkas [5], Reinhold E. Schmidt [2,5], Georg M. N. Behrens [2,5], Christian Dopfer [1,3,†] and Alexandra Jablonka [2,5,*,†]

1. Department of Pediatric Pneumology, Allergology, and Neonatology, Hannover Medical School, 30625 Hannover, Germany; wetzke.martin@mh-hannover.de (M.W.); happle.christine@mh-hannover.de (C.H.); dopfer.christian@mh-hannover.de (C.D.)
2. German Center for Infection Research (DZIF), Partner Site Hannover-Braunschweig, 38124 Braunschweig, Germany; Schmidt.Reinhold.Ernst@mh-hannover.de (R.E.S.); behrens.georg@mh-hannover.de (G.M.N.B.)
3. German Center for Lung Research, Biomedical Research in End Stage and Obstructive Lung Disease/BREATH Hannover, 30625 Hannover, Germany
4. Hannover Medical School, 30625 Hannover, Germany; Annabelle.Schaell@stud.mh-hannover.de
5. Department of Clinical Immunology and Rheumatology, Hannover Medical School, 30625 Hannover, Germany; ernst.diana@mh-hannover.de (D.E.); sogkas.georgios@mh-hannover.de (G.S.)
* Correspondence: jablonka.alexandra@mh-hannover.de; Tel.: +49-511-532-5337; Fax: +49-511-532-5324
† These authors contributed equally to this work.

Received: 12 June 2018; Accepted: 26 September 2018; Published: 1 October 2018

Abstract: During the current period of immigration to Western Europe, national healthcare systems are confronted with high numbers of asylum seekers with largely unknown health status. To improve care taking strategies, we assessed healthcare utilization in a large, representative cohort of newly arriving migrants consisting of $n = 1533$ residents of a reception center in Northern Germany in 2015. Most asylum seekers were young, male adults, and the majority came from the Eastern Mediterranean region. Overall, we observed a frequency of 0.03 visits to the onsite primary healthcare ward per asylum seeker and day of camp residence (IQR 0.0–0.07, median duration of residence 38.0 days, IQR 30.0–54.25). Female asylum seekers showed higher healthcare utilization rates than their male counterparts, and healthcare utilization was particularly low in asylum seekers in their second decade of life. Furthermore, a significant correlation between time after camp entrance and healthcare utilization behavior occurred: During the first week of camp residence, 37.1 visits/100 asylum seekers were observed, opposed to only 9.5 visits/100 asylum seekers during the sixth week of camp residence. This first data on healthcare utilization in a large, representative asylum seeker cohort entering Western Europe during the current crisis shows that primary care is most needed in the first period directly after arrival. Our dataset may help to raise awareness for refugee and migrant healthcare needs and to adapt care taking strategies accordingly.

Keywords: healthcare; migration; refugee; asylum seeker; medical service; migrant; medical care; doctor; Europe; Germany

1. Introduction

At the height of the current refugee and migrant crisis, in 2015, more than 24 million migrants were on the move worldwide. Many of them entered Western Europe, with Germany being the leading destination for asylum seekers from countries such as Syria, Afghanistan, Somalia and others [1]. Appropriate medical care for this growing population of refugees and migrants represents an enormous challenge to the receiving population. During their migration, the vast majority of refugees and migrants had only irregular access to medical services and good sanitation, leaving them at high risk of communicable and non-communicable diseases [2–6]. Many refugees have experienced political and personal trauma such as war, detainment, torture, forced migration, and separation or death from family members and friends [7–9]. Depending on gender, age, or nationality, refugees may have different health status and health-seeking behaviors [10]. Although the current extent of immigration to Western Europe is considered to be the largest of our generation thus far [11], national healthcare systems across Europe are still struggling to provide appropriate care and meet the needs of immigrating refugees and migrants. Especially in the summer of 2015, when Western European countries were first confronted with a massive influx of persons with unclear health status and healthcare needs [12], national caregivers were comparably ill-prepared. It took a long time to harmonize efforts for the set-up of primary care structures that were effective, cost-sensitive and, most importantly, met the refugees' and migrants' needs [13,14]. However, there is still little knowledge on general healthcare utilization among refugees and migrants during the current crisis, and updated information on the specific demand for emergency onsite healthcare in refugee camps is scarce. To treat and prevent further disease burden in this vulnerable population, and to improve primary care in extreme humanitarian situations similar to the current situation, we aimed to analyze primary healthcare utilization behavior in a well characterized, representative cohort of asylum seekers in a Northern German refugee camp during the current exodus.

2. Methods

2.1. Study Population

For the description of healthcare utilization in asylum seekers, data on all residents (n = 1533) of a reception center in Celle, Northern Germany in September–December 2015 were analyzed. All subjects had been allocated to Lower Saxony based on a federal state specific German allocation key (Königssteiner Schlüssel) and were sent to a reception center in Celle based on space availability. They were not preselected in any fashion. All residents were asylum seekers and registered upon arrival and their departure date was documented. For asylum seekers leaving the center without notice to camp authorities, last contact documentation of the camp staff (for example, medical service, food service, transportation) was used as date of departure. Parts of this cohort have been described previously [15–17].

2.2. Medical Service and Analysis of Healthcare Utilization

A 24 h-onsite medical ward was available to all residents of the center. This ward offered medical services at primary medical care level with constant paramedical emergency service and daily consultation hours by medical doctors for general medical treatment. For medical problems exceeding general medical care, further referral to specialists was arranged whenever needed. All visits to the onsite medical center were documented in electronic form. Mandatory primary check-ups of asylum seekers upon arrival, as required by asylum law, were not included in the data set for this analysis. Health care utilization was determined by analyzing individual presentations to the onsite medical ward in relation to personal days of residence at the reception center.

2.3. Data Analysis

All information was collected in routine clinical care. Proband specific information on age, gender, country of origin, attendance dates, and visits to the medical center was extracted from an electronic database. All data had been fully anonymized by the Order of Malta (Malteser Hilfsdienst) before scientific analysis.

2.4. Statistics

Analyses were conducted employing SPSS version 24.0 (IBM, Armonk, NY, USA) and Graphpad Prism version 5.02 (GraphPad Software, La Jolla, CA, USA). Descriptive statistics were assessed using median and range or interquartile range (IQR) for non-normally distributed variables and using mean ± SD for normally distributed variables or a combination of both. Group differences with categorical items were evaluated by Mann-Whitney-U or one-way ANOVA/Kruskal-Wallis testing and p values below 0.05 were considered significant.

2.5. Ethics Compliance

All analyses were approved by local authorities (Institutional Review Board of Hannover Medical School approval #2972-2015). All patient information was anonymized prior to analysis.

3. Results

Data of healthcare utilization of n = 1533 asylum seekers was included in the analysis. For n = 45 asylum seekers, information on nationality and for n = 36, information on age was missing. Overall, 71.8% of asylum seekers were male. The median age of all probands was 22 years (male asylum seekers 23 years, range 0–73 years; female asylum seekers 21 years, range 0–62 years, Figure 1). The vast majority of probands (80.5%) came from the Eastern Mediterranean region, followed by two smaller proportions from Europe (7.7%) and Africa (7.7%) and only few persons from Southeast Asia (1.2%) or of unknown origin (2.9%).

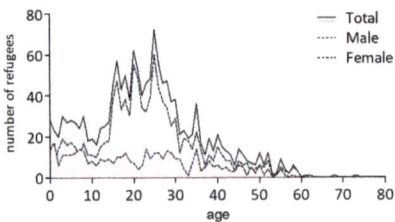

Figure 1. Age and gender distribution within the analyzed cohort.

During their stay at the reception center, overall 47.4% of the asylum seekers utilized medical care at the ward. 47.2% of male refugees and 48% of female refugees presented at the primary healthcare unit of the shelter (Figure 2A,B). Out of all patients that visited the primary healthcare unit, male patients sought medical help up to 27 times (median 2 (QR 1–4), mean 3.2 ± SD 3.1), and female patients paid up to 18 visits to the onsite clinical team (median 2 (IQR 1–4), mean 2.9 ±SD 2.5), Figure 2C,D). Irrespective of gender, the vast majority of patients paid between 1 and 5 visits to the medical ward, and the median visit number was 2 (IQR 1–4, mean 3.1 ± SD 3.0) visits per patient.

Next, we analyzed individual factors possibly influencing healthcare utilization in asylum seekers. For n = 1094 asylum seekers, exact entrance and exit dates of camp residence were available. They had a median duration of camp inhabitation of 38.0 (IQR 30–54.25, mean 41.3 ± 0.7) days. We observed a median visit frequency of 0.03 per asylum seeker and day of camp residence (IQR 0.0–0.07). The highest rate of healthcare utilization occurred in asylum seekers above the age of 60 years, and a particularly low rate of medical visits per day in the age group of 10–19 years in our cohort was found. Children below the age of ten years and adults in their fourth, fifth and sixth decade of life showed significantly higher healthcare utilization rates. In addition, young adults aged 20–29 years spent significantly less visits to the onsite medical ward than those aged 30–39 years (Figure 3A). When we compared male and female asylum seekers in our cohort, we found a significantly higher rate of healthcare utilization in females (Figure 3B). With regard to the asylum seekers' origins, no significant influence on health care utilization behavior was observed: WHO regions of origin had no significant effect on the percentage of refugees seeking help at the onsite ward, and were also not associated with significantly different frequencies of healthcare utilization per day of camp residence (Figure 3C,D, Table S1). When focusing on the top five most prevalent nationalities within the cohort, the frequency of visits per day were also not significantly different between asylum seekers from Afghanistan, Syria, Iraq, Pakistan, or Sudan (Figure 3E). For relative visit numbers from other nations of this cohort, please refer to Supplementary Figure S1.

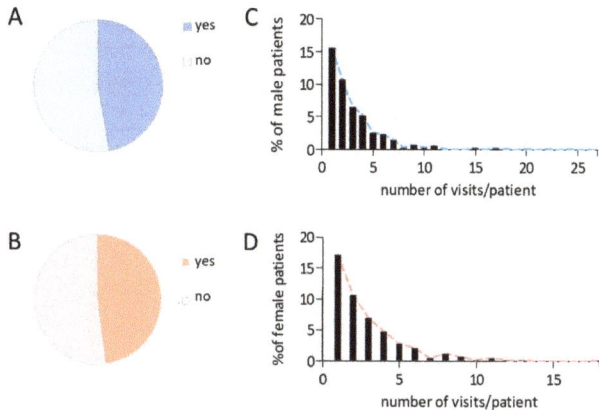

Figure 2. Healthcare utilization within the analyzed refugee cohort. (**A,B**) Proportion of male and female probands seeking help (yes) or not (no) in the medical ward. (**C,D**) visit number distribution in male and female patients [HCU: healthcare utilization].

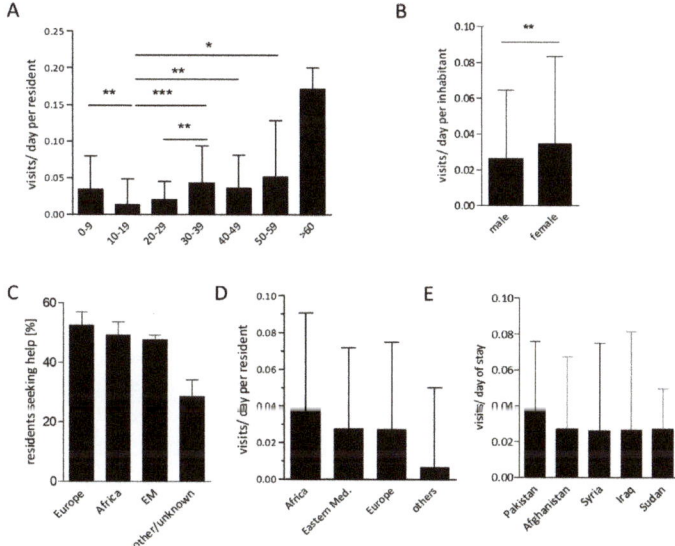

Figure 3. Factors influencing healthcare utilization in the analyzed cohort. Visits to the onsite medical ward per day of camp residence in age specific subgroups (**A**) and males vs. females (**B**). Percentage of asylum seekers utilizing medical help amongst all camp residents from this WHO region of origin (**C**). Medical consultations per day of camp residence in asylum seekers from different regions of origin (**D**) or from the top five most prevalent nations within the cohort (**E**) (bars display mean + IQR (A,B,D,E) and mean ± 95%CI (C), * $p \leq 0.05$, ** $p \leq 0.01$, *** $p \leq 0.005$).

The timepoint of stay at the camp had clear influence on the probability of overall healthcare utilization within the cohort. Most patients visited the medical ward during their first week of stay, and fewest during their last week of camp inhabitation (Figure 4A). During the first week of personal camp residence, 37.1 visits per 100 asylum seekers occurred, whereas only 9.5 visits per 100 asylum seekers were noted in week six of inhabitance at the reception center. A significant correlation between duration of camp residence in days and relative number of visits occurred, with clearly higher rates of healthcare utilization on the day of arrival at the camp (10.1 visits per 100 residents) compared to only 0.1 visits per 100 residents on day 67 and no visits on day 70 of personal camp inhabitance (Figure 4B). Overall, the proportion of asylum seekers that had not sought medical help at the reception center at all declined over time, whilst the percentage of probands with one, two to five or more than five visits gradually increased (Figure 4C).

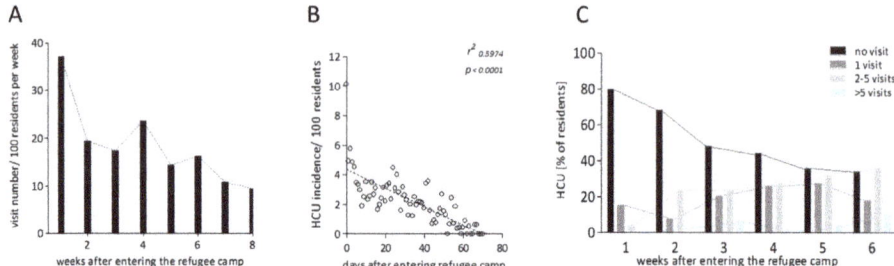

Figure 4. Time of refugee center inhabitance influences health care utilization. (**A**) Healthcare utilization rates per 100 camp residents per week after entering the shelter. (**B**) Correlation of healthcare utilization rates per 100 residents with residence duration in days. (**C**) Overall healthcare utilization depending on personal week of stay at the center (HCU: healthcare utilization).

4. Discussion

To the best of our knowledge, we present here the first comprehensive data on age, gender and origin dependent healthcare utilization behavior in a large cohort of newly arriving asylum seekers in Western Europe during the current refugee and migrant crisis. The fact that the largest proportion of asylum seekers in our cohort were young, male adults and many of them came from the Eastern Mediterranean region is in accordance with current pan-European immigration statistics [18–20].

Primary medical service for refugees and migrants is a corner stone of humanitarian care during the current crisis [11]. Political conflicts and wars in the Middle East and Africa as well as economic imbalances in Eastern Europe and many other parts of the world have led to extensive migration towards Western Europe. In 2015, more than 24 million people worldwide were fleeing, and Germany represented a top destination for many asylum seekers [1]. As such, the German healthcare system has been particularly challenged in taking primary care of newly arriving asylum seekers of unknown health status [1,12,21]. Despite this enormous challenge—which is experienced by most healthcare systems in Europe—primary healthcare needs of arriving immigrants has thus far received little attention. This is a dilemma, as provision of easily accessible healthcare to asylum seekers upon arrival, on transit or even for longer periods at onsite medical wards is essential to appropriately manage this humanitarian situation [11].

In this context, we aimed to compile an initial data set describing the health care utilization experience after setting up onsite primary medical care at an asylum seeker reception center in Northern Germany in 2015. In our cohort, a high percentage of asylum seekers sought onsite medical help, with almost half of all migrants seeking medical exceeding the initial mandatory checkup visit. The time after entering the refugee camp appeared to have a strong effect on personal healthcare utilization. An inverse correlation of visit frequency with days of camp inhabitance occurred, and the probability of presentation at the medical ward was significantly higher in the first compared to the last day of camp residence. In the first week after entering the refugee camp, more than 37 visits per 100 camp residents were noted, whereas during week five and six of camp inhabitation, only 10.8 and 9.45 visits per 100 asylum seekers occurred. This observation may have significant impact on the planning of primary healthcare setup in future situations of similar nature.

Our data clearly shows that primary medical care is most needed when a group of asylum seekers arrive, and it could make sense to intensify personnel and medical supplies for an onsite medical ward in preparation for newly arriving cohorts. Our data supports the notion that, after an initial rush of patients (in our cohort around 10 visits per day and 100 asylum seekers on the day of camp entry), the need for primary care gradually declines (in our cohort 75% reduction with 2.25 visits per 100 migrants after around one month).

Of note, the visit frequency described in our cohort was much higher than that described by Hermans et al. in their brief report on healthcare utilization at two Greek refugee sites: here the authors observed only 3.6 patient visits per person years in n = 298 newly arriving refugees in Lesbos [22]. We can only speculate on why rates were much lower in this Greek cohort and assume that different study design, primary care accessibility, overall organization in the reception centers, and possibly other factors such as nationality were considerably different from our setting.

However, certain limitations need to be taken into account when interpreting our dataset. Our results cannot be extrapolated too far, as the current refugee situation is complex and our cohort, albeit representative according to overall demographic data, is just a small specimen of the large extent of migrants currently entering Western Europe. Furthermore, this cohort is unique with regard to the fact that onsite general practitioner care was offered on a daily basis and that specialists (e.g., pediatricians, surgeons, psychiatrists) were available for referral. An interpreter service was available whenever needed and present for most consultations. All medical appointments as well as medication were free of charge. These structural circumstances were designed to facilitate easy access to care and may therefore have resulted in rather high utilization. We used this dataset to describe refugee healthcare utilization, because the underlying cohort constituted of a large and unselected specimen of newly arriving asylum seekers with well-documented inhabitance duration at the initial migrant residence in Germany. The provision of full time primary medical care at an onsite ward of the asylum seeker residence—with patient specific documentation of visit time and frequency—was unique to the here presented cohort and ideal for the conducted analysis. In other cohorts thus far analyzed by our team, similar analysis is hampered by limited data extraction of residence time and medical records that could only be obtained by a proportion of asylum seekers or were collected in a different fashion than in the here described cohort [15–17,19,20,23,24]. Currently, however, we aim at harmonizing and analyzing further large asylum seeker cohorts of a similar kind to see whether our results can be confirmed in a greater specimen of migrants entering Western Europe during the current crisis. For example, our observed statistical independence of country of origin from healthcare seeking behavior may very well be based on the low number of probands from single countries. This prohibits comprehensive statistical analyses and should be further analyzed in larger cohorts or meta-analyses of probands with several thousand migrants thus far not available to us.

Refugees and migrants are not a homogenous population, and depending on home countries, personal history, motivation to emigrate, and experiences of violence and neglect, the medical needs of persons on the run may vary considerably [22,23,25]. In addition, age is a clear factor influencing an asylum seeker's medical needs, with children being particularly vulnerable to neglect and insufficient healthcare [19,26,27]. Indeed, we found higher healthcare utilization rates in young children below the age of ten years compared to older children, adolescents and young adults and observed the highest rate of medical demand in the oldest refugee group above the age of 60 years. Furthermore, women in our cohort displayed higher healthcare utilization rates than males. These findings are in line with previous reports on the high risk of elder refugees and females for increased migration associated morbidity [1,5]. Our future analyses will focus on pediatric primary healthcare utilization and age-dependent complaints in different refugee and migrant cohorts.

Taken together, this data emphasize the high demand of migrants for primary care when first arriving to a destination country with high socioeconomic standard and stress their strong need for high accessibility and affordability of health services during the first period after arrival. As such, our data may help to plan and organize primary healthcare facilities for arriving migrants in countries with high economic resources according to the patient needs.

The UNHCR has recently stated that optimal refugee care during the current humanitarian crisis demands a "multidimensional and comprehensive approach in public health and nutrition, and will require funding and donations of both technical support and commodities/funds beyond the normal programming needs" [28]. The European Commission has recognized the demand for structured analysis of refugee medical needs and setup the "3rd Health Programme by the Consumers, Health, Agriculture and Food Executive Agency (CHAFEA)" to fund projects aiming at assessing healthcare needs of refugees reaching Europe, and development, improvement, and testing of health educational tools for this population [11].

The growing population of refugees and migrants currently entering Europe poses enormous challenges to the receiving communities and their healthcare systems and, in accordance with the UNHCR vision and the World Health Organization, requires effective onsite healthcare programs based on reliable epidemiological data [29]. In this context, we would like to emphasize the particular need for primary care demand in newly arriving refugees and migrants and hope that our initial analysis helps to better estimate needs in the vulnerable migrating population, and to adapt care taking strategies accordingly.

Supplementary Materials: The following are available online at http://www.mdpi.com/1660-4601/15/10/2163/s1. Figure S1: Visits per day of refugee center inhabitance depending on country of origin [median ± IQR], Table S1: WHO regions of origin.

Author Contributions: Research design: R.E.S., G.M.N.B., C.H., A.J.; sample collection and analyses: routine clinical care; data analysis: M.W., A.V., D.E., G.S., C.H., C.D., A.J.; writing and contributing to writing of the manuscript: all authors.

Funding: Martin Wetzke was funded by the Young Academy Clinician/Scientist program of Hannover Medical School, Germany and the DZIF clinical leave stipend of the German Center for Infection Research. Alexandra Jablonka was funded by the Young Academy Clinician/Scientist program of Hannover Medical School, Germany. Christine Happle received funding from the Young Academy Clinician/Scientist foundation and HiLF funding of Hannover Medical School, Germany. This project was supported by the German Center for Infection Research by funding of infrastructure.

Acknowledgments: The authors would like to thank all doctors and medical personnel involved in medical care of the asylum seekers for their exceptional work. We would furthermore like to thank the Order of Malta (Malteser Hilfsdienst) for the provision of data and Nexave for the extraction from the electronic database.

Conflicts of Interest: The authors declare no conflict of interest.

Abbreviations

CI	confidence interval
HCU	healthcare utilization
IQR	interquartile range
SEM	standard error mean
WHO	world health organization

References

1. UNHCR. Global Trends—Forced Displacement in 2015. 2016. Available online: http://www.unhcr.org/576408cd7.pdf (accessed on 30 April 2018).
2. Lam, E.; McCarthy, A.; Brennan, M. Vaccine-preventable diseases in humanitarian emergencies among refugee and internally-displaced populations. *Hum. Vaccines Immunother.* **2015**, *11*, 2627–2636. [CrossRef] [PubMed]
3. Castelli, F.; Tomasoni, L.R.; El Hamad, I. Migration and chronic noncommunicable diseases: Is the paradigm shifting? *J. Cardiovasc. Med. (Hagerstown)* **2014**, *15*, 693–695. [CrossRef] [PubMed]

4. Castelli, F.; Sulis, G. Migration and infectious diseases. *Clin. Microbiol. Infect.* **2017**, *23*, 283–289. [CrossRef] [PubMed]
5. Henjum, S.; Barikmo, I.; Strand, T.A.; Oshaug, A.; Torheim, L.E. Iodine-induced goitre and high prevalence of anaemia among Saharawi refugee women. *Public Health Nutr.* **2012**, *15*, 1512–1518. [CrossRef] [PubMed]
6. Blanck, H.M.; Bowman, B.A.; Serdula, M.K.; Khan, L.K.; Kohn, W.; Woodruff, B.A. Angular stomatitis and riboflavin status among adolescent Bhutanese refugees living in southeastern Nepal. *Am. J. Clin. Nutr.* **2002**, *76*, 430–435. [CrossRef] [PubMed]
7. White, C.C.; Solid, C.A.; Hodges, J.S.; Boehm, D.H. Does Integrated Care Affect Healthcare Utilization in Multi-problem Refugees? *J. Immigr. Minor. Health* **2015**, *17*, 1444–1450. [CrossRef] [PubMed]
8. Adams, K.M.; Gardiner, L.D.; Assefi, N. Healthcare challenges from the developing world: Post-immigration refugee medicine. *BMJ* **2004**, *328*, 1548–1552. [CrossRef] [PubMed]
9. The Lancet. Our responsibility to protect the Rohingya. *Lancet* **2018**, *390*, 2740.
10. Wangdahl, J.; Lytsy, P.; Martensson, L.; Westerling, R. Poor health and refraining from seeking healthcare are associated with comprehensive health literacy among refugees: A Swedish cross-sectional study. *Int. J. Public Health* **2018**, *63*, 409–419. [CrossRef] [PubMed]
11. Lionis, C.; Petelos, E.; Mechili, E.A.; Sifaki-Pistolla, D.; Chatzea, V.E.; Angelaki, A.; Rurik, I.; Pavlic, D.R.; Dowrick, C.; Dückers, M.; et al. Assessing refugee healthcare needs in Europe and implementing educational interventions in primary care: A focus on methods. *BMC Int. Health Hum. Rights* **2018**, *18*, 11. [CrossRef] [PubMed]
12. Nicolai, T.; Fuchs, O.; von Mutius, E. Caring for the Wave of Refugees in Munich. *N. Engl. J. Med.* **2015**, *373*, 1593–1595. [CrossRef] [PubMed]
13. Campos-Matos, I.; Zenner, D.; Smith, G.; Cosford, P.; Kirkbride, H. Tackling the public health needs of refugees. *BMJ* **2016**, *352*, i774. [CrossRef] [PubMed]
14. Arnold, F.; Katona, C.; Cohen, J.; Jones, L.; McCoy, D. Responding to the needs of refugees. *BMJ* **2015**, *351*, h6731. [CrossRef] [PubMed]
15. Jablonka, A.; Happle, C.; Wetzke, M.; Dopfer, C.; Merkesdal, S.; Schmidt, R.E.; Behrens, G.M.N.; Solbach, P. Measles, Rubella and Varicella IgG Seroprevalence in a Large Refugee Cohort in Germany in 2015: A Cross-Sectional Study. *Infect. Dis. Ther.* **2017**, *6*, 487–496. [CrossRef] [PubMed]
16. Jablonka, A.; Solbach, P.; Happle, C.; Hampel, A.; Schmidt, R.E.; Behrens, G.M.N. Hepatitis A immunity in refugees in Germany during the current exodus. *Med. Klin. Intensivmed. Notfmed.* **2017**, *112*, 347–351. [CrossRef] [PubMed]
17. Grote, U.; Schleenvoigt, B.T.; Happle, C.; Dopfer, C.; Wetzke, M.; Ahrenstorf, G.; Holst, H.; Pletz, M.W.; Schmidt, R.E.; Behrens, G.M.N.; et al. Norovirus outbreaks in German refugee camps in 2015. *Z. Gastroenterol.* **2017**, *55*, 997–1003. [CrossRef] [PubMed]
18. Buber-Ennser, I.; Kohlenberger, J.; Rengs, B.; Al Zalak, Z.; Goujon, A.; Striessnig, E.; Potančoková, M.; Gisser, R.; Testa, M.R.; Lutz, W. Human Capital, Values, and Attitudes of Persons Seeking Refuge in Austria in 2015. *PLoS ONE* **2016**, *11*, e0163481. [CrossRef] [PubMed]
19. Jablonka, A.; Happle, C.; Grote, U.; Schleenvoigt, B.T.; Hampel, A.; Dopfer, C.; Hansen, G.; Schmidt, R.E.; Behrens, G.M.N. Measles, mumps, rubella, and varicella seroprevalence in refugees in Germany in 2015. *Infection* **2016**, *44*, 781–787. [CrossRef] [PubMed]
20. Jablonka, A.; Behrens, G.M.; Stange, M.; Dopfer, C.; Grote, U.; Hansen, G.; Schmidt, R.E.; Happle, C. Tetanus and diphtheria immunity in refugees in Europe in 2015. *Infection* **2017**, *45*, 157–164. [CrossRef] [PubMed]
21. Sothmann, P.; Schmedt auf der Gunne, N.; Addo, M.; Lohse, A.; Schmiedel, S. Medical care for asylum seekers and refugees at the University Medical Center Hamburg-Eppendorf—A case series. *Dtsch. Med. Wochenschr.* **2016**, *141*, 34–37. [PubMed]
22. Hermans, M.P.J.; Kooistra, J.; Cannegieter, S.C.; Rosendaal, F.R.; Mook-Kanamori, D.O.; Nemeth, B. Healthcare and disease burden among refugees in long-stay refugee camps at Lesbos, Greece. *Eur. J. Epidemiol.* **2017**, *32*, 851–854. [CrossRef] [PubMed]
23. Semere, W.; Agrawal, P.; Yun, K.; Di Bartolo, I.; Annamalai, A.; Ross, J.S. Factors Associated with Refugee Acute Healthcare Utilization in Southern Connecticut. *J. Immigr. Minor. Health* **2018**, *20*, 327–333. [CrossRef] [PubMed]

24. Dopfer, C.; Vakilzadeh, A.; Happle, C.; Kleinert, E.; Müller, F.; Ernst, D.; Schmidt, R.E.; Behrens, G.M.N.; Merkesdal, S.; Wetzke, M.; Jablonka, A. Pregnancy Related Health Care Needs in Refugees-A Current Three Center Experience in Europe. *Int. J. Environ. Res. Public Health* **2018**, *15*, 1934. [CrossRef] [PubMed]
25. Doocy, S.; Lyles, E.; Akhu-Zaheya, L.; Burton, A.; Burnham, G. Health service access and utilization among Syrian refugees in Jordan. *Int. J. Equity Health* **2016**, *15*, 108. [CrossRef] [PubMed]
26. Carrasco-Sanz, A.; Leiva-Gea, I.; Martin-Alvarez, L.; Del Torso, S.; van Esso, D.; Hadjipanayis, A.; et al. Migrant children's health problems, care needs, and inequalities: European primary care paediatricians' perspective. *Child Care Health Dev.* **2018**, *44*, 183–187. [CrossRef] [PubMed]
27. Abbott, K.L.; Woods, C.A.; Halim, D.A.; Qureshi, H.A. Pediatric care during a short-term medical mission to a Syrian refugee camp in Northern Jordan. *Avicenna J. Med.* **2017**, *7*, 176–181. [PubMed]
28. UNHCR. *UNHCR Strategic Plan for Anaemia Prevention, Control and Reduction*; Reducing the Global Burden of Anaemia in Refugee Populations; UNHCR: Geneva, Switzerland, 2008–2010.
29. WHO. Population Movement Is a Challenge for Refugees and Migrants as well as for the Receiving Population. 2015. Available online: http://www.euro.who.int/en/health-topics/health-determinants/migration-and-health/news/news/2015/09/population-movement-is-a-challenge-for-refugees-and-migrants-as-well-as-for-the-receiving-population (accessed on 30 April 2018).

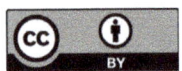

© 2018 by the authors. Licensee MDPI, Basel, Switzerland. This article is an open access article distributed under the terms and conditions of the Creative Commons Attribution (CC BY) license (http://creativecommons.org/licenses/by/4.0/).

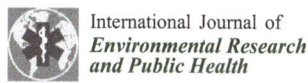

Article

Fruit and Vegetable Consumption among Immigrants in Portugal: A Nationwide Cross-Sectional Study

Liliane Costa [1,*], Sónia Dias [2] and Maria do Rosário O. Martins [1]

1. Global Health and Tropical Medicine, GHTM, Instituto de Higiene e Medicina Tropical, IHMT, Universidade Nova de Lisboa, UNL, Rua da Junqueira 100, 1349-008 Lisboa, Portugal; mrfom@ihmt.unl.pt
2. Escola Nacional de Saúde Pública, Centro de Investigação em Saúde Pública, Universidade NOVA de Lisboa & Global Health and Tropical Medicine, GHTM, Instituto de Higiene e Medicina Tropical, Universidade Nova de Lisboa, 1600-560 Lisboa, Portugal; sonia.dias@ensp.unl.pt
* Correspondence: liliane.lilocosta@gmail.com; Tel.: +351-96-633-5522

Received: 27 August 2018; Accepted: 17 October 2018; Published: 19 October 2018

Abstract: This study aims to compare adequate fruit and vegetable (F&V) intake between immigrants and natives in Portugal, and to analyse factors associated with consumption of F&V among immigrants. Data from a population based cross-sectional study (2014) was used. The final sample comprised 17,410 participants ($\geq$20 years old), of whom 7.4% were immigrants. Chi-squared tests and logistic regression models were conducted to investigate the association between adequate F&V intake, sociodemographic, anthropometric, and lifestyle characteristics. Adequate F&V intake was more prevalent among immigrants (21.1% (95% CI: 19.0–23.4)) than natives (18.5% (95% CI: 17.9–19.1)), (p = 0.000). Association between migrant status and adequate F&V intake was only evident for men: immigrants were less likely to achieve an adequate F&V intake (OR = 0.67, 95% CI = 0.66–0.68) when compared to Portuguese. Among immigrants, being female, older, with a higher education, and living in a low urbanisation area increased the odds of having F&V consumption closer to the recommendations. Adjusting for other factors, length of residence appears as a risk factor (15 or more years vs. 0–9 years: OR = 0.52, 95% CI = 0.50–0.53), (p = 0.000) for adequate F&V intake. Policies aiming to promote adequate F&V consumption should consider both populations groups, and gender-based strategies should address proper sociodemographic, anthropometric, and lifestyle determinants.

Keywords: fruit; vegetable; immigrant; Portuguese; health

---

1. Introduction

Fruit and vegetables are important components of a healthy diet and could help prevent major diseases, such as cardiovascular diseases, obesity, type 2 diabetes, and certain cancers, especially if integrated in an active and healthy lifestyle [1,2]. Therefore, fruit and vegetable (F&V) consumption is used worldwide as an important diet quality indicator [3]. F&V are rich sources of dietary fibre, vitamins, minerals, and phytochemicals, which may explain these positive effects on health [4]. A prospective cohort study conducted during 7.4 years, in 18 low-income, middle-income, and high-income countries from the five continents, among 135,335 individuals, showed that total F&V intake was associated with lower noncardiovascular mortality and total mortality, in a multivariable adjusted model [5,6]. The risk estimate for all-cause mortality, cardiovascular disease, and cancer, decreases by 10% and 11%, with consumption above 250–300 grams per day (g/d) of fruit and 300 g/d of vegetables, respectively [6]. According to World Health Organization (WHO), an adequate quantity of F&V of 400 to 500 g/d or five portions is recommended [1,2]. Worldwide, mean intakes of F&V were below current recommendations, and higher consumption was observed among women and older adults [7]. The National Food and Physical Activity Survey 2015–2016 (IAN-AF) revealed that one in two Portuguese do not consume the quantities of F&V recommended by the WHO [8].

Migration is a worldwide phenomenon and may contribute as an important experimental framework for investigate the effects of environmental factors on diet and health disparities. According to the Statistical Office of the European Communities (EUROSTAT), at the beginning of 2016, there were 35.1 million immigrants living in a European Union (EU) member state that were born outside of the EU-28, and 19.3 million were born in a different EU member state [9]. In Portugal, between 1995 and 2013 foreign-born immigrants rose from 5.2% to 8.2% of the population [10].

Migration has been associated with dietary changes, although generalisations must be carefully taken due to different individual, social, and economic factors affecting immigrants before and after arriving in the new country [11–13]. When arriving at the host country, immigrants may retain, adapt, or exclude traditional foods, and adopt the eating patterns/food choices in part or in whole, through a process called "dietary acculturation" [14]. This is a multidimensional and dynamic process that may have either positive or negative implications for health. Length of residence in the host country is often a measure of acculturation, and has been reported as an important determinant of immigrants' health [15,16]. In the literature, dietary intake has been associated with length of residence, with mixed benefits [17]. However, in general, detrimental effects on diet have been observed among immigrants and racial/ethnic minorities [18,19].

Immigration has known to have a strong impact on dietary practices and also on health disparities among immigrants and between minority groups and natives [13,19,20]. Therefore studies among foreign-born and comparisons with natives would likely be of interest for disparities research. Most studies on adult immigrants' frequency and determinants of F&V intake were conducted in the United States of America (USA) mostly among racial and ethnic groups [21–24]. In Canada, studies between immigrants and natives concluded that more information would be needed about nutritional health and immigration-related dietary changes [15]. In Europe, few studies are available on adequate F&V consumption and they mainly focus on immigrants from low- and middle-income countries [25–27]. In Portugal, scarce information is available on frequency, distribution, and determinants of adequate F&V consumption among adults and immigrants, and little is known about differences between native and immigrant food habits.

A more comprehensive understanding on adherence of F&V intake to dietary recommendations, and factors that influence its consumption, may provide important insights for health promotion and disease prevention of immigrants, as they are becoming a large share of the population over the world. Knowledge about dietary habits of both populations groups would contribute to address health disparities, an important public health concern for policy makers and health services.

Therefore, the main purpose of this study is to investigate the adequacy of F&V intake among immigrants living in Portugal, and identify the main determinants of F&V consumption. Additionally, this study extends findings by differentiating the primary outcome between immigrants and Portuguese adult populations.

2. Materials and Methods

2.1. Population and Sample

Data used in this study come from the National Health Survey (NHS) 2014, the fifth in Portugal since 1987, promoted by the Health Ministry [28]. The NHS 2014 was conducted by the Statistics Portugal Institute (INE) in collaboration with the National Institute of Health Doctor Ricardo Jorge [29]. The microdata database used for the present study was provided under protocol between INE, Directorate-General for Education and Science Statistics (DGEEC), and the Foundation for Science and Technology (FCT). The NHS 2014 is a population-based survey and collected information from the resident population aged 15 and over, on self-assessment health status, health care, and determinants related to lifestyles. This survey followed methodological guidelines and practices regulated at EU level (Commission Regulation (EU) No 141/2013), in order to enable an international comparison of the results. National questions were also included, with a view to obtaining data on relevant issues for characterising the population health status (namely reproductive health, food consumption, satisfaction with life, and long-term disability). INE carried out for the first time the collection of data on the Internet, from a sample survey of households and individuals. Results from the NHS 2014 correspond to estimates of residents, regardless of their nationality or migrant status, in the whole country between September and December 2014. This population-based survey included a total of 22,538 family housing units and the interview completion rate was 80.8% nationwide. The main methodological and conceptual features used in the NHS 2014 have been previously described elsewhere [30]. This study was reported according to the STROBE checklist for observational studies in epidemiology (Supplementary file 1) [31]. Country of birth was used to determine immigrant population and only the adult population, aged 20 and over, was consider for the present study. The final sample size comprised 17,410 participants of whom 7.4% were immigrants (Figure 1).

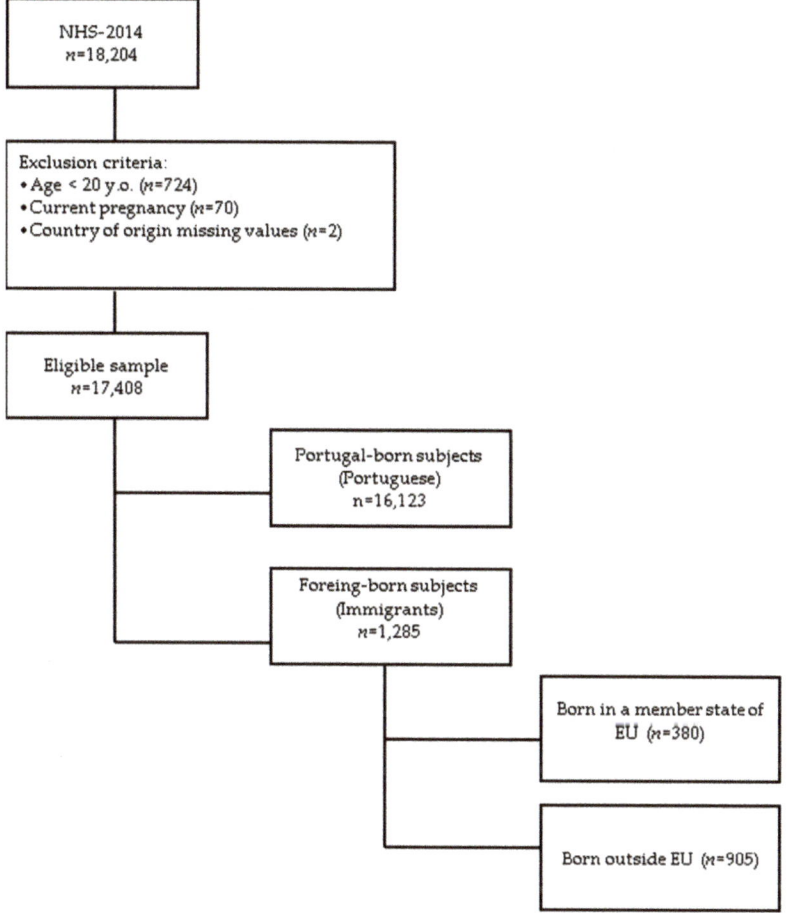

Figure 1. Flowchart for selection of study participants. Legend: NHS: National Health Survey; y.o.: years old; EU: European Union.

2.2. Variables

The outcome variable of the present study was five or more daily servings of fruit and vegetables (F&V ≥ 5). The formulation of consumption of F&V questions followed the guidelines established by the European Health Interview Survey (EHIS wave 2) Methodological manual [32]. Participants were asked to report the frequency of F&V intake, separately: "once or more a day"; "4 to 6 times a week"; "1 to 3 times a week"; "less than once a week"; or "never". The question concerning the consumption of fruit was "How often do you eat fruit, including juices squeezed from fresh fruit, and excluding juice made from concentrate? Canned and dried fruit are excluded." For vegetables intake the question was "How often do you eat vegetables or salad, excluding potatoes and juice made from concentrate? Juices squeezed from fresh or canned vegetables, as well as legumes (beans, lentils), soups (warm and cold), and vegetarian dishes are included." Those who revealed a daily frequency, "one or more times a day", were invited to estimate the number of servings per day. One serving was defined as more or less one handful for fruits and three or four tablespoons of vegetables. A show card of examples of fruit, vegetables, and standard portions were used. Ultimately, these variables were joined together to create a dummy variable for adequate F&V consumption.

Sociodemographic (sex, age, education level, legal marital status, job status, urbanisation degree, country of origin, and length of residence), anthropometric (being overweight), and lifestyle (physical activity, smoking, and alcohol habits) characteristics were assessed in the present study as covariates variables.

Education level was divided into three categories: none or basic, secondary, and higher education. Basic education consists of 9 years of school, starting at age six; secondary education spans 3 years, for students aged 15 to 18 years old; and higher education includes post-secondary-level technological specialised courses and university or polytechnic education. Legal marital status was recorded as married or not married. Job status was divided into two categories: employed and not employed. The employed category includes those participants who worked for family without a salary, those with temporary medical incapacity for work or parental leave, and those in vocational training, apprenticeships, or paid traineeships. The "not employed" category includes unemployed, pensioners, students, housewives, permanently incapacitated, unpaid internship or other status. The degree of urbanisation of place of residence was classified on three types of areas: densely populated area (the same as cities or large urban area); intermediate density area (the same as towns and suburbs or small urban area); and thinly-populated area (alternative name: rural area).

The country of origin was not available in database used for the present study. Instead, immigrants were grouped in two categories: inside EU (born in another member state of the European Union) and outside EU (born in another country outside the European Union). Length of residence in Portugal was categorised as follows, 1 to 4; 5 to 9; 10 to 14; and 15 or more years. Similar categories were used in previous research among immigrants in Portugal [33]. Due to simple size constraints the first two categories were amalgamated resulting in only three categories.

Body mass index (BMI) was calculated based on self-reported height and weight data, and for statistical analyses overweight classification was used as a dummy variable (0 = <25.0 kg/m^2; 1 = ≥25.0 kg/m^2) [34]. Lifestyle variables included in this study were smoking habits (current smoker if smoke daily or occasionally; never/former if never smoked or stopped smoking); alcohol drinking classes (regular drinking if drink alcohol every day or once or twice a week; light drinkers if consume alcohol one to three times a month; and occasional drinkers if did not consume last year or less than once a month); and physical activity (active and sedentary were assumed if engaged/not engaged in at least 150 minutes a week of any leisure time or sports exercises, respectively).

2.3. Statistical Analysis

The statistical analyses included univariate, bivariate, and multivariate analysis. The Chi-square test was carried out to assess differences in proportions for sociodemographic, anthropometric, and lifestyle characteristics between immigrants and natives and between men and women from each group. Using adequate recommended F&V intake (1 if it is adequate or 0 if otherwise) as a dependent variable, we estimated the unadjusted and adjusted odds ratio (OR) using logistic regression. The model was estimated using sample weights provided by the NHS2014 and included all relevant covariates, namely sex, age, education level, legal marital status, job status, urbanisation degree, country of origin, length of residence, BMI, physical activity, smoking status, and drinking classes. Separate models were estimated for men and women. We considered a 5% confidence level and 95% confidence interval (CI). The data analysis was performed using IBM SPSS®Statistics for Windows, version 23.0 (IBM Corp., Armonk, NY, USA).

3. Results

Sociodemographic, anthropometric, and lifestyle characteristics of the Portuguese and immigrant populations are described in Table 1. Among the immigrant population, 74.9% were born outside the EU and the median length of residence was 28 years.

Table 1. Characteristics of Portuguese and immigrant adult study population living in Portugal.

Variables	Portuguese			Immigrants		
	T % (95% CI)	M % (95% CI)	F % (95% CI)	T % (95% CI)	M % (95% CI)	F % (95% CI)
	n = 16,123	n = 7037	n = 9086	n = 1285	n = 539	n = 746
Age (years)						
20–30	21.1 (20.4–25.9)	22.6 (21.6–23.6)	19.9 (19.1–21.7)	22.5 (20.2–24.8)	25.8 (22.1–29.5)	19.8 (16.9–22.7)
35–49	26.6 (25.9–27.3)	27.7 (26.7–28.7)	25.5 (24.6–26.4)	45.5 (42.8–48.2)	44.0 (39.8–41.2)	46.8 (43.2–50.4)
50–64	25.5 (24.8–26.2)	25.7 (24.7–26.7)	25.3 (24.4–26.2)	23.4 (21.1–25.7)	24.8 (21.2–28.4)	22.1 (19.1–25.1)
65+	26.8 (26.1–27.5)	24.0 (23.0–25.0)	29.3 (28.4–30.2)	8.6 (7.1–10.1)	5.4 (3.5–7.3)	11.3 (9.0–13.6)
p value	0.000 *	0.000 **			0.000 **	
Education level						
None or basic	64.4 (63.7–65.1)	65.6 (64.5–66.7)	63.4 (62.4–64.4)	38.9 (36.2–41.6)	40.0 (35.9–44.1)	37.9 (34.4–41.4)
Secondary	17.2 (16.6–17.8)	18.4 (17.5–19.3)	16.2 (15.4–17.0)	31.7 (29.2–34.2)	34.4 (30.4–38.4)	29.4 (26.1–32.7)
Higher education	18.4 (17.8–19.0)	16.0 (15.1–16.9)	20.4 (19.6–21.2)	29.4 (26.9–31.9)	25.6 (21.9–29.3)	32.6 (29.2–36.0)
p value	0.000 *	0.000 **			0.000 **	
Legal marital status						
Married	60.3 (59.5–61.1)	64.0 (62.9–65.1)	56.9 (55.9–57.9)	54.9 (52.2–57.6)	55.7 (51.5–59.9)	54.2 (50.6–57.8)
p value	0.000 *	0.000 **			0.000 **	
Job status						
Employed	48.6 (47.8–49.4)	54.0 (52.8–55.2)	43.9 (42.9–44.9)	62.2 (59.5–64.9)	69.4 (65.5–73.3)	56.0 (52.4–59.6)
p value	0.000 *	0.000 **			0.000 **	
Urbanisation degree						
Densely	42.2 (41.4–43.0)	41.4 (40.2–42.6)	42.9 (41.9–43.9)	56.6 (53.9–59.3)	54.8 (50.6–59.0)	58.1 (54.6–61.6)
Intermediate	30.1 (29.4–30.8)	30.2 (29.1–31.3)	30.0 (29.1–30.9)	24.8 (22.4–27.2)	27.5 (23.7–31.3)	22.6 (19.6–25.6)
Thinly	27.7 (27.0–28.4)	28.4 (27.3–29.5)	27.1 (26.2–28.0)	18.6 (16.5–20.7)	17.7 (14.5–20.9)	19.3 (16.5–22.1)
p value	0.000 *	0.000 **			0.000 **	
Anthropometric						
Overweight	54.4 (53.6–55.2)	58.8 (58.0–60.0)	50.6 (50.0–51.6)	47.4 (44.7–50.1)	51.3 (47.1–55.5)	44.1 (40.5–47.7)
p value	0.000 *	0.000 **			0.000 **	
F&V intake						
≥5 servings/day	18.5 (17.9–19.1)	15.7 (14.8–16.5)	21.0 (20.2–21.8)	21.1 (19.0–23.4)	16.6 (13.5–19.7)	25.0 (21.9–28.1)
p value	0.000 *	0.000 **			0.000 **	
Physical activity						
Active	63.4 (62.7–64.1)	65.8 (66.9–69.1)	60.5 (59.5–61.5)	62.8 (60.2–65.4)	64.5 (60.5–68.5)	60.5 (57.0–64.0)
p value	0.000 *	0.000 **			0.000 **	
Smoke status						
Current	20.3 (19.7–20.9)	28.8 (27.7–29.9)	12.8 (12.1–13.5)	23.7 (21.4–26.0)	28.8 (25.0–32.6)	19.4 (16.6–22.2)
p value	0.000 *	0.000 **			0.000 **	
Drinking classes						
Regular	46.1 (45.3–46.9)	68.0 (66.9–69.1)	26.9 (26.0–27.8)	39.9 (37.2–42.6)	57.5 (53.3–61.7)	24.8 (21.7–27.9)
Light	13.8 (13.3–14.3)	12.6 (11.8–13.4)	14.8 (14.1–15.5)	18.5 (16.4–20.6)	16.3 (13.2–19.4)	20.4 (17.5–23.3)
Occasional	40.1 (39.3–40.9)	19.4 (18.5–20.3)	58.3 (57.3–59.3)	41.6 (38.9–44.3)	26.2 (22.5–29.9)	54.7 (51.1–58.3)
p value	0.000 *	0.000			0.000	

p value from chi-square tests; T: Total; M: Male; F: Female; CI: Confidence intervals; *: differences in proportions between populations; **: differences in proportions between sexes.

Compared with natives, immigrants were younger (68.0% (95% CI: 65.4–70.6) vs. 47.7% (95% CI: 46.9–48.5) being 20 to 49 years old), and more immigrants than Portuguese have attained higher education (29.4% (95% CI: 26.9–31.9) vs. 18.4% (95% CI: 17.8–19.0)). A greater proportion of foreign-born than natives were employed (62.2% (95% CI: 59.5–64.9) vs. 48.6% (95% CI: 47.8–49.4)) and lived in more densely populated areas (56.6% (95% CI: 53.9–59.3) vs. 42.2% (95% CI: 41.4–43.0) lived in cities or urban areas). In both groups, more men than women were overweight, whose prevalence was higher in the Portuguese population (54.4% (95% CI: 53.6–55.2)).

Adequate F&V intake was more prevalent among immigrants (21.1% (95% CI: 19.0–23.4)) than natives (18.5% (95% CI: 17.9–19.1)). Consuming five or more servings of F&V on a daily basis were more frequent among women, in both population groups.

Results of the association between adequate F&V intake and migrant status, and after adjustment for all relevant variables (Model 1) are shown in Figure 2.

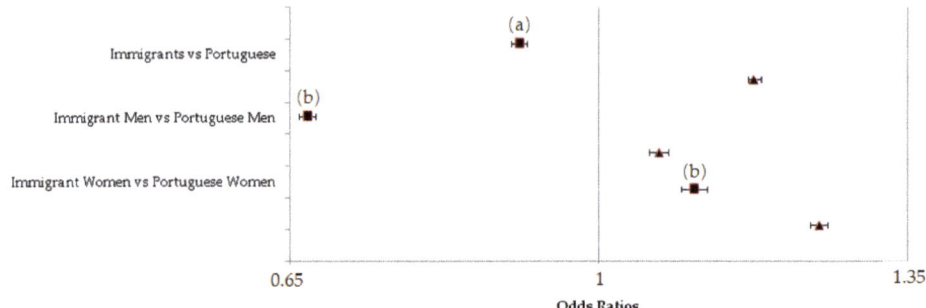

Figure 2. Adjusted (■) and unadjusted (▲) association of migrant status with adequate F&V intake. Legend: (a) adjusted for sex, age, educational level, legal marital status, job status, urbanisation degree, body mass index, physical activity, smoking status, and drinking classes; (b) adjusted for age, educational level, legal marital status, job status, urbanisation degree, body mass index, physical activity, smoking status, and drinking classes.

For Model 1, unadjusted results revealed that being an immigrant was positively associated with adequate F&V intake (OR = 1.18, 95% CI = 1.17–1.18), especially for women (OR = 1.25, 95% CI = 1.24–1.26). However, for the adjusted model, association between migrant status and recommended F&V consumption was only evident for men: immigrants were less likely to achieve an adequate fruit and vegetable intake (OR = 0.67, 95% CI = 0.66–0.68), when compared to Portuguese (Figure 2).

The Model 2 logistic regression (Table 2) considers only the subsample of the immigrant population; the dependent variable is adequate F&V consumption and results are disaggregated by sex.

For the subsample of immigrants (model 2), adequate F&V intake (≥ 5 servings/day) was significantly associated with sex, age, and education level, after adjustment for all covariates. Women had 3.6-fold higher odds (95% CI = 3.54–3.70) of having an adequate F&V consumption, than men (Table 2). Immigrants between 35 and 39 years old had 3.3-fold higher odds (OR = 3.35, 95% CI = 3.26–3.45) of achieving F&V recommendations, compared to younger immigrants. Higher education level appears to be a protective factor for adequate F&V intake (OR = 2.44, 95% CI = 2.37–2.51). In both sexes, for the adjusted model, adequate F&V intake was also positively associated with a low urbanisation degree (thinly vs. densely: OR = 1.76, 95% CI = 1.71–1.81). Compared to immigrants from another member state of the EU, immigrants from outside the EU had lower odds of achieving F&V recommendations (OR = 0.64, 95% CI = 0.63–0.66). Time living in Portugal was found to be a risk factor for adequate F&V consumption, after adjustment for all covariates (15 or more years vs. 0–9 years: OR = 0.52, 95% CI = 0.50–0.53). Being overweight (OR = 0.59, 95% CI = 0.58–0.61), a current smoker (OR = 0.46, 95% CI = 0.45–0.47), and an occasional alcohol drinker (occasional vs. regular: OR = 0.63, 95% CI = 0.61–0.64) decrease the odds of adequate F&V. An active lifestyle among immigrants, compared to sedentary behaviour, increased the odds of meeting the recommendations for these two food groups (OR = 1.43, 95% CI = 1.40–1.46).

Table 2. Correlates of adequate F&V consumption for the subsample of 1285 immigrants: logistic regression results.

Variables	F&V ≥ 5 Servings per Day					
	Total		Men		Women	
	Unadjusted	Adjusted †	Unadjusted	Adjusted ‡	Unadjusted	Adjusted ‡
Sociodemographic						
Sex						
Men	1	1	1	1	1	1
Women	1.67 (1.65–1.69) *	3.62 (3.54–3.70) *	n.a	n.a	n.a	n.a
Age						
20–34y	1	1	1	1	1	1
35–39y	2.50 (2.46–2.55) *	3.35 (3.26–3.45) *	2.70 (2.62–2.77) *	3.44 (3.27–3.62) *	2.25 (2.20–2.31) *	4.44 (4.26–4.63) *
50–64y	1.81 (1.77–1.85) *	2.00 (1.93–2.08) *	1.10 (1.93–2.06) *	3.20 (3.00–3.41) *	1.65 (1.60–1.69) *	2.02 (1.93–2.12) *
65+ y	3.60 (3.51–3.69) *	8.10 (7.75–8.47) *	4.83 (4.64–5.04) *	21.19 (19.63–22.87) *	2.73 (2.65–2.81) *	5.69 (5.34–6.06) *
Education level						
None or basic	1	1	1	1	1	1
High school	1.32 (1.30–1.34) *	1.94 (1.88–1.99) *	1.49 (1.46–1.53) *	1.62 (1.56–1.69) *	1.25 (1.22–1.27) *	1.61 (1.55–1.68) *
Higher educ.	2.19 (2.16–2.22) *	2.44 (2.37–2.51) *	2.64 (2.58–2.71) *	0.99 (0.95–1.03)	1.88 (1.85–1.92) *	3.66 (3.52–3.81) *
Legal marital status						
Not married	1	1	1	1	1	1
Married	1.16 (1.15–1.18) *	0.61 (0.60–0.63) *	1.28 (1.26–1.31) *	0.78 (0.75–0.81) *	1.11 (1.09–1.13) *	0.48 (0.46–0.49) *
Job status						
Not Employed	1	1	1	1	1	1
Employed	1.24 (1.23–1.26) *	1.28 (1.25–1.31) *	1.79 (1.75–1.84) *	1.76 (1.68–1.85) *	1.17 (1.15–1.19) *	0.91 (0.88–0.94) *
Urbanisation degree						
Densely	1	1	1	1	1	1
Intermediate	0.59 (0.58–0.60) *	1.67 (1.63–1.71) *	1.66 (1.62–1.70) *	2.34 (2.25–2.42) *	0.98 (0.97–1.00)	1.59 (1.54–1.65) *
Thinly	0.69 (0.68–0.70) *	1.76 (1.71–1.81) *	2.51 (2.45–2.58) *	3.73 (3.56–3.91) *	1.33 (1.31–1.36) *	1.22 (1.18–1.26) *
Country of origin						
Inside EU	1	1	1	1	1	1
Outside EU	0.69 (0.68–0.70) *	0.79 (0.77–0.81) *	0.57 (0.56–0.58) *	0.67 (0.64–0.69) *	0.79 (0.77–0.80) *	0.73 (0.71–0.75) *
Length of residence						
0–9 years	1	1	1	1	1	1
10–14 years	1.23 (1.10–1.15) *	0.20 (0.19–0.21) *	1.00 (0.97–1.04)	0.05 (0.05–0.05) *	1.27 (1.23–1.31) *	0.46 (0.43–0.49) *
15+ years	1.32 (1.29–1.34) *	0.52 (0.50–0.53) *	0.72 (0.70–0.74) *	0.27 (0.26–0.29) *	2.10 (2.04–2.16) *	1.03 (0.98–1.09)
Anthropometric						
Body mass index						
<25 kg/m2	1	1	1	1	1	1
≥25 kg/m2	0.83 (0.82–0.84) *	0.59 (0.58–0.61) *	1.05 (1.03–1.07) *	0.64 (0.62–0.66) *	0.75 (0.73–0.76) *	0.62 (0.61–0.64) *
Lifestyle						
Physical activity						
Sedentary	1	1	1	1	1	1
Active	1.24 (1.22–1.26) *	1.43 (1.40–1.46) *	1.72 (1.67–1.78) *	1.50 (1.44–1.55) *	1.11 (1.08–1.14) *	1.13 (1.10–1.16) *
Smoking status						
Never/ former	1	1	1	1	1	1
Current	0.49 (0.48–0.50) *	0.46 (0.45–0.47) *	0.36 (0.35–0.37) *	0.19 (0.18–0.20) *	0.67 (0.66–0.69) *	0.72 (0.69–0.74) *
Drinking classes						
Regular	1	1	1	1	1	1
Light	1.12 (1.10–1.14) *	0.70 (0.68–0.72) *	1.12 (1.09–1.15) *	1.42 (1.36–1.48) *	0.90 (0.88–0.92) *	0.57 (0.55–0.59) *
Occasional	0.99 (0.97–1.00)	0.63 (0.61–0.64) *	0.67 (0.66–0.69) *	0.48 (0.46–0.50) *	0.84 (0.83–0.86) *	0.81 (0.78–0.84) *

OR: Odds Ratio; CI: Confidence Intervals; 1: reference group; n.a: not applicable; * $p < 0.05$. † Adjusted for sex, age, education level, legal marital status, job status, urbanisation degree, country of origin, length of residence, body mass index, physical activity, smoking status, and drinking classes. ‡ Adjusted for age, education level, legal marital status, job status, urbanisation degree, country of origin, length of residence, body mass index, physical activity, smoking status, and drinking classes.

Stratified by sex, the results showed that the determinants of adequate F&V intake are different among immigrant men and women (Table 2). In men, being employed (OR = 1.76, 95% CI = 1.68–1.85), living in a thinly urbanised area (OR = 3.73, 95% CI = 3.56–3.91), and engaging in an active lifestyle

(OR = 1.5, 95% CI = 1.44–1.55) were more likely to consume adequate F&V (Table 2). Length of residence was negatively associated with adequate F&V intake, after adjustment for other factors, especially for men immigrants living in Portugal for 10 to 14 years (OR = 0.05, 95% CI = 0.05–0.05). For long term immigrants (15 or more years) the odds of adequate F&V consumption was 73% lower for men (OR = 0.27, 95% CI = 0.26–0.29), but not significant for women (OR = 1.03, 95% CI = 0.98–1.09) compared to those arriving in Portugal less than 10 years ago. Among women, those who have attained a higher education level were 3.7 times more likely to achieve the WHO recommendation for F&V consumption (OR = 3.66, 95% CI = 3.52–3.81), compared with their counterparts who had none or only basic education.

4. Discussion

The main objectives of this study were to investigate the adequacy of F&V intake among immigrants living in Portugal, and identify the main determinants of consumption. Only 21% of immigrants reported an adequate consumption of ≥5 F&V on a daily basis. Among immigrants, sex, age, education, place of residence, and country of origin were found to be important determinants of a healthy diet.

Among immigrants, women were more likely to attain daily adequate servings of F&V compared with men, after adjustment for all covariates. This finding is in line with the work of Volken and colleagues, who studied immigrants in Switzerland and found that women exhibited a lower risk of an inadequate F&V consumption [35]. Kumar and colleagues showed evidence that women reported a higher intake of this food group in all groups of migrants [36]. Sex-differences in food consumption (vegetables, fruit, and berries) suggested that women had a healthier food intake among Russian, Somali, and Kurdish immigrants in Finland [37]. Despite these results, female migrants were, traditionally, at higher risk of the negative effects of migration and dietary acculturation [13]. A work review on changes in food habits among immigrant women showed that a busier lifestyle, higher level of stress, low socialisation, children's preferences, unavailability of traditional foods, food insecurity, and taste may result in low consumption of F&V and other unfavourable dietary changes that can in turn cause chronic diseases [13]. However, this negative impact seems to be more evident in USA and Canada, whereas in Europe, studies showed less minor negative or even positive impacts. It is possible that in Europe, and particularly in Portugal, those social and environmental factors identifying as having a negative impact in adequate F&V consumption may not be present among immigrant women, or have a minor expression.

In this study, older age and lower urbanisation degree were found to be positively associated with recommended F&V consumption, for both sexes and after adjustment for all variables. Health reasons, cooking skills, and lack of time were found to be some of the age-related factors that may influence dietary habits [24]. It is possible that older immigrants had more awareness of F&V health benefits, more cooking skills and more available time to spend preparing dishes with these food groups. Among immigrants in Switzerland, the relative risk of low F&V intake decreased with age, but no significant association was found between specific dwelling zones (rural/urban) and low or medium F&V intake, compared with the recommendations [35]. Urbanisation may have a positive influence on availability and diversity of fruits and vegetables, but seasonality and prices determine access [26]. In low- and middle-income countries, living in urban areas, alongside with increasing income have been associated to a higher intake of F&V, in part because of the high cost and limited access to fresh-food markets and stores in rural areas [38]. In the present study, immigrants living in rural areas were more likely to consume the recommended daily servings of F&V, compared with those living in densely urban areas. The inhabitants of rural areas in Portugal traditionally have a small area devoted to the production of fresh vegetables and fruits for their own consumption and to share with neighbours. It is possible that immigrants who choose less densely urbanised places to live adopt the traditional growing of one's own produce. Because the majority of immigrants in the present study were employed, lack of time to achieve and to prepare meals may explain disparities in F&V consumption, for those living in densely urban areas.

In our study, after adjustment for all covariates, factors that were positively associated with adequate F&V intake, in the general immigrant population, revealed different directions when data was disaggregated by sex. Among immigrant women, education was positively associated with adequate daily F&V consumption. Among immigrant men, being employed and engaged in a more active lifestyle increased the odds of attaining recommendations of F&V. These results highlight the need for different gender-based approaches to changing eating habits, for men and women.

Length of residence has been controversially associated with F&V intake. In Canada, the longer South Asians lived in the host country, the greater their consumption of nonstarchy vegetables, but no significant association was found with the fruit group [39]. In the United Kingdom, a study conducted, also with South Asians, found no changes in F&V intake, between recent ($\leq$5 years) and long-term immigrants (>10 years) [40]. A systematic review of the relationship between acculturation and diet, among Latinos in USA, concluded that total F&V consumption were negatively associated with acculturation [41]. Findings from our study were in line with these results. Length of residence may not fully capture the acculturation process and data from age at arrival could add new insight for this discussion, however no such data was available in the database disposable for the present study. Notwithstanding, length of residence has been used as a measure of acculturation in many studies [15,16,42].

Data from the country of origin was not available for the present study. Instead, countries of birth were aggregated into two large groups, with a great heterogeneity among them with regard to sociodemographic factors. This constitutes a limitation to understand how the bond to country of origin and more traditional foodways may influence F&V adequacy. Nevertheless, in this study, results showed that immigrants from outside EU member states were less likely to attain F&V recommendations.

In Portugal, by 2014, two of the main immigrant groups of non-EU origin came from Brazil and China: Brazilians were the main foreign resident community in Portugal (22.1%), and Chinese, although representing only 5.4% of the immigrant population, had a numerical increment of 14.8% over the prior year [43]. These two countries faced a rapid shift in diet, physical activity and morbidity over the past decades [44,45]. This phenomenon is known as "nutrition transition" and is negatively linked with nutrition-related noncommunicable diseases, because of the reduction of F&V consumption, and the reduction of physical activity in work and leisure [46]. By 2011, fruit supply in Brazil and vegetable supply in China were higher than in Europe [47]. Notwithstanding, only 23.6% of the adult Brazilian population consumed the recommended daily F&V servings [48], and the Chinese diet shifted from a traditional diet abundant with vegetables, to a more Westernised dietary pattern, with low F&V consumption, especially in the low-income groups [47,49].

Furthermore, after adjustment for all covariates, immigrant's poor lifestyle habits (sedentary and current smoker) and overweight were associated with inadequate F&V consumption. Regarding alcohol drinking habits, findings from the present study were consistent with international research, which show that men drink alcoholic beverages more regularly than women [50]. It has been suggested in the literature that wine drinkers tended to consume more F&V, while preference for other alcoholic beverages (beer and spirits) was associate with less healthy dietary habits [51]. Portugal is a wine producer country and consuming this beverage during meals is an acceptable social behaviour, which may explain that drinking occasionally appears to be a risk factor for inadequate F&V intake, for both sexes and compared to regular drinkers. However, for men, but not for women, light drinking seems to be a protector factor for F&V adequacy. On the one hand, those immigrants who are engaged in poor health habits, like drinking, may try to compensate unhealthy outcomes by improving diet behaviour. On the other hand, regular alcohol consumption is traditionally attributed to men and a reduction in the frequency of alcohol drinking, from regular to light, may indicate greater health vigilance and consequently a greater quality dietary improvement. Among women, being a light drinker may indicate a different pattern of alcohol consumption, with regard to the alcoholic beverage preference and the absolute alcohol intake, which have been associated in previous research with dietary pattern [51,52]. It is possible that for women who do not drink alcohol beverages on a regular basis, alcoholic consumption takes place outside meals, and may be a substitute for meals or food choices. Additionally, we cannot exclude under-reporting of intake, especially from those who know to have unhealthy dietary habits. Differential patterns of alcohol consumption between men and women and its effects on diet suffer influenced by biological, social and cultural factors, which are not part of the scope of this study [53]. It would be valuable to future research with immigrant population, to consider additional alcohol exposure variables besides frequency, namely type of alcohol beverages and absolute consumption. It is important to highlight that an inadequate diet in combination with other poor lifestyle choices may increase the risk of immigrants' unhealthy outcomes and constitute a serious burden on the health services.

Another purpose of the present study was to verify disparities in adequate F&V consumption between natives and immigrants. Results showed a healthier F&V consumption among immigrants than Portuguese, although for men, being an immigrant was negatively associated with F&V$\geq$5 intake. One possible explanation for differences in F&V consumption between natives and immigrants is that they may have better nutritional knowledge and at least equal F&V accessibility and availability than Portuguese. Immigrants were younger, well-educated, and most of them were employed and inhabitants of densely urban areas, which may indicate a low level of food insecurity. Despite that this factor has not been evaluated in the present study, it is known that the predominant barriers to F&V consumption include inaccessibility, cost, and low income [24,27]. Additionally, participants from the NHS were selected from accommodation units and so the sample may potentially favour well-integrated and well-educated immigrants, and not consider vulnerable groups with different socioeconomic characteristics. Comparisons between immigrant and native groups in previous studies revealed mixed results. The Canadian Community Health Survey showed two different outcomes: data from 2009 revealed that immigrants consumed less F&V than those born in Canada [54], while data from 2007 found no statistically significant difference in F&V intake between immigrants and Canadians [55]. In two other studies conducted in the Netherlands, results showed that South Asian (Surinamese and Pakistanis) generally reported lower frequency of fruit and vegetables compared with the Dutch population [56,57]. The Oslo Immigrant Health Profile from 2008, showed that Vietnamese men had the lowest and Turkish women the highest consumption of F&V, while Norwegians were neither the end nor the beginning of spectrum [36]. Conflicting results may be explained by the use of different methodologies to define and measure F&V, and because of the variety of subjects' ethnic and social backgrounds used in the studies. Literature shows strong evidence that in European countries there are considerable differences between traditional dietary habits among ethnic populations [12].

Findings from the present study revealed that the majority of both Portuguese and immigrant populations do not likely to attain the recommendations of WHO for an adequate F&V consumption. These results are particularly curious because Portugal, as a South European country, was expected to have a food pattern closer to the Mediterranean style, which is characterised by high consumption of fruit and vegetables [58,59]. However, according to the Portuguese Food Balance Sheet (BAP), an analytical instrument of statistical nature that allows the portrait and trend of food availability, Portugal has been progressively moving away from the Mediterranean food standard. Notwithstanding some improvements in the last decade, F&V availability still does not reach the recommendations [60].

Some limitations of the present study should be considered. First, the measuring of F&V intake was based on memory, thus recall problems are involved. Second, NHS included fruit juices and legumes, which is controversial [61,62]. Pure fruit juices can provide most of the nutrient substances that are present in the original fruit, but with less fibre and sometimes with added sugar [62]. Although legumes, often termed beans or pulses, share some bioactive compounds and fibre with vegetables, they are also a protein source, unlike vegetables. In Europe, recent studies have not included legumes when analysing vegetable consumption [63]. Another limitation was social desirability, which may be considered when F&V intake is assessed [62]. Although not within the scope of this study, disparities in the definition of fruit and vegetable food groups, measures and units were observed between studies and make comparisons difficult. Cultural-based perceptions on food groups and portions may influence reported consumption because they may not coincide with the host country's classification [63]. In order to minimise methodological differences, standardised approaches and tools to collect and quantify information should be developed [61]. Another limitation is that, because part of the information used for this study was collected via computer-assisted web interviewing, some individuals, without internet or with lower computer literacy, may have been excluded. Additionally, we had to merge two classes from the length of residence variable, for sample size constraints, in order to estimate OR and have better precision. Despite this limitation, is our view that the categories of length of residence used in this study are more suitable for comparisons with other studies. Finally, future studies should consider vulnerable groups, namely refugees or illegal immigrants, with different socioeconomic characteristics and health outcomes.

5. Conclusions

This study showed that the WHO recommendation of five or more portions of F&V, on a daily basis, was attained by only 21.1% of immigrants and 18.5% of Portuguese population. Despite of this immigrant status, especially among women, increased the odds of achieve the WHO recommendations. Among immigrants, sex, age, education, and place of residence were found to be important determinants of a healthy diet.

The findings from this study on adequacy and disparities of F&V intake, of both native and foreign-born groups of the Portuguese community, highlight the need for strategies to increase F&V consumption for both communities and provide a starting point for more robust investigations. The main strength of the present study is to contribute with knowledge about the main drivers of a healthy diet among immigrants. Effective gender-based strategies to attain recommendations of daily F&V intake should be considered, and particular attention should be given for immigrant men. Future works should explore the role of the urbanisation degree of the place of residence as an important driver for healthy food consumption. More effective measures of dietary acculturation and food insecurity should be included in future studies about health of immigrants.

Supplementary Materials: The following are available online at http://www.mdpi.com/1660-4601/15/10/2299/s1, File S1: STROBE Statement—Checklist of items that should be included in reports of cross-sectional studies.

Author Contributions: All authors made substantial contributions to study conception, analysis, and the interpretation of data. L.C. was involved in drafting the manuscript. M.d.R.O.M. contributed to the statistical analysis and critical review. S.D. was involved in critically revising the important intellectual content. All authors read and approved the final version of the manuscript.

Funding: FCT for funds to GHTM—UID/Multi/04413/2013. The funders had no role in study design, data, collection and analysis, decision to publish or preparation of the manuscript.

Acknowledgments: The data that support the findings of this study are available from Statistics Portugal. Restrictions apply to the availability of these data, which were used under license for the current study, and so are not publicly available.

Conflicts of Interest: The authors declare no conflicts of interest.

References

1. World Health Organization. Diet, Nutrition and the Prevention of Chronic Diseases: Report of a Joint WHO/FAO Expert Consultation. Available online: http://apps.who.int/iris/bitstream/10665/42665/1/WHO_TRS_916.pdf?ua=1 (accessed on 20 May 2017).
2. World Health Organization. Fruit and Vegetable Promotion Initiative: A Meeting Report, 25–27 August, Geneva. Available online: http://apps.who.int/iris/bitstream/10665/68395/1/WHO_NMH_NPH_NNP_0308.pdf (accessed on 20 May 2017).
3. Gil, Á.; Martinez de Victoria, E.; Olza, J. Indicators for the evaluation of diet quality. *Nutr. Hosp.* **2015**, *31* (Suppl. 3), 128–144. [PubMed]
4. Slavin, J.L.; Lloyd, B. Health benefits of fruits and vegetables. *Adv. Nutr.* **2012**, *3*, 506–516. [CrossRef] [PubMed]

5. Miller, V.; Mente, A.; Dehghan, M.; Rangarajan, S.; Zhang, X.; Swaminathan, S.; Dagenais, G.; Gupta, R.; Mohan, V.; Lear, S.; et al. Fruit, vegetable, and legume intake, and cardiovascular disease and deaths in 18 countries (PURE): A prospective cohort study. *Lancet* **2017**, *390*, 2037–2049. [CrossRef]
6. Schwingshackl, L.; Schwedhelm, C.; Hoffmann, G.; Lampousi, A.M.; Knüppel, S.; Iqbal, K.; Bechthold, A.; Schlesinger, S.; Boeing, H. Food groups and risk of all-cause mortality: A systematic review and meta-analysis of prospective studies. *Am. J. Clin. Nutr.* **2017**, *105*, 1462–1473. [CrossRef] [PubMed]
7. Ng, M.; Fleming, T.; Robinson, M.; Thomson, B.; Graetz, N.; Margono, C.; Mullany, E.C.; Biryukov, S.; Abbafati, C.; Abera, S.F.; et al. Global, regional, and national prevalence of overweight and obesity in children and adults during 1980–2013: A systematic analysis for the Global Burden of Disease Study 2013. *Lancet* **2014**, *384*, 776–781. [CrossRef]
8. Lopes, C.; Torres, D.; Oliveira, A.; Severo, M.; Alarcão, V.; Guiomar, S.; Mota, J.; Teixeira, P.; Rodrigues, S.; Lobato, L.; et al. Inquérito Alimentar Nacional e de Atividade Física 2015–2016. Available online: https://ian-af.up.pt/ (accessed on 3 October 2017).
9. Eurostat. Migration and Migrant Population Statistics—Statistics Explained. Available online: http://ec.europa.eu/eurostat/statistics-explained/index.php/Migration_and_migrant_population_statistics (accessed on 23 August 2017).
10. OECD. Foreign-Born Population (indicator). Available online: https://data.oecd.org/migration/foreign-born-population.htm (accessed on 23 August 2017).
11. Wandel, M.; Råberg, M.; Kumar, B.; Holmboe-Ottesen, G. Changes in food habits after migration among South Asians settled in Oslo: The effect of demographic, socio-economic and integration factors. *Appetite* **2008**, *50*, 376–385. [CrossRef] [PubMed]
12. Gilbert, P.A.; Khokhar, S. Changing dietary habits of ethnic groups in Europe and implications for health. *Nutr. Rev.* **2008**, *66*, 203–215. [CrossRef] [PubMed]
13. Popovic-Lipovac, A.; Strasser, B. A Review on Changes in Food Habits among Immigrant Women and Implications for Health. *J. Immigr. Minor. Health* **2015**, *17*, 582–590. [CrossRef] [PubMed]
14. Satia-Abouta, J. Dietary acculturation: Definition, process, assessment, and implications. *Int. J. Hum. Ecol.* **2003**, *4*, 71–86.
15. Sanou, D.; O'Reilly, E.; Ngnie-Teta, I.; Batal, M.; Mondain, N.; Andrew, C.; Newbold, B.K.; Bourgeault, I.L. Acculturation and nutritional health of immigrants in Canada: A scoping review. *J. Immigr. Minor. Health* **2014**, *16*, 24–34. [CrossRef] [PubMed]
16. Goulão, B.; Santos, O.; Carmo, I.D. The impact of migration on body weight: A review. *Cad Saude Publica.* **2015**, *31*, 229–245.
17. Talegawkar, S.A.; Kandula, N.R.; Gadgil, M.D.; Desai, D.; Kanaya, A.M. Dietary intakes among South Asian adults differ by length of residence in the USA. *Public Health Nutr.* **2016**, *19*, 348–355. [CrossRef] [PubMed]
18. Satia-Abouta, J. Dietary acculturation and the nutrition transition: An overview. *Appl. Physiol. Nutr. Metab.* **2010**, *35*, 219–223.
19. Leung, G.; Stanner, S. Diets of minority ethnic groups in the UK: Influence on chronic disease risk and implications for prevention. *Nutr. Bull.* **2011**, *36*, 161–198. [CrossRef]
20. Raza, Q.; Snijder, M.B.; Seidell, J.C.; Peters, R.J.G.; Nicolaou, M. Comparison of cardiovascular risk factors and dietary intakes among Javanese Surinamese and South-Asian Surinamese in the Netherlands. The HELIUS study. *BMC Res. Notes* **2017**, *10*, 23. [CrossRef] [PubMed]
21. Wang, K. Availability and Consumption of Fruits and Vegetables among Non-Hispanic Whites, Blacks, Hispanics, and Asians in the USA: Findings from the 2011–2012 California Health Interview Adult Survey. *J. Racial Ethn. Health Disparities* **2017**, *4*, 497–506. [CrossRef] [PubMed]
22. Tichenor, N.; Conrad, Z. Inter- and independent effects of region and race/ethnicity on variety of fruit and vegetable consumption in the USA: 2011 Behavioral Risk Factor Surveillance System (BRFSS). *Public Health Nutr.* **2016**, *19*, 104–113. [CrossRef] [PubMed]
23. Satia, J.A. Diet-related disparities: Understanding the problem and accelerating solutions. *J. Am. Diet. Assoc.* **2009**, *109*, 610–615. [CrossRef] [PubMed]
24. Yeh, M.-C.; Ickes, S.B.; Lowenstein, L.M.; Shuval, K.; Ammerman, A.S.; Farris, R.; Katz, D.L. Understanding barriers and facilitators of fruit and vegetable consumption among a diverse multi-ethnic population in the USA. *Health Promot. Int.* **2008**, *23*, 42–51. [CrossRef] [PubMed]

25. Landman, J.; Cruickshank, J.K. A review of ethnicity, health and nutrition-related diseases in relation to migration in the United Kingdom. *Public Health Nutr.* **2001**, *4*, 647–657. [CrossRef] [PubMed]
26. Holmboe-Ottesen, G.; Wandel, M. Changes in dietary habits after migration and consequences for health: A focus on South Asians in Europe. *Food Nutr. Res.* **2012**, *56*. [CrossRef] [PubMed]
27. Osei-Kwasi, H.A.; Nicolaou, M.; Powell, K.; Terragni, L.; Maes, L.; Stronks, K.; Lien, N.; Holdsworth, M. Systematic mapping review of the factors influencing dietary behaviour in ethnic minority groups living in Europe: A DEDIPAC study. *Int. J. Behav. Nutr. Phys. Act.* **2016**, *13*, 85. [CrossRef] [PubMed]
28. Dias, C.M. 25 anos de Inquérito Nacional de Saúde em Portugal. Available online: https://run.unl.pt/handle/10362/4409 (accessed on 10 April 2017).
29. INE, INSA. Inquérito Nacional de Saúde 2014. Available online: https://www.ine.pt/xportal/xmain?xpid=INE&xpgid=ine_publicacoes&PUBLICACOESpub_boui=263714091&PUBLICACOEStema=55538&PUBLICACOESmodo=2 (accessed on 10 April 2017).
30. Chkotua, S.; Peleteiro, B. Mammography Use in Portugal: National Health Survey 2014. *Prev. Chronic. Dis.* **2017**, *14*, E100. [CrossRef] [PubMed]
31. Von Elm, E.; Altman, D.G.; Egger, M.; Pocock, S.J.; Gøtzsche, P.C.; Vandenbroucke, J.P.; Strobe, I. Strengthening the Reporting of Observational Studies in Epidemiology (STROBE) statement: Guidelines for reporting observational studies. *BMJ* **2007**, *335*, 806–808. [CrossRef] [PubMed]
32. European Commission. European Health Interview Survey (EHIS wave 2)—Methodological manual. Available online: https://ec.europa.eu/eurostat/documents/3859598/5926729/KS-RA-13-018-EN.PDF/26c7ea80-01d8-420e-bdc6-e9d5f6578e7c (accessed on 13 January 2018).
33. Da Costa, L.P.; Dias, S.F.; Martins, M.R.O. Association between length of residence and overweight among adult immigrants in Portugal: A nationwide cross-sectional study. *BMC Public Health* **2017**, *17*, 316. [CrossRef] [PubMed]
34. The Asia-Pacific Perspective: Redefining Obesity and Its Treatment. Obesity: Preventing and Managing the Global Epidemic Geneva: WHO. 2000. Available online: http://www.wpro.who.int/nutrition/documents/docs/Redefiningobesity.pdf (accessed on 25 January 2016).
35. Volken, T.; Rüesch, P.; Guggisberg, J. Fruit and vegetable consumption among migrants in Switzerland. *Public Health Nutr.* **2013**, *16*, 156–163. [CrossRef] [PubMed]
36. Kumar, B.N.; Grøtvedt, L.; Meyer, H.E.; Søgaard, A.-J.; Strand, B.H. The Oslo Immigrant Health Profile. Available online: https://brage.bibsys.no/xmlui/bitstream/handle/11250/220525/Kumar_2008_The.pdf?sequence=3 (accessed on 22 May 2017).
37. Adebayo, F.A.; Itkonen, S.T.; Koponen, P.; Prättälä, R.; Härkänen, T.; Lamberg-Allardt, C.; Erkkola, M. Consumption of healthy foods and associated socio-demographic factors among Russian, Somali and Kurdish immigrants in Finland. *Scand. J. Public Health* **2017**, *45*, 277–287. [CrossRef] [PubMed]
38. Mayén, A.-L.; Marques-Vidal, P.; Paccaud, F.; Bovet, P.; Stringhini, S. Socioeconomic determinants of dietary patterns in low- and middle-income countries: A systematic review. *Am. J. Clin. Nutr.* **2014**, *100*, 1520–1531. [CrossRef] [PubMed]
39. Kandola, K.; Sandhu, S.; Tang, T. Immigration and dietary patterns in South Asian Canadians at risk for diabetes. *J. Diabetes Complicat.* **2016**, *30*, 1462–1466. [CrossRef] [PubMed]
40. Garduño-Diaz, S.D.; Khokhar, S. South Asian dietary patterns and their association with risk factors for the metabolic syndrome. *J. Hum. Nutr. Diet.* **2013**, *26*, 145–155. [CrossRef] [PubMed]
41. Ayala, G.X.; Baquero, B.; Klinger, S. A systematic review of the relationship between acculturation and diet among Latinos in the United States: Implications for future research. *J. Am. Diet. Assoc.* **2008**, *108*, 1330–1344. [CrossRef] [PubMed]
42. Alegria, M. The Challenge of Acculturation Measures: What are we missing? A commentary on Thomson & Hoffman-Goetz. *Soc. Sci. Med.* **2009**, *69*, 996–998. [PubMed]
43. Oliveira, C.R.D.; Gomes, N. Indicadores de Integração de Imigrantes. Relatório Estatístico Anual. Outubro de 2016, Coleção Imigração em Números. Observatório das Migrações. Available online: http://www.om.acm.gov.pt/publicacoes-om/colecao-imigracao-em-numeros/relatorios-anuais (accessed on 28 May 2017).
44. Conde, W.L.; Monteiro, C.A. Nutrition transition and double burden of undernutrition and excess of weight in Brazil. *Am. J. Clin. Nutr.* **2014**, *100*, 1617S–1622S. [CrossRef] [PubMed]
45. Popkin, B.M. Synthesis and Implications: China's Nutrition Transition in the Context of Changes Across other Low and Middle Income Countries. *Obes. Rev.* **2014**, *15*. [CrossRef] [PubMed]

46. Popkin, B.M. The shift in stages of the nutrition transition in the developing world differs from past experiences! *Public Health Nutr.* **2002**, *5*, 205–214. [PubMed]
47. Gill, M.; Feliciano, D.; Macdiarmid, J.; Smith, P. The environmental impact of nutrition transition in three case study countries. *Food Secur.* **2015**, *7*, 493–504. [CrossRef]
48. Malta, D.C.; Silva , J.B.D., Jr. O Plano de Ações Estratégicas para o Enfrentamento das Doenças Crônicas Não Transmissíveis no Brasil e a Definição das Metas Globais para o Enfrentamento Dessas Doenças até 2025: Uma Revisão. *Epidemiologia Serviços Saúde* **2013**, *22*, 151–164. [CrossRef]
49. Du, S.; Lu, B.; Zhai, F.; Popkin, B.M. A new stage of the nutrition transition in China. *Public Health Nutr.* **2002**, *5*, 169–174. [CrossRef] [PubMed]
50. Chaiyasong, S.; Huckle, T.; Mackintosh, A.-M.; Meier, P.; Parry, C.D.H.; Callinan, S.; Cuong, P.V.; Kazantseva, E.; Gray-Phillip, G.; Parker, K.; et al. Drinking patterns vary by gender, age and country-level income: Cross-country analysis of the International Alcohol Control Study. *Drug Alcohol Rev.* **2018**, *37*, S53–S62. [CrossRef] [PubMed]
51. Sluik, D.; Bezemer, R.; Sierksma, A.; Feskens, E. Alcoholic Beverage Preference and Dietary Habits: A Systematic Literature Review. *Crit. Rev. Food Sci. Nutr.* **2016**, *56*, 2370–2382. [CrossRef] [PubMed]
52. Breslow, R.A.; Guenther, P.M.; Smothers, B.A. Alcohol Drinking Patterns and Diet Quality: The 1999–2000 National Health and Nutrition Examination Survey. *Am. J. Epidemiol.* **2006**, *163*, 359–366. [CrossRef] [PubMed]
53. Erol, A.; Karpyak, V.M. Sex and gender-related differences in alcohol use and its consequences: Contemporary knowledge and future research considerations. *Drug Alcohol Depend.* **2015**, *156*, 1–13. [CrossRef] [PubMed]
54. Meshefedjian, G.A.; Leaune, V.; Simoneau, M.-È.; Drouin, M. Disparities in Lifestyle Habits and Health Related Factors of Montreal Immigrants: Is Immigration an Important Exposure Variable in Public Health? *J. Immigr. Minor. Health* **2014**, *16*, 790–797. [CrossRef] [PubMed]
55. Azagba, S.; Sharaf, M.F. Disparities in the frequency of fruit and vegetable consumption by socio-demographic and lifestyle characteristics in Canada. *Nutr. J.* **2011**, *10*, 118. [CrossRef] [PubMed]
56. Raza, Q.; Nicolaou, M.; Dijkshoorn, H.; Seidell, J.C. Comparison of general health status, myocardial infarction, obesity, diabetes, and fruit and vegetable intake between immigrant Pakistani population in the Netherlands and the local Amsterdam population. *Ethn. Health* **2017**, *22*, 551–564. [CrossRef] [PubMed]
57. Raza, Q.; Nicolaou, M.; Snijder, M.B.; Stronks, K.; Seidell, J.C. Dietary acculturation among the South-Asian Surinamese population in the Netherlands: The HELIUS study. *Public Health Nutr.* **2017**, *20*, 1983–1992. [CrossRef] [PubMed]
58. Shen, J.; Wilmot, K.A.; Ghasemzadeh, N.; Molloy, D.L.; Burkman, G.; Mekonnen, G.; Gongora, M.C.; Quyyumi, A.A.; Sperling, L.S. Mediterranean Dietary Patterns and Cardiovascular. *Health. Annu. Rev. Nutr.* **2015**, *35*, 425–449. [CrossRef] [PubMed]
59. Sofi, F.; Cesari, F.; Abbate, R.; Gensini, G.F.; Casini, A. Adherence to Mediterranean diet and health status: Meta-analysis. *BMJ* **2008**, *337*, a1344. [CrossRef] [PubMed]
60. Lisboa, Portugal: Instituto Nacional de Estatística, I.P. Portuguese Food Balance Sheet 2012–2016. Available online: https://www.ine.pt/xportal/xmain?xpid=INE&xpgid=ine_publicacoes&PUBLICACOESpub_boui=290053341&PUBLICACOESmodo=2&xlang=en (accessed on 9 June 2017).
61. Pomerleau, J.; Lock, K.; McKee, M.; Altmann, D.R. The Challenge of Measuring Global Fruit and Vegetable Intake. *J. Nutr.* **2004**, *134*, 1175–1180. [CrossRef] [PubMed]
62. Agudo, A. Measuring Intake of Fruit and Vegetables. Workshop on Fruit and Vegetables for Health, 1–3 September 2004, Kobe, Japan. Available online: http://www.who.int/dietphysicalactivity/publications/f&v_intake_measurement.pdf. (accessed on 9 June 2017).
63. Roark, R.A.; Niederhauser, V.P. Fruit and vegetable intake: Issues with definition and measurement. *Public Health Nutr.* **2013**, *16*, 2–7. [CrossRef] [PubMed]

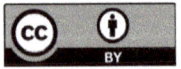

© 2018 by the authors. Licensee MDPI, Basel, Switzerland. This article is an open access article distributed under the terms and conditions of the Creative Commons Attribution (CC BY) license (http://creativecommons.org/licenses/by/4.0/).

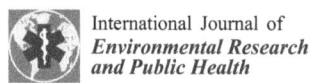

Article

Exploring Risk Factors Affecting the Mental Health of Refugee Women Living with HIV

Agata Vitale [1],* and Judy Ryde [2]

[1] College of Liberal Arts (CoLA), Bath Spa University, Newton Park, Bath BA29BN, UK
[2] Trauma Foundation South West, Barrow Castle, Rush Hill, Bath BA22QR, UK; judy.ryde@barrowcastle.co.uk
* Correspondence: a.vitale@bathspa.ac.uk; Tel.: +44-(0)1225-875-480

Received: 25 September 2018; Accepted: 16 October 2018; Published: 22 October 2018

Abstract: Little is known about how the intersection of being a forced migrant and living with HIV can contribute to the development or exacerbation of pre-existing mental conditions. This study is set in this context and it aims to explore specific risk factors affecting the mental health of refugee women living with HIV. A total of eight refugee women living with HIV took part in the study; they were individually interviewed, and their transcripts were thematically analyzed. The overall findings indicated that participants' mental health was impaired by multiple stressors associated with their conditions, such as racial discrimination, HIV-related stigma, including from health professionals, loneliness, and resettlement adversities. These all represent threats to public health, as they discourage individuals from engaging with adequate health/mental health services. Despite their situation, participants had not received psychological interventions and their healthcare was reduced to managing the physical symptoms of HIV. Participants indicated their need to take part in group interventions that could promote their mental health and social recovery. These findings are relevant to raising awareness about the specific risk factors affecting refugee women living with HIV and to provide evidence for public health interventions based on this specific population's need.

Keywords: refugees women; HIV; mental health; stigma; discrimination

1. Introduction

Implementing effective strategies to promote the mental health of refugee women living with HIV represents a complex public health issue as it needs to address simultaneously the challenges that this specific population experience as forced migrants, as well as dealing with the physical/psychological sequalae of having contracted the virus. It is therefore imperative to identify specific risk factors to which refugee women living with HIV are exposed, and to provide evidence for the development and the implementation of effective mental health interventions that enable them to improve their living conditions.

1.1. Background

The Human Immunodeficiency Virus (HIV) is transmitted when infected body fluids are in contact either with mucous membranes or damaged tissues or are directly injected into the bloodstream from a needle [1]. Once in the system, HIV attacks and becomes part of the CD4 cells (a type of white blood cell in the immune system); when these cells multiply to fight infections, they make more copies of HIV, to the point that the body cannot react to opportunistic infections, cancers and diseases. This in turn can lead to AIDS (Acquired Immunodeficiency Syndrome), which represents the last stage of HIV infection [2].

Up until the mid-1990s, individuals with HIV could progress to AIDS within a few years, however, with the introduction of antiretroviral therapy (ART), mortality and the morbidity rates of individuals living with HIV have significantly improved [3] and those who start ART in a timely way and who comply with it adequately can have a long life expectancy [4]. However, according to recent statistics, out of the approximately 36.9 million individuals who are affected currently by HIV globally, only about 20.9 million are receiving adequate treatment [1]. HIV, therefore, represents one of the most destructive infectious disease epidemics in recorded history [5] and recent statistics indicated that, in 2016, it killed one million individuals [1]. This shows that, despite the enormous investment in the HIV response over the past 20 years which is paying off, the epidemics continues to pose serious public health threats in all regions and predominantly to the most vulnerable groups, including those who are affected by forced migration, gender based-violence, social inequalities, stigmatization, and discrimination [6,7]. Women and young girls (who overall represent more than half of the global population affected by HIV) are among the most vulnerable to contracting the virus in many communities, especially in the high-burden epidemics of sub-Saharan Africa [7]. HIV, therefore, remains a cause of death, particularly in disadvantaged populations, and as the World Health Organization (WHO) Draft global health sector strategies HIV, 2016–2021 [8] indicates, providing immediate and effective treatment will remain an important public health priority globally.

1.2. HIV, Gender, and Mental Health

HIV does not only attack and debilitate the immune system but, in turn, has detrimental consequences for individuals' health and mental health [9–14]. Specifically, mood disorders, anxiety disorders, and post-traumatic stress disorder (PTSD) have been identified as the most prevalent mental health disorders among individuals living with HIV [15]. Depression in particular, seems to be twice as common in people living with HIV (especially when symptomatic) than in uninfected individuals [16,17].

Furthermore, self-harm and suicide attempts and/or completion rates are also high in individuals affected by HIV [18–20]. The high comorbidity of mental disorders in individuals living with HIV can be explained by many psychological and environmental risk factors, particularly in those from disadvantaged backgrounds, including unemployment, poor housing, food insecurity, stigma, and fear of disclosing their condition and of interacting with the health care system [21].

Furthermore, gender inequalities play a significant role not only in HIV transmission, but also in the course of HIV and its comorbidity rates with mental disorders [22].

In this regard, a PubMed search conducted by Orza et al. cited nearly 800 peer-reviewed articles about the high comorbidity of mental health disorders in women who are HIV positive [23]. Women living with HIV from disadvantaged backgrounds seem particularly at risk of having co-occurring mental disorders. This might be related to multiple gender-related risk factors, such as gender dynamics that result in power imbalances, marginalization from access to goods and opportunities which power ensures [22], unprotected sex, trading sex for money or other goods, having sex with high-risk partners, substance misuse gender-based violence [23–25], sexual and reproductive health complications, and human rights [26], their poor access and adherence to healthcare and medications [27], and stressors during pregnancy [28]. Above all, women of color living with HIV show particularly high rates of mental disorders, and this might be due to the cumulative effect of stigma, racial discrimination, poverty, and immigration status, if they are living abroad [29]. As expected, the comorbidity of HIV and mental disorders often leads to poor compliance and adherence to antiretroviral therapy [30] and/or to the lack of adequate engagement with relevant health/mental health services [31–35]. This, in turn, further reduces the quality of life of women affected by HIV, including poorer psychological adjustment to a chronic, progressive and life-threatening illness, worse HIV treatment adherence and outcomes [36,37], and an increased risk of HIV transmission [31,38].

1.3. HIV, Gender and Refugees

Due to the adverse pre-migratory conditions and often the adverse journey, refugees represent a high-risk group for contracting HIV [39]. This might be due to multiple risk factors, including the

HIV prevalence in refugees' country of origin, the lack of health services available to them [40,41], and the abuses and violence they might be exposed to during their journey and in refugee camps. HIV-related symptoms can be further worsened in refugee populations by the fact that some of the host countries might be overburdened by the impact of AIDS and, therefore, they can be unable or unwilling to provide adequate treatment for them [42]. Refugee women and girls might be at greater risk of contracting HIV (both in their country of origin and, in some cases in the host country) which might be due to gender inequalities [39]. There is, in fact, plenty of evidence indicating that refugee women are disproportionately impacted by economic, legal, cultural, and social disadvantages, food insecurity, unequal distribution of goods and by the destruction of the community and family structures that usually protect them [43,44]. Furthermore, refugee women are often the main target of all forms of violence in their country of origin, during the journey and in refugee camps [45]. Since the normal social safety nets are absent during conflicts, refugee women might be also forced to exchange sexual services for money, food, or protection.

Furthermore, rape is often used as a weapon of war and refugee women might be subject to sexual violence and exploitation in refugee settings [39,40]. Refugee women living with HIV might face several challenges during their resettlement process as they deal with their multiple health/mental health stressors associated with having contracted the virus, as well as trying to understand and navigate a new health system [46,47].

1.4. Refugees, Gender, and Mental Health

As for other refugee populations, refugee women's mental health might be impaired by multiple pre and post-migratory psychological and environmental factors, including, in some cases, by being forced to leave their country of origin because of war, genocide, discrimination and the violation of human rights [48,49], they might be exposed to inhumane conditions during their journey [50,51], and/or they might be facing several cultural, economic and language barriers during their resettlement process [50–55]. Furthermore, among refugees, women are frequently identified in humanitarian reports as being particularly exposed to physical and mental health difficulties; refugee women might be at greater risk of violence in their country of origin and during their journey [56]. In addition, during their resettlement, refugee women might face several challenges associated with their gender, including carrying the burden of raising their children in a new country, adjusting to changes in family dynamics and to the new expectations about their roles [56,57]. In some cases, refugee women's mental health might be impaired by the fact that they have lost their previous family and community support (which is essential in collectivist cultures) and they might be left on their own to adjust to their new gender-related roles [56].

However, despite the multiple risk factors, refugee women have often proved to be resilient and to adapt well to post-migratory stressors [58], especially if they perceive adequate community support in the host country [59].

1.5. Rationale for the Study

Despite the existing evidence on the link that mental health has with HIV, gender, and forced migration, little is known about how their intersection (i.e., being affected simultaneously by the sequelae of having contracted the virus as well as by the challenges associated with being refugees) might affect refugee women living with HIV. The current study therefore is set in this context and it aims is to provide some support to the scarce literature in this field. The objectives of this study are to explore the risk factors that refugee women living with HIV are exposed to, the type of support available to them and their view of taking part in a narrative, group-based intervention. This latter objective will provide the basis to the longer study that the authors will conduct at a subsequent stage with the same population by exploring the effectiveness of a group-based narrative intervention to support their mental health and social recovery.

For the purpose of this study *mental health* does not simply refer to the lack of psychological symptoms attached to a diagnostic category [60]; but, in line with the World Health Organization (WHO), it is considered *a state of wellbeing in which an individual realizes his or her own abilities, can cope with the normal stresses in life, can work productively and fruitfully* ([61], p. 1). In addition, within this study, *mental health promotion*, refers to *the process of enhancing the capacity of individuals and communities to take control over their lives and improve their mental health* [62].

Furthermore, in line with 1951 Geneva Convention [63], in this study, the term refugee refers to a person who has a 'well-founded fear of being persecuted in his or her country of origin for reasons of race, religion, nationality, membership of a particular social group, or political opinion'.

2. Materials and Method

Due to the exploratory nature of the research, a qualitative study design was employed [64,65]. This design is considered well suited for health and wellbeing investigations, as it offers a rich insight into the direct experience of individuals who are struggling with specific health/mental health conditions [66]. Furthermore, qualitative methods are considered highly appropriate when conducting research with refugees, as they allow the researcher to listen directly to their voices [67]. This enables researchers to build 'a refugee centred perspective' where the diverse narratives told by participants are organized to tell their collective story directly rather than this being filtered by stakeholders [68]. Specifically, for this study, semi-structured interviews were used; those are considered the most suitable method of data collection when investigating sensitive topics with refugee populations [69].

2.1. Materials

This consisted, in the following order, of: an information sheet, a consent form, a demographic form (to gather generic demographic details), and the interview script; this latter contains questions aiming at fostering discussion around the research topics, including of living with HIV, being a refugee and the type of health/ mental support available to them.

A digital recorder was used to record the interviews.

2.2. Ethical Considerations

Ethical approval was granted by the Ethics Committee from the first author's institution. The interview process was in line with the British Psychological Society's (BPS) guidelines for professional practice [70] and the Ethical Guidelines for Good Research Practice with Refugee Studies [71]. The ethical principles of *respect for persons, beneficence*, and of *informed consent* were observed [72,73].

In line with these ethical principles and prior to the interview, the overall process was explained to participants in detail, including the research aims and objectives, the confidentiality of the study, the freedom not to answer any questions that they did not feel comfortable with, and of withdrawing at any time without any consequences.

Furthermore, it was essential to take extra ethical considerations for this specific study. Some refugees fear interviews, as they may recall traumatic memories of interrogations they could have had within their home countries, or, despite the interviews with immigration officers offering the possibility of gaining residence, it might be in fact distressing for some specific people to be in an interview situation [68,74].

To address this concern, the mental health implications for those who may have been traumatized through being exposed and/or witnessing horrifying events, were not approached in the study, even if this might mean that participants' mental health was likely not to fully emerge from the data [75]. Furthermore, the contact details of specific organizations that could provide support to participants who might have found the experience of being interviewed distressing, were provided in the information sheet and they were restated verbally by the researcher prior to the interview.

2.3. Selection Criteria

These were: being female, aged over 18, being a forced migrant, having a level of English that could sustain a conversation and being able to give informed consent.

2.4. Accessing the Sample

All participants were recruited from those attending a non-profit organisation providing support to individuals *living* with HIV in the South West of England. Potential participants were identified and approached by a migrant key worker from this non-profit organisation to ascertain if they were willing to take part in the study. To facilitate this process, the first author provided the manager with a leaflet containing some generic information about the study, along with the researchers' contact details. Individuals who showed an interest in the research and who fitted the selection criteria met the first author on an individual basis for more detailed information. Out of nine individuals who were asked to take part in the study, eight agreed and the one declined for family reasons. The size of this sample is in line with the literature in this field, which indicates that, in conducting research with refugees, having small samples is relatively normal, as refugees are a difficult to reach, mobile population [76,77]. A small sample is also considered suitable for explorative studies, as the thoroughness of the close investigation enhances the validity of in-depth inquiry [78].

2.5. Procedure

To facilitate participants' comfort in taking part in the research [76], they were individually interviewed in a room free of distraction at the HIV organization from which they were recruited. However, it was made clear, through the ethic forms, that the study was not commissioned or linked in any manner to that organization. Prior to starting the interviews, participants were given the information sheet and were asked to sign the consent form. It was deemed important to help the interviewees talk freely about topics they raised, and additional questions were only asked to seek clarification, illustration, or further exploration [79]. The interviews took approximately 45 min each and were audio-recoded with the participants' permission.

2.6. Data Analysis

Interview transcripts were analysed via thematic analysis. This method is not tied to a predetermined theoretical perspective and/or predefined ideas [80], but it rather situates the coding process in the realm of evidence [81] and it is considered well suited for health and wellbeing investigations [65]. The analysis was primarily conducted by the first author; however, to ensure its trustworthiness and consistency, the second author independently analysed a sample of transcripts by using a coding template to ensure inter code agreement [81,82]. There were not many differences between the analysis undertaken by the two authors, and they agreed on the final themes.

3. Results

3.1. Overview of the Sample

The sample for the study consisted of eight women aged between 30 and 55 years. Seven participants were from Africa and one from Jamaica. The length of time that participants lived in the UK varied between nine and 18 years. Six participants had already obtained their Leave to Remain (i.e., residency), while the remaining two had temporary leave status. In line with the UK National Health Service policy, all participants were entitled to and benefited from primary and secondary care (i.e., these are free to asylum seekers and refugees in the UK) [83].

Except for one participant (who stated that she had a partner but that they were not cohabitating), all remaining ones were single at the time of the interviews. Six participants had secondary level education, one primary and the remaining one had a tertiary level education. Six participants had adult children, and one had young children who lived with her. Except for one participant, who worked as a carer for older people, the remaining participants stated that they were currently not working, mostly for 'health related reasons'. All participants stated that they were receiving treatment for their HIV, however, other than the practical and emotional support offered by the non-profit organization they linked to, none of them was in receipt of psychological treatment by psychologists, psychotherapists or counsellors within 12 months of the interviews.

3.2. Qualitative Analysis

Participants provided a rich description of how the intersection of being HIV positive and refugees affected their mental health, including facing HIV-related stigma, racial discrimination, isolation, and feeling disempowered by the relationship they had with some of the health professionals involved in their care. The themes are organised in a manner that could facilitate the understanding of participants' struggles with being HIV positive, as well as with being refugees. The final analysis contains both broad and more focused themes, and this is in line with the specific analytic method employed [84].

Theme 1: The intersection of the HIV related symptoms and the practical challenges of being refugees

Participants indicated that the quality of their life was significantly impaired by dealing with the sequelae of having contracted the virus, as well as with the practical challenges they faced as refugees, including their struggle to meet basic needs and their poor living conditions.

In particular, the lack of suitable accommodation represented one of the main concerns for all participants. Due to their financial restrictions, as well as their HIV-related symptoms, they were in fact often confined indoors with very little to entertain themselves. For instance, when talking about her financial struggle, P.7 said: *I am so poor, but this month I don't think I can pay the rent because I am not working*; whereas P.5 indicated: *You're limited on what you can do because you're a refugee sometimes*. Furthermore, when talking about her daily routine, P.6 (who lived in a small council flat, in a block that she described as quite dull and unpleasant), said: *If I am not working and I don't have an appointment then I stay home. I don't go anywhere ... First thing I pray. And yes, that is it. Maybe I may do cleaning, cleaning and doing other things, it is just inside (the house)*.

In addition, P.1 (who lived in a shared catholic accommodation, with 13 residents) indicated: *I'm worried that my heart can stop at any time ... So, I'm always in the house ... I am limited in the activities I can do. If there is no one in the house, I spend the day sleeping because there is nothing to do ...* P.1 also indicated she had to live under strict catholic rules, including that she did not even have the freedom to choose the television programs she wanted to watch: *As a Community House we are not allowed to watch television ... we watch a few movies not like action movies, they would be sort of like censored movies*.

Furthermore, when talking about her financial situation P.2 stated: *The money they give us is not enough to rely on a week. Because I have to use transport, we have to eat healthy*. Her conditions were also aggravated by the lack of predictability of her HIV related symptoms: *So, my days aren't predictable. I can get up this morning and I just felt fine and I can wake up tomorrow morning and feel quite sick ...* As a result, P.2 indicated that she was forced to spend most of her time, indoors, in a small hostel room that she shared with her two young children: *Sometimes I just find it very difficult just to ... because now I'm in one room with my children, because I'm still bidding for a house, I just find it challenging, waking up in the morning, at night I don't have my own time, I have to go to bed when they have to go to bed, I don't sit there to just reflect on myself*.

Furthermore, when talking about how HIV-related symptoms affected her, P.8 said: *It's painful for me, it's not letting me do anything. If I stand too long it's a problem. I need to be only on the bed*. She added that being confined in a home was quite challenging for her, as she shared an over-crowded accommodation with other female refugees: *I share the house with the other ladies, it is very difficult. You know people from* different countries and it's really difficult to manage ... We don't have privacy, no privacy in the house and very, very difficult you know it's very difficult for me to manage.

The intersection of dealing with the sequelae of the HIV, as well as facing practical challenges associated with their condition, seemed to affect participants' mental health, as they mostly complained about anxiety, insomnia, fatigue and lack of motivation. In this regard, P.1 *I tend not to do a lot because of my condition, because I get tired too early;* Or, P.3, who indicated: *My sleep is not very good, so I wake up still tired and sometimes I want to stay in bed. I don't feel like doing anything, lack of motivation;* and P.5, who stated: *I don't feel like doing anything. I'm tired, fatigued, (I have) chest infections.*

Theme 2: Care received by health professionals: 'I'm the one carrying the body'

Participants indicated that, despite their circumstances, the type of care they were receiving was mostly related to reducing the physical symptoms of HIV, rather than taking a holistic approach that could address both their health/mental health needs. This was well exemplified by P.3 who, when talking about her mental conditions said: *Medication, I get it from the GPs (General Practitioners). Psychological help, nothing really.* Participants had mixed experiences of receiving care from the health professionals. The only exception was represented by P.4, who indicated: *Yeah, health professionals, they are quite fine. They don't treat me in any way different. They treat me quite fine, so I can express myself to them.* However, P.4 was elusive in explaining the reasons of her satisfaction. From her interview and her demographic form, it was difficult to understand the causes of her satisfaction, as it not did seem related to having a better situation than the rest of the sample.

The remaining participants indicated that their General Practitioner (i.e., family doctor), who they saw regularly for routine cheek-ups and for the referrals to secondary care, was quite supportive and empathetic towards them. For instance, P.1 said that she was able to build a relationship overtime with her General Practitioner and that she could talk freely about her concerns: *We have a very good communication with my GP, I feel more happier whenever I go and sit with her, just to talk to her, explain to her how I feel.* This was echoed by P.8, who indicated: *If I feel down, I have my GP who I can talk to;* Or, for instance, by P.2, who stated: *He (the General Practitioner) treats me well.*

However, participants felt that they were not treated with the same respect by other health professionals involved in their care. For instance, when they had to book a last-minute appointment at their family practice (which happened quite often because of their HIV-related symptoms) they felt disempowered by some of the General Practitioners on duty. This is well exemplified by P.1, who stated:

There are times when you book an appointment and you see just any other doctor, they don't want to listen. There are times when I say, "You are not listening to me, you are telling me but I'm the one carrying the body that you're working on and you need to listen to what I'm saying that I'm feeling. Yes, I know it's part and parcel of the condition but at the same time, I'm not well, you have to listen that I'm saying I'm not well." But sometimes they'll say, "Oh there's nothing else we can do."

In addition, some participants felt that other health professionals (not from the HIV clinic) involved in their care, might fear contracting HIV from them. In this regard, P.1. said: *They (the doctors) think they might be at risk of getting HIV from me.* Or P.6 discussed how some health professionals reacted when she disclosed being HIV positive, for the fear of being contaminated: *When you mention you (to some doctors) are HIV sometimes their face drops. They are like careful in this and that way, so when I go, "Yes I am HIV but it is undetectable if you treat me".*

In addition, P.6 talked about her struggle when disclosing to a dentist she was referred to that she was HIV positive. P.6 said that she indicated in the pre-assessment form that she was HIV positive and this generated fear of contracting the virus in the dentist. P.6 felt that the long wait after she handed back her form at the reception was due to the dentist not knowing how to handle her situation: *But as soon as I signed that on the form my time I waited was up to almost five hours. She (the dentist) could not touch me.* P.6 then explained: *It took time and I was the last one* (in the waiting room). *But I knew that it was not the first one that if they don't understand about HIV.* P.6 indicated that she reported this episode to her key worker from the HIV organization, who then wrote a letter to the dental clinic to find out what happened: *I asked my support worker and she wrote to the dental clinic and they wrote back and said 'Oh, we are very sorry, some people don't know how to take this but we need to train them'*. This experience discouraged P.6 to return to that dental clinic: *So I never went back*.

Theme 3: Facing multiple forms of intolerance

Overall participants indicated that, they were exposed simultaneously to the stigma of living with HIV, as well as racism as refugees and discrimination as migrants. These sub-themes are described below.

3.3. Facing HIV Stigma: 'It's the Sickness of Shame'

All participants struggled with the stigma associated with living with HIV, first in their countries of origin (where they contracted the virus) and then in the UK. The stigma affected their self-esteem and led to isolation from their family and/or community networks. When talking about how the stigma of living with HIV affected women in their countries, participants indicated that this was mostly associated with them having low moral standards and with promiscuous sexual behaviour. Specifically, when talking about people's attitude towards women living with HIV in her country, P.4 said: *If they (people in her country) discover that you're HIV, they try to shun you and try to keep to their friends*. Or, P.5, explained how being HIV positive is considered a moral fault in her country:

Yeah, you're perceived as like you've been not a good person for you to contract HIV. You're made to feel like it's your fault all the time and, unless you talk to someone and you hear their story, you don't know how they got it and it's a shame because we then paint it with just one brush, you've all been not looking after yourself or you've been sleeping around or yeah. So it's really sad.

The feeling of shame because of the HIV was also echoed by P.3, who stated:

In Africa when somebody has got it, it's a disgrace, it's shame, you know, you have to be left to die and things like that. So when I was diagnosed with this sickness, I'm thinking okay, it's sickness of shame and now I'm going to die, nobody will want me, nobody will want to talk to me.

Furthermore, participants indicated that the fear that disclosing their HIV condition in the UK could also lead to social isolation and with being negatively judged. This was well illustrated by P.2. when said:

There's a stigma (in the UK), because I can't just wake up in the morning and say to my fellow colleagues or people I walk around with that I'm HIV, no, I can't. This is something they'll try to isolate you, because it has ever happened to me, one of my friends just discovered that I was HIV positive, she stopped bringing her children to my house. So at the end of the day you don't just wake up and say you're HIV, there's a lot of stigma around.

In addition, P.8 said that she was forced to leave the UK city where she lived for many years after her neighbours found out she was HIV positive ... *Because I tried in XXX they start pointing with their finger, this lady she is HIV positive, nobody wants to be approachable. I say oh my god and I decided to change the city, so I can start.*

However, some participants indicated the stigma associated with being HIV positive was due, in part, to peoples' lack of understanding and education about how the virus spreads, including its transmission. In this regard, P.3 stated: *But some people are still ignorant about these things ... A lot of people don't know. People that I know, there's a lot of people I know, not like friends but we talk to, but they don't know.*

Furthermore, P.6 indicated that she could not find a partner because men in general have a poor understanding of the HIV transmission and, as soon as she disclosed it, they ran away: *Because some people they don't know how to go about this HIV because they think, 'Oh HIV I am dying, that women gave me HIV.* In addition, P.2 stated that she was surprised about her experience of communicating to the police (who intervened in a domestic dispute) that she is HIV positive, as the police was not aware of the difference between HIV and AIDS: *I said yes then I did tell her I was HIV positive, and she looked at me, she threw down the pen and she said you're HIV positive? Do you have AIDs? I said no, it is HIV positive.* However, P.6 said that the police were willing to find out more on HIV transmission: *So I had to start explaining to her what HIV positive was, how you live, then she said oh my god, I need to learn more about this.*

3.4. Feeling Unwelcomed: 'You Are Not Supposed to Be Here'

All participants indicated that they were exposed to racism as refugees as well as discrimination as migrants living in the UK. Specifically, when talking about her situation as a refugee, P.3 indicated: *Up to now, I'm still struggling with that issue (being unwelcome because she is a refugee), but I hope it's going to be okay.* Furthermore, P.5 said:

> It's hard and hard sometimes. Sometimes there are situations that always remind you that you're a refugee ... I mean once they know that you're a refugee they sort of look look down upon you and they make you feel rubbish and nothing.

When talking about the discrimination she faces as a migrant, P.1 she said:

> They (people in general) are welcoming in a way, but there is still that thing, no one will be able to break it. People might say, "Oh, things are changing in the UK." Things are not changing, people are suppressing what they think, but it's still there, even racism. People might say, "Racism is not there anymore." Racism is still there ... you still have got, these negative things about immigrants and other people from different cultures. She also described the discrimination she experienced from the residents in her community home: *Because even when I'm living in a Christian Community, you still have got, these negative things about immigrants and other people from different cultures.*

In addition, P.6 felt that the Brexit referendum increased discrimination towards migrants:

> It is after Brexit that is where I have seen, it is just becoming like wildfire because of Brexit, 'You foreigners, you have to leave.' I think that is what they thought when it was Brexit. As soon as it is Brexit everyone will have to go. P.6 also described her experience of racial discrimination at work: *But people take it in the wrong way and they will make you uncomfortable. They will really make you uncomfortable. Sometimes at work yes you can ask someone, 'Look can I help you?' And they say, 'No I don't want you, go back to your country.'*

Theme 4: Building social networks: 'I have nobody to go'

The multiple risk factors significantly impaired their ability to integrate and to build social networks. This included the way that participants were exposed to the practical challenges of being refugees as well as their health conditions and being exposed to HIV related stigma, racism, and discrimination.

However, according to all participants, their sense of loneliness was only eased by the staff members of the HIV organization from where they were recruited. These professionals were described by participants as very understanding, supportive and helpful, including dealing with practical issues and in helping them in feeling valued. In this regard, for instance, P.2 stated: *... they are welcoming and they have a heart*; and P.3 said *... they make me feel like it's nothing, you know, it's nothing*; or, when talking about her key worker P.4 indicated: *For me even to get that flat it was my support worker she really worked hard.* For the rest, participants discussed the detrimental effects that their sense of solitude and isolation had on them. In this regard, P.2 stated: *If I don't have an appointment then I stay home. I don't go anywhere, I stay just indoors.* OR P.1 indicated: *So, I'm always in the house ... Like some people organise to go out for drinks. I don't go out for drinks because of my condition, I can't walk very far, so I get left behind because I can't do much.* In addition, P.8 said: *I have nobody to go to visit, I stay home doing nothing. That's it..., I don't have friends in XXX (name of the city where she lives).* Or P.7 indicated: *Sometimes I can stay in* the house for one week and I haven't seen anybody. Everybody is busy ... I don't live with anybody and because of this situation (being HIV positive). In addition, P.6 said that, because of her mental health conditions, she feared meeting people: *It is partly because of I have a mental health problem as well so I have so much anxiety meeting other people and because of what happened before.* As indicated, the lack of social relations did affect their mental health, and this was well illustrated by P.3, who stated: *The only thing I don't want is to be by myself and because as soon as I'm alone I start thinking about a lot of things.*

Theme 5: The need to take part in narrative based-interventions

Participants indicated their need and willingness to take part in group-based interventions that could promote their mental health. This might be explained by several factors, including the fact that none of them was receiving any form of psychological intervention at the time of the interviews. Furthermore, participants indicated the need to take part in an intervention that could help them share stories with women who are in a similar situation. In this regard, P.2 said: *... to encourage us, we need encouragement, we need ... encourage, to encourage us. you need to sit together, come together, sit, talk about how you feel, share it with somebody.* This feeling of having a safe space to share their experience and receiving support from women in their situation was echoed by the remaining participants. For instance, for P.7:

> *You see. I will not be taking because it's not being alone, people also have the same problems and it's like it will keep me going. I just want to keep myself freely to be a human being. I don't want to sit isolated and just take care of this ... To me, I wish I will meet people so I will be happy.*

Or said P.6 *... and then maybe if I join a group I am seeing other woman and I will feel I am not the only one. It will motivate me, that is another way, that's how I feel.* Furthermore, P.3 stated: *It (the intervention) sounded like fun. Something to do to get together to run away from thinking of problem ... I try to be busy because once I'm alone I start thinking and I'm stressed.*

Additionally, for P.5, indicated that taking part in the intervention could help her, as well as other women in her situation, to be resilient and, as she indicated, not to be defined by the HIV:

> *I think for women living with HIV, one thing that they must always try and maintain is looking after themselves and you know, reminding themselves that they're beautiful and making themselves look ... Yes and worth it and you've still got a lot to give. HIV is not going to define who you are.*

Furthermore, P.6 discussed how talking directly about her multiple traumas might be difficult for her and, therefore, she might benefit by taking part in an art-based intervention:

> *I used to go to a therapist because half of the time if I start saying how I feel and so on and so on it makes me umm, how shall I say it, emotional. Yes. So I would rather draw how I feel but some talk. So I draw how I feel at the end of the session they will ask either do I want to share? If I don't want to share.*

4. Discussion

Overall, the findings of this study indicated that participants were affected by the intersection of living with HIV and being refugees, including struggling with the sequalae of having contracted the virus, feeling disempowered by some of health professionals, not being able to meet their basic needs, being exposed to multiple forms of discrimination, and feeling isolated; all these risk factors seemed to impair their mental health, their ability to build social networks, and to integrate in the UK. Furthermore, participants indicated their willingness to take part in group-based psychological interventions that could promote their mental health, build resilience and strengthen their social connections.

The intersection of HIV and social and health inequalities, such housing and food insecurity, seemed to have affected participants mental health [21,23–29].

Housing in particular represented one of the main concerns for participants; this might represent a threat to their mental health, as they were deprived of living space and routine, and affected the individual's sense of safety and overall sense of identity [85,86]. The meaning that refugees give to 'home' is extremely important at this difficult time when they are attempting to settle into the community, and/or when they feel detached from their previous networks [87,88]. In this regard, a study conducted by Vitale and Ryde [75] indicated that one of the main sources of stress for male refugees is not having a 'home' where they feel protected while they are starting to build their social networks, including the ability to invite people to their home, especially as they have very limited means of socializing outside their houses. This particularly applied to the participants of this study, as the lack of suitable accommodation has been proven to exacerbate the physical and psychological symptoms of their HIV [89], as the individuals find it difficult to manage their chronic conditions. They might struggle to follow medication schedules, to secure and prepare nutritious meals and to rest adequately [89,90]. This specific finding of this study, therefore, supports the need to further develop our understanding of the role that housing plays in women living with HIV from socio-economic disadvantaged background, including refugees [91].

Another finding that emerged from the analysis was that participants were exposed simultaneously to prejudice, racial discrimination and the stigma of living with HIV.

Participants in fact experienced prejudice as refugees, as they reported feelings *unwelcomed, looked down on,* and *like rubbish,* and as migrants. This represented a threat to their mental health and might have contributed to the exacerbation of their health/mental health conditions [92].

Participants were exposed to HIV-related stigma, which means that they are devalued and discriminated against based on actual or perceived HIV-positive serostatus [93]. They also specified that they contracted HIV in their countries of origin, where they said the virus is still considered a *sickness of shame* and *a cause of disgrace*. As expected, the internalized HIV stigma contributed to negative beliefs about themselves and to low self-esteem [94]. Participants indicated that women with HIV are discriminated against in their countries of origin because they are considered to have low morals and/or promiscuous sexual behaviour; this happens even though female refugees living with HIV often contract the virus as the result of gender-based violence [7,46,54]. As expected, the HIV-related stigma they experienced in their countries had devastating effects on their mental health, including for the fact that they belong to collectivist cultures where being singled out could also have consequences for their survival [43]. In addition, participants indicated that, because of the HIV-related stigma, they feared losing the already weak social networks that they were attempting to build in the UK and this also represented a risk factor to their mental health [94]. As expected, the intersection of racial discrimination, social inequalities, resettlement adversities and HIV stigma might lead participants to being socially isolated and disconnected [95], which, in turn, might have impaired their mental health [95–97].

Social ties and networks are in fact considered essential in promoting and maintaining good mental health [98]; this particularly applies to refugees, as being able to build networks increases their sense of belonging in the new country and therefore strengthens their new sense of identity [48,99,100]. In addition, social support, including emotional and instrumental assistance has been shown to promote better health and to buffer against the negative effects of stressors on health in individuals living with HIV [101], including increased coping skills and treatment success [102].

As participants suggested, to reduce isolation for individuals living with HIV, it is important to educate others, including health professionals, about the virus and its transmission. Health services in fact represent one of the main settings for HIV-related stigma and this might be due to a lack of awareness in health professionals of the importance of not perpetuating stigma and/or their fear that casual contact with patients might pass on the disease [103].

HIV-related stigma from health professionals therefore represents a significant public health concern and is one of the main barriers to individuals with HIV accessing adequate treatment [93].

Furthermore, when talking about barriers to accessing healthcare, participants indicated that, they felt disempowered by the relationship they had with some of their health professionals, and particularly from those who were not directly involved in their HIV care. This indicates the importance of health professionals listening to the refugees' voice. Empowering individuals to make decisions about their own care is considered one of the key factors in supporting the recovery of individuals experiencing mental distress [104–106]; it is also in line with the WHO Global Health Strategy [8] which recommends enabling individuals with HIV to be important partners in their treatment.

However, the findings from the current study indicated that the participants felt empowered and did have a voice in the care provided by their General Practitioners; this supports the need to provide adequate support for General Practitioners in their role of managing patients with chronic diseases [107,108]. This is also in line with the current WHO: Global Health Sector Strategy on HIV [8], which stresses the need for individuals living with HIV to have a continuum of care across health services, starting with primary care.

Another finding from this study is that, despite the need for mental health interventions, participants were simply receiving treatment for the health conditions associated with HIV. This represents a public health concern, as there is plenty of evidence which indicated that poor mental health also leads to physical health conditions and faster disease progression [13,14,109–111], as it is becoming increasingly clear that physical health cannot be detached from psychological well-being [15]. It is important, therefore, that refugee women living with HIV have appropriate access to comprehensive HIV treatment, care, and support [7,8].

The crossing of multiple adversities that participants experienced, therefore, might have aggravated participants' mental health, which might have been already impaired by the pre-migratory risk factors that generally affect refugees [49–53], as well as the trauma of having contracted HIV through gender-based violence [22].

It is, therefore, important to provide effective care for refugee women living with HIV, which has a holistic approach to their health/mental health needs and can foster their social recovery [112], and community integration [113]. In turn, social recovery promotes, cohesion, their personal and social identity [104,105], and promote resilience in refugee women [60]. This is in line with the findings of the current study, which indicated that participants were willing to take part in interventions that could support their ability to cope with their condition as well as their social recovery, and their ability to share their experience and build cohesiveness with other individuals in their situation. These factors are considered essential in supporting in the quality of life and the overall social recovery following a diagnosis of HIV [114,115].

5. Conclusions

The risk factors affecting refugee women living with HIV are complex as these are strengthened by the intersection of the health and psychological sequalae of having contracted the virus, as well as the poor living conditions which are often associated with being forced migrants. This is an extremely vulnerable population, as they might be exposed to social and gender inequalities, as well as racial discrimination as refugees and migrants, and HIV-related stigma, including in health care settings. The risk factors they experience represent a threat to public health, as it might discourage refugee women living with HIV from seeking adequate treatment. In line with the current WHO Global Health Strategy on HIV, the findings of the current study suggest that the emphasis of the treatment and care of these individuals should shift from the management of the physical symptoms of HIV, to comprehensive and multidisciplinary care that addresses the multiple risk factors associated with their conditions. In addition, refugee women living with HIV should have a voice in decisions about their care and they should be involved in interventions that promote their mental health, integration, and their overall social recovery.

Author Contributions: A.V. and J.R. designed the project, including the surveying material. A.V. conducted the fieldwork and she analyzed the data; J.R. cross-analyzed the data. Both authors were engaged in writing the current article.

Funding: This research did not receive external funding. This study has been funded by the Global Academy of Liberals Arts at Bath Spa University. The costs for publishing in open access have been covered by the Department of Psychology at Bath Spa University.

Acknowledgments: The authors are grateful the participants of this study and to the staff members of the HIV organization who facilitated the fieldwork.

Conflicts of Interest: The authors declare no conflict of interest.

References

1. World Health Organization (WHO). Fact Sheet on HIV/AIDS, 2018. Available online: http://www.who.int/news-room/fact-sheets/detail/hiv-aids (accessed on 13 June 2018).
2. HIV.gov. What Are HIV and AIDS? Available online: https://www.hiv.gov/hiv-basics/overview/about-hiv-and-aids/what-are-hiv-and-aids (accessed on 13 June 2018).
3. Quinn, T.C. HIV Epidemiology and the Effects of Antiviral Therapy on Long-Term Consequences. *AIDS* **2008**, *22*, S7–S12. [CrossRef] [PubMed]
4. Calmy, A.; Ford, N.; Meintjes, G. The Persistent Challenge of Advanced HIV Disease and AIDS in the Era of Antiretroviral Therapy. *Clin. Infect. Dis.* **2018**, *66* (Suppl. S2), S103–SS105. [CrossRef] [PubMed]
5. AIDS/WHO. AIDS Epidemic Update: 2005. Geneva, Switzerland. Available online: http://data.unaids.org/publications/irc-pub06/epi_update2005_en.pdf (accessed on 13 June 2018).
6. Gayle, H.D.; Gena, L.; Hill, G.L. Global Impact of Human Immunodeficiency Virus and AIDS. *Clin. Microbiol. Rev.* **2001**, *14*, 327–335. [CrossRef] [PubMed]
7. UNAIDS. Empowering Young Women and Adolescent Girls: UNAIDS & the African Union/Reference/2015 Fast-Tracking the End of the AIDS Epidemic in Africa. 2015. Available online: http://www.unaids.org/sites/default/files/media_asset/JC2746_en.pdf (accessed on 16 June 2018).
8. WHO. Global Health Sector Strategy on HIV 2016–2021—Towards Ending AIDS. Geneva, Switzerland, 2016. Available online: http://apps.who.int/iris/bitstream/handle/10665/246178/WHO-HIV-2016.05-eng.pdf;jsessionid=89158F2C8ED9847F25A28F5AAB258D5A?sequence=1 (accessed on 20 June 2018).
9. Angelino, A.F. Impact of Psychiatric Disorders on the HIV Epidemic. *Top. HIV Med.* **2008**, *16*, 99–103. [PubMed]
10. Bing, E.G.; Burnam, A.; Longshore, D.; Fleishman, J.A.; Sherbourne, C.D.; London, A.S.; Turner, B.J.; Eggan, F.; Beckman, R.; Vitiello, B.; et al. Psychiatric Disorders and Drug Use among Human Immunodeficiency Virus-Infected Adults in the United States. *Arch. Gen. Psychiatry* **2001**, *58*, 721–728. [CrossRef] [PubMed]
11. Blank, M.B.; Eisenberg, M.M. Tailored Treatment for HIV? Persons with Mental Illness: The Intervention Cascade. *J. Acquir. Immune Defic. Syndr.* **2013**, *63*, S44–S48. [CrossRef] [PubMed]
12. Chibanda, D.; Cowan, F.; Gibson, L.; Weiss, H.A.; Lund, C. Prevalence and Correlates of Probable Common Mental Disorders in a Population with High Prevalence of HIV in Zimbabwe. *BMC Psychiatry* **2016**, *16*, 55. [CrossRef] [PubMed]
13. Yehia, B.R.; Stephens-Shield, A.J.; Momplaisir, F.; Taylor, L.; Gross, R.; Dubé, B.; Glanz, K.; Brady, K.A. Health Outcomes of HIV-Infected People with Mental Illness. *AIDS Behav.* **2015**, *19*, 1491–1500. [CrossRef] [PubMed]
14. Sherbourne, C.D.; Hays, R.D.; Fleishman, J.A.; Vitiello, B.; Magruder, K.M.; Bing, E.G.; McCaffrey, D.; Burnam, A.; Longshore, D.; Eggan, F.; et al. Impact of Psychiatric Conditions on Health-Related Quality of Life in Persons with HIV Infection. *Am. J. Psychiatry* **2000**, *157*, 248–254. [CrossRef] [PubMed]
15. Reif, S.S.; Pence, B.W.; Legrand, S.; Wilson, E.S.; Swartz, M.; Ellington, T.; Whetten, K. In-Home Mental Health Treatment for Individuals with HIV. *AIDS Patient Care STDS* **2012**, *26*, 655–661. [CrossRef] [PubMed]
16. Maj, M.; Janssen, R.; Starace, F.; Zaudig, M.; Satz, P.; Sughondhabirom, B.; Luabeya, M.A.; Riedel, R.; Ndetei, D.; Calil, H.M.; et al. WHO Neuropsychiatric AIDS Study, Cross-Sectional Phase I. Study Design and Psychiatric Findings. *Arch. Gen. Psychiatry* **1994**, *51*, 39–49. [CrossRef] [PubMed]
17. Owe-Larsson, B.; Säll, L.; Salamon, E.; Allgulander, C. HIV Infection and Psychiatric Illness. *Afr. J. Psychiatry* **2009**, *12*, 115–128. [CrossRef]

18. Carrico, A.W.; Johnson, M.O.; Morin, S.F.; Remien, R.H.; Charlebois, E.D.; Steward, W.T.; Chesney, M.A.; NIMH Healthy Living Project Team. Correlates of Suicidal Ideation among HIV-Positive Persons. *Aids* **2007**, *2*, 1199–1203. [CrossRef] [PubMed]
19. Catalan, J.; Harding, R.; Sibley, E.; Clucas, C.; Croome, N.; Sherr, L. HIV Infection and Mental Health: Suicidal Behaviour—Systematic Review. *Psychol. Health Med.* **2011**, *16*, 588–611. [CrossRef] [PubMed]
20. Kalichman, S.C.; Heckman, T.; Kochman, A.; Sikkema, K.; Bergholte, J. Depression and Thoughts of Suicide among Middle-Aged and Older Persons Living with HIV-AIDS. *Psychiatr. Serv.* **2000**, *51*, 903–907. [CrossRef] [PubMed]
21. Collins, P.Y.; Holman, A.R.; Freeman, M.; Patel, V. What is the Relevance of Mental Health to HIV/AIDS Care and Treatment Programs in Developing Countries? A Systematic Review. *AIDS* **2006**, *20*, 1571–1582. [CrossRef] [PubMed]
22. Farmer, P.; Connors, M.; Simmons, J. *Women, Poverty, and AIDS: Sex, Drugs, and Structural Violence*, 2nd ed.; Series in Health and Social Justice; Common Courage Press: Monroe, ME, USA, 2011.
23. Orza, L.; Bewley, S.; Logie, C.H.; Tyler Crone, E.; Moroz, S.; Strachan, S.; Vazquez, M.; Welbourn, A. How Does Living with HIV Impact on Women's Mental Health? Voices from a Global Survey. *J. Int. AIDS Soc.* **2015**, *18*, 20289. [CrossRef] [PubMed]
24. Meade, C.S.; Sikkema, K.J. HIV Risk Behavior among Adults with Severe Mental Illness: A Systematic Review. *Clin. Psychol. Rev.* **2005**, *25*, 433–457. [CrossRef] [PubMed]
25. Otto-Salaj, L.L.; Kelly, J.A.; Stevenson, L.Y. Implementing Cognitive-Behavioral AIDS/HIV Risk Reduction Group Interventions in Community Mental Health Settings that Serve People with Serious Mental Illness. *Psychiatr. Rehabil. J.* **1998**, *21*, 394–404. [CrossRef]
26. Cottingham, J.; Kismodi, E.; Martin-Hilber, A.; Lincetto, O.; Stahlhofer, M.; Gruskin, S. Using Human Rights for Sexual and Reproductive Health: Improving Legal and Regulatory Frameworks. *Bull. World Health Organ.* **2010**, *88*, 551–555. [CrossRef] [PubMed]
27. Clucas, C.; Sibley, E.; Harding, R.; Liang, L.; Catalan, J.; Sherr, L. A Systematic Review of Intervention for Anxiety in People with HIV. *Psychol. Health Med.* **2011**, *16*, 528–547. [CrossRef] [PubMed]
28. Kapetanovic, S.; Dass-Brailsford, P.; Nora, D.; Talisman, N. Mental Health of HIV-Seropositive Women during Pregnancy and Postpartum Period: A Comprehensive Literature Review. *AIDS Behav.* **2014**, *18*, 1152–1173. [CrossRef] [PubMed]
29. Murray, C.; Naghavi, M.; Wang, H.; Lozano, R. Global, Regional, and National Age-Sex Specific All-Cause and Cause-Specific Mortality for 240 Causes of Death, 1990–2013: A Systematic Analysis for the Global Burden of Disease Study 2013. *Lancet* **2015**, *385*, 117–171. [CrossRef]
30. Shubber, Z.; Mills, E.J.; Nachega, J.B.; Vreeman, R.; Freitas, M.; Bock, P.; Nsanzimana, S.; Martina Penazzato, M.; Appolo, T.; Doherty, M.; et al. Patient-Reported Barriers to Adherence to Antiretroviral Therapy: A Systematic Review and Meta-Analysis. *PLoS Med.* **2016**, *13*. [CrossRef] [PubMed]
31. Kaaya, S.; Eustache, E.; Lapidos-Salaiz, I.; Musisi, S.; Psaros, C.; Wissow, L. Grand Challenges: Improving HIV Treatment Outcomes by Integrating Interventions for Co-Morbid Mental Illness. *PLoS Med.* **2013**, *10*. [CrossRef] [PubMed]
32. Sherr, L.; Clucas, C.; Harding, R.; Sibley, E.; Catalan, J. HIV and Depression: A Systematic Review of Interventions. *Psychol. Health Med.* **2011**, *16*, 493–527. [CrossRef] [PubMed]
33. Rao, D.; Kekwaletswe, T.C.; Hosek, S.; Martinez, J.; Rodriguez, F. Stigma and Social Barriers to Medication Adherence with Urban Youth Living with HIV. *AIDS Care* **2007**, *19*, 28–33. [CrossRef] [PubMed]
34. Wagner, G.J.; Goggin, K.; Remien, R.H.; Rosen, M.I.; Simoni, J.; Bangsberg, D.R.; Liu, H. A Closer Look at Depression and Its Relationship to HIV Antiretroviral Adherence. *Ann. Behav. Med.* **2011**, *42*, 352–360. [CrossRef] [PubMed]
35. Whetten, K.; Reif, S.; Whetten, R.; Murphy-McMillan, L.K. Trauma, Mental Health, Distrust, and Stigma among HIV-Positive Persons: Implications for Effective Care. *Psychosom Med.* **2008**, *70*, 531–538. [CrossRef] [PubMed]
36. Hinkin, C.H.; Castellon, S.A.; Atkinson, J.H.; Goodkin, K. Neuropsychiatric Aspects of HIV Infection among Older Adults. *J. Clin. Epidemiol.* **2001**, *54*, S44–S52. [CrossRef]
37. Mayston, R.; Kinyanda, E.; Chishinga, N.; Prince, M.; Patel, V. Mental Disorder and the Outcome of HIV/AIDS in Low-Income and Middle-Income Countries: A Systematic Review. *AIDS* **2012**, *26*, S117–S135. [CrossRef] [PubMed]

38. Shuper, P.A.; Neuman, M.; Kanteres, F.; Baliunas, D.; Joharchi, N.; Rehm, J. Causal Considerations on Alcohol and HIV/AIDS—A Systematic Review. *Alcohol* **2010**, *45*, 159–166. [CrossRef] [PubMed]
39. Hankins, C.A.; Friedman, S.R.; Zafar, T.; Strathdee, S.A. Transmission and Prevention of HIV and Sexually Transmitted Infections in War Settings: Implications for Current and Future Armed Conflicts. *AIDS* **2002**, *16*, 2245–2252. [CrossRef]
40. Spiegel, P.B. HIV/AIDS among Conflict-Affected and Displaced Populations: Dispelling Myths and Taking Action. *Disasters* **2004**, *28*, 322–339. [CrossRef] [PubMed]
41. Khaw, A.J.; Salama, P.; Burkholder, B.; Dondero, T.J. HIV Risk and Prevention in Emergency-Affected Populations: A review. *Disasters* **2000**, *24*, 181–197. [CrossRef] [PubMed]
42. McGinn, T.; Purdin, S.; Krause, S.; Jones, R. The Effects of Forced Migration on HIV/AIDS/STI Transmission and Policy and Program Responses. UCSF HIV InSite Knowledge Base. 2001. Available online: http://hivinsite.ucsf.edu/InSite?page=kb-08-01-08 (accessed on 15 June 2018).
43. Amowitz, L.L.; Reis, C.; Lyons, K.H.; Vann, B.; Mansaray, B.; Akinsulure-Smith, A.M.; Taylor, L.; Iacopino, V. Prevalence of War-Related Sexual Violence and Other Human Rights Abuses among Internally Displaced Persons in Sierra Leone. *JAMA* **2002**, *30*, 513–521. [CrossRef]
44. Spiegel, P.; Nankoe, A. HIV/AIDS and Refugees: Lessons Learned. *Forc. Migr. Rev.* **2004**, *19*, 21–23.
45. ANAIDS and UNHCR. HIV and Policy. Policy Brief. 2007. Available online: http://data.unaids.org/pub/briefingnote/2007/policy_brief_refugees.pdf (accessed on 15 June 2018).
46. Declaration of Commitment to HIV/AIDS United Nations General Assembly Special Session on HIV/AIDS—25–27 June 2001. Available online: http://data.unaids.org/publications/irc-pub03/aidsdeclaration_en.pdf (accessed on 15 June 2018).
47. Ives, N. More Than a "Good Back": Looking for Integration in Refugee Resettlement. *Refuge* **2007**, *24*, 54–63.
48. Burnett, A.; Peel, M. Health Needs of Asylum Seekers and Refugees. *BMJ* **2001**, *3*, 544–547. [CrossRef]
49. Stompe, T.; Holze, D.; Friedmann, A. Pre-Migration and Mental Health of Refugees. In *Mental Health of Refugees and Asylum Seekers*; Bhugra, D., Craig, T., Bhui, K., Eds.; Oxford University Press: New York, NY, USA, 2010; pp. 23–38.
50. Porter, M.; Haslam, N. Pre-Displacement and Post-Displacement Factors Associated with Mental Health of Refugees and Internally Displaced Persons: A Meta-Analysis. *JAMA* **2005**, *294*, 602–612. [CrossRef] [PubMed]
51. Tribe, R. Mental Health of Refugees and Asylum Seekers. *Adv. Psychiatr. Treat.* **2002**, *8*, 240–247. [CrossRef]
52. Watter, C. The Need for Understanding. *Health Matters* **1999**, *39*, 12–13.
53. Colic-Peisker, V.; Tilbury, F. 'Active' and 'Passive' Resettlement: The influence of Host Culture, Support Services, and Refugees' Own Resources on the Choice of Resettlement Style. *Int. Migr.* **2003**, *41*, 61–91. [CrossRef]
54. Mann, C.M.; Fazil, Q. Mental Illness in Asylum Seekers and Refugees. *Primary Care Ment. Health* **2006**, *4*, 57–66.
55. Freedman, J. Sexual and Gender-Based Violence against Refugee Women: A Hidden Aspect of the Refugee "Crisis". *Reprod. Health Matters* **2016**, *24*, 18–26. [CrossRef] [PubMed]
56. Blitz, B.K.; d'Angelo, A.; Kofman, E.; Nicola Montagna, N. Health Challenges in Refugee Reception: Dateline Europe 2016. *Int. J. Environ. Res. Public Health* **2017**, *14*, 1484. [CrossRef] [PubMed]
57. Donnelly, T.T.; Hwang, J.J.; Este, D.; Ewashen, C.; Adair, C.; Clinton, M. If I Was Going to Kill Myself, I Wouldn't Be Calling You. I Am Asking for Help: Challenges Influencing Immigrant and Refugee Women's Mental Health. *Issues Ment. Health Nurs.* **2011**, *32*, 279–290. [CrossRef] [PubMed]
58. Jsuthasan, J.; Sönmez, E.; Abels, I.; Kurmeyer, C.; Gutermann, J.; Kimbel, R.; Krüger, A.; Niklewski, G.; Richter, K.; Stangier, U.; et al. Near-Death Experiences, Attacks by Family Members, and Absence of Health Care in Their Home Countries Affect the Quality of Life of Refugee Women in Germany: A Multi-Region, Cross-Sectional, Gender-Sensitive Study. *BMC Med.* **2018**, *16*, 15. [CrossRef] [PubMed]
59. Rachael, D.; Goodman, R.D.; Vesely, C.K.; Letiecq, B.; Cleaveland, C.L. Trauma and Resilience among Refugee and Undocumented Immigrant Women. *J. Couns. Dev.* **2017**, *95*, 309–315.
60. Pulvirenti, M.; Mason, G. Resilience and Survival: Refugee Women and Violence. *Curr. Issues Crim. Justice* **2011**, *23*, 37–52.
61. Kashdan, T.B. Psychological Flexibility as a Fundamental Aspect of Health. *Clin. Psychol. Rev.* **2010**, *30*, 865–878. [CrossRef] [PubMed]

62. World Health Organization (WHO). *Strengthening Mental Health Promotion*; World Health Organization: Geneva, Switzerland, 2001.
63. Joubert, N.; Taylor, L.; Williams, I. *Mental Health Promotion: The Time Is Now*; Mental Health Promotion Unit: Ottawa, ON, Canada, 1996.
64. United Nation General Assembly. *Convention Related to the Status of Refugee*; United Nation Treaty Series No. 2545; United Nation General Assembly: New York, NY, USA, 1951; Volume 189.
65. Denzin, N.K.; Lincoln, Y.S. Introduction: The Discipline and Practice of Qualitative Research. In *Handbook of Qualitative Research*; Denzin, N.K., Lincoln, Y.S., Eds.; Sage: Thousand Oaks, CA, USA, 2000; pp. 1–28.
66. Taylor, S.J.; Bogdan, R. *Introduction to Qualitative Research Methods: The Search for Meanings*; John Wiley & Sons: New York, NY, USA, 1998.
67. Braun, V.; Clarke, V. What Can Thematic Analysis Offer Health and Wellbeing Researchers? *Int. J. Qual. Stud. Health Well-Being* **2014**, *9*. [CrossRef] [PubMed]
68. Eastmond, M. Stories as Lived Experience: Narratives in Forced Migration Research. *J. Refug. Stud.* **2007**, *20*, 248–264. [CrossRef]
69. Dona, G. The Microphysics of Participation in Refugee Research. *J. Refug. Stud.* **2007**, *20*, 210–229. [CrossRef]
70. Vitale, A.; Judy, R. Conducting Individual Semi-Structured Interviews with Male Refugees on Their Mental Health and Integration. In *SAGE Research Methods Cases Part 2*; SAGE: Newcastle, UK, 2018. [CrossRef]
71. The British Psychological Society. Code of Human Research Ethics. 2010. Available online: www.bps.org.uk/sites/default/files/documents/code_of_human_research_ethics.pdf (accessed on 10 June 2018).
72. Refugee Studies Centre. Ethical Guidelines for Good Research Practice. *Refug. Surv. Q.* **2007**, *26*, 162–172. [CrossRef]
73. LoBiondo-Wood, G.; Haber, G. *Nursing Research: Methods, Critical Appraisal and Utilization*, 8th ed.; CV. Mosby: Saint Louis, MO, USA, 2014.
74. Mauthner, M.; Birch, M.; Jessop, J.; Miller, T. (Eds.) *Ethics in Qualitative Research*; SAGE Publications: London, UK, 2002.
75. Hynes, T. *The Issue of 'Trust' or 'Mistrust' in Research with Refugees: Choices, Caveats and Considerations for Researchers*; United Nations High Commissioner for Refugees (UNHCR): Geneva, Switzerland, 2003; Available online: http://www.refworld.org/pdfid/4ff2ad742.pdf (accessed on 20 June 2018).
76. Vitale, A.; Ryde, J. Promoting Male Refugees' Mental Health after They Have Been Granted Leave to Remain (Refugee Status). *Int. J. Ment. Health Promot.* **2016**, *18*, 106–125. [CrossRef]
77. Gabriel, P.; Kaczorowski, J.; Berry, N. Recruitment of Refugees for Health Research: A qualitative study to add refugees' perspectives. *Int. J. Environ. Res. Public Health* **2017**, *14*, 125. [CrossRef] [PubMed]
78. Harrell-Bond, B.; Voutira, E. In Search of 'Invisible Actors': Barriers to Access in Refugee Research. *J. Refug. Stud.* **2007**, *20*, 281–298. [CrossRef]
79. Crouch, M.; McKenzie, H. The Logic of Small Samples in Interview-Based Qualitative Research. *Soc. Sci. Inf.* **2006**, *45*, 483–499. [CrossRef]
80. Parahoo, K. *Nursing Research: Principles, Process and Issues*, 2nd ed.; McMilliam: Hampshire, UK, 2006.
81. Braun, V.; Clarke, V. Thematic Analysis. In *The Handbook of Research Methods in Psychology*; Cooper, H., Ed.; American Psychological Association: Washington, DC, USA, 2012.
82. Ragin, C.C.; Amoroso, L. *Constructing Social Research: The Unity and Diversity of Methods*, 2nd ed.; Pine Forge Press: Los Thousand Oak, CA, USA, 2011.
83. Bernard, H.R.; Ryan, G.W. *Analyzing Qualitative Data: Systematic Approaches*; Sage: Los Angeles, CA, USA, 2010.
84. NHS. Entailments Migrant Health Guided. Available online: https://www.gov.uk/guidance/nhs-entitlements-migrant-health-guide (accessed on 22 June 2018).
85. Ryan, G.W.; Bernard, H. Techniques to Identify Themes. *Field Methods* **2003**, *15*, 85–109. [CrossRef]
86. Clapham, D. *The Meaning of Housing: A Pathways Approach*; The Policy Press: Bristol, UK, 2005.
87. Kisson, P. From Persecution to Destitution: A Snapshot of Asylum Seekers' Housing and Settlement Experiences in Canada and United Kingdom. *J. Immigr. Refug. Stud.* **2010**, *8*, 4–31. [CrossRef]
88. Netto, G. Identity Negotiation, Pathways to Housing and "Place": The Experience of Refugees in Glasgow. *Hous. Theory Soc.* **2011**, *28*, 123–143. [CrossRef]
89. Hummon, D.M. Community Attachment: Local Sentiment and Sense of Place. In *Place Attachment*; Altman, I., Low, S., Eds.; Plenum Press: New York, NY, USA, 1992; pp. 253–278.

90. Leaver, C.A.; Bargh, G.; Dunn, J.R.; Hwang, S.W. The Effect of Housing Status on Health-Related Outcomes in People Living with HIV: A Systematic Review of Literature. *Aids Behav.* **2007**, *11*, 85–100. [CrossRef] [PubMed]
91. Logie, C.H.; Jerkinson, J.R.; Earnshaw, V.; Tharao, W.; Loufty, M. A Structural Equation Model of HiV-Related Stigma, Racial Discrimination, Housing, Insecurity and Wellbeing among African and Carribean Black Women Living with HIV in Ontario. *PLoS ONE* **2016**, *11*, e01622826. [CrossRef] [PubMed]
92. Dolwick Grieb, S.M.; Davey-Rothwell, M.; Latkin, C.A. Housing Stability, Resident Transience, and HIV Testing among Low-Income African Americans. *AIDS Educ. Prev.* **2012**, *25*, 430–444. [CrossRef] [PubMed]
93. Kastrup, K. The Impact of Racism and Discrimination on Mental Health of Refugees and Asylum Seekers. *Eur. Psychiatry* **2016**, *33*, S43. [CrossRef]
94. UNAIDS. *Reducing HIV Stigma and Discrimination: A Critical Part of National AIDS Programmes*; UNAIDS: Geneva, Switzerland, 2007; Available online: http://www.unaids.org/sites/default/files/media_asset/jc1521_stigmatisation_en_0.pdf (accessed on 22 June 2018).
95. Simbayi, L.C.; Kalichman, S.C.; Strebel, A.; Cloete, A.; Henda, N.; Mqeketo, A. Disclosure of HIV Status to Sex Partners and Sexual Risk Behaviours among HIV-Positive Men and Women, Cape Town, South Africa. *Sex. Transm. Infect.* **2007**, *83*, 29–34. [CrossRef] [PubMed]
96. Zeng, C.; Li, L.; Hong, Y.A.; Zhang, H.; Babbitt, A.W.; Liu, C.; Li, L.; Qiao, J.; Guo, Y.; Cai, W. A Structural Equation Model of Perceived and Internalized Stigma, Depression, and Suicidal Status among People Living with HIV/AIDS. *BMC Public Health* **2018**, *15*, 138. [CrossRef] [PubMed]
97. Logie, C.H.; James, L.L.; Tharao, W.; Loutfy, M.R. HIV, Gender, Race, Sexual Orientation, and Sex Work: A Qualitative Study of Intersectional Stigma Experienced by HIV-Positive Women in Ontario, Canada. *PLoS. Med.* **2011**, *8*, e1001124. [CrossRef] [PubMed]
98. Parker, R.; Aggleton, P. HIV and AIDS-Related Stigma and Discrimination: A Conceptual Framework and Implications for Action. *Soc. Sci. Med.* **2003**, *57*, 13–24. [CrossRef]
99. Mushtaq, S.; Shoib, S.; Shah, T.; Mushtaq, S. Relationship between Loneliness, Psychiatric Disorders and Physical Health? A Review on the Psychological Aspects of Loneliness. *J. Clin. Diagn. Res.* **2014**, *8*, WE01–WE04. [CrossRef] [PubMed]
100. Berkman, L.F.; Glass, T. Social Integration, Social Networks, Social Support and Health. In *Social Epidemiology*; Berkman, L.F., Kawachi, I., Eds.; Oxford University Press: New York, NY, USA, 2000; pp. 158–162.
101. Sales, R. The Deserving and the Undeserving? Refugees, Asylum Seekers and Welfare in Britain. *Crit. Soc. Policy* **2002**, *22*, 456–478. [CrossRef]
102. Kawachi, I.; Kennedy, B.P. Socioeconomic Determinants of Health: Health and Social Cohesion—Why Care about Income Inequality? *BMJ* **1997**, *314*, 1037–1040. [CrossRef] [PubMed]
103. Antelman, G.; Kaaya, S.; Wei, R.; Mbwambo, J.; Msamanga, G.; Fawzi, W.; Fawzi, M. Depressive Symptoms Increase Risk of HIV Disease Progression and Mortality among Women in Tanzania. *J. Acquir. Immune Defic. Syndr.* **2007**, *44*, 470–477. [CrossRef] [PubMed]
104. Nyblade, L.; Stangl, A.; Weiss, E.; Ashburn, K. Combating HIV Stigma in Health Care Settings: What works? *J. Int. AIDS Soc.* **2009**, *12*, 15. [CrossRef] [PubMed]
105. Corrigan, P.W. Empowerment and Serious Mental Illness: Treatment Partnership and Community Opportunities. *Psychiatr. Q.* **2002**, *73*, 2017–2228. [CrossRef]
106. Lee, A.; Irwin, R. *Psychopathology: A Social Neuropsychological Perspective*; Cambridge University Press: Cambridge, UK, 2018; pp. 200–220. ISBN 9780521279024.
107. Wallcraft, J. Recovery from Mental Breakdown. In *Social Perspective in Mental Health: Developing Social Models of Understanding and Work with Mental Distress*; Tew, J., Ed.; Jessica Kingsley: London, UK, 2005; pp. 200–2015.
108. Kitahata, M.M.; Koepsell, T.D.; Deyo, R.A.; Maxwell, C.L.; Dodge, W.T.; Wagner, E.H. Physicians' Experience with the Acquired Immunodeficiency Syndrome as a Factor in Patients' Survival. *N. Engl. J. Med.* **1996**, *14*, 701–706. [CrossRef] [PubMed]
109. Landon, B.E.; Wilson, I.B.; McInnes, K.; Landrum, M.B.; Hirschhorn, L.R.; Marsden, P.V.; Cleary, P.D. Physician Specialization and the Quality of Care for Human Immunodeficiency Virus Infection. *Arch. Intern. Med.* **2005**, *165*, 1133–1139. [CrossRef] [PubMed]
110. Mavronicolas, H.A.; Laraque, F.; Shankar, A.; Campbell, C. Factors Influencing Collaboration among HIV PCPs and Case Managers Remain to be Studied. *J. Interpof. Care* **2017**, *3*, 368–375. [CrossRef] [PubMed]

111. Mkanta, W.; Mejia, M.; Duncan, R. Race, Outpatient Mental Health Service Use and Survival after an AIDS Diagnosis in the Highly Active Antiretroviral Therapy Era. *AIDS Patient Care STDs* **2010**, *24*, 31–37. [CrossRef] [PubMed]
112. Ohl, M.; Landon, B.; Cleary, P.; LeMaster, J. Medical Clinic characteristics and Access to Behavioral Health Services for Persons with HIV. *Psychiatr. Serv.* **2008**, *59*, 400–407. [CrossRef] [PubMed]
113. Sikkema, K.J.; Watt, M.H.; Drabkin, A.S.; Meade, C.S.; Hansen, N.B.; Pence, B.W. Mental Health Treatment to Reduce HIV Transmission Risk Behavior: A Positive Prevention Model. *AIDS Behav.* **2010**, *14*, 252–262. [CrossRef] [PubMed]
114. Davis, B.A.; Townley, G.; Kloos, B. The Roles of Clinical and Nonclinical Dimensions of Recovery in Promoting Community Activities for Individuals with Psychiatric Disabilities. *Psychiatr. Rehabil. J.* **2013**, *36*, 51–53. [CrossRef] [PubMed]
115. Marino, C.K. To Belong, Contribute, and Hope: First Stage Development of a Measure of Social Recovery. *J. Ment. Health* **2015**, *24*, 68–72. [CrossRef] [PubMed]

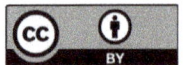

© 2018 by the authors. Licensee MDPI, Basel, Switzerland. This article is an open access article distributed under the terms and conditions of the Creative Commons Attribution (CC BY) license (http://creativecommons.org/licenses/by/4.0/).

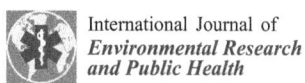

Review

Accessibility and Acceptability of Infectious Disease Interventions Among Migrants in the EU/EEA: A CERQual Systematic Review

Matt Driedger [1], Alain Mayhew [1], Vivian Welch [2], Eric Agbata [3], Doug Gruner [2], Christina Greenaway [4,5], Teymur Noori [6], Monica Sandu [1], Thierry Sangou [1], Christine Mathew [1], Harneel Kaur [1], Manish Pareek [7] and Kevin Pottie [2,*]

1. Bruyère Research Institute, 85 Primrose Ave, Annex E, Ottawa, ON K1R 6M1, Canada; matt.driedger@uottawa.ca (M.D.); amayhew@bruyere.org (A.M.); sandumonique@yahoo.com (M.S.); thiesang@gmail.com (T.S.); cmath054@uottawa.ca (C.M.); hkaur006@uottawa.ca (H.K.)
2. Departments of Family Medicine & Epidemiology and Community Medicine, University of Ottawa, Ottawa, ON K1H 8M5, Canada; vivian.welch@uottawa.ca (V.W.); gruner18@yahoo.ca (D.G.)
3. Department of Paediatrics, Obstetrics, Gynaecology and Preventive Medicine, Universität Autònoma de Barcelona, 08193 Barcelona, Spain; ericagbata@gmail.com
4. Division of Infectious Diseases, Jewish General Hospital, McGill University, Montreal, QC H3T 1E2, Canada; ca.greenaway@mcgill.ca
5. Centre for Clinical Epidemiology of the Lady Davis Institute for Medical Research, Jewish General Hospital, Montreal, QC H3T 1E2, Canada
6. European Centre for Disease Prevention and Control, 16973 Stockholm, Sweden; teymur.noori@ecdc.europa.eu
7. Department of Infection, Immunity and Inflammation, University of Leicester, Leicester LE1 7RH, UK; mp426@le.ac.uk
* Correspondence: kpottie@uottawa.ca

Received: 31 July 2018; Accepted: 18 October 2018; Published: 23 October 2018

Abstract: In the EU/EEA, subgroups of international migrants have an increased prevalence of certain infectious diseases. The objective of this study was to examine migrants' acceptability, value placed on outcomes, and accessibility of infectious disease interventions. We conducted a systematic review of qualitative reviews adhering to the PRISMA reporting guidelines. We searched MEDLINE, EMBASE, CINAHL, DARE, and CDSR, and assessed review quality using AMSTAR. We conducted a framework analysis based on the Health Beliefs Model, which was used to organize our preliminary findings with respect to the beliefs that underlie preventive health behavior, including knowledge of risk factors, perceived susceptibility, severity and barriers, and cues to action. We assessed confidence in findings using an adapted GRADE CERQual tool. We included 11 qualitative systematic reviews from 2111 articles. In these studies, migrants report several facilitators to public health interventions. Acceptability depended on migrants' relationship with healthcare practitioners, knowledge of the disease, and degree of disease-related stigma. Facilitators to public health interventions relevant for migrant populations may provide clues for implementation. Trust, cultural sensitivity, and communication skills also have implications for linkage to care and public health practitioner education. Recommendations from practitioners continue to play a key role in the acceptance of infectious disease interventions.

Keywords: access to care; disease prevention; public health; stigma; refugees; migrants

1. Introduction

Migrant populations often come from or travel through low- and middle-income countries where the prevalence and burden of infectious diseases differs from the European Union/European

Economic Area (EU/EEA) [1]. Migrant populations include immigrants, refugees, asylum-seekers, displaced persons, undocumented migrants, and other foreign-born residents. In the EU/EEA, for example, subgroups of migrants have a higher prevalence of HIV, tuberculosis (TB), hepatitis B (HBV), and hepatitis C (HCV), and have lower rates of childhood vaccinations compared to native-born populations [1].

Evidence-based guidelines can direct public health and healthcare practitioners in the screening and treatment of such diseases. These guidelines include information on testing and vaccination and may also consider culturally sensitive ways to approach migrants. For example, existing guidelines for HIV among migrant populations [2–4] synthesize evidence on benefits, harms and cost effectiveness, and also provide some interpretation on qualitative data relevant to HIV related stigma and strategies to link patients for treatment. To implement public health guidelines, an understanding of migrant populations' perceptions and fears is needed [5]. Thus, to ethically offer interventions, we need to understand the perspective of migrants regarding the acceptability of interventions, value placed on outcomes, and accessibility of screening and treatment of infectious disease interventions in the EU/EEA [6,7].

The acceptability of infectious disease interventions influences the readiness of migrants and clinicians to incorporate guidelines into practice, as seen in the case of HIV screening [8]. Insufficient knowledge among clinicians about the acceptability of interventions may inhibit them from offering screening to migrants [9]. How patients value the disease-related outcomes of interventions (e.g., perception of risk of disease, diagnoses, symptoms, or disease resolution), or other outcomes (e.g., time away from work, stigma, side effects, or adverse events) can create barriers to the uptake of guideline recommendations [5]. For example, one qualitative study on developing decision aids for HIV testing for newly arrived Sub-Saharan African women to Canada demonstrated how the provision of accurate HIV information can reduce stress [10]. Existing strategies to improve access to healthcare for migrants include support for transportation, interpreters, and cultural brokers [11].

The objective of this study is to understand the acceptability, the value placed on outcomes and the accessibility of infectious disease interventions and other health services among recently arrived EU/EEA migrants. We focused specifically on tuberculosis, HIV, HBV, HCV, vaccine-preventable diseases (VPD), and parasitic diseases; diseases that were selected during an ECDC consensus meeting in Stockholm [12]. We also aimed to explore how the GRADE CERQual tool can appraise qualitative research on implementation considerations.

2. Materials and Methods

2.1. Search Strategy and Selection Criteria

We conducted a systematic review of qualitative reviews, and adhered to the Preferred Reporting Items for Systematic Reviews and Meta-Analyses (PRISMA) reporting guideline [13]. A team of experts with qualitative research expertise developed a protocol that considered implementation for public health interventions relevant to migrant populations in EU/EEA. We registered the protocol on Prospero (CRD42016045798) and published our detailed review methods in BMJ Open [12,14].

We searched MEDLINE, MEDLINE In-Process, MEDLINE Ahead of Print, EMBASE, CINAHL, DARE, and CDSR for articles published between 1 January 2010 and 29 July 2016. The full search strategy is provided in Supplementary File S1. We also searched grey literature for published reports that met our inclusion criteria from the CDC, ECDC, UNAIDS, EU, and WHO, and scanned references to identify additional qualitative systematic reviews. We included qualitative systematic reviews that reported on values, perceptions on access, and acceptability of infectious disease interventions (see Appendix A). We restricted our inclusion to studies published in English. We included reviews if search and selection strategy methods were explicitly provided, and if the review included qualitative evidence. We focused on migrant and forcibly displaced populations, including children, adolescents, pregnant women, and adults. See Appendix B for full inclusion and exclusion criteria.

2.2. Study Selection and Data Extraction

Three independent team members (MD, MS, TS) screened title and abstracts in duplicate, followed by full-text assessments for eligibility. Conflicts were resolved through discussion or the involvement of a fourth reviewer (AM). Data were downloaded into EndNote reference software [15]. We assessed the methodological quality of included reviews using the Assessing Methodological Quality of Systematic Reviews tool (AMSTAR) [16] but did not exclude any studies based on quality.

The same team members extracted data from the included reviews in duplicate. We used a calibration exercise prior to data extraction and discrepancies were resolved through discussion. We designed our data extraction form using the Jacob's accessibility framework [17]. The Jacob's accessibility framework highlights barriers to accessing health services from both the supply and demand side, and as such recognizes that determinants of geographic accessibility, acceptability, availability, and affordability play a critical role in access. The framework focusses more on accessibility rather than appraising the acceptability and attitudes towards these services. However, adapting this framework to create an inclusive data extraction form (see Appendix C) allowed us to capture all relevant data, which was subsequently contextualized with respect to our research objectives.

2.3. Data Synthesis

We contextualized the preliminary findings on migrant populations using the Health Belief Model framework (HBM) [18]. The HBM is a commonly used model of the beliefs, expectations, and values that underlie preventive health behavior [19], and was therefore selected for its clear alignment with our stated research objectives involving the values and acceptability of interventions. HBM suggests that six factors predict health behavior: perceived susceptibility, perceived severity, benefits to action, barriers to action, self-efficacy, and cues to action [18].

We applied a qualitative lens considering saturation (200 studies were identified within the reviews) and triangulation of data between different diseases, migrant populations, and destination countries to identify preliminary findings. We consulted clinicians (KP, MP, DG, CG) with expertise and experience in migrant health to identify and corroborate the credibility, transferability, confirmability, and dependability to establish the trustworthiness of these findings. Of note, while many reviews discussed how knowledge of risk factors influences health behavior, only two reviews [20,21] commented specifically on how susceptibility, in itself, determines health behavior, which is how "perceived susceptibility" is classically theorized in the HBM [18]. Given the strong cognitive component of susceptibility within the HBM [22], we opted to include the knowledge data in our main findings, yet we typified this as "knowledge of risk factors" to maintain accuracy.

Five of the 12 preliminary findings were selected as "key findings" to be further analyzed with the Confidence in the Evidence from Reviews of Qualitative research (CERQual) tool. These were selected by consensus among three authors (MD, KP, AM), based on their respective strength of evidence, the number of reviews supporting the finding, the level of variability in review findings, and the significance of the findings as stated in the included reviews.

We used the CERQual tool to assess the confidence of our findings. CERQual is a new method for assessing the confidence of qualitative review evidence, similar to how the GRADE approach assesses the certainty of quantitative evidence [23]. CERQual bases this evaluation on four criteria: (a) methodological limitations of included studies supporting a review finding, (b) the relevance of included studies to the review question, (c) the coherence of the review finding, and (d) the adequacy of the data contributing to a review finding. To our knowledge, CERQual has not been used in a review of reviews to date. To apply the principles of CERQual to a review of reviews, we needed to make minor adjustments, such as considering the number of primary studies within a given review to assess the adequacy criterion.

3. Results

3.1. Study Selection

The formal search identified 2108 articles. Reference scanning identified three additional reviews. We screened 87 full-text articles and 11 qualitative systematic reviews met our inclusion criteria. All reviews examined populations migrating from low- and middle-income countries to high-income countries. See PRISMA Flow Sheet showing selection, Figure 1.

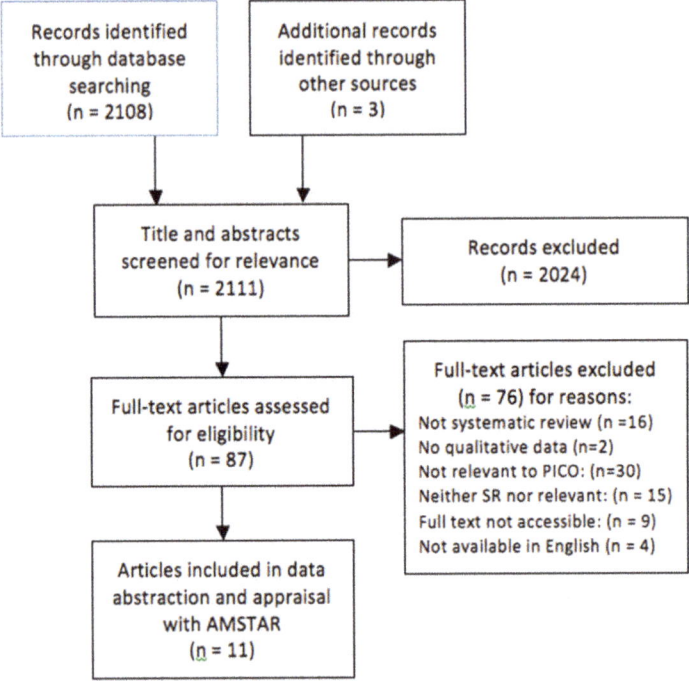

Figure 1. PRISMA Flow Diagram.

Three of the systematic reviews focused exclusively on migrant populations [24–26]. Other reviews examined migrant populations as subgroups within the general populations [21,27,28]. The host population countries were predominantly in Western Europe and the United States. Participants mostly consisted of Latino, Hispanic, or sub-Saharan African migrants, but also included South-East Asian and Middle-Eastern migrants. Most reviews included both quantitative data from cohort and cross-sectional studies as well as qualitative data from focus groups and interviews. Three reviews focused on HIV, three on HBV/HCV, and five on TB. No reviews specifically addressed vaccine-preventable or parasitic diseases. See characteristics of included studies in Table 1.

Table 1. Characteristics of Included Studies.

Citation	Years Searched	Population	Intervention/ Service Setting	Analysis/ Synthesis Approach	EU/EEA Settings Included?	1' Study Design	# of 1' Studies	AMSTAR Score (/11)
Alvarez-del Arco et al. [20]	2005–2009	Migrants and ethnic minorities populations living in high-income countries Migrants were largely from sub-Saharan Africa and Latin America, (1) and other regions.	HIV testing and/or counselling in health and community settings	None specified-Narrative	Yes	Quantitative (25); mixed-methods (2); qualitative (6); literature reviews (4)	37	1
Blondell et al. [24]	1997–2014	Foreign-born: African, particularly Sub-Saharan, and Hispanic/Latino migrants were the most studied populations.	HIV screening, testing	None specified - narrative	Yes	quantitative (n = 21) (descriptive/non-randomized) and qualitative (n = 10).	31	3
de Vries et al. [29]	2010–2017 (OECD countries); or 1990–2017 (EU, EEA, EU candidate countries)	Hard-to-reach populations including homeless, migrants, travelers (including Roma), refugees, others. 7/10 studies were of migrants only. One study included homeless, migrants, and drug users.	TB services of any kind	Thematic and content analysis	Yes	Qualitative: Interviews (6), focus groups (2), both Interviews and Focus groups (3) multi-method participatory research (1)	12	7
Do et al. [30]	2002–2009	Asian Americans and Pacific Islanders (69% foreign-born).	Health education, screening, and vaccination for HBV	None specified - narrative	No	Cross-sectional (13); RCT (1); quasi-experimental (1); Longitudinal (1)	20	1
Greenaway et al. [27]	1950 to 17 December 2008) *	Immigrants (subgroup).	Screening and treatment of latent TB	Summary of findings table (GRADE)	Not specified	SRs (7) and guidelines (2)	9	2
Mitchell et al. [28]	1985–April 2011	30 individual risk groups * Data extracted from two groups only—Internally Displaced Populations (IDPs), and "Migrants/Immigration"	TB screening (CXR, Mantoux TST)	Metasynthesis	Yes	Qualitative and Quantitative literature.	21	2

Table 1. Cont.

Citation	Years Searched	Population	Intervention/ Service Setting	Analysis/ Synthesis Approach	EU/EEA Settings Included?	1' Study Design	# of 1' Studies	AMSTAR Score (/11)
Nguyen-Truong et al. [31]	1998–2012	Vietnamese Americans—most studies report that majority of sample are immigrants, but most aggregated immigrant and native-born.	Screening (HBV and Colorectal cancer)	None specified	No	Descriptive (15); Interventional (2); Qualitative (3); Chart/medical record review (2); Mixed-method (1)	23	2
Owiti et al. [25]	1970–2014 **	High-risk 1st- or 2nd-gen immigrants from high-prevalence countries or intermediate prevalence countries who migrated to traditionally low prevalence countries.	Knowledge of HBV and/or HCV infections and/or with targeted screening, vaccination, and treatment	Narrative synthesis	Yes	Quantitative surveys (39) and qualitative studies (11); mixed-methods (1)	51	6
Pottie et al. [21]	1995–2008	Immigrants and refugees (subgroup).	HIV Screening and treatment	Summary of findings table (GRADE)	Not specified	SRs (7) and guidelines (2)	8	4
Tankimovich et al. [32]	1998–2012	Homeless and immigrants with TB.	TB detection and treatment (active and latent)	None specified—narrative	Yes	Quantitative (17); Qualitative (5); Intervention studies (10)	22	2
Tomas et al. [26]	1995–2011	Immigrants, and intra-national migrants and including migrants, asylum-seekers, refugees.	Screening and treatment of TB (active and latent)	Meta-ethnographyRes	Yes	In-depth interviews (24); focus groups (12); participant observation (5); case studies (1); Other (6) Many combined qualitative and quantitative methods.	30	3

* Includes primary studies from 1995 onwards; ** Includes primary studies from 1999 onwards.

3.2. Methodological Quality

We assessed methodological quality using the AMSTAR tool. AMSTAR was originally designed for quantitative reviews but many of the criteria are applicable to qualitative reviews, such as, a priori design, duplicate selection, comprehensive search, criteria, and characteristics of included and excluded studies and consideration of scientific quality. The authors have used AMSTAR for qualitative systematic reviews [33,34]. AMSTAR scores were distributed fairly evenly between one and seven points out of a possible 11, with a median score of 2/11. AMSTAR items varied significantly with respect to the proportion of reviews meeting that item.

3.3. Migrants' Perceptions of Acceptability

We organized the findings using the Health Beliefs Model (HBM) [19]. Through our framework analysis, we identified 12 preliminary findings from the data. See Table 2 for a detailed description of these findings.

Three reviews reported on acceptability of interventions [25,26,28]. Tomas et al. found that the TB screening process was generally well-received among migrants [26]. According to Mitchell et al. [28], the overall acceptability of TB screening among migrants was considered to be high, yet migrants' perception of TB as a severe disease was associated with screening refusal. Owiti et al., reported that some migrants expressed motivation to or actively sought screening for HBV/HCV, and that certain populations were receptive to HBV vaccination [25].

Furthermore, peer support and the influence of family members promotes self-efficacy in seeking healthcare and improves the acceptability of interventions, yet there are also instances in which these social connections may introduce other barriers [20,24,25]. For example, family support would improve adherence to TB treatment, but the need for women, at times, to request their partner's approval to seek screening acted as a barrier [20,24]. Cultural and family beliefs that differ from those of the host nation may present a perceived barrier, and may lead to other barriers, such as disease-related stigma, that can influence acceptability of care [21,26,27,30–32]. In addition, various attitudes towards an intervention itself, especially side effects and cultural taboos, may influence its acceptability among migrants [24,26,27].

The patient-practitioner relationship was consistently emphasized as an important cue to action in seeking further care. Trust, cultural sensitivity, and communication skills can greatly improve the acceptability of infectious disease interventions [20,25–31]. Therefore, recommendations from healthcare practitioners can influence migrants' health seeking behavior [25,30,31].

Social determinants also influenced the acceptability of interventions. The number of years of formal education was positively correlated with HIV screening [21,24], HBV/HCV knowledge [25], testing and vaccination [30] and TB screening and treatment [27]. In one review, older age was associated with HBV/HCV knowledge [25], but another review, among Asian Americans/Pacific Islanders [30] showed younger age was associated with HBV/HCV knowledge. Gender also played a role, as females were more receptive to HIV screening [20,24], but males were more likely to be screened for HBV [30,31].

3.4. Migrants' Values on Outcomes of Interventions

Traditional beliefs of migrants may play a role in the value placed on outcomes of infectious disease interventions. The reviews report that migrants' perceived severity of and susceptibility to infectious diseases influences their uptake of testing and treatment interventions. Reviews of TB, HIV and hepatitis reported a low level of western knowledge and understanding of risk factors and transmission of disease among migrants, and this may make them less likely to seek screening, vaccination, or treatment [20,21,24,25,27,29–31]. While the degree of knowledge varied among studies, it was consistently associated with the uptake of interventions.

Migrants reported certain perceived benefits as valued outcomes of screening, vaccination, and treatment. The most consistently valued outcomes included reassurance of disease-free status and thus prevention of transmission to others [21,24,26,30]. Uptake of interventions was associated with perceptions of negative disease-related outcomes among migrants. Stigma, and its related connotation, acts as a large barrier to screening and treatment [20,21,24–27,29,32]. Indirect costs, such as loss of employment and loss of migration status and social status, reduced the value placed on interventions [20,24,25,29,32]. For example, certain migrants feared that a positive test result would have a negative impact on their immigration status or refugee claim. Symptoms were consistently reported as an important cue for health actions; for example, migrants value screening or treatment of symptomatic diseases over asymptomatic diseases and often wait until they are symptomatic before seeking care [24,26,29–31].

3.5. Accessibility of Health Services

Barriers to accessibility were reported at both structural and community levels. Structural barriers to care for migrants include cultural and language barriers [35], inadequate practitioner cultural competencies [36], disease-related stigma and discrimination [20], perceptions of health and healthcare [37], and legal status of migrants [24]. Community-level barriers include the availability and awareness of services such as transportation, economic barriers including healthcare coverage and cost of services, and policy barriers such as the healthcare system capacity and coverage. These barriers interact with poverty, inequality, and power, further exacerbating the poor health of the migrants [38]. Time spent accessing healthcare can incur a significant opportunity cost for migrants, especially when they have insecure employment or cannot meet basic needs during their settlement process [20,24,26–29]. Furthermore, barriers related to the migration process, including language proficiency, cultural barriers, and navigation of the healthcare system, can make interventions less acceptable or accessible for migrants [20,21,24–27,29,30]. While interpreters may improve accessibility, their presence may introduce new potential barriers surrounding confidentiality [24,26,30].

3.6. Confidence in Findings

We analyzed the confidence of our five findings using CERQual (see Table 3). Three findings were assigned a moderate confidence rating, and two were assigned a low confidence rating. See Table 4 for a detailed explanation of confidence ratings.

Table 2. Preliminary Findings from Health Belief Model Framework Analysis.

Main Theme		Reviews Cited (Lead Authors)	Disease-Specific Supporting Examples
Knowledge of Risk Factors	Low level of knowledge of risk factors and transmission of disease may make migrants less likely to seek screening, immunization, or treatment.	(5) de Vries, Owiti, Lee, Nguyen, Blondell	TB: • Underestimated risk of acquiring TB due to poor understanding of transmission and false beliefs, e.g. that TB is not present in US. (de Vries) HBV/HCV • HBV screening is associated with better knowledge of HBV and specific modes of transmission (Owiti, Lee, Nguyen) HIV: • Migrants with greater knowledge of HIV and its risk factors were more likely to be screened (Blondell)
Perceived Susceptibility	Low perceived personal risk of acquiring an infectious disease may make migrants less likely to seek screening	(3) Greenaway, Pottie, Alvarez	• Perceived low risk of progressing from latent to active infection is a barrier to screening/treatment of latent TB (Greenaway) HIV • Low perceived personal risk is a barrier to screening (Pottie, Alvarez)
Perceived Severity	The severity and consequences (medical, social, economic) of diseases varied between studies, were generally well understood. However, the literature is divided on whether this is a motivating factor, or a perceived barrier to screening (i.e. risk of realizing the negative consequences through screening).	(4) Blondell, Lin, de Vries, Owiti	Tuberculosis: • TB was thought to be important, potentially fatal disease; participants afraid of disease's severity (Tomas) • Varying perception on TB severity included: very serious, lethal disease, a long-lasting but curable disease, fear of dying from incurable disease (de Vries) HBV/HCV: • Perceived outcomes of HepB and C: Poor health; discrimination/stigma; loss of income; loss of social status; liver disease (Owiti) • On the other hand, belief that HBV infection is transient could lead to it not being taken seriously (Owiti) HIV: • Concerns regarding the logistical consequences of living with a positive status, and fear of a future with a positive result, reduced the acceptability of screening among African migrants (Blondell)

423

Table 2. Cont.

Main Theme	Reviews Cited (Lead Authors)	Disease-Specific Supporting Examples
Perceived Benefits Several distinct, tangible benefits to screening, vaccination, and treatment were reported by reviews, especially reassurance of negative status and prevention of spread to others.	(4) Tomas, Do, Pottie, Blondell,	Tuberculosis: • In some communities, benefits of treating latent TB were well understood, including efficacy of medication, avoidance of stigma, and reducing risk of transmission to others (Tomas) HBV/HCV: • Primary motivations for hepatitis B vaccination were protection of future health and avoidance of hepatitis B (Do) HIV: • "Just wanted to find out" was a motivator among Latino migrants; "ensure they were healthy and clean" (Blondell) • Refugees and refugee claimants might be reluctant to accept screening tests because they fear limited access to antiretroviral treatment and thus do not see a perceived benefit to screening (Pottie)
Perceived Barriers Stigma is an overarching barrier to screening and treatment that was reflected in most diseases and reviews. Stigma is also related to other perceived barriers (e.g. confidentiality issues with interpreters, hesitancy to report symptoms to family/healthcare providers)	(8) Tomas, Tankunovich, de Vries, Greenaway, Pottie, Owiti, Blondell, Alvarez,	Tuberculosis: • Feelings of stigma influenced immigrants' attitudes towards prevention and diagnosis and could prevent them from sharing relevant information with their doctors. Medical interpreters often posed a problem due to the perceived sensitivity of the information, loss of privacy, and stigmatization (Tomas) HBV/HCV: • Shame and stigma of hepatitis may negatively uptake screening; may dissuade migrants from disclosing test results (Owiti) HIV: • Stigma, discrimination related to HIV described as most important impediment to HIV testing, treatment (Pottie) • Stigma is not significant across all studies, which may be explained by population characteristics or definitions of stigma. The few quantitative studies on stigma failed to show a statistically significant association with testing (Blondell)

Table 2. Cont.

Main Theme	Reviews Cited (Lead Authors)	Disease-Specific Supporting Examples
Time spent accessing healthcare can incur a significant opportunity cost on migrants, especially when they are in a precarious employment situation or do not have basic needs met in their settlement process.	(6) Tomas, Greenaway, de Vries, Mitchell, Blondell, Alvarez	Tuberculosis: • Missed days at work is a barrier to TB screening and treatment adherence (Greenaway) • Reasons for refusing TB screening were predominantly a lack of time (Mitchell) HIV: • Provision of rapid testing outside normal working hours may improve uptake by eliminating the opportunity cost of missed work (Blondell, Alvarez)
Indirect costs that may be unique to migrants can reduce the value placed on these screening and treatment interventions. The most prominent of these was that a positive test result may have a negative impact on the migrant's immigration status or refugee claim.	(5) Lin, Tankimovich, Blondell, Alvarez de Vries,	Tuberculosis: • Undocumented status was consistently correlated with non-adherence to treatment (Lin) • Migrants may not seek treatment due to fear of revealing their illegal immigration status (Tankimovich) HIV: • Migrants placed their legal status as among their highest priorities, and fears on the implications of testing positive on their visa/residency application or deportation were main barriers in several studies (Alvarez). However, this was not a barrier in all studies (Blondell)
Factors inherent to the migration process, including language proficiency, cultural barriers, and navigation of the healthcare system, can create barriers for migrants. However, reviews reported conflicting results regarding the influence of acculturation and language proficiency	(9) Tomas, Lin, Do, Owiti, Pottie, Blondell, Greenaway, de Vries, Alvarez,	Tuberculosis • Years spent in host country inconsistently associated with treatment completion/outcomes. Two studies found that immigrants with better English proficiency were at increased risk of not completing treatment (Lin) • Lack of familiarity with the local language was a barrier to screening (Tomas) HBV/HCV • Access to interpreter services increased odds of testing (Do, Owiti) • One study reported an association between lower English proficiency and higher likelihood of being tested for HBV, while another found that not needing an interpreter was associated with getting tested (Owiti) HIV • Non-integration of health services was a key barrier to HIV screening • Inability to communicate in the host country's language was a prominent barrier to screening (Pottie) • While language services increase uptake, translators may introduce confidentiality concerns (Blondell)

Table 2. Cont.

Main Theme	Reviews Cited (Lead Authors)	Disease-Specific Supporting Examples
Various attitudes and expectations of the intervention itself (the procedure or its side effects) may influence its acceptability among migrants	(4) Greenaway, Lin, Blondell, Tomas	**Tuberculosis** • Barriers to TB screening included fear of a painful test (Tomas) and venipuncture (Greenaway) • Side effects are inconsistently associated with treatment adherence. Quantitative studies found no significant correlations in multivariate analysis (Lin) **HIV** • Some African migrants felt that too much blood was taken during screening (Blondell)
Recommendation from healthcare providers can influence healthcare seeking by migrant patients.	(3) Owiti, Do, Nguyen	**HBV/HCV** • Recommendation by healthcare professionals was positively associated with uptake of screening and vaccination (Owiti, Do, Nguyen)
The importance of the patient-physician relationship was consistently emphasized. Trust, cultural sensitivity, and communication skills can act as facilitators to the acceptability of infectious disease interventions, whereas a negative relationship can serve as a barrier.	(7) Tomas, Greenaway, Mitchel, de Vries, Do, Nguyen, Owiti	**Tuberculosis** • Using a dedicated nurse and cultural interpreter to provide a "transcultural" approach increased screening acceptability within one year (Mitchell) • Health staff can improve adherence to treatment by providing personal advice with sensitivity and "the ability to establish a personal relation on the same cultural terms". Positive relationships with health staff are perceived as "a crucial element" (Tomas) **HCV/HBV** • Poor patient-doctor communication, and reliance on professional opinion, discouraged testing and vaccine uptake (Do, Nguyen)

Cues to Action

The presence of symptoms can be a necessary cue to seeking healthcare among migrants who may not understand or value the importance of treating asymptomatic disease	(5) Tomas, Do, Blondell, de Vries, Nguyen	**TB** • A lack of symptoms despite contact with infected persons can lead migrants to place less value on prevention and screening (Tomas) **HBV/HCV** • Apparent good health and personal preferences of migrants may discourage screening and vaccination (Do) **HIV** • African and Latin migrants reported waiting until health crises, symptoms, or being extremely sick before seeking formal healthcare (Blondell) • Feeling healthy and a lack of symptoms were consistently cited as barriers to HIV screening (Blondell)

Table 3. GRADE CERQual Evidence Profile.

Key Finding	Studies Supporting Key Finding	Methodological Quality	Relevance-Research Question	Relevance-Population	Coherence	Adequacy-Reviews	Adequacy-Primary Studies	Overall Assessment of Confidence	Explanation of Judgement
Subjects may be reluctant to undergo screening due to negative indirect costs of having a positive result—on employment status, immigration status, and social status	[20,21,24,26,29,32]	Moderate methodological concerns	No relevance concerns Full (6/6)	Moderate relevance concerns Full (3/6) partial (3/6)	Minor coherence concerns Coherent (5/6) Among Latino migrants in Spain, legal and administrative fears were not found to be significant barriers [29]	Minor adequacy concerns 6 reviews	20 studies	Low confidence	Lack of adequate evidence, including contradictory evidence, in addition to methodological concerns among reviews reporting this finding.
Patients value testing and treatment less if they are asymptomatic	[24,26,29–31]	Moderate methodological concerns	Minor relevance concerns Full (4/5) Indirect (1/5)	Moderate relevance concerns Full (2/5) Partial (3/5)	No coherence concerns Coherent (5/5)	Minor adequacy concerns 5 reviews	25 studies	Low confidence	Methodological concerns, indirect/partial relevance of reviews supporting key finding.
Incorrect knowledge of infectious diseases and low self-perceived risk are barriers to acceptability of screening and vaccination	[20,21,24–32]	Moderate methodological concerns	Minor relevance concerns Full (8/11) Indirect (3/11)	Moderate relevance concerns Full (8/11) Partial (3/11)	Minor coherence concerns Coherent (10/11) Perceiving tuberculosis as a severe disease (OR 0.29, 95% CI 0.09-0.91) was associated with refusal of TST screening [28]	Minor adequacy concerns 11 reviews	81 studies	Moderate confidence	Some reviews have significant methodological concerns, yet the key finding is consistently supported by directly relevant data in reviews with only minor methodological concerns.
The acceptability of screening and treatment interventions is highly dependent on the cultural sensitivity and relationship with healthcare professionals	[20,21,24–32]	Moderate methodological concerns	Minor relevance concerns Full (10/11) Indirect (1/11)	Minor relevance concerns Full (8/11) Partial (3/11)	No coherence concerns Coherent (11/11)	Minor adequacy concerns 11 reviews	67 studies	Moderate confidence	Supported by all reviews. Although some reviews have significant methodological concerns, reviews with few methodological concerns report directly relevant data.

Table 3. Cont.

Key Finding	Studies Supporting Key Finding	Methodological Quality	Relevance- Research Question	Relevance- Population	Coherence	Adequacy- Reviews	Adequacy- Primary Studies	Overall Assessment of Confidence	Explanation of Judgement
Stigma associated with infectious diseases is a barrier to the acceptability of screening interventions	[20,21,24–27, 29]	Moderate methodological concerns	No relevance concerns Full (7/7)	Minor relevance concerns Full (6/7) Partial (1/7)	Minor coherence concerns Coherent (6/7) Stigma is not a significant factor in all studies. Two quantitative studies on stigma found it was not a significant deterrent to testing	Minor adequacy concerns 7 reviews	71 studies	Moderate confidence	Well-supported by review data that is directly relevant. Direct support from reviews with few methodological concerns.

Objective: To identify, appraise and synthesize review level evidence on values and preferences for infectious disease interventions among migrants in Europe. Perspectives: Experience and attitudes of migrant population regarding ID interventions in the EU/EEA? Included programs: Reviews of programs of testing and prevention of infectious diseases in migrants where values and preferences are evaluated.

Table 4. Summary CERQual Confidence Ratings.

Key Finding	CERQual Assessment Rating for Assessment of Confidence	Explanation of Confidence Rating
Incorrect knowledge of infectious diseases and low self-perceived risk are barriers to acceptability of screening and vaccination	Moderate confidence	Some reviews have significant methodological concerns, yet the key finding is consistently supported by directly relevant data in reviews with only minor methodological concerns.
The acceptability of screening and treatment interventions is highly dependent on the cultural sensitivity and sense of trust in healthcare professionals and their recommendations	Moderate confidence	Supported by all reviews. Although some reviews have significant methodological concerns, reviews with few methodological concerns report directly relevant data.
Stigma associated with infectious diseases is a barrier to the acceptability of screening interventions	Moderate confidence	Well-supported by review data that is directly relevant. Direct support from reviews with only mild methodological concerns.
Subjects may be reluctant to undergo screening due to negative indirect costs of having a positive result—on employment status, immigration status, and social status	Low confidence	Lack of adequate evidence, including contradictory evidence, in addition to methodological concerns among reviews reporting this finding.
Patients value testing and treatment less if they are asymptomatic	Low confidence	Methodological concerns, indirect/partial relevance of reviews supporting key finding.

4. Discussion

We identified 11 systematic reviews that addressed factors influencing acceptability, the value placed on outcomes, and accessibility of screening and treatment of infectious diseases among migrants. Using the framework of the Health Belief Model, we found factors that influenced healthcare engagement and intervention uptake in each disease group, i.e., TB, HIV, HBV, and HCV. This analysis supports the role of the HBM in identifying and organizing implementation considerations in public health guidelines for migrants. We also assessed the confidence in five key findings using the CERQual tool. Three findings were rated as moderate confidence, and two were rated as low confidence (See GRADE CERQual Table 4).

The findings of this review suggest that disease-related stigma, and inaccurate knowledge related to certain infectious diseases, continue to be major deterrents for screening among migrants. However, ongoing education of migrant patients and their physicians may increase adherence to TB screening and treatment [27]. Stigma relates to traditional and western beliefs concerning disease outcomes, and these beliefs interact with longstanding cultural and social barriers [37]. Stigma can manifest in family and community life and may impact employment as well as healthcare. Addressing stigma will require a multi-faceted approach that involves engagement of affected communities as well as efforts to reduce structural barriers [24], as exemplified by the integration efforts taking place in Germany [39].

Migrant populations face screening at the political, public health and primary health care levels. We found that migrants consider the indirect costs that potentially accompany disease results, such as loss of employment and loss of migration status and social status. These negative outcomes may vary across the EU/EEA. On the contrary, migrants value screening, post hoc, when they do not have a disease.

Migrants consistently identify trust in practitioners as a key determinant to accepting infectious disease interventions [40]. Various organizations have developed cultural competency [41], cultural humility [42] programs to build trust for newly arrived migrants. In the context of cultural sensitivity, practitioners' approach may play an important role for linkage to care for migrants. More research, including participatory research, is needed to engage migrants in implementation strategies [43,44]. For example, one qualitative study used interviews with migrant leaders in community health to not only identify barriers to disease screening, but also identify innovative approaches to mitigate barriers by combining screening for all relevant diseases into one standardized check-up, thereby improving accessibility and further reducing disease-related stigma [45].

4.1. Implications for Practice

The qualitative data from our 11 reviews reports a compelling story of migrant access to care issues and acceptability issues related to stigma, indirect costs, and health system barriers. When migrants experienced disease symptoms or were able to perceive benefits from screening and/or trusted their practitioners, they were more likely to value, accept, and access infectious disease interventions. These findings tap into the lived experience of many migrants and may have relevance for screening programs; however, these findings cannot be generalized across all populations and diseases.

4.2. Strengths and Limitations

Traditionally, the GRADE CERQual tool is used to assess confidence in the evidence of synthesized qualitative studies. This paper is the first to adapt the CERQual tool to assess the confidence of systematic review level qualitative evidence. We also directed our findings and applied our confidence ratings as evidence in the ECDC Guidance development process, including values on intervention outcomes and acceptability of screening and treatment interventions of infectious diseases among migrant populations. These findings were implemented into evidence to decision tables and helped to develop ECDC guidance and implementation considerations for migrants.

According to the AMSTAR scores, the quality of eligible systematic reviews was low, highlighting a need for more rigorous evidence on the acceptability and accessibility of interventions among migrants. Specifically, the methods used to combine findings were generally appropriate, yet only two reviews [24,29] assessed and documented the quality of the primary studies included. While this may impact the validity of our findings, we demonstrated how the CERQual methodology can be used to account for the quality of the included reviews to generate sound assessments of the strength of qualitative evidence.

Our systematic review of reviews approach allowed us to use data that summarized findings from over 200 primary studies and supported the assessment of adequacy, consistency, and coherence. However, this approach also created some methodological challenges. We were obliged to report the findings without additional interviews and triangulation. Second, while we used the number of reviews and primary studies supporting a finding as evidence for the robustness of a finding, the precise relevance of these findings varied.

We began with six infectious disease interventions, which were consistent with those prioritized by the EU/EEA guidance work. This allowed us to consider consistencies across different individual diseases and provided more data to synthesize into findings. However, examining the data in aggregate may mask differences between these diseases. For example, most of the evidence on stigma comes from reviews on HIV and TB, and thus may not be generalizable to HBV or HCV or diseases not represented in the included reviews. We were unable to find qualitative systematic reviews that addressed vaccine-preventable diseases or intestinal parasites. While some of the evidence is likely relevant to these diseases, we accept that some of the barriers may be different. For example, VPDs are likely more relevant for migrant children and parents/caregivers, for whom the barriers and facilitators differ from adult migrants.

We were able to look at the findings from various migrant population and destination country perspectives. We chose to group the priority infectious diseases together, demonstrating that migrant perspectives varied across these diseases. We were unable to effectively rule out outliers on all the priority conditions and our findings are more aligned with migrant populations than destination countries.

5. Conclusions

Our review highlights migrants' perspectives on screening and treatment of infectious diseases, and as such, provides insight as to why migrants may accept or reject screening and treatment. Addressing disparities in prevalence and treatment rates of diseases between and within migrant populations will require implementation strategies that address migrant and practitioner knowledge, fear, and access barriers to health services. The acceptability, value of main outcomes and accessibility of screening and treatment interventions among migrants is highly dependent on the cultural sensitivity, relationship with healthcare professionals, disease-related stigma, and the degree of knowledge and self-perceived risk of diseases. Migrants may fear negative outcomes of screening including indirect costs related to the employment and immigration status, and they value screening and treatment less when asymptomatic. While our findings demonstrate similarities and differences across several infectious diseases, the available data was not sufficient for a complete analysis of factors that are specific to individual diseases or to migrant sub-populations. This highlights a need for ongoing implementation research involving individual populations and diseases to address this important public health and primary care topic.

Supplementary Materials: The following are available online at http://www.mdpi.com/1660-4601/15/11/2329/s1, Table S1: Search Strategy.

Author Contributions: Conceptualization, K.P., M.D., V.W.; Methodology, K.P., M.D., and V.W.; Validation, M.D., A.M., T.S., M.S., K.P.; Formal Analysis, M.D., E.A., A.M., D.G., T.N., M.S., T.S., K.P. Investigation, M.D., A.M., T.S., M.S.; Writing-Original Draft Preparation, M.D., K.P.; Writing-Review and Editing, M.D., C.G., V.W., M.P., T.N., C.M., H.K., K.P.; Supervision, K.P.

Funding: This research received no external funding.

Acknowledgments: We would like to acknowledge the work of Astrid Lykke Pedersen, who contributed to the data abstraction process.

Conflicts of Interest: Pareek is supported by the National Institute for Health Research (NIHR Post-Doctoral Fellowship, PDF-2015-08-102). The views expressed in this publication are those of the author(s) and not necessarily those of the NHS, the National Institute for Health Research or the Department of Health. Pareek reports an institutional grant (unrestricted) for project related to blood-borne virus testing from Gilead Sciences outside the submitted work. No other conflicts of interests declared.

Appendix A Determinants of Interest

We analyzed data on three overarching determinants of intervention uptake—values of main outcomes, acceptability, and accessibility. These are defined below:

Values of Main Outcomes of Infectious Disease Interventions:

- The importance placed upon the main outcomes of an intervention. These outcomes include those directly related to the disease (e.g., cure, symptom reduction, diagnosis), or costs or benefits resulting from the downstream effects of the intervention (e.g., side effects, time spent at the hospital, stigma, disclosure of disease status, cultural beliefs)

Acceptability of Infectious Disease Interventions:

- The willingness of the patient to request or adhere to the intervention based on their subjective attitudes and preferences towards the intervention itself or the process of receiving it (e.g., adherence challenges, social/cultural attitudes, fears about the procedure)

Accessibility of Infectious Disease Interventions:

- The ease with which patients use an infectious disease intervention. Determinants of accessibility include policies, community factors, healthcare service organization, or the delivery of the intervention itself.

Appendix B Determinants of Interest

- Study design: Systematic reviews (qualitative or qualitative/quantitative) defined as any review that includes selection criteria, search strategy, and use of at least one database
- Time: Published after 1 January 2010
- Language: English language
- Relevant to the PICO question:

    - Population: Migrants from Low- and Middle-Income Countries residing in High-Income Countries (i.e., permanent resettlement countries)
    - Intervention: Prevention, screening, and treatment interventions for infectious diseases (tuberculosis, hepatitis, VPDs, HIV, parasitic diseases)
    - Comparison: No intervention
    - Outcome: Valuation of outcomes, views about acceptability and accessibility of interventions

Appendix C Data Abstraction Tables

Table A1. Value of Outcomes.

Citation
Disease
Knowledge of Disease Status
Behavioral Prevention
Vaccination
Treatment of Asymptomatic Disease
Cure of Symptomatic Disease

Table A2. Acceptability.

Citation
Demand-Side Determinants
User's attitudes and Expectations
Household attitudes and expectations
Information on healthcare choice/providers
Disease-related knowledge
Intervention-related knowledge
Stigma
Indirect costs
Acculturation
SocialSupply-Side Determinants
Characteristics of the Health Services
Management/Staff Efficiency
Technology
Staff Interpersonal Skills, Including Trust
Wages and Quality of Staff
Language Barriers

Table A3. Accessibility.

Citations
Demand-Side Determinants
Indirect costs to household (e.g. transport, legal status)
Household income and willingness to pay
Opportunity costs
Means of transport available
System navigation
Low self-esteem and little assertivenessSupply-Side Determinants
Service/household location
Availablity of health workers, drugs, equipment
Direct price of service, including informal fees
Waiting time
Unqualified health woerks, absenteeism
Non-integration of health services
Lack of opportunity (exclusion from services)
Late or no referral

References

1. Mladovsky, P.; Shadwick, R.; Odone, A.; Ingleby, D.; Tillman, T.; Rechel, B.; McKee, M. *Assessing the Burden of Key Infectious Diseases Affecting Migrant Populations in the EU/EEA*; European Centre for Disease Prevention and Control: Stockholm, Sweden, 2014.

2. Pottie, K.; Greenaway, C.; Feightner, J.; Welch, V.; Swinkels, H.; Rashid, M.; Narasiah, L.; Kirmayer, L.J.; Ueffing, E.; MacDonald, N.E. Evidence-based clinical guidelines for immigrants and refugees. *CMAJ* **2011**, *183*, E824–E925. [CrossRef] [PubMed]
3. Chaves, N.; Biggs, B.A.; Thambiran, A.; Smith, M.; Williams, J.; Gardiner, J.; Davis, J.S. *Recommendations for Comprehensive Post-Arrival Health Assessment for People from Refugee-Like Backgrounds*; Australasian Society for Infectious Diseases and Refugee Health Network: Surrey Hills, Australia, 2016.
4. HPSC Scientific Advisory Committee. *Infectious Disease Assessment for Migrants*; Health Protection Surveillance Centre: Dublin, Ireland, 2015.
5. Alonso-Coello, P.; Oxman, A.D.; Moberg, J.; Brignardello-Petersen, R.; Akl, E.A.; Davoli, M.; Treweek, S.; Mustafa, R.A.; Vandvik, P.O.; Meerpohl, J. Grade evidence to decision (ETD) frameworks: A systematic and transparent approach to making well informed healthcare choices. 2: Clinical practice guidelines. *BMJ* **2016**, *353*, i2089. [CrossRef] [PubMed]
6. Agudelo-Suárez, A.A.; Gil-González, D.; Vives-Cases, C.; Love, J.G.; Wimpenny, P.; Ronda-Pérez, E. A metasynthesis of qualitative studies regarding opinions and perceptions about barriers and determinants of health services' accessibility in economic migrants. *BMC Health Serv. Res.* **2012**, *12*, 461. [CrossRef] [PubMed]
7. Gil-González, D.; Carrasco-Portino, M.; Vives-Cases, C.; Agudelo-Suarez, A.A.; Castejón Bolea, R.; Ronda-Pérez, E. Is health a right for all? An umbrella review of the barriers to health care access faced by migrants. *Ethn. Health* **2015**, *20*, 523–541. [CrossRef] [PubMed]
8. World Health Organization. Consolidated Guidelines on HIV Testing Services. Available online: http://www.who.int/hiv/pub/guidelines/hiv-testing-services/en/ (accessed on 1 August 2016).
9. Lawson, E.; Calzavara, L.; Husbands, W.; Myers, T.; Tharao, W.E. *HIV/AIDS Stigma, Denial, Fear and Discrimination: Experiences and Responses of People from African and Carribean Communities in Toronto*; African and Carribean Council on HIV/AIDS in Ontario (AACHO): Toronto, ON, Canada, 2006.
10. Mitra, D.; Jacobsen, M.; O'Connor, A.; Pottie, K.; Tugwell, P. Assessment of the decision support needs of women from HIV endemic countries regarding voluntary HIV testing in Canada. *Patient Educ. Couns.* **2006**, *63*, 292–300. [CrossRef] [PubMed]
11. Ahmed, S.; Shommu, N.S.; Rumana, N.; Barron, G.R.; Wicklum, S.; Turin, T.C. Barriers to access of primary healthcare by immigrant populations in Canada: A literature review. *J. Immigr. Minor. Health* **2016**, *18*, 1522–1540. [CrossRef] [PubMed]
12. Pottie, K.; Morton, R.; Greenaway, C.; Akl, E.; Rahman, P.; Zenner, D.; Pareek, M.; Tugwell, P.; Welch, V.; Meerpohl, J.; et al. Prevention and assessment of infectious diseases among children and adult migrants arriving to the European Union/European Economic Association: A protocol for a suite of systematic reviews for public health and health systems. *BMJ Open* **2017**, *7*, e014608. [CrossRef] [PubMed]
13. Moher, D.; Shamseer, L.; Clarke, M.; Ghersi, D.; Liberati, A.; Petticrew, M.; Shekelle, P.; Stewart, L.A. Preferred reporting items for systematic review and meta-analysis protocols (PRISMA-P) 2015 statement. *Syst. Rev.* **2015**, *4*, 1. [CrossRef] [PubMed]
14. Schünemann, H.J.; Wiercioch, W.; Brozek, J.; Etxeandia-Ikobaltzeta, I.; Mustafa, R.A.; Manja, V.; Brignardello-Petersen, R.; Neumann, I.; Falavigna, M.; Alhazzani, W. GRADE evidence to decision (ETD) frameworks for adoption, adaptation, and de novo development of trustworthy recommendations: Grade-adolopment. *J. Clin. Epidemiol.* **2017**, *81*, 101–110. [CrossRef] [PubMed]
15. Endnote Clarivate Analytics. Available online: endnote.com (accessed on 15 May 2016).
16. Shea, B.J.; Hamel, C.; Wells, G.A.; Bouter, L.M.; Kristjansson, E.; Grimshaw, J.; Henry, D.A.; Boers, M. AMSTAR is a reliable and valid measurement tool to assess the methodological quality of systematic reviews. *J. Clin. Epidemiol.* **2009**, *62*, 1013–1020. [CrossRef] [PubMed]
17. Jacobs, B.; Bigdeli, M.; Annear, P.L.; Van Damme, W. Addressing access barriers to health services: An analytical framework for selecting appropriate interventions in low-income Asian countries. *Health Policy Plan* **2011**, *27*, 288–300. [CrossRef] [PubMed]
18. Rosenstock, I.M.; Strecher, V.J.; Becker, M.H. The health belief model and HIV risk behavior change. *Springer* **1994**, *2*, 5–24. [CrossRef]
19. Glanz, K.; Bishop, D.B. The role of behavioral science theory in development and implementation of public health interventions. *Annu. Rev. Public Health* **2010**, *31*, 399–418. [CrossRef] [PubMed]

20. Alvarez-del Arco, D.; Monge, S.; Azcoaga, A.; Rio, I.; Hernando, V.; Gonzalez, C.; Alejos, B.; Caro, A.; Perez-Cachafeiro, S.; Ramirez-Rubio, O.; et al. HIV testing and counselling for migrant populations living in high-income countries: A systematic review. *Eur. J. Public Health* **2013**, *23*, 1039–1045. [CrossRef] [PubMed]
21. Pottie, K.; Vissandjée, B.; Grant, J. Human immunodeficiency virus. Evidence review for newly arriving immigrants and refugees. *CMAJ* **2010**. [CrossRef]
22. Rosenstock, I.M. Historical origins of the health belief model. *Health Educ. Monogr.* **1974**, *4*, 328–335. [CrossRef]
23. Lewin, S.; Glenton, C.; Munthe-Kaas, H.; Carlsen, B.; Colvin, C.J.; Gülmezoglu, M.; Noyes, J.; Booth, A.; Garside, R.; Rashidian, A. Using qualitative evidence in decision making for health and social interventions: An approach to assess confidence in findings from qualitative evidence syntheses (GRADE-CERQual). *PLoS Med.* **2015**, *12*, e1001895. [CrossRef] [PubMed]
24. Blondell, S.J.; Kitter, B.; Griffin, M.P.; Durham, J. Barriers and facilitators to HIV testing in migrants in high-income countries: A systematic review. *AIDS Behav.* **2015**, *19*, 2012–2024. [CrossRef] [PubMed]
25. Owiti, J.A.; Greenhalgh, T.; Sweeney, L.; Foster, G.R.; Bhui, K.S. Illness perceptions and explanatory models of viral hepatitis b & c among immigrants and refugees: A narrative systematic review. *BMC Public Health* **2015**, *15*, 151. [CrossRef]
26. Tomás, B.A.; Pell, C.; Cavanillas, A.B.; Solvas, J.G.; Pool, R.; Roura, M. Tuberculosis in migrant populations: A systematic review of the qualitative literature. *PLOS ONE* **2013**, *8*, e82440.
27. Greenaway, C.; Sandoe, A.; Vissandjee, B.; Kitai, I.; Gruner, D.; Wobeser, W.; Pottie, K.; Ueffing, E.; Menzies, D.; Schwartzman, K. Tuberculosis: Evidence review for newly arriving immigrants and refugees. *CMAJ* **2011**, *183*, E939–E951. [CrossRef] [PubMed]
28. Mitchell, E.M.; Shapiro, A.; Golub, J.; Kranzer, K.; Portocarrero, A.V.; Najlis, C.A.; Ngamvithayapong-Yanai, J.; Lönnroth, K. *Acceptability of TB Screening among At-Risk and Vulnerable Groups: A Systematic Qualitative/Quantitative Literature Metasynthesis*; World Health Organization: Geneva, Switzerland, 2012.
29. de Vries, S.G.; Cremers, A.L.; Heuvelings, C.C.; Greve, P.F.; Visser, B.J.; Bélard, S.; Janssen, S.; Spijker, R.; Shaw, B.; Hill, R.A. Barriers and facilitators to the uptake of tuberculosis diagnostic and treatment services by hard-to-reach populations in countries of low and medium tuberculosis incidence: A systematic review of qualitative literature. *Lancet Infect Dis.* **2017**, *17*, e128–e143. [CrossRef]
30. Do, T.N.; Nam, S. Knowledge, awareness and medical practice of Asian Americans/Pacific Islanders on chronic hepatitis B infection: Review of current psychosocial evidence. *Pogon Sahoe Yongu* **2011**, *31*, 341. [PubMed]
31. Nguyen-Truong, C.K.; Lee-Lin, F.; Gedaly-Duff, V. Contributing factors to colorectal cancer and Hepatitis B screening among Vietnamese Americans. *Oncol. Nurs. Forum* **2013**, *40*, 238–251. [CrossRef] [PubMed]
32. Tankimovich, M. Barriers to and interventions for improved tuberculosis detection and treatment among homeless and immigrant populations: A literature review. *J. Community Health Nurs.* **2013**, *30*, 83–95. [CrossRef] [PubMed]
33. Zhang, Z.; Cheng, J.; Liu, Z.; Ma, J.; Li, J.; Wang, J.; Yang, K. Epidemiology, quality and reporting characteristics of meta-analyses of observational studies published in chinese journals. *BMJ Open* **2015**, *5*. [CrossRef] [PubMed]
34. Kung, J.; Chiappelli, F.; Cajulis, O.O.; Avezova, R.; Kossan, G.; Chew, L.; Maida, C.A. From systematic reviews to clinical recommendations for evidence-based health care: Validation of revised assessment of multiple systematic reviews (R-AMSTAR) for grading of clinical relevance. *Open Dent. J.* **2010**, *4*, 84–91. [CrossRef] [PubMed]
35. Kleinman, A.; Benson, P. Anthropology in the clinic: The problem of cultural competency and how to fix it. *PLoS Med.* **2006**, *3*, e294. [CrossRef] [PubMed]
36. Mota, L.; Mayhew, M.; Grant, K.J.; Batista, R.; Pottie, K. Rejecting and accepting international migrant patients into primary care practices: A mixed method study. *Int. J. Migr. Health Soc. Care* **2015**, *11*, 108–129. [CrossRef]
37. Helman, C.G. *Culture, Health and Illness*, 5th ed.; CRC Press: Boca Raton, FL, USA, 2007.
38. Farmer, P. *Pathologies of Power: Health, Human Rights, and the New War on the Poor*; University of California Press: Berkeley, CA, USA, 2004; ISSN 0520931475.

39. Asylverfahrensbeschleunigungsgesetz (Act on the Acceleration of Asylum Procedures). Available online: http://www.bgbl.de/xaver/bgbl/start.xav?startbk=Bundesanzeiger_BGBl&jumpTo=bgbl115s1722.pdf (accessed on 20 July 2016).
40. Kleinman, A.; Eisenberg, L.; Good, B. Culture, illness, and care: Clinical lessons from anthropologic and cross-cultural research. *Ann. Intern. Med.* **1978**, *88*, 251–258. [CrossRef] [PubMed]
41. Beach, M.C.; Price, E.G.; Gary, T.L.; Robinson, K.A.; Gozu, A.; Palacio, A.; Smarth, C.; Jenckes, M.W.; Feuerstein, C.; Bass, E.B.; et al. Cultural competency: A systematic review of health care provider educational interventions. *Med. Care* **2005**, *43*, 356–373. [CrossRef] [PubMed]
42. Wallerstein, N.; Duran, B. Community-based participatory research contributions to intervention research: The intersection of science and practice to improve health equity. *Am. J. Public Health* **2010**, *100*, S40–S46. [CrossRef] [PubMed]
43. Beach, M.C.; Gary, T.L.; Price, E.G.; Robinson, K.; Gozu, A.; Palacio, A.; Smarth, C.; Jenckes, M.; Feuerstein, C.; Bass, E.B. Improving health care quality for racial/ethnic minorities: A systematic review of the best evidence regarding provider and organization interventions. *BMC Public Health* **2006**, *6*, 104. [CrossRef] [PubMed]
44. Grol, R. Improving the quality of medical care: Building bridges among professional pride, payer profit, and patient satisfaction. *JAMA* **2001**, *286*, 2578–2585. [CrossRef] [PubMed]
45. Seedat, F.; Hargreaves, S.; Friedland, J.S. Engaging new migrants in infectious disease screening: A qualitative semi-structured interview study of UK migrant community health-care leads. *PLOS ONE* **2014**, *9*, e108261. [CrossRef] [PubMed]

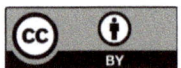

© 2018 by the authors. Licensee MDPI, Basel, Switzerland. This article is an open access article distributed under the terms and conditions of the Creative Commons Attribution (CC BY) license (http://creativecommons.org/licenses/by/4.0/).

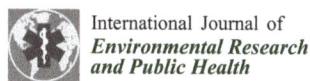

Article

Perspectives on the Measles, Mumps and Rubella Vaccination among Somali Mothers in Stockholm

Asha Jama [1], Mona Ali [1], Ann Lindstrand [1], Robb Butler [2] and Asli Kulane [3],*

[1] Unit for Vaccination Programmes, The Public Health Agency of Sweden, SE-171 82 Solna, Sweden; asha.jama@folkhalsomyndigheten.se (A.J.); mona.m.ali1987@gmail.com (M.A.); Ann.Lindstrand@folkhalsomyndigheten.se (A.L.)
[2] Division of Communicable Diseases and Health Security, WHO Regional Office for Europe, DK-2100 Copenhagen, Denmark; butlerr@who.int
[3] Equity and Health Policy Research Group, Department of Public Health Sciences, Karolinska Institute, Tomtebodavägen 18, 171 77 Stockholm, Sweden
* Correspondence: Asli.Kulane@ki.se; Tel.: +46-08-524-833-88

Received: 20 September 2018; Accepted: 19 October 2018; Published: 1 November 2018

Abstract: *Background*: Vaccination hesitancy and skepticism among parents hinders progress in achieving full vaccination coverage. Swedish measles, mumps and rubella (MMR) vaccine coverage is high however some areas with low vaccination coverage risk outbreaks. This study aimed to explore factors influencing the decision of Somali parents living in the Rinkeby and Tensta districts of Stockholm, Sweden, on whether or not to vaccinate their children with the measles, mumps and rubella (MMR) vaccine. *Method*: Participants were 13 mothers of at least one child aged 18 months to 5 years, who were recruited using snowball sampling. In-depth interviews were conducted in Somali and Swedish languages and the data generated was analysed using qualitative content analysis. Both written and verbal informed consent were obtained from participants. *Results*: Seven of the mothers had not vaccinated their youngest child at the time of the study and decided to postpone the vaccination until their child became older (delayers). The other six mothers had vaccinated their child for MMR at the appointed time (timely vaccinators). The analysis of the data revealed two main themes: (1) barriers to vaccinate on time, included issues surrounding fear of the child not speaking and unpleasant encounters with nurses and (2) facilitating factors to vaccinate on time, included heeding vaccinating parents' advice, trust in nurses and trust in God. The mothers who had vaccinated their children had a positive impact in influencing other mothers to also vaccinate. *Conclusions*: Fear, based on the perceived risk that vaccination will lead to autism, among Somali mothers in Tensta and Rinkeby is evident and influenced by the opinions of friends and relatives. Child Healthcare Center nurses are important in the decision-making process regarding acceptance of MMR vaccination. There is a need to address mothers' concerns regarding vaccine safety while improving the approach of nurses as they address these concerns.

Keywords: MMR vaccination; measles; vaccine hesitancy; autism; Rinkeby; Tensta

1. Introduction

Vaccines are one of the safest and most effective medical interventions in history; yet there has been a surge in concerns related to vaccination, leading parents to become hesitant to immunize their children [1]. Vaccine hesitancy refers to delay in acceptance or refusal of vaccines despite availability of vaccination services [2]. Vaccine hesitancy is a global challenge to the achievement of full vaccination coverage [3].

The most commonly reported reason for vaccine hesitancy is concern regarding the safety of one or more vaccines [4], and most common is the fear of presumed side-effects of the MMR vaccine [5]. Autism, immune system overload, and other presumed adverse reactions have often been cited [6].

Some parents do not recognize the full benefits of childhood immunizations, and can be especially skeptical of routine schedules that call for multiple immunizations given simultaneously on a strict timeline. Other reasons for not vaccinating include belief that a child is too young or too sick to receive a vaccine. Parents who accept vaccines are generally confident that immunization is a proven method to prevent disease [7].

Vaccine hesitancy varies greatly with context and across time, place and vaccines [8,9]. According to the Strategic Advisory Group of Experts (SAGE) working group matrix for vaccination hesitancy, several individual and contextual issues play a role in addition to the vaccine-specific issues [10]. The impact of social networks can also not be ignored [11]. These networks form a cohort of influencers that drive opinions on immunization [12].

Growing hesitancy related to MMR vaccination existed even among parents who have vaccinated their children [13]. Studies have shown that even parents who have previously consented to vaccination can be negatively influenced by rumours and ongoing debates [14].

MMR vaccine hesitancy has been found to be more prevalent among some faith based group or ethnic minorities and this has increased interest in identifying prevailing attitudes toward MMR vaccination [15–17]. The ethnic minorities include Somali parents living in Birmingham (UK) who perceived that there is a link between autism and MMR vaccine [18]. Similarly the Somali community in Minnesota (USA) have low MMR vaccine coverage and attribute it to concerns regarding the higher than average prevalence of autism spectrum disorder in the community [19].

In Sweden, MMR vaccine is offered at Child Healthcare Center at age 18 months and at age 6–8 years in schools. Overall, MMR vaccination coverage in Sweden at age 2 years is 97.5% [20] however several communities have vaccine coverage below 95%, the level needed to maintain herd immunity for measles. Child Health Centres (CHCs) in the Rinkeby and Tensta districts of Stockholm have reported MMR coverage of 71.5% and 69.7% respectively in 2012 [20]. The two districts have high percentage of residents with foreign background and approximately 30% with a Somali origin (20). The vaccination coverage has remained low since the late 1990s, when Wakefield published the later refuted article on a presumed link between autism and the MMR vaccine [20,21]. The current study aimed to identify factors influencing the decision of Somali parents living in Rinkeby and Tensta on whether or not to vaccinate their children with the MMR vaccine.

2. Materials and Methods

2.1. Study Design and Setting

This study is a part of larger project using the tailoring immunization programmes (TIP) methodology developed by the World Health Organisation (WHO) to find motivators and barriers to vaccination [22]. The study design is explorative with inductive qualitative approach. In depth interviews were used [23]. The study was conducted in Rinkeby and Tensta, districts located in the northwest part of Stockholm with a high percentage of residents with foreign backgrounds. The population in Rinkeby district was 16,047 in 2013, including 1638 children under five years (8.9%). The population of Tensta was 18,866, including 1673 children under five years (10.2%). An estimated 30% of this population is of Somali origin. This sub-population was chosen for the study based on concerns expressed by health workers regarding vaccine hesitancy specifically among Somali parents, and low MMR vaccination coverage in these districts [20].

2.2. Participants

Parents of children aged 18 months to 5 years were recruited for this study through different routes. A community stakeholders group consisting of local Somali nongovernmental organizations (NGOs), parent groups and mosque leaders assisted in the recruitment process. The leaders of these community groups were approached to inform potential participants, who in turn invited others who met the inclusion criteria in a process of snowball sampling. In addition, written invitations were available and posters pinned at the CHCs, but no participants were recruited through this channel. Thirteen mothers volunteered to be interviewed. Recruitment was stopped after 13 participants when no more new information was coming from the interviews [24]. All of the invited fathers declined. One father was present during the interview with his wife but declined to comment.

2.3. Data Collection

In-depth interviews (IDIs) were used to collect data because interviewing is the best-suited method to gain insight into parents' experiences and perspectives in deciding about vaccination for their children [24]. All interviews were conducted during June to September 2013. The participants chose the venues for the interviews. Most interviews took place at the interviewee's home, one took place at the CHC and three were conducted by phone. In most cases, only the interviewer, the note taker, the mother and her child were present, ensuring that confidentiality was maintained. The interviewer used probing and question rephrasing techniques to clarify questions and obtain details from the participants. The interviews were conducted by the first two authors (AJ & MA) and the last author (AK) in either Swedish or Somali, depending on the participant's choice. Each individual interview lasted around 30 to 60 min, with the exception of one that lasted 15 min.

2.4. Data Analysis and Interpretation

The interviews were transcribed verbatim and the researchers read all of the obtained data. The results were interpreted using a qualitative content analysis method as described by Graneheim and Lundman [25]. This method helps researchers to interpret and understand both the manifest and latent or hidden meanings. The researchers developed codes for the meaning units and also coded data within the same content area to identify differences and similarities. Codes and similarities were then put together in a category to show manifest meaning, from which themes emerged. Peer debriefing was conducted, in which the preliminary results were shared with the rest of the team and thereafter member checking was conducted to ensure credibility [26].

2.5. Research Ethics

The study was approved by the Regional Ethics Committee, Stockholm, Sweden (Dnr 2013/678-31/3). All participants were given information about the study and its objectives prior to giving their verbal consent to participate. Verbal consent was chosen for anonymity of the participants and was was approved by the ethics board. The information provided to participants covered the aim of the study, voluntariness, confidentiality and the option to discontinue participation at any time during the study. The participants were also provided with the contact information of the responsible researchers. All collected data was coded to ensure anonymity and kept within the research group's locked facilities.

3. Results

The 13 mothers were aged 25 to 42 years. Two of them had two children, six had three children, one had four children, two had five children, one had six children and one had seven children.

Seven of the mothers had not vaccinated their youngest child within the selected age group for MMR and had decided to postpone the first dose of this vaccination until their child became older (delayers). The remaining six mothers had vaccinated their child for MMR at the appointed time (timely vaccinators).

The analysis of the data revealed two main themes: (1) barriers to vaccinate on time, consisting of two categories (*issues surrounding fear of child not speaking* and *unpleasant encounters with nurses*) and (2) facilitating factors to vaccinate on time, consisting of three categories *heeding vaccinating parents' advice*, *trust in nurses* and *trust in God*.

3.1. Barriers to Vaccinate on Time

3.1.1. Issues Surrounding Fear of Child Not Speaking

Parents who chose to delay their child's vaccination had experienced peer pressure from other parents in their social network, including parents they did not known personally. This peer pressure created a perception among the delaying mothers that they would put their children's ability to speak at risk if they accepted the vaccine. The parents met these people in many settings, such as gatherings where women meet to listen to religious leaders and other social events, but most often at the CHCs as illustrated in this quote:

"No I don't meet anyone [them] here in the playground, it's the CHC centre where we meet". Delayer 6

It is at the CHCs where mothers obtain advice about their children's health however the mothers expressed that they often sought additional advice from other mothers before the routine child care visits. They made phone calls to mothers whom they perceived to have more experience in raising children and had older children who had gone through these routine programmes.

"I ask other mothers who have had children and have more experience". Delayer 3

If they spoke to other mothers who had delayed vaccination, this fueled their suspicion that vaccination at 18 months was not advisable. The messages and opinions received during these conversations were given serious consideration by mothers who eventually chose to delay vaccination.

"It was an aunt, an older woman whose child had received it[vaccine] and then became ill of it and since then I know about it. It has happened, so that is why one thinks, no thanks". Delayer 11

Some parents believe that vaccinations prevent diseases, but they delay vaccination beyond the age of 18 months to avoid the perceived risk of vaccine side effects, especially related to speech development. They preferred to wait until the child could speak fluently as illustrated below.

"I would like to get more information about this 18 months vaccine. It is the one people say makes "children stop talking". I waited to see if this child stopped talking by himself. I wanted to see him start talking". Delayer 6

Vaccine hesitant parents in the area who are worried about the MMR vaccine convey their fears to parents who want to vaccinate their children on time. This was reported to create peer pressure, and mothers who have vaccinated their children on time may begin to doubt their earlier decisions.

"I would like to add that parents who are worried forward their worries to parents who want to vaccinate. It happens very often". Timely vaccinator 2

Uncertainty about vaccine safety fueled by these rumours makes some mothers reluctant to have their children vaccinated for MMR, and leads them to delay the vaccination.

"One becomes afraid as a parent . . . when there is so much talk about how bad it [the MMR vaccine] is. Of course they say it has nothing to do with the vaccination and it's proven, but you still don't know. One doesn't want to have a bad conscience later in life as a parent . . . That's how I reasoned, but you never know what's bad or good really". Delayer 13

The delaying mothers mentioned the fear of other development disorders and that they did not want to risk their children developing any type of mental disorders by giving the MMR vaccine. Some did not understand the reasons for vaccinating against MMR.

"Why should one take it if your child is not in need of it, if she doesn't take it nothing happens but if she does there is a risk". Delayer 11

Others doubted the effectiveness of the vaccine and used this reason to delay or avoid the decision.

"I'm worried because one cannot say that all vaccines work for all children. I believe that maybe some react differently than others do. In special cases, not in the majority of course but I believe that some get ill from it. I really believe it has to do with something in that child's genes. One never knows if one's child is like that and that is the fear I believe. I don't know how they will react, if they will react positively to it". Delayer 7

Parents' negative attitudes toward vaccinations are particularly against the MMR vaccine. The participants said that other mothers told them not to vaccinate for MMR, however it was fine to receive other vaccines because they prevent deadly diseases and are safe.

"You can take the other vaccines. They are for the six diseases for example against polio, pneumonia, cold and also malaria". Delayer 1

3.1.2. Unpleasant Encounters with Nurses

Some mothers who had had negative experiences related to how they were received at the CHC were compelled to delay vaccination. The negative experiences, which had even caused some to change centres to those outside their areas of residence, were a driving force for these mothers' hesitancy. These experiences included how the mothers were greeted at the CHCs by the nurses and how they were addressed with information in regard to vaccination.

"It was bad information I think and also this nurse, she was tired of the work and maybe had worked there too long and seen too many faces. I felt the encounter was very boring. It was a burden for me to go there so I stopped going". Delayer 11

The mothers further shared nurses' perceptions of Somali parents who had not vaccinated their children. The mothers felt they were judged, had no chance of explaining their worries, and were denied the opportunity to get information about the vaccine.

"When I went there she said that all Somalis avoided this vaccine and why don't you want to vaccinate. She already had her own answers. She didn't want to know my reason. I understood that she had her own answers and I from Somalia am already being judged. "Yes yes, I know all of you don't want this vaccine and avoid it and you think you can get autism". I just was quiet and listened. Do you think so? I asked. " Yes, we believe so", she responded. I replied "Okay I am the mother of [name of the child] and I am going to wait [to vaccinate], then it was only goodbye". Delayer 13

This feeling of resentment and the perceived lack of interest in what they had to say drove these mothers away from the vaccination encounter, even though they acknowledged that the nurses appeared to be overwhelmed by their work.

"The staff are a little stressed, because they have a staff shortage and they have had it forever because [name of centre] is responsible for the whole of [name of area]. So the staff are not many, and it is not enough I think. But they do what they can". Delayer 12

3.2. Facilitating Factors to Vaccinate on Time

3.2.1. Heeding Vaccinating Parents' Advice

All parents shared that they had friends and relatives who told them about their perceptions regarding autism being caused by the MMR vaccine. Even the parents who decided to vaccinate on time said everyone around them was talking about autism; however, those who got positive feedback from their friends went ahead to vaccinate their children.

" . . . One of them is my best friend who is my only friend who came to this country before me and knows the language, works and knows much about health issues. She has one son and vaccinated her son". Timely vaccinator 2

These mothers were able to dismiss claims about the perceived negative side effects of the MMR vaccine because of the positive influence of their colleagues or friends who were vaccinating on time.

> "Sometimes there are places where a lot of people gather for religious events where mothers with young children can talk to each other. They usually ask how old is your child? Have you vaccinated him for one and a half year old vaccine? Yes. Has he not stopped talking? No, I answer.[Laughter]. I don't think that is true". Timely vaccinator 4

3.2.2. Trust in Nurses

Parents who had more trust in the nurses vaccinated on time, asked more questions and believed the answers they received from the nurses.

> "Now I ask advice from the nurse. Before it was the Somali talk I used to listen to ... Nowadays I take what the nurse says". Timely vaccinator 1

Some timely vaccinating mothers discredited the rumours and had their children vaccinated on time following positive discussions with the nurses. A couple of mothers who did not vaccinate their older children for the MMR vaccine but later changed their minds and vaccinated their younger children said that the nurse had an impact on their decision to vaccine on time.

> "I have received all information, but all this talk about the vaccine is not true she said. And I have observed and there are no differences that I have noticed on children either". Timely vaccinator 5

These timely vaccinators strongly believed that the healthcare providers would never do anything to harm their children but rather had an interest in keeping their children healthy. They put the health of their children first and entrusted the nurses with the duty of protecting their children's health.

> "I have never seen that someone who has been vaccinated stops talking. I often say that these are doctors and healthcare workers, I don't believe they would do anything to harm children". Timely vaccinator 4

3.2.3. Trust in God

All mothers who vaccinated for MMR on time had confidence in their decision to vaccinate their children. Their motivation was that they trusted God and believed anything that happened to their children was according to the will of God. They shared that if their child became ill then it was the will of God and no one could do anything to prevent it.

> "I believe that God has given you your child yesterday and can as quickly give him something tomorrow. He can give him something after twenty years or when he is little. One should believe in God, that is very important". Timely vaccinator 2

4. Discussion

This study found that concerns about MMR vaccine is evident among the Somali mothers in the Rinkeby and Tensta districts in Stockholm, Sweden. These results echo the opinions expressed by Somali women residing in the United Kingdom [18]. The strong component of mistrust and fear of MMR vaccine side effects was illustrated in both studies. The perceived side effect feared most is that the child may stop speaking. Other previous studies in this setting in Sweden [21], mothers skipped information meetings at CHCs and relied on receiving that information from the one or few mothers who did attend, relying more on mother's advice than nurses' advice.

Many mothers interviewed in this study are suspicious of the MMR vaccine. One of the reasons for this is that the MMR is provided at the time children usually develop speech. Therefore, when parents see or hear that other children have stopped speaking after receiving the vaccine, they assume that it is a MMR vaccine side effect and a sign of autism. Even though some mothers already know that this is not true, they don't want to take the risk of living with permanent guilt if their children end up being autistic. It is the fear of this risk that has compelled them to rather delay the vaccination until an age they believe is safe.

The peer pressure not to vaccinate at 18 months from other members of the community was strong and drove many to delay the vaccination. This is consistent with results from Downs et. al. who found that even the parents who favoured vaccination would be confused by ongoing debates, which would make them question their choices [14]. In this study, many mothers had simple and unchallenged beliefs about the vaccine, which could make them more vulnerable to anti-vaccination information. The negative impact that the social network can have on parents has been highlighted in other studies [11]. The mothers in the current study reported to the CHC that their friends and relatives had informed them about the alleged MMR side effects and this greatly influenced their decision to delay.

This study highlights that mothers who chose not to vaccinate had a greater fear of autism than measles, mumps and rubella. Unlike in previous studies in which Somali mothers expressed greater anxiety about their children catching infectious diseases [27], for some mothers in this study the fear of autism overshadowed fear of the infectious diseases. In line with other studies, they believed that the diseases the vaccine is intended to prevent are mild and uncommon compared to the risk of autism [28]. In addition in this study we find that both advice from peer parents and trust and distrust in nurses seem to be influencing the decision to vaccinate on time or not.

Trust in the nurses was an essential element for the mothers who vaccinated their children. The parents' reporting of positive relations with the CHC nurses highlights the important role the nurses play in the parents' decision to vaccinate [29]. Trust in healthcare providers and the information they provide facilitates the decision to vaccinate. Parents who vaccinated their children on time had the universal understanding that vaccines were beneficial to their children's health and they trusted nurses, whom they regarded as being responsible for their children's health.

The safety of the MMR vaccine has been amply tested and demonstrated [30] and its association with autism dispelled [31,32]. There is no evidence that the risk of autism is higher in children vaccinated with MMR [33], yet the rumours questioning its safety continue. The mothers interviewed in this study found the process of deciding whether to have their children vaccinated difficult and stressful because of the ongoing debate, as expressed in other studies [34]. Interventions should therefore focus on communication mechanisms and decision-making pathways that would contribute to improving immunization coverage with the MMR vaccination in this target population.

Methodological Considerations

Several steps were taken to ensure trustworthiness of the information. Interviews were conducted in the participants language of choice and tape-recorded to capture as much detail as possible and allow for an engaging discussion. Individual interviews were conducted with a female interviewer to permit open discussion and room for more probing for deeper understanding. Triangulation was done in analysing data and sharing the preliminary findings with child health experts to increase the credibility of the data. A member check with the mothers was also conducted. In this study, all parents who did not vaccinate described themselves as delayers and not decliners and this made it difficult to identify those who declined entirely [35,36]. Great efforts were made by the research team to contact potential participants through gatekeepers. They presented the project at different venues such as local NGO meetings and open day care and used the snowball method to recruit additional participants. In this study all participants who volunteered to be interviewed were either parents who vaccinate on time and those who delayed to vaccinate on time. Therefore, we do not have the views and experiences of parents who reject the MMR vaccine, which may have re-enforced our study findings or introduced new findings.

5. Conclusions

Fear that the MMR vaccine can cause autism persists among Somali mothers in Tensta and Rinkeby who participated in this study and is fueled by rumours spread by their friends and relatives. Relieving this source of anxiety among the mothers should be the cornerstone of interventions by MMR vaccination programmes. The positive attitude of CHC nurses can compel mothers to vaccinate their children, due to the strong trust accorded to them. CHC nurses are the first contact between mothers and the primary health care system and this could be a strong avenue through which to improve vaccination coverage. This study informs and suggests some opportunities for tailored interventions for improving vaccination coverage and ultimately eliminating measles and rubella.

Author Contributions: The interviews were conducted by the first two authors (A.J. & M.A.) and the last author (A.K.). All authors (A.J., M.A., A.L., R.B., A.K.) were involved in the study design, data analysis and writing of the manuscript. All authors have read through, consented and agreed to the publication of this manuscript.

Funding: The study was funded by WHO Regional Office for Europe.

Conflicts of Interest: The authors had no competing interests in this work.

References

1. Bloom, B.R.; Marcuse, E.; Mnookin, S. Addressing vaccine hesitancy. *Science* **2014**, *344*, 339. [CrossRef] [PubMed]
2. MacDonald, N.E. SAGE Working Group on Vaccine Hesitancy. Vaccine hesitancy: Definition, scope and determinants. *Vaccine* **2015**, *33*, 4161–4164. [CrossRef] [PubMed]
3. Larson, H.J.; de Figueiredo, A.; Xiahong, Z.; Schulz, W.S.; Verger, P.; Johnston, I.G.; Cook, A.R.; Jones, N.S. The State of Vaccine Confidence 2016: Global Insights Through a 67-Country Survey. *EBioMedicine* **2016**, *12*, 295–301. [CrossRef] [PubMed]
4. Gilkey, M.B.; McRee, A.L.; Brewer, N.T. Forgone vaccination during childhood and adolescence: Findings of a statewide survey of parents. *Prev. Med.* **2013**, *56*, 202–206. [CrossRef] [PubMed]
5. Gowda, C.; Schaffer, S.E.; Kopec, K.; Markel, A.; Dempsey, A.F. Does the relative importance of MMR vaccine concerns differ by degree of parental vaccine hesitancy?: An exploratory study. *Hum. Vaccines Immunother.* **2013**, *9*, 430–436. [CrossRef]
6. Luthy, K.E.; Beckstrand, R.L.; Callister, L.C. Parental hesitation in immunizing children in Utah. *Public Health Nurs.* **2010**, *27*, 25–31. [CrossRef] [PubMed]
7. Frew, P.M.; Hixson, B.; del Rio, C.; Esteves-Jaramillo, A.; Omer, S.B. Acceptance of pandemic 2009 influenza A (H1N1) vaccine in a minority population: Determinants and potential points of intervention. *Pediatrics* **2011**, *127* (Suppl. 1), S113–S119. [CrossRef] [PubMed]
8. Larson, H.J.; Jarrett, C.; Eckersberger, E.; Smith, D.M.; Paterson, P. Understanding vaccine hesitancy around vaccines and vaccination from a global perspective: A systematic review of published literature, 2007–2012. *Vaccine* **2014**, *32*, 2150–2159. [CrossRef] [PubMed]
9. Hickler, B.; Guirguis, S.; Obregon, R. Vaccine Special Issue on Vaccine Hesitancy. *Vaccine* **2015**, *33*, 4155–4156. [CrossRef] [PubMed]
10. WHO. *SAGE Working Group on Vaccine Hesitancy*; WHO: Geneva, Switzerland, 2014; pp. 8–10.
11. Brunson, E.K. The impact of social networks on parents' vaccination decisions. *Pediatrics* **2013**, *131*, e1397-1404. [CrossRef] [PubMed]
12. Brunson, E.K. How parents make decisions about their children's vaccinations. *Vaccine* **2013**, *31*, 5466–5470. [CrossRef] [PubMed]
13. Casiday, R.; Cresswell, T.; Wilson, D.; Panter-Brick, C. A survey of UK parental attitudes to the MMR vaccine and trust in medical authority. *Vaccine* **2006**, *24*, 177–184. [CrossRef] [PubMed]
14. Downs, J.S.; de Bruin, W.B.; Fischhoff, B. Parents' vaccination comprehension and decisions. *Vaccine* **2008**, *26*, 1595–1607. [CrossRef] [PubMed]
15. Brown, K.F.; Shanley, R.; Cowley, N.A.; van Wijgerden, J.; Toff, P.; Falconer, M.; Ramsay, M.; Hudson, M.J.; Green, J.; Vincent, C.A.; et al. Attitudinal and demographic predictors of measles, mumps and rubella (MMR) vaccine acceptance: Development and validation of an evidence-based measurement instrument. *Vaccine* **2011**, *29*, 1700–1709. [CrossRef] [PubMed]
16. Bystrom, E.; Lindstrand, A.; Likhite, N.; Butler, R.; Emmelin, M. Parental attitudes and decision-making regarding MMR vaccination in an anthroposophic community in Sweden—A qualitative study. *Vaccine* **2014**, *32*, 6752–6757. [CrossRef] [PubMed]

17. Woudenberg, T.; van Binnendijk, R.S.; Sanders, E.A.; Wallinga, J.; de Melker, H.E.; Ruijs, W.L.; Hahne, S.J. Large measles epidemic in the Netherlands, May 2013 to March 2014: Changing epidemiology. *Eurosurveill* **2017**, *22*. [CrossRef] [PubMed]
18. Tomlinson, N.; Redwood, S. Health beliefs about preschool immunisations: An exploration of the views of Somali women resident in the UK. *Divers. Equal. Health Care* **2013**, *10*, 101–113.
19. Bahta, L.; Ashkir, A. Addressing MMR Vaccine Resistance in Minnesota's Somali Community. *Minn. Med.* **2015**, *98*, 33–36. [PubMed]
20. Folkhälsomyndigheten. *Barriers Motivating Factors MMR Vaccination Communities Low Coverage Sweden*; The Public Health Agency: Stockholm, Sweden, 2014; ISBN 978-91-7603-451-4.
21. Kulane, A.J.A.; Robleh, I.; Bågenholm, G. *Somali Parents' Acceptance of MMR Vaccinations for Their Children. An Exploratory Study*; Report for Stockholm County: Stockholm, Sweden, 2007.
22. Butler, R.; MacDonald, N.E.; SAGE Working Group on Vaccine Hesitancy. Diagnosing the determinants of vaccine hesitancy in specific subgroups: The Guide to Tailoring Immunization Programmes (TIP). *Vaccine* **2015**, *33*, 4176–4179. [CrossRef] [PubMed]
23. Holloway, I. *Qualitative Research in Health Care*; Open University Press: Maidenhead, UK, 2005.
24. Boyce, C.; Neale, P. *Conducting in-Depth Interviews: A Guide for Designing and Conducting in-Depth Interviews for Evaluation Input*; Pathfinder International: Watertown, MA, USA, 2006.
25. Graneheim, U.H.; Lundman, B. Qualitative content analysis in nursing research: Concepts, procedures and measures to achieve trustworthiness. *Nurse Educ. Today* **2004**, *24*, 105–112. [CrossRef] [PubMed]
26. Dahlgren, L.; Emmelin, M.; Winkvist, A. *Qualitative Methodology for International Public Health*; Umeå University: Umeå, Sweden, 2007.
27. Condon, L. Maternal attitudes to preschool immunisations among ethnic minority groups. *Health Educ. J.* **2002**, *61*, 180–189. [CrossRef]
28. Brown, K.F.; Kroll, J.S.; Hudson, M.J.; Ramsay, M.; Green, J.; Long, S.J.; Vincent, C.A.; Fraser, G.; Sevdalis, N. Factors underlying parental decisions about combination childhood vaccinations including MMR: A systematic review. *Vaccine* **2010**, *28*, 4235–4248. [CrossRef] [PubMed]
29. Levi, B.H. Addressing parents' concerns about childhood immunizations: A tutorial for primary care providers. *Pediatrics* **2007**, *120*, 18–26. [CrossRef] [PubMed]
30. Institute of Medicine Immunization Safety Review, C. *Immunization Safety Review: Measles Mumps Rubella Vaccine and Autism*; Stratton, K., Gable, A., Shetty, P., McCormick, M., Eds.; National Academies Press (US): Washington, DC, USA, 2001.
31. Maglione, M.A.; Das, L.; Raaen, L.; Smith, A.; Chari, R.; Newberry, S.; Shanman, R.; Perry, T.; Goetz, M.B.; Gidengil, C. Safety of vaccines used for routine immunization of U.S. children: A systematic review. *Pediatrics* **2014**, *134*, 325–337. [CrossRef] [PubMed]
32. Hensley, E.; Briars, L. Closer look at autism and the measles-mumps-rubella vaccine. *Am. Pharm. Assoc. JAPhA* **2010**, *50*, 736–741. [CrossRef] [PubMed]
33. Miller, E. Measles-mumps-rubella vaccine and the development of autism. *Semin. Pediatr. Infect. Dis.* **2003**, *14*, 199–206. [CrossRef]
34. Evans, M.; Stoddart, H.; Condon, L.; Freeman, E.; Grizzell, M.; Mullen, R. Parents' perspectives on the MMR immunisation: A focus group study. *Br. J. Gen. Pract.* **2001**, *51*, 904–910. [PubMed]
35. Holloway, I.; Todres, L. The status of method: Flexibility, consistency and coherence. *Qual. Res.* **2003**, *3*, 345–357. [CrossRef]
36. Golafshani, N. Understanding reliability and validity in qualitative research. *Qual. Rep.* **2003**, *8*, 597–606.

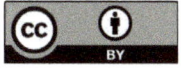

© 2018 by the authors. Licensee MDPI, Basel, Switzerland. This article is an open access article distributed under the terms and conditions of the Creative Commons Attribution (CC BY) license (http://creativecommons.org/licenses/by/4.0/).

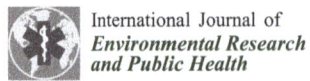

Article

Health-Related Lifestyle Behavior and Religiosity among First-Generation Immigrants of Polish Origin in Germany

Eva Morawa * and Yesim Erim

Department of Psychosomatic Medicine and Psychotherapy, University Hospital of Erlangen, Friedrich-Alexander-University Erlangen-Nürnberg (FAU), 91054 Erlangen, Germany; yesim.erim@uk-erlangen.de
* Correspondence: eva.morawa@uk-erlangen.de; Tel.: +49-9131-8535-951; Fax: +49-9131-8535-952

Received: 17 September 2018; Accepted: 9 November 2018; Published: 13 November 2018

Abstract: *Background*: Health-related lifestyle behaviors such as smoking, alcohol consumption, physical inactivity and obesity are major cardiovascular risk factors. Previous studies have mostly demonstrated a favorable association between religiosity and these cardiovascular risk factors; however, no studies have investigated this relationship in Polish immigrants. The aim of this cross-sectional study was to examine the association between health-related lifestyle behaviors and religiosity in Polish immigrants in Germany. *Methods*: The smoking patterns, frequency of alcohol consumption, physical activity, and presence of overweight/obesity were assessed in 257 first-generation immigrants of Polish origin living in Germany. Religiosity was measured with the Centrality of Religiosity Scale (CRS, Huber, 2003) consisting of 15 items that categorized the respondents into intrinsically, extrinsically, and not/marginally religious. *Results*: After adjusting for various sociodemographic, migration, and health-related characteristics, intrinsic religiosity was significantly associated with a lower risk of being a smoker (odds ratios (OR) = 0.34, confidence intervals (CI) = 0.15–0.76) and was also associated with a lower risk of alcohol consumption (OR = 0.33, CI = 0.15–0.71), but a higher risk of being overweight/obese (OR = 2.53, CI = 1.15–5.56) in comparison with extrinsic/marginal religiosity. No significant relationship was found between religiosity and physical activity. *Conclusions*: In Polish immigrants, intrinsic religiosity acts as a protective factor against some cardiovascular risk factors (smoking and alcohol consumption).

Keywords: immigrants; Polish; religiosity; lifestyle behavior; smoking; alcohol consumption; physical activity; overweight; obesity

1. Introduction

There has been increasing interest in examining the relationships between religious, spiritual, and health variables in medical and psychological research during the last decades. Despite scientific progress, the role of religion/religiosity is still substantial for a large proportion of humankind. According to the Global Index of Religion and Atheism from 2012 [1] (including 51,927 people from 57 countries in five continents), 59% of all people regard themselves as being religious. Religious beliefs and practices provide not only a sense of meaning in the lives of human beings but are also an important source of rules for (moral) behaviors.

1.1. The Religious Landscape in Poland and Germany

Religion plays an essential role in the lives of Poles. In Poland, 96% of the population declare their affiliation with the Roman Catholic Church [2], whereas only 28.5% of the citizens in Germany are Roman Catholics [3]. The high identification of the Poles with the Catholic faith as well as the religious, cultural, and political influence of the Catholic Church through the centuries until now are grounded in the history of Poland [4]. During times of foreign oppression, the Catholic Church contributed substantially to the preservation of the identity of the Polish nation, the Polish language, and traditions, as well as to the national resistance and fight for independence.

The statistics indicate not only the formal declaration of being Catholic of most Poles but also the high proportion of religious people in this nation. Eighty-one percent of Poles and 51% of the Germans describe themselves as religious [1]. According to the Centre for Public Opinion Research in Poland [5], 93% of all citizens in Poland consider themselves to be believers (85% believers and 8% strong believers). This trend of the Polish religiosity has remained stable over the last 20 years (between 92% and 97%). In 2016, on average, 50% of Catholics in Poland participated in the Sunday mass [5] compared to only 10.2% of Catholics in Germany [6].

In Germany, no statistics are available for the mass attendance of Polish immigrants. Many immigrants of Polish origin participate in Polish-speaking religious services in the "Polish Catholic Missions" in almost every large city in Germany. In these Polish pastoral centers, it is not only church services that take place but also religious education in Polish, Polish classes, and activities of various religious and cultural groups [4]. Therefore, the local Catholic Polish communities are places where the immigrants can maintain their indigenous language as well as religious and cultural traditions and thus preserve their identity [6].

1.2. Immigrants of Polish Origin in Germany

In Germany, more than every fifth person (22%) has a migration background, either having personally moved there or having at least one parent who moved [7]. There are approximately two million immigrants of Polish origin [8], one of the three largest immigration groups in German society today, the other two being Turkish and Russian origins. Polish immigrants are a heterogeneous group with a high percentage of ethnic German resettlers who have an official status as German citizens (for further information on the history of Polish immigration to Germany and the characteristics of Polish immigrants, see [4,9]).

1.3. Definition and Measures of Religiosity

Although religion/religiosity is a universal human phenomenon, there is no consensus among researchers regarding a definition for this concept. Religion is a complex and multidimensional construct that is generally associated with specific beliefs, practices, and rituals that are related to a sacred or transcendent (God, higher power, or ultimate truth/reality) and take place within a community but can also be practiced in private [10]. Religion is founded in an established tradition of common beliefs of a group concerning the sacred and is linked to formal institutions such as churches, synagogues, mosques, and temples. Religiosity is considered to be the personal form of the transcendent-related beliefs, experiences, and behaviors [11].

The terms religiosity and spirituality are often used interchangeably in the literature; however, despite some similarities between them, they do not mean the same thing. Spirituality is more difficult to define than religiosity. It is a broader concept than religiosity and is not restricted to religious traditions. Spirituality can be regarded as the individual experience characterized by a quest for meaning in life and the relationship with the sacred or transcendent that can, but does not have to be, connected to formal religious communities and institutions [12]. Another important aspect of religiosity described in the literature is religious coping, whereby religion is used as a coping strategy to manage stressors and critical life events [13].

A wide variety of operationalizations of religion/religiosity exist. More than 125 measurement instruments were identified by Hill and Hood [14]. Several studies have assessed only one aspect of religion using single item scales, for example, asking for the frequency of attendance of religious services or prayer, or the importance of religion in one's life. However, the reliability and validity of one-item measurement scales is debatable. A multidimensional approach to religion seems to be more adequate.

Two classical theoretical approaches to religion are worth mentioning: the conceptualizations of Allport [15] and Glock [16]. Allport's concept of intrinsic and extrinsic religiousness has had the greatest impact on the empirical psychology of religion [17]. Glock [16] defined five main dimensions of religion that depict the overall religious life and constitute the frame of reference for empirical research: intellect (interest on religious themes), ideology (beliefs of a religious tradition), religious experience (experiencing the transcendence), and private (e.g., prayer) and public (e.g., participation on public religious services) practices.

The questionnaire applied in the present study to measure religiosity (the Centrality of Religiosity Scale [18]) is a synthesis of these classical approaches. The centrality is conceptualized as the degree of importance or salience of religiosity in the personality of an individual assessed based on the intensity of the five core dimensions of religiosity in one's life: the more religious a person is, the greater the intensity [19].

1.4. Religiosity, (Mental) Health and Health-Related Lifestyle Behaviors

Scientific evidence for the association between religion and mental health is largely based on the Handbook of Religion and Health [12] which is the most comprehensive systematic review ever performed in the field of psychology of religion discussing more than 1200 studies published in the 20th century. A systematic review [20] largely based on this handbook and including additional publications between 2000 and 2005 summarized the main results on the relationship between religiosity and several indicators of mental health and psychological well-being as follows: the majority of studies have shown higher levels of religiosity to be associated with less risk of depression, less suicidal thoughts and behaviors, less alcohol/drug use/abuse, and higher well-being (life satisfaction, happiness, positive affectivity, optimism, hope, self-esteem, sense of meaning in life, internal locus of control, and social support). These beneficial associations remain significant after controlling for important sociodemographic variables and even after adjusting for social support, and they are similar in populations from different countries, religions, ethnic backgrounds, and ages. However, they are more robust among people under stressful circumstances such as those with a medical illness or disability, and among elderly individuals. Also, a systematic evidence-based review [21] including original research published in the top 25% of psychiatry and neurology journals between 1990–2010 found good empirical evidence for the association between religious involvement and less risk of depression, less substance abuse, and less suicide.

Although most of the research on religiosity and health has been conducted in the USA in Christian samples, in recent years, studies from other countries and religions have mostly supported the protective function of religiosity observed in U.S. surveys [20,22].

Despite the growing research interest in the examination of the health status of immigrants as well as the association between religiosity and various indicators of health, the literature on the relationship between religiosity and health-related lifestyle behaviors among immigrants is very scarce, and no investigation has been conducted on the population of Polish immigrants. Most of the studies on this topic have been conducted in the USA in Latino and Asian Indian immigrants. In sum, the scarce literature on the association between religiosity and health-related behaviors in immigrants has consistently shown an inverse relationship between religiosity and tobacco [23–25] as well as alcohol consumption or alcohol use disorders ([25–28]; a positive association between religiosity and physical activity (however, only one study has examined this topic [25]); and mixed results concerning religiosity and being overweight/obese—one survey reported no significant relationship [25] and one [29] demonstrated a positive association (found only for Asian Indians practicing Hinduism or Sikhism, but not for Muslims).

In a recently published systematic review on religion and body weight [30] including 85 studies (49% of the studies included mixed race/ethnicity), a significant association was detected between a higher level of religiosity and a higher body weight in both cross-sectional and prospective investigations—in bivariate analyses but less so in multivariate analyses. Only one of five longitudinal multivariate analyses demonstrated a statistically significant relationship between religiosity and body weight.

1.5. Possible Explanations for the Positive Effects of Religiosity on (Mental) Health and Health-Related Lifestyle Behaviors

Several mechanisms have been proposed as explanations for the impact of religion/religiosity on human health, namely, healthy behaviors and lifestyle, cognitive framework, social support, religious practices, spiritual direction, coping, alternative values, and positive emotions [20,31,32]. Religion may improve health by discouraging or even forbidding behaviors that may harm health, such as alcohol (abuse) and drugs, and encouraging people to live in a healthy way (e.g., keeping a day of rest, eating moderately, having peaceful relationships). In addition, religious doctrines that promote attitudes such as forgiveness and empathy, or virtues such as compassion, gratitude, humility, etc., may reduce feelings of anger and hostility and are therefore beneficial for health. Belonging to a religious organization may provide social cohesion and support that promotes health. Religious practices such as prayer and meditation may be forms of relaxation that contribute to reduced stress levels. Religion can provide meaning, orientation, and a sense of control in life as well as helping individuals to cope successfully with stressful and critical life circumstances, such as a severe illness. Furthermore, religious belief systems often emphasize socially critical, alternative values, such as social engagement and humility, and thus, may relieve an individual from the pressure to perform and compete and, consequently, reduce stress. Finally, it is also possible that religion might have a beneficial contribution to health by increasing positive emotions such as happiness and gratitude.

The relationship between religiosity and health has also aroused scientific interest in the field of neuroscience, for example, brain activity during prayer and meditation has been investigated [33]. Also, several physiological mechanisms concerning the central nervous system, neurotransmitters, and the endocrine and immune systems have been proposed to mediate the favorable effects of religiosity on health [34].

Although a large body of studies has generally demonstrated a positive effect of religiosity on various parameters of health, it is important to mention that religion/religiosity (i.e., special religious doctrines and practices) may also have negative effects on human health in some cases, e.g., if a religious group forbids blood transfusions or medications, or leads to social isolation, etc. [31].

Since religion/religiosity is a multidimensional phenomenon, it can be postulated that not the single mechanisms but rather their combination contributes to the favorable effects of religion/religiosity on health.

1.6. Study Aims

The homogenous structure of the religious affiliation among the Polish immigrants provides a favorable basis to analyze the impact of (Christian, mostly Catholic) religiosity on health-related lifestyle behaviors.

The aims of the study were:

1. To examine the frequency of health-related lifestyle behaviors (smoking, alcohol consumption, physical activity, and obesity) and categories of religiosity (intrinsic, extrinsic, and no/marginal religiosity) in immigrants of Polish origin in Germany.
2. To investigate the association between religiosity and the four health-related lifestyle behaviors, with adjustment for various important sociodemographic, migration, and health-related characteristics in immigrants of Polish origin.

Based on previous research, we postulated high religiosity to be associated with a lower risk of being a smoker and for alcohol consumption but hypothesized that there is no relationship between religiosity and physical activity or being overweight/obese.

2. Materials and Methods

2.1. Participants

The recruitment took place in Germany (immigrants of Polish origin) and in Poland (autochthone Poles). The present study focuses only on Polish immigrants. The data obtained have already been used for other publications [9,35–37].

In Germany, participants were recruited in centers in the Ruhr area (North Rhine Westphalia, West Germany) where Polish communities had been established, e.g., after Polish language mass, in religious and cultural groups in Polish churches, in non-religious places promoting Polish culture as well as among students from Polish migration backgrounds at the Ruhr University Bochum in Germany. In addition, probands were also recruited by the "snowball" method. This method can be regarded as an alternative sampling strategy if the examined target population is difficult to reach or identify [38], which is the case with immigrants of Polish origin who have German citizenship. Most of the Polish immigrants living in Germany are formally German citizens and thus rank as Germans in statistics; a random sample would, therefore, not include them, whereas data collection within the Polish community made it possible to recruit both immigrants of Polish origin with German as well as immigrants with Polish citizenship.

The inclusion criteria for the study were age of consent (minimum of 18 years), agreement to participate in the study, adequate knowledge of the Polish language due to the fact that the questionnaire was applied only in Polish, residence in the Ruhr area or in neighboring cities, and the status of a Polish immigrant according to the definition applied in epidemiological research in Germany [7], i.e., having immigrated themselves or having at least one parent who immigrated. Therefore, immigrants as well as resettlers were included in the study, regardless of having German citizenship or not.

Four hundred and nine questionnaires were distributed, and 264 were returned (response rate: 56.3%). Two participants were excluded based on the exclusion criteria (residence not in the Ruhr area). Because only five people belonged to the second generation of immigrants (born in Germany), they were excluded from the analyses, so a total sample of $n = 257$ first-generation immigrants were included in the present study.

2.2. Procedure and Setting

Data were collected between August 2009 and October 2010 in the abovementioned recruitment centers. Participants completed the self-report questionnaire in Polish language at home.

2.3. Ethics Statement

The present study was conducted in accordance with the Declaration of Helsinki, and the protocol was approved by the Ethics Committee of the Medical Faculty of the University of Duisburg-Essen (Project identification code: 11-4723). Written informed consent was obtained from all participants.

2.4. Measures

2.4.1. Sociodemographic and Migration-Specific Variables

The following sociodemographic and migration-specific items were assessed: gender, age, marital status, education level, employment status, subjectively perceived income, citizenship, length of residence in Germany, and German language proficiency.

2.4.2. Health-Related Lifestyle Behaviors

Four health-related lifestyle behaviors were measured:

1. The smoking status: current smoker or non-smoker and the number of smoked cigarettes per day: <5, 5–10, 11–20, 21–40, >40.
2. Alcohol consumption: never, seldom, once a month, several times a month, once a week, several times a week, every day.
3. Physical activity per week (sport): never, <1 h, 1–2 h, 2–4 h, >4 h.
4. Body mass index (BMI) category (kg/m^2): <18.5 (underweight), 18.5–24.9 (normal weight), 25.0–29.9 (overweight), ≥30 (obese). Obesity was defined according to the World Health Organization (WHO) as BMI ≥ 30 kg/m^2 [39].

2.4.3. Depressive Symptoms

Depressive symptoms were measured by the Beck Depression Inventory (BDI) [40] which consists of 21 items representing the most important symptoms of depression. Scores range between 0 and 63. A total score of 18 points and above indicates clinically relevant depression. In this study, a validated Polish version of the BDI used in clinical studies of the Silesian Medical University [41] was employed, which obtained a Cronbach's alpha score of 0.90 in the present sample.

2.4.4. Anxiety Symptoms

Anxiety symptoms were assessed by the Beck Anxiety Inventory (BAI) [42] which comprises 21 items (13 related to somatic anxiety symptoms, 5 to cognitive aspects of anxiety, and 3 items measure both cognitive and somatic symptoms). Scores between 0 and 63 can be achieved. In the present sample, the Cronbach's alpha score of the validated Polish version [41] was 0.91. A cut-off-value of 26 indicates clinically relevant anxiety.

2.4.5. Somatic Symptoms

The brief form of the Giessen Subjective Complaints List (GBB-24) [43], which consists of 24 items, was employed to assess somatic symptoms. Scores range between 0 and 96. Four subscales ("exhaustion", "stomach complaints", "pain in the extremities" and "heart complaints") and a total score can be calculated ("symptom pressure"). In the present study, a validated Polish version developed by the research group of the Department of Medical Psychology and Medical Sociology at the University of Leipzig [44] was used. The Cronbach's alpha score in the examined sample was 0.93.

2.4.6. Perceived Discrimination

Subjectively perceived discrimination was assessed by means of four self-constructed items on a 1–5 Likert scale (higher scores indicating higher perceived discrimination) concerning the categories "neighborhood", "shopping", "administrative office", and "working life" (see [36]). A total score was created as an index for the discrimination (there was a Cronbach's alpha score of 0.78. in the present study).

2.4.7. Sense of Coherence

The Sense of Coherence Scale (SOC-29) is a self-report questionnaire consisting of 29 items on a seven-point Likert scale designed to assess the extent of coherence [45] which represents the basic human orientation consisting of three components: comprehensibility, manageability, and meaningfulness. A higher score indicates a higher SOC. In the present study, an adapted Polish version of the SOC-29 was applied that has been proven to have high internal consistency with Cronbach's alpha coefficients ranging from 0.81 to 0.91 for the global scale and the subscales [46]. In the present study, the Cronbach's alpha score for the validated Polish version was 0.92.

2.4.8. Religiosity

The Centrality of Religiosity Scale (CRS) [18] was applied to assess religiosity. It comprises 15 items that categorize the respondents into not/marginally religious (0–15 points), extrinsically (16–44), and intrinsically religious (45–60). The CRS has been employed in more than 100 studies in 25 countries and has excellent psychometric properties (Cronbach's alpha = 0.92–0.96) [19]. The Cronbach's alpha score of the validated Polish version [47] in the study sample was 0.96.

2.5. Statistical Analysis

Data analyses were conducted with SPSS V. 21 (IBM, Armonk, NY, USA). Missing values in the questionnaires were replaced with the expectation-maximization algorithm (max. 20% missing data per questionnaire was accepted, otherwise the case was excluded from the analysis). The following descriptive statistics were computed to profile the sociodemographic and migration-specific sample characteristics and the lifestyle behaviors: means, standard deviations, ranges, and frequencies. To test for differences between women and men for categorical data, parametric tests (χ^2-tests or Fisher's exact test) were performed and for continuous data, t-tests for independent samples were computed. Pearson's correlation analyses among the main psychological variables were calculated prior to estimating regressions to test multicollinearity (by inspection of a pairwise correlation matrix). If the correlation coefficients were higher than 0.70 [48], one of the variables was excluded from the logistic regression models. Multicollinearity was also checked by calculating the variance inflation factors. Binary logistic regression analyses were conducted with the enter method to examine the influence of sociodemographic, migration- and health-related variables and religiosity on smoking, alcohol consumption, physical activity, and being overweight/obese. The three non-categorical lifestyle behaviors and the religiosity were dichotomized: frequency of alcohol (no/seldom consumption vs. all other categories), physical activity (no activity/<1 h vs. all other categories), BMI (under/normal weight vs. overweight/obesity) and religiosity (intrinsic vs. extrinsic/marginal). For the predictors, we report odds ratios (ORs) and 95% confidence intervals (CIs). A level of significance of $p < 0.05$ was predetermined.

3. Results

3.1. Sociodemographic and Migration-Specific Data

In Table 1, the main sociodemographic and migration-specific characteristics are presented for the total sample as well as for women and men of Polish origin living in Germany. Approximately two-thirds (64.6%) of the participants were women. Immigrant women were significantly younger than immigrant men ($p = 0.004$), were more likely to be unemployed ($p = 0.001$), to have a (very) low income ($p = 0.001$) but a higher education ($p < 0.001$), to have lived for a shorter period of time in Germany than the men ($p = 0.027$), and they more frequently had Polish citizenship ($p = 0.001$).

Table 1. Sociodemographic, socio-economic, and immigrant-specific sample characteristics, and differences by gender.

Variables		Total Sample (n = 257)	Women (n = 166)	Men (n = 91)	p-Value
Age	mean	42.8	41.0	46.2	
	SD *	14.0	13.6	14.0	0.004 [a]
	range	18-84	18-76	20-84	
Marital status	married	155 (60.3%)	94 (56.6%)	61 (67.0%)	
	single	68 (26.5%)	50 (30.1%)	18 (19.8%)	0.174 [b]
	divorced/widowed	33 (12.8%)	22 (13.3%)	11 (12.1%)	
	no data	1 (0.4%)	0	1 (1.1%)	
Education	low	76 (29.6%)	41 (24.7%)	35 (38.5%)	
	middle (university entrance diploma)	114 (44.4%)	69 (41.6%)	45 (49.5%)	<0.001 [b]
	high (university degree)	64 (24.9%)	54 (32.5%)	10 (11.0%)	
	no data	3 (1.2%)	2 (1.2%)	1 (1.1%)	

Table 1. Cont.

Variables		Total Sample (n = 257)	Women (n = 166)	Men (n = 91)	p-Value
Employment status	employed	149 (58.0%)	84 (50.6%)	65 (71.4%)	0.001 [b]
	unemployed (housewife/jobless/pensioner/student)	105 (40.9%)	80 (48.2%)	25 (27.5%)	
	no data	3 (1.2%)	2 (1.2%)	1 (1.1%)	
Subjectively perceived income	no income/very low/low	115 (44.7%)	88 (53.0%)	27 (29.7%)	0.001 [b]
	middle	131 (51.0%)	71 (42.8%)	60 (65.9%)	
	high/very high	9 (3.5%)	6 (3.6%)	3 (3.3%)	
	no data	2 (0.8%)	1 (0.6%)	1 (1.1%)	
Citizenship	German	100 (38.9%)	59 (35.5%)	41 (45.1%)	0.011 [b]
	Polish	76 (29.6%)	60 (36.1%)	16 (17.6%)	
	German and Polish	75 (29.2%)	45 (27.1%)	30 (33.0%)	
	no data	6 (2.3%)	2 (1.2%)	4 (4.4%)	
Length of residence in Germany	mean	18.0	17.2	19.3	0.027 [a]
	SD *	7.6	8.2	6.4	
	range	<1–53	<1–53	<1–29	
Language proficiency	excellent	37 (14.4%)	27 (16.3%)	10 (11.0%)	0.382 [b]
	very good	38 (14.8%)	28 (16.9%)	10 (11.0%)	
	good	96 (37.4%)	62 (37.3%)	34 (37.4%)	
	moderate	65 (25.3%)	37 (22.3%)	28 (30.8%)	
	little	11 (4.3%)	7 (4.2%)	4 (4.4%)	
	no data	10 (3.9%)	5 (3.0%)	5 (5.5%)	

* SD = Standard deviation; [a] t-test; [b] χ^2-test.

3.2. Frequency and Gender-Specific Differences Regarding Health-Related Lifestyle Behaviors and Religiosity Levels

Table 2 shows the frequency of smoking, alcohol consumption, physical activity, BMI, and religious categories in the examined sample. Immigrant men were less frequently smokers ($p = 0.022$) but more frequently were overweight/obese ($p < 0.001$) than immigrant women. Regarding the number of smoked cigarettes per day, the frequency of alcohol consumption, and the physical activity level as well as the level of religiosity, no significant gender-specific differences were found.

Table 2. Frequency of cigarette smoking, alcohol consumption, physical activity, body mass index (BMI), and religiosity categories in immigrants of Polish origin in Germany.

Variables	Total (n = 257)	Women (n = 166)	Men (n = 91)	p-Value
Smoking status, n (%)				
Non-smoker	177 (68.9)	106 (63.9)	71 (78.0)	0.022 [b]
Current smoker	79 (30.7)	59 (35.5)	20 (22.0)	
No data	1 (0.4)	1 (0.6)	-	
Smoked cigarettes per day *, n (%)				
<5	12 (15.2)	10 (16.9)	2 (10.0)	0.341 [c]
5–10	25 (31.6)	21 (35.6)	4 (20.0)	
11–20	32 (40.5)	22 (37.3)	10 (50.0)	
21–40	10 (12.7)	6 (10.2)	4 (20.0)	
Alcohol consumption, n (%)				
Never	14 (5.4)	9 (5.4)	5 (5.5)	0.278 [c]
Seldom	143 (55.6)	100 (60.2)	43 (47.3)	
Once a month	10 (3.9)	6 (3.6)	4 (4.4)	
Several times a month	46 (17.9)	25 (15.1)	21 (23.1)	
Once a week	27 (10.5)	18 (10.8)	9 (9.9)	
Several times a week	11 (4.3)	6 (3.6)	5 (5.5)	
Everyday	4 (1.6)	1 (0.6)	3 (3.3)	
No data	2 (0.8)	1 (0.6)	1 (1.1)	

Table 2. Cont.

Variables	Total (n = 257)	Women (n = 166)	Men (n = 91)	p-Value
Physical activity per week, n (%)				
None	100 (38.9)	68 (41.0)	32 (35.2)	
<1 h	63 (24.5)	40 (24.1)	23 (25.3)	
1–2 h	42 (16.3)	29 (17.5)	13 (14.3)	0.423 [b]
2–4 h	28 (10.9)	17 (10.2)	11 (12.1)	
>4 h	23 (8.9)	11 (6.6)	12 (13.2)	
No data	1 (0.4)	1 (0.6)	-	
BMI categories (kg/m^2), n (%)				
<18.5 (underweight)	5 (1.9)	5 (3.0)	0	
18.5–24.9 (normal weight)	125 (48.6)	104 (62.7)	21 (23.1)	<0.001 [c]
25.0–29.9 (overweight)	97 (37.7)	44 (26.5)	53 (58.2)	
≥30 (obesity)	24 (9.3)	8 (4.8)	16 (17.6)	
No data	6 (2.3)	5 (3.0)	1 (1.1)	
BMI, Mean (SD)	24.94 (3.90)	23.69 (3.60)	27.19 (3.40)	<0.001
Religiosity, n (%)				
Intrinsically religious	71 (27.6)	48 (28.9)	23 (25.3)	
Extrinsically religious	141 (54.9)	88 (53.0)	53 (58.2)	0.646 [b]
Not/marginally religious	39 (15.2)	27 (16.3)	12 (13.2)	
No data	6 (2.3)	3 (1.8)	3 (3.3)	
Mean (SD)	34.20 (15.0)	33.94 (15.44)	34.69 (14.24)	0.709 [a]

* n = 79 current smokers (59 women and 20 men); SD = Standard deviation; [a] t-test; [b] χ^2-test; [c] Fisher's exact test.

3.3. Correlations between Potential Psychological Predictors

To avoid multicollinearity, bivariate correlations were computed among the main psychological variables. The correlation coefficients are presented in Table 3. Correlation coefficients higher than 0.70 indicate potential multicollinearity [48]. In such cases, one of the two variables was not included in the logistic regression models. Two correlations showed a correlation coefficient >0.70: between depressive symptoms and sense of coherence (r = −0.74) and between anxiety and somatic symptoms (r = 0.73). Due to this fact, sense of coherence and somatic symptoms were excluded from the logistic regressions.

Table 3. Pearson's correlation coefficients between central study variables in immigrants of Polish origin in Germany.

Variables	1	2	3	4	5	6
1. Depressive symptoms (BDI)	1	0.61 ***	0.67 ***	0.33 ***	−0.74 ***	0.02
2. Anxiety symptoms (BAI)	-	1	0.73 ***	0.35 ***	−0.59 ***	0.11
3. Somatic symptoms (GBB-24)	-	-	1	0.37 ***	−0.57 ***	0.18 **
4. Perceived discrimination (self-constructed items)	-	-	-	1	−0.35 ***	0.04
5. Sense of Coherence (SOC-29)	-	-	-	-	1	0.05
6. Religiosity (CRS)	-	-	-	-	-	1

** $p \leq 0.01$, *** $p \leq 0.001$; BDI: Beck Depression Inventory, BAI: Beck Anxiety Inventory, GBB-24: Giessen Subjective Complaints List, SOC-29: Sense of Coherence Scale, CRS: Centrality of Religiosity Scale.

3.4. Predictors of Health-Related Lifestyle Behaviors

The odds ratios for the total sample are depicted in Table 4. After adjusting for various sociodemographic, migration, and health-related characteristics, intrinsic religiosity was significantly associated with a lower risk of being a smoker (OR = 0.34, CI = 0.15–0.76, p = 0.009) and also a lower risk of alcohol consumption (OR = 0.33, CI = 0.15–0.71, p = 0.005) in comparison with extrinsic/marginal/non-religiosity. No relationship was found between religiosity and physical activity. Highly religious immigrants were more likely to be overweight/obese than extrinsically, marginally, and non-religious immigrants (OR = 2.53, CI = 1.15–5.56, p = 0.021).

Table 4. Odds Ratios (OR) with 95% confidence intervals (CI) for smoking, alcohol consumption, physical activity, and overweight/obesity in immigrants of Polish origin.

Independent Variables	Smoking Predictors: OR [95% CI], p-Value	EV	Alcohol Predictors: OR [95% CI], p-Value	EV	Physical Activity Predictors: OR [95% CI], p-Value	EV	Weight/Obesity Predictors: OR [95% CI], p-Value	EV
Model 1: Socio-demographic variables	1. gender: 1.99 [1.06–3.74], p = 0.033 2. age: 0.99 [0.97–1.01], p = 0.381 3. education: 0.94 [0.50–1.76], p = 0.848 4. employment: 1.16 [0.63–2.14], p = 0.637 5. income: 0.96 [0.52–1.79], p = 0.900	3.6	1. gender: 0.44 [0.24–0.81], p = 0.008 2. age: 0.95 [0.93–0.98], p < 0.001 3. education: 1.08 [0.59–2.01], p = 0.797 4. employment: 1.43 [0.76–2.72], p = 0.271 5. income: 0.98 [0.53–1.83], p = 0.956	13.7	1. gender: 0.56 [0.30–1.02], p = 0.057 2. age: 0.96 [0.94–0.98], p < 0.001 3. education: 1.65 [0.92–2.99], p = 0.095 4. employment: 0.76 [0.42–1.40], p = 0.383 5. income: 1.60 [0.87–2.95], p = 0.132	12.4	1. gender: 0.15 [0.08–0.30], p < 0.001 2. age: 1.06 [1.04–1.09], p < 0.001 3. education: 0.74 [0.38–1.45], p = 0.382 4. employment: 1.07 [0.55–2.07], p = 0.846 5. income: 1.14 [0.59–2.22], p = 0.698	37.1
Model 2: Socio-demographic + migration-specific variables + discrimination	1. gender: 2.28 [1.17–4.47], p = 0.016 2. age: 0.97 [0.94–1.0], p = 0.082 3. education: 0.86 [0.45–1.67], p = 0.660 4. employment: 1.21 [0.61–2.41], p = 0.585 5. income: 1.05 [0.53–2.07], p = 0.892 6. length of residence: 1.05 [0.99–1.1], p = 0.112 7. language: 0.83 [0.57–1.22], p = 0.350 8. discrimination: 1.05 [0.95–1.16], p = 0.374	6.7	1. gender: 0.52 [0.28–0.98], p = 0.044 2. age: 0.94 [0.91–0.98], p = 0.001 3. education: 1.10 [0.57–2.13], p = 0.772 4. employment: 1.73 [0.84–3.54], p = 0.137 5. income: 0.86 [0.43–1.70], p = 0.665 6. length of residence: 1.05 [0.99–1.10], p = 0.087 7. language: 0.99 [0.68–1.44], p = 0.967 8. discrimination: 0.92 [0.83–1.03], p = 0.131	15.6	1. gender: 0.60 [0.31–1.14], p = 0.115 2. age: 0.97 [0.94–1.0], p = 0.072 3. education: 1.77 [0.94–3.31], p = 0.075 4. employment: 0.82 [0.42–1.63], p = 0.575 5. income: 1.42 [0.72–2.79], p = 0.306 6. length of residence: 1.01 [0.96–1.07], p = 0.710 7. language: 1.34 [0.93–1.95], p = 0.119 8. discrimination: 1.01 [0.92–1.12], p = 0.787	14.0	1. gender: 0.14 [0.07–0.28], p < 0.001 2. age: 1.05 [1.01–1.09], p = 0.010 3. education: 0.70 [0.34–1.43], p = 0.330 4. employment: 0.99 [0.47–2.08], p = 0.970 5. income: 1.29 [0.62–2.71], p = 0.500 6. length of residence: 1.02 [0.96–1.08], p = 0.512 7. language: 0.91 [0.60–1.38], p = 0.653 8. discrimination: 1.0 [0.89–1.12], p = 0.962	38.3
Model 3: Socio-demographic + migration-specific variables + discrimination + health-related variables	1. gender: 2.3 [1.14–4.64], p = 0.019 2. age: 0.97 [0.94–1.01], p = 0.091 3. education: 1.03 [0.52–2.06], p = 0.933 4. employment: 1.26 [0.63–2.55], p = 0.515 5. income: 1.13 [0.56–2.26], p = 0.738 6. length of residence: 1.05 [0.99–1.11], p = 0.106 7. language: 0.84 [0.57–1.24], p = 0.386 8. discrimination: 1.03 [0.92–1.15], p = 0.621 9. depressive symptoms: 1.06 [1.01–1.12], p = 0.025 10. anxiety symptoms: 0.98 [0.94–1.02], p = 0.241	9.1	1. gender: 0.44 [0.23–0.87], p = 0.017 2. age: 0.94 [0.91–0.98], p = 0.001 3. education: 1.03 [0.52–2.03], p = 0.929 4. employment: 1.81 [0.87–3.76], p = 0.110 5. income: 0.91 [0.45–1.83], p = 0.793 6. length of residence: 1.05 [0.99–1.10], p = 0.095 7. language: 1.01 [0.70–1.47], p = 0.955 8. discrimination: 0.89 [0.79–1.0], p = 0.053 9. depressive symptoms: 0.99 [0.94–1.04], p = 0.666 10. anxiety symptoms: 1.04 [1.0–1.08], p = 0.068	17.8	1. gender: 0.54 [0.28–1.06], p = 0.074 2. age: 0.97 [0.94–1.01], p = 0.110 3. education: 1.61 [0.84–3.08], p = 0.155 4. employment: 0.84 [0.42–1.69], p = 0.626 5. income: 1.33 [0.66–2.65], p = 0.425 6. length of residence: 1.01 [0.95–1.06], p = 0.836 7. language: 1.36 [0.94–1.97], p = 0.108 8. discrimination: 1.01 [0.90–1.13], p = 0.867 9. depressive symptoms: 0.96 [0.91–1.01], p = 0.133 10. anxiety symptoms: 1.03 [0.99–1.07], p = 0.213	15.1	1. gender: 0.13 [0.06–0.26], p < 0.001 2. age: 1.05 [1.01–1.09], p = 0.013 3. education: 0.83 [0.39–1.75], p = 0.618 4. employment: 1.03 [0.48–2.21], p = 0.946 5. income: 1.51 [0.71–3.24], p = 0.288 6. length of residence: 1.02 [0.96–1.09], p = 0.460 7. language: 0.92 [0.60–1.40], p = 0.682 8. discrimination: 0.97 [0.86–1.10], p = 0.656 9. depressive symptoms: 1.08 [1.02–1.15], p = 0.013 10. anxiety symptoms: 0.98 [0.94–1.03], p = 0.46	40.9

Table 4. Cont.

Independent Variables	Smoking Predictors *: OR [95% CI], p-Value	EV #	Alcohol Predictors: OR [95% CI], p-Value	EV	Physical Activity Predictors: OR [95% CI], p-Value	EV	Weight/Obesity Predictors: OR [95% CI], p-Value	EV
Model 4: Socio-demographic + migration-specific variable + discrimination + health-related variable + religiosity	1. **gender: 2.57 [1.25–5.29], p = 0.01** 2. age: 0.98 [0.95–1.02], p = 0.398 3. education: 1.07 [0.53–2.16], p = 0.849 4. employment: 1.22 [0.59–2.51], p = 0.599 5. income: 1.14 [0.55–2.35], p = 0.721 6. length of residence: 1.03 [0.97–1.09], p = 0.294 7. language: 0.83 [0.57–1.23], p = 0.363 8. discrimination: 1.03 [0.91–1.15], p = 0.682 9. **depressive symptoms: 1.05 [1.0–1.11], p = 0.049** 10. anxiety symptoms: 0.98 [0.95–1.02], p = 0.418 11. **religiosity: 0.34 [0.15–0.76], p = 0.009**	13.7	1. **gender: 0.43 [0.22–0.86], p = 0.017** 2. **age: 0.95 [0.92–0.99], p = 0.012** 3. education: 1.11 [0.56–2.21], p = 0.772 4. employment: 1.83 [0.86–3.91], p = 0.117 5. income: 0.89 [0.43–1.83], p = 0.746 6. length of residence: 1.03 [0.98–1.09], p = 0.247 7. language: 1.0 [0.68–1.46], p = 0.985 8. **discrimination: 0.88 [0.78–1.0], p = 0.042** 9. depressive symptoms: 0.98 [0.93–1.03], p = 0.430 10. **anxiety symptoms: 1.05 [1.0–1.09], p = 0.032** 11. **religiosity: 0.33 [0.15–0.71], p = 0.005**	22.2	1. gender: 0.56 [0.28–1.09], p = 0.089 2. age: 0.97 [0.94–1.01], p = 0.090 3. education: 1.57 [0.82–3.02], p = 0.176 4. employment: 0.84 [0.42–1.70], p = 0.627 5. income: 1.35 [0.67–2.74], p = 0.405 6. length of residence: 1.01 [0.96–1.06], p = 0.769 7. language: 1.35 [0.93–1.96], p = 0.115 8. discrimination: 1.01 [0.90–1.14], p = 0.820 9. depressive symptoms: 0.96 [0.91–1.01], p = 0.153 10. anxiety symptoms: 1.03 [0.98–1.07], p = 0.234 11. religiosity: 1.23 [0.61–2.47], p = 0.561	15.0	1. **gender: 0.11 [0.05–0.24], p < 0.001** 2. **age: 1.04 [1.0–1.08], p = 0.047** 3. education: 0.85 [0.39–1.82], p = 0.668 4. employment: 1.25 [0.56–2.76], p = 0.587 5. income: 1.18 [0.54–2.60], p = 0.678 6. length of residence: 1.04 [0.97–1.10], p = 0.276 7. language: 0.91 [0.59–1.41], p = 0.672 8. discrimination: 0.97 [0.85–1.11], p = 0.668 9. **depressive symptoms: 1.09 [1.02–1.15], p = 0.01** 10. anxiety symptoms: 0.98 [0.93–1.02], p = 0.331 11. **religiosity: 2.53 [1.15–5.56], p = 0.02**	44.0

Model 1: adjusted for age, gender (men (ref.) vs. women), education (low (ref.) vs. middle/high), employment status (unemployed (ref.) vs. employed), subjectively perceived income (no income/very low/low (ref.) vs. middle/high/very high); Model 2: additionally adjusted for length of residence in Germany, language proficiency (higher scores = higher proficiency); discrimination (higher scores = higher discrimination); Model 3: additionally adjusted for depressive and anxiety symptoms; Model 4: additionally adjusted for religiosity (extrinsic/marginal/non-religious (ref.) vs. intrinsic); * significant predictors are marked in bold; # EV: explanation of variance (%).

Other significant predictors for smoking were gender and depression: women and more depressed individuals had a higher risk of being a smoker. Concerning alcohol consumption, younger age, masculine gender, lower discrimination levels, and higher anxiety were further significant predictors. For physical activity, significant tendencies were only detected for gender ($p = 0.089$) and age ($p = 0.09$): older individuals and women were more likely to be physically inactive. In the full model for overweight/obesity, gender, depression, and age were also significant predictors: masculine gender, older age and a higher depression level were risk factors for being overweight/obese. The explanation of variance for the full model was 13.7% for smoking, 22.2% for alcohol consumption, 15.0% for physical activity, and 44.0% for overweight/obesity, respectively.

4. Discussion

To the best of our knowledge, this is the first study to examine the association between religiosity and various indicators of health-related behaviors in immigrants of Polish origin.

The main result of the present investigation is the significantly lower risk of being a current smoker and for drinking alcohol in highly religious individuals in comparison with less religious or non-religious people. This result is consistent with findings from previous studies with immigrant samples ([23–28]) and with the results of the Polish General Social Survey ($n = 1526$) [49] and the Survey of Health, Ageing, and Retirement in Europe ($n = 16,557$) ([50]). Several possible explanations can be provided for the protective role of religiosity against substance consumption. It can be postulated, in accordance with Huber [18], that highly religious people have internalized the moral norms, values, and believes of their religion. Thus, they are more likely to also follow lifestyle-related religious prohibitions with detrimental effects to their health such as smoking and drinking alcohol. Furthermore, it can be postulated that the sense of meaning and control in life provided by a religion as well as social support from the religious community can contribute to the successful management of problems and adverse life circumstances in high religious individuals, so they do not use nicotine or alcohol as self-medications for emotion regulation. A further possible explanation is a stress-reducing effect of religious practices such as prayer, meditation, worships, etc., which is supported by several studies [51]. Thus, highly religious involved people who regularly perform these practices can benefit from them as a "by-product". In addition, the internalized attitudes of highly religious people, such as forgiveness or compassion, are related to decreased unhealthy feelings of anger and hostility and may also have a stress-reducing impact [52]. Religiosity may also influence the personality towards self-control and emotional stability/ positive affectivity [20]. Finally, it could be possible that the positive emotions associated with religiosity make artificial "mood lifters" such as smoking and alcohol superfluous.

Our results suggest that a high level of religiosity may not have the same beneficial effects on physical activity and on weight as it does on smoking and drinking. A possible reason for this is that the Catholic religion has a more negative attitude towards substance abuse than towards inactivity and being overweight. In particular, alcohol abuse is regularly denounced, and abstinence is promoted by the Catholic Church. Different religious programs are promoted by priests, such as total abstinence in August for adults or total abstinence for adolescences for a year. Such large engagement for other (un)healthy lifestyle behaviors is not realized.

Highly religious people showed an increased risk of being overweight/obese. This result was also demonstrated in a study with immigrants from the USA [29]. One explanation could be that high religiosity is associated with a lower risk of being a smoker. As a result, highly religious people cannot benefit from nicotine as an appetite suppressant. According to the review on religion and bodyweight mentioned above [30], the relationship between religiosity and higher body weight is still unclear. Other determinants not examined in this study could have mediated the association between religiosity and being overweight/obese and should be explored in future investigations to allow a better understanding of the underlying mechanisms.

An important finding of our study is the high smoking rate (35.5%) in women. Also, the regression model provided support for the conclusion that immigrant women of Polish origin are a risk group for cigarette smoking. This gender difference found in our study does not match trends, as (immigrant) men are more likely to smoke than (immigrant) women [53–55]. A possible explanation for the high rate of tobacco use in immigrant women is that tobacco consumption may be used as a strategy to deal with (acculturative) stress, various burdens, and multiple experiences of discrimination (as women, immigrants, and frequently low-paid workers). In addition, the high probability of women to be smokers may be partially explained by the level of acculturation. An increased smoking prevalence was observed to be associated with increased acculturation among Hispanic women and Asian women in the USA [56,57]. In our sample, more than 70% of the immigrant women assessed their own German language proficiency (one of the best indicators of acculturation) as being at least as good and thus can be regarded as highly acculturated and hence, more strongly influenced by practices of the host society than less acculturated individuals [53]. As a result, their smoking patterns may converge to those of the host society, as has been shown for resettlers from the Former Soviet Union in Germany [58]. This could also be partially postulated for the women in the present study: a lower smoking prevalence was observed for women in Poland (23% [54]) than those in our study (35.5%). However, among the immigrant women, a higher proportion of smokers was found than among women in Germany (27% [55]). Thus, other influencing factors on the high smoking rate and the increased risk of being a smoker in immigrant women as compared with the men can be assumed and these should be investigated in future research.

Another important gender-related difference in this study was the significantly higher proportion of overweight/obese men than women. The male gender was also found to be a risk factor for being overweight/obese in the regression analysis. The higher probability of being overweight/obese among immigrant men is in line with the results of some prior studies [29,59], while other studies reported a higher prevalence in immigrated women in relation to men [60]. One plausible explanation for the increased odds ratio of overweight/obese men in our investigation may be the high prevalence of smokers among women. Smoking has been shown to be negatively linked to the probability of obesity in different immigrant groups in the USA [61]. The high odds for being overweight/obese in men could also be explained by their lower education level as compared with the women. The protective function of high educational attendance has been demonstrated in immigrants [61] as well as in populations of different countries [62]. It may contribute to a healthier lifestyle in the form of, e.g., healthier dietary practices.

It is notable that a large proportion of our sample are physically inactive and are also overweight/obese. Almost two-thirds of the immigrants do not participate in any sport activity or participate for less than 1 h per week. According to the WHO, at least 150 min of moderate intensity physical activity per week is recommended to receive benefits on health [63]. However, less than 20% of the examined immigrants stated that they follow this recommendation. In the multivariable analysis, there was a tendency for higher age and female gender to be associated with an increased risk of physical inactivity. The poor health of the older adults could prevent them from sport participation [64]. Women may be involved in less sport activities because of their multiple roles, stressors, and responsibilities meaning they have less time for leisure activities.

In the present study, high levels of depressive or anxiety symptoms were associated with a higher risk of smoking, alcohol consumption, and being overweight/obese. This finding is in line with empirical evidence supporting the association between worse lifestyles and depressive and anxiety symptoms [65]. It can be postulated that people with mental health problems use smoking, drinking, and/or eating as dysfunctional "coping strategies" against negative mood states.

Strengths and Limitations

The primary strength of the present study is that we applied a multidimensional, well conceptualized, reliable, and valid measurement of religiosity in a relatively large, religiously homogenous population of immigrants of Polish origin. Furthermore, we were able to include individuals who are difficult to identify for surveys (immigrants of Polish origin with German citizenship) and people who are often excluded from participation in studies in Germany because of insufficient language competencies (immigrants of Polish origin with insufficient German language proficiency). In addition, we included many potential moderator factors of religiosity in the regression models; thus, we were able to control for several confounding variables when examining the impact of religiosity on the indicators of health-related lifestyle behaviors.

The results of our study should be interpreted in light of some limitations. The cross-sectional design of the study did not allow causal conclusions regarding the influence of the variables examined on the health-related behavior to be drawn. Prospective studies are therefore needed to investigate the associations found in the study and to detect underlying mechanisms. Another limitation was the low response rate (56.3%), which may have led to a selection bias, possibly with healthier immigrants being included in the sample. The "snowball method" could also have biased the results. Thus, the findings should be viewed as exploratory and cannot be generalized to the population of all immigrants of Polish origin living in Germany or to other ethnic minorities. Moreover, the non-objective, self-reported estimates of the four health-related lifestyle behaviors may also have been a source of bias because (some) respondents may not have reported the real data due to social desirability or shame (especially for body weight or the frequency of alcohol consumption). Studies indicate that women may underestimate their body weight, while men may overestimate their height [66]. Finally, the item used to measure the physical activity (sport) is not precise and thus is of questionable validity. Valid measures such as MVPA (moderate to vigorous physical activity) should be applied in future research to ensure valid evaluation of physical activity levels. Future studies should examine the association between religiosity and health-related behavior in representative samples that also include second generation immigrants, taking into account other important psychological (e.g., self-esteem), psychosocial (e.g., social support), lifestyle (e.g., dietary habits) or acculturation-related (e.g., acculturative stress) variables that were not examined in this study, and separate analyses should be performed for men and women.

5. Conclusions

Due to the limitations in the study design (cross-sectional, snowball method) and the low response rate, the findings should be interpreted with caution. Several conclusions can be drawn from the results that provide important implications for public health. First, our findings indicate that high religiosity can be regarded as a protective factor against tobacco and alcohol consumption in immigrants of Polish origin. This should be considered in prevention programs. Secondly, immigrant Polish women present a risk group for smoking and should be targeted in preventive gender and immigration-specific anti-smoking programs. Thirdly, highly religious people and men are at a higher risk of being overweight/obese. Religious leaders and local religious communities should therefore be involved in preventive programs to promote not only abstinence from smoking and drinking but also a healthy lifestyle with physical activity and a healthy diet. Fourth, depressive and anxiety symptoms were shown to increase the likelihood for smoking, drinking, and being overweight/obese. Psychological support should be offered to immigrants with mental health problems to avoid dysfunctional coping with cigarettes or alcohol. Finally, religiosity can still be regarded as the "forgotten factor" in the research of (mental) health [21], so it remains a desideratum for researchers and healthcare providers to take this variable into account in their studies and clinical practice.

Author Contributions: Conceptualization, E.M. and Y.E.; Data curation, E.M.; Formal analysis, E.M.; Methodology, E.M. and Y.E.; Project administration, E.M.; Supervision, Y.E.; Validation, Y.E.; Visualization, E.M.; Writing—original draft, E.M.; Writing—review and editing, E.M. and Y.E.

Funding: This research received no external funding.

Conflicts of Interest: The authors declare no conflict of interest.

References

1. Global Index of Religion and Atheism 2012. Available online: https://sidmennt.is/wp-content/uploads/Gallup-International-um-tr%C3%BA-og-tr%C3%BAaleysi-2012.pdf (accessed on 17 September 2018).
2. Central Statistical Office. National, Ethnic, Language and Religious Structure of the Population in Poland. National Population and Housing Census 2011. Available online: https://stat.gov.pl/files/gfx/portalinformacyjny/pl/defaultaktualnosci/5670/22/1/1/struktura_narodowo-etniczna.pdf (accessed on 17 September 2018).
3. Secretariat of the German Bishops' Conference. Eckdaten Kirchliches Leben 2016—Deutsche Bischofskonferenz. Available online: https://www.dbk.de/fileadmin/redaktion/diverse_downloads/presse_2017/2017-121a-Flyer-Eckdaten-Kirchenstatistik-2016.pdf (accessed on 17 September 2018).
4. Morawa, E. Patriots, Masters of Survival, Chaotic Types?—Introduction into the Specifics of the Polish Identity and Culture. In *Clinical Intercultural Psychotherapy*; Erim, Y., Ed.; Kohlhammer: Stuttgart, Germany, 2009; pp. 263–277.
5. Centre for Public Opinion Research. The Membership of the Poles in Religious Associations and Communities. Available online: https://www.cbos.pl/SPISKOM.POL/2017/K_084_17.PDF (accessed on 17 September 2018).
6. German Bishops' Conference. Catholic Church in Germany. Numbers and Facts 2016/2017. Available online: https://www.dbk.de/fileadmin/redaktion/Zahlen%20und%20Fakten/Kirchliche%20Statistik/Allgemein_-_Zahlen_und_Fakten/AH294_Zahlen-und-Fakten-2016-2017_web.pdf (accessed on 17 September 2018).
7. Federal Statistical Office. Population and Employment. Available online: https://www.destatis.de/DE/Publikationen/Thematisch/Bevoelkerung/MigrationIntegration/Migrationshintergrund2010220147004.pdf?__blob=publicationFile (accessed on 17 September 2018).
8. Embassy of the Republic of Poland in Berlin. Available online: http://berlin.msz.gov.pl/de/bilaterale_zusammenarbeit/auslandspolen_127/ (accessed on 17 September 2018).
9. Morawa, E.; Erim, Y. Health-related quality of life and sense of coherence among Polish immigrants in Germany and indigenous Poles. *Transcult. Psychiatry* **2015**, *52*, 376–395. [CrossRef] [PubMed]
10. Koenig, H.G. Research on religion, spirituality, and mental health: A review. *Can. J. Psychiatry* **2009**, *54*, 283–291. [CrossRef] [PubMed]
11. Grom, B. Religion. In *Lexicon of Theology and the Church*; Kasper, W., Ed.; Herder-Verlag: Freiburg im Breisgau, Germany, 1999.
12. Koenig, H.G.; MacCullough, M.E.; Larson, D.B. *Handbook of Religion and Health*; Oxford University Press: New York, NY, USA, 1998.
13. Pargament, K.I. *The Psychology of Religion and Coping: Theory, Research, Practice*; Guilford Press: New York, NY, USA, 1997.
14. Hill, P.C.; Hood, R.W. *Measures of Religiosity*; Religious Education Press: Birmingham, AL, USA, 1999.
15. Allport, G.W. *The Individual and His Religion: A Psychological Interpretation*; Mac Milan: New York, NY, USA, 1950.
16. Glock, C.Y. On the study of religious commitment. *Relig. Educ.* **1962**, *57*, 98–110. [CrossRef]
17. Donahue, M.J. Intrinsic and extrinsic religiousness: Review and meta-analysis. *J. Pers. Soc. Psychol.* **1985**, *48*, 400–419. [CrossRef]
18. Huber, S. *Centrality and Content—A New Multidimensional Measurement of Religiosity*; Leske and Budrich: Opladen, Germany, 2003.
19. Huber, S.; Huber, O.W. The Centrality of Religiosity Scale (CRS). *Religions* **2012**, *3*, 710–724. [CrossRef]
20. Moreira-Almeida, A.; Neto, F.L.; Koenig, H.G. Religiousness and mental health: A review. *Rev. Bras. Psiquiatr.* **2006**, *28*, 242–250. [CrossRef] [PubMed]
21. Bonelli, R.M.; Koenig, H.G. Mental disorders, religion and spirituality 1990 to 2010: A systematic evidence-based review. *J. Relig. Health* **2013**, *52*, 657–673. [CrossRef] [PubMed]
22. AbdAleati, N.S.; Mohd Zaharim, N.; Mydin, Y.O. Religiousness and Mental Health: Systematic Review Study. *J. Relig. Health* **2016**, *55*, 1929–1937. [CrossRef] [PubMed]
23. Baron-Epel, O.; Havlv-Messika, A.; Tamır, D.; Nıtzan-Kaluski, D.; Green, M. Multiethnic differences in smoking in Israel: Pooled analysis from three national surveys. *Eur. J. Public Health* **2004**, *14*, 384–389. [CrossRef] [PubMed]

24. Patel, M.; Mistry, R.; Maxwell, A.E.; Divan, H.A.; McCarthy, W.J. Contextual Factors Related to Conventional and Traditional Tobacco Use Among California Asian Indian Immigrants. *J. Community Health* **2018**, *43*, 280–290. [CrossRef] [PubMed]
25. Shapiro, E. Places of Habits and Hearts: Church Attendance and Latino Immigrant Health Behaviors in the United States. *J. Racial Ethn. Health Disparities* **2018**. [CrossRef] [PubMed]
26. Daniel-Ulloa, J.; Reboussin, B.A.; Gilbert, P.A.; Mann, L.; Alonzo, J.; Downs, M.; Rhodes, S.D. Predictors of Heavy Episodic Drinking and Weekly Drunkenness Among Immigrant Latinos in North Carolina. *Am. J. Mens Health* **2014**, *8*, 339–348. [CrossRef] [PubMed]
27. Sanchez, M.; Dillon, F.R.; Concha, M.; De La Rosa, M. The Impact of Religious Coping on the Acculturative Stress and Alcohol Use of Recent Latino Immigrants. *J. Relig. Health* **2015**, *54*, 1986–2004. [CrossRef] [PubMed]
28. Meyers, J.L.; Brown, Q.; Grant, B.F.; Hasin, D. Religiosity, race/ethnicity, and alcohol use behaviors in the United States. *Psychol. Med.* **2017**, *47*, 103–114. [CrossRef] [PubMed]
29. Bharmal, N.; Kaplan, R.M.; Shapiro, M.F.; Kagawa-Singer, M.; Wong, M.D.; Mangione, C.M.; Divan, H.; McCarthy, W.J. The association of religiosity with overweight/obese body mass index among Asian Indian immigrants in California. *Prev. Med.* **2013**, *57*, 315–321. [CrossRef] [PubMed]
30. Yeary, K.H.K.; Sobal, J.; Wethington, E. Religion and body weight: A review of quantitative studies. *Obes. Rev.* **2017**, *18*, 1210–1222. [CrossRef] [PubMed]
31. Klein, C.; Albani, C. Religiousness and mental health. An overview about findings, conclusions, and consequences for clinical practice. *Psychiatr. Prax.* **2007**, *34*, 58–65. [PubMed]
32. Zimmer, Z.; Jagger, C.; Chiu, C.T.; Ofstedal, M.B.; Rojo, F.; Saito, Y. Spirituality, religiosity, aging and health in global perspective: A review. *SSM Popul. Health* **2016**, *2*, 373–381. [CrossRef] [PubMed]
33. Newberg, A.B.; d'Aquili, E. *Why God Won't Go Away: Brain Science and the Biology of Belief*; Ballantine Books: New York, NY, USA, 2001.
34. Seybold, K.S. Physiological mechanisms involved in religiosity/spirituality and health. *J. Behav. Med.* **2007**, *30*, 303–309. [CrossRef] [PubMed]
35. Morawa, E.; Senf, W.; Erim, Y. Mental health of Polish immigrants compared to that of the Polish and German populations. *Z. Psychosom. Med. Psychother.* **2013**, *59*, 209–217. [PubMed]
36. Morawa, E.; Erim, Y. The interrelation between perceived discrimination, depressiveness, and health related quality of life in immigrants of Turkish and Polish origin. *Psychiatr. Prax.* **2014**, *41*, 200–207. [PubMed]
37. Morawa, E.; Erim, Y. Traumatic Events, Posttraumatic Stress Disorder and Utilization of Psychotherapy in Immigrants of Polish Origin in Germany. *Psychother. Psychosom. Med. Psychol.* **2016**, *66*, 369–376. [PubMed]
38. Lamnek, S. *Qualitative Social Research*, 5th ed.; Beltz: Weinheim, Germany, 2010.
39. World Health Organization. Body Mass Index-BMI. Available online: http://www.euro.who.int/en/health-topics/disease-prevention/nutrition/a-healthy-lifestyle/body-mass-index-bmi (accessed on 17 September 2018).
40. Beck, A.T.; Ward, C.H.; Mendelson, M.; Mock, J.; Erbaugh, J. An inventory for measuring depression. *Arch. Gen. Psychiatry* **1961**, *4*, 561–571. [CrossRef] [PubMed]
41. Drosdzol, A.; Skrzypulec, V. Depression and anxiety among Polish infertile couples—An evaluative prevalence study. *J. Psychosom. Obstet. Gynaecol.* **2009**, *30*, 11–20. [CrossRef] [PubMed]
42. Beck, A.T.; Epstein, N.; Brown, G.; Steer, R.A. An inventory for measuring clinical anxiety: Psychometric properties. *J. Consult. Clin. Psychol.* **1988**, *56*, 893–897. [CrossRef] [PubMed]
43. Gunzelmann, T.; Schumacher, J.; Brähler, E. Physical complaints in old age: Standardization of the Giessen Complaint Questionnaire GBB-24 in over 60-year-old patients. *Z. Gerontol. Geriatr.* **1996**, *29*, 110–118. [PubMed]
44. Wittig, U.; Lindert, J.; Merbach, M.; Brähler, E. Mental health of patients from different cultures in Germany. *Eur. Psychiatry* **2008**, *23*, 28–35. [CrossRef]
45. Antonovsky, A. *Unraveling the Mystery of Health: How People Manage Stress and Stay Well*; Jossey-Bass: San Francisco, CA, USA, 1987.
46. Dudek, B.; Makowska, Z. Psychometric characteristics of the Orientation to Life Questionnaire measuring sense of coherence. *Pol. Psychol. Bull.* **1993**, *24*, 309–318.
47. Zarzycka, B. Centrality of Religiosity Scale by S. Huber. *Rocz. Psychol.* **2007**, *10*, 133–157.
48. Tabachnick, B.; Fidell, L. *Using Multivariate Statistics*, 5th ed.; Allyn & Bacon/Pearson Education: Boston, MA, USA, 2007.

49. Szaflarski, M. Gender, self-reported health, and health-related lifestyles in Poland. *Health Care Women Int.* **2001**, *22*, 207–227. [CrossRef] [PubMed]
50. Linardakis, M.; Papadaki, A.; Smpokos, E.; Sarri, K.; Vozikaki, M.; Philalithis, A. Are religiosity and prayer use related with multiple behavioural risk factors for chronic diseases in European adults aged 50+ years? *Public Health* **2015**, *129*, 436–443. [CrossRef] [PubMed]
51. Goncalves, J.P.; Lucchetti, G.; Menezes, P.R.; Vallada, H. Religious and spiritual interventions in mental health care: A systematic review and meta-analysis of randomized controlled clinical trials. *Psychol. Med.* **2015**, *45*, 2937–2949. [CrossRef] [PubMed]
52. Lutjen, L.J.; Silton, N.R.; Flannelly, K.J. Religion, forgiveness, hostility and health: A structural equation analysis. *J. Relig. Health* **2012**, *51*, 468–478. [CrossRef] [PubMed]
53. Kabir, Z.; Clarke, V.; Currie, L.M.; Zatonski, W.; Clancy, L. Smoking characteristics of Polish immigrants in Dublin. *BMC Public Health* **2008**, *8*, 428. [CrossRef] [PubMed]
54. Centre for Public Opinion Research. Attitudes towards Smoking. Available online: https://www.cbos.pl/SPISKOM.POL/2012/K_107_12.PDF (accessed on 17 September 2018).
55. Robert Koch Institut. Health in Germany. Available online: https://www.rki.de/DE/Content/Gesundheitsmonitoring/Gesundheitsberichterstattung/GesInDtld/gesundheit_in_deutschland_2015.pdf?__blob=publicationFile (accessed on 17 September 2018).
56. Bethel, J.W.; Schenker, M.B. Acculturation and smoking patterns among Hispanics: A review. *Am. J. Prev. Med.* **2005**, *29*, 143–148. [CrossRef] [PubMed]
57. Choi, S.; Rankin, S.; Stewart, A.; Oka, R. Effects of acculturation on smoking behavior in Asian Americans: A meta-analysis. *J. Cardiovasc. Nurs.* **2008**, *23*, 67–73. [CrossRef] [PubMed]
58. Reiss, K.; Spallek, J.; Razum, O. 'Imported risk' or 'health transition'? Smoking prevalence among ethnic German immigrants from the Former Soviet Union by duration of stay in Germany—Analysis of microcensus data. *Int. J. Equity Health* **2010**, *9*, 15. [CrossRef] [PubMed]
59. Petrelli, A.; Di Napoli, A.; Rossi, A.; Spizzichino, D.; Costanzo, G.; Perez, M. Overweight and obesity among adult immigrant populations resident in Italy. *Epidemiol. Prev.* **2017**, *41*, 26–32. [PubMed]
60. Gele, A.A.; Mbalilaki, A.J. Overweight and obesity among African immigrants in Oslo. *BMC Res. Notes* **2013**, *6*, 119. [CrossRef] [PubMed]
61. Wen, M.; Kowaleski-Jones, L.; Fan, J.X. Ethnic-immigrant disparities in total and abdominal obesity in the US. *Am. J. Health Behav.* **2013**, *37*, 807–818. [CrossRef] [PubMed]
62. Devaux, M.; Sassi, F. Social inequalities in obesity and overweight in 11 OECD countries. *Eur. J. Public Health* **2013**, *23*, 464–469. [CrossRef] [PubMed]
63. World Health Organization. Global Recommendations on Physical Activity for Health. Available online: http://apps.who.int/iris/bitstream/handle/10665/44399/9789241599979_eng.pdf;jsessionid=F025A36BD5BAD47FFD88DDA6564F25E3?sequence=1 (accessed on 17 September 2018).
64. Jenkin, C.R.; Eime, R.M.; Westerbeek, H.; O'Sullivan, G.; van Uffelen, J.G.Z. Sport and ageing: A systematic review of the determinants and trends of participation in sport for older adults. *BMC Public Health* **2017**, *17*, 976. [CrossRef] [PubMed]
65. Penninx, B.W. Depression and cardiovascular disease: Epidemiological evidence on their linking mechanisms. *Neurosci. Biobehav. Rev.* **2017**, *74*, 277–286. [CrossRef] [PubMed]
66. Nyholm, M.; Gullberg, B.; Merlo, J.; Lundqvist-Persson, C.; Rastam, L.; Lindblad, U. The validity of obesity based on self-reported weight and height: Implications for population studies. *Obesity* **2007**, *15*, 197–208. [CrossRef] [PubMed]

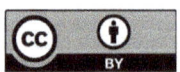

© 2018 by the authors. Licensee MDPI, Basel, Switzerland. This article is an open access article distributed under the terms and conditions of the Creative Commons Attribution (CC BY) license (http://creativecommons.org/licenses/by/4.0/).

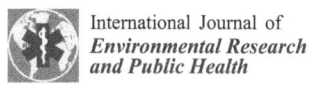

Review

Effectiveness of Screening and Treatment Approaches for Schistosomiasis and Strongyloidiasis in Newly-Arrived Migrants from Endemic Countries in the EU/EEA: A Systematic Review

Eric N. Agbata [1,2,*], Rachael L. Morton [3], Zeno Bisoffi [4,5], Emmanuel Bottieau [6], Christina Greenaway [7], Beverley-A. Biggs [8,9], Nadia Montero [10], Anh Tran [3], Nick Rowbotham [3], Ingrid Arevalo-Rodriguez [10,11], Daniel T. Myran [12], Teymur Noori [13], Pablo Alonso-Coello [14], Kevin Pottie [15] and Ana Requena-Méndez [16]

1. Faculty of Health Science, University of Roehampton London, London SW15 5PU, UK
2. Department of Paediatrics, Obstetrics, Gynaecology and Preventive Medicine, Universitat Autònoma de Barcelona, Bellaterra, 08193 Barcelona, Spain
3. NHMRC Clinical Trials Centre, University of Sydney, Camperdown, NSW 2050, Australia; Rachael.morton@ctc.usyd.edu.au (R.L.M.); anh.tran@ctc.usyd.edu.au (A.T.); rowbothamn@gmail.com (N.R.)
4. Centre for Tropical Diseases (CTD), IRCCS Sacro Cuore Don Calabria Negrar, Negrar, 37024 Verona, Italy; zeno.bisoffi@sacrocuore.it
5. Department of Diagnostics and Public Health, University of Verona, 37134 Verona, Italy
6. Department of Clinical Sciences, Institute of Tropical Medicine, 155 Nationalestraat, 2000 Antwerp, Belgium; EBottieau@itg.be
7. Division of Infectious Diseases and Clinical Epidemiology, Sir Mortimer B. Davis-Jewish General Hospital, McGill University, Montreal, QC H3A 0G4, Canada; ca.greenaway@mcgill.ca
8. Department of Medicine at the Doherty Institute, University of Melbourne, Parkville, VIC 3010, Australia; babiggs@unimelb.edu.au
9. Victorian Infectious Diseases Service, The Royal Melbourne Hospital RMH, Parkville, VIC 3050, Australia
10. Centro de Investigación en Salud Pública y Epidemiología Clínica (CISPEC), Facultad de Ciencias de la Salud Eugenio Espejo, Universidad Tecnológica Equinoccial, Quito 170509, Ecuador; nadiamonteromd@gmail.com (N.M.); inarev7@yahoo.com (I.A.-R.)
11. Clinical Biostatistics Unit, Hospital Universitario Ramon y Cajal (IRYCIS); CIBER Epidemiology and Public Health (CIBERESP), 28034 Madrid, Spain
12. Bruyere Research Institute, University of Ottawa, Ottawa, ON K1N 6N5, Canada; daniel.myran@gmail.com
13. European Centre for Disease Prevention and Control, Gustav III: s Boulevard 40, 169 73 Solna, Sweden; Teymur.Noori@ecdc.europa.eu
14. Iberoamerican Cochrane Center, Biomedical Research Institute Sant Pau (IIB Sant Pau-CIBERESP), 08025 Barcelona, Spain; PAlonso@santpau.cat
15. Centre for Global Health Institute of Population Health, University of Ottawa, Ottawa, ON K1N 6N5, Canada; kpottie@uottawa.ca
16. ISGlobal, Barcelona Institute for Global Health (ISGlobal-CRESIB, Hospital Clínic-University of Barcelona), E-08036 Barcelona, Spain; ana.requena@isglobal.org
* Correspondence: eric.agbata@roehampton-online.ac.uk

Received: 15 September 2018; Accepted: 17 December 2018; Published: 20 December 2018

Abstract: We aimed to evaluate the evidence on screening and treatment for two parasitic infections—schistosomiasis and strongyloidiasis—among migrants from endemic countries arriving in the European Union and European Economic Area (EU/EEA). We conducted a systematic search of multiple databases to identify systematic reviews and meta-analyses published between 1 January 1993 and 30 May 2016 presenting evidence on diagnostic and treatment efficacy and cost-effectiveness. We conducted additional systematic search for individual studies published between 2010 and 2017. We assessed the methodological quality of reviews and studies using the AMSTAR, Newcastle–Ottawa Scale and QUADAS-II tools. Study synthesis and assessment of the certainty of the evidence was performed using GRADE (Grading of Recommendations Assessment, Development and Evaluation) approach. We included 28 systematic reviews and individual studies in this review. The GRADE certainty of evidence was low for the effectiveness of screening techniques and moderate to high for treatment efficacy. Antibody-detecting serological tests are the most effective screening tests for detection of both schistosomiasis and strongyloidiasis in low-endemicity settings, because they have higher sensitivity than conventional parasitological methods. Short courses of praziquantel and ivermectin were safe and highly effective and cost-effective in treating schistosomiasis and strongyloidiasis, respectively. Economic modelling suggests presumptive single-dose treatment of strongyloidiasis with ivermectin for all migrants is likely cost-effective, but feasibility of this strategy has yet to be demonstrated in clinical studies. The evidence supports screening and treatment for schistosomiasis and strongyloidiasis in migrants from endemic countries, to reduce morbidity and mortality.

Keywords: migrant populations; schistosomiasis/schistosoma; strongyloidiasis/strongyloides; screening/diagnosis; treatment; public health; GRADE

1. Introduction

The public health importance of schistosomiasis and strongyloidiasis has increased in non-endemic regions as a result of growing global migration [1,2]. Schistosomiasis is caused by species of the trematode *Schistosoma* spp. *Sc. mansoni* is the most prevalent in Africa, the Americas, the Middle East and the West Indies, followed by *Sc. haematobium* in Africa and the Middle East and *Sc. japonicum* in east and south-east Asia [3]. Sub-Saharan African countries account for 90% of reported cases globally [3]. Prevalence rates of 10–50% for *Sc. haematobium* infections have been reported in some countries in sub-Saharan Africa and the Middle East [4], and prevalence rates of 1–40% have been reported for *Sc. mansoni* in sub-Saharan Africa and South America and for *Sc. japonicum* in Indonesia, parts of China and south-east Asia [5].

Strongyloidiasis is caused by the nematode *Strongyloides stercoralis* and, although it generally occurs in sub-tropical and tropical countries, it can be present in temperate countries where conditions are favourable [6]. The global burden of both diseases has been underestimated because of the poor sensitivity of diagnostic methods used in low-resource settings [6], but recent estimates indicate that around 370 million people are infected with *St. stercoralis* [7] and more than 200 million are infected with schistosomiasis causing a loss of more than 1.53 million disability-adjusted life years (DALYs) [4,5,8,9].

Few studies have assessed the prevalence schistosomiasis in European countries, but recent data show rates above 17% in migrants from sub-Saharan Africa [10]; prevalence of strongyloidiasis among refugee populations originating from south-east Asia and Africa was reported to be between 0.8% and 4.3% using microscopy; higher rates of between 9% and 77% using antibody detection assays were reported among refugees from south-east Asia [11]. Prevalence rates of 3.3%, 4.2% and 5.6% were reported in Italy, Spain and France, respectively, mainly in migrant populations or expatriates, without specifying diagnostic methods [6].

From all parasitic infections that may be highly prevalent among migrants, schistosomiasis and strongyloidiasis have several characteristics which support the rationale for screening based on the classical principles of Wilson and Jungner [12]. First, both infections are of particular importance, besides being as highly prevalent as other parasitic infections, they can cause long-term complications and severe consequences. Schistosomiasis is associated with chronic urogenital, hepato-intestinal and central nervous system complications [9,13–15]. *St. stercoralis* can cause disseminated infections or hyper infections with fatal outcomes in immunosuppressed patients (e.g., transplant recipients, those on corticosteroid therapy, with malignancies or co-infections with human T-cell lymphotropic virus-1 (HTLV-1)) [16]. In addition, there is a potential risk of transmission in the EU/EEA, either through organ transplantation in the case of strongyloidiasis [17] or through a favourable environment for the intermediate host, as in recent autochthonous cases of urinary schistosomiasis in Corsica, France which is not the case from many other parasitic infections [11,18]. Second, most infections are asymptomatic [13,19,20] and those infected are either unaware of their infection [19] or have very mild unspecific symptoms [3]. Third, both are chronic infections if untreated [19]. Schistosomiasis can remain as a sub-clinical infection for many years [3], and *St. stercoralis* replicates indefinitely inside the human host, causing lifelong infection if untreated [19].

Fourth, screening could be based on a simple and widely accessible technology, including commercially available serological test with a reasonable cost. In this sense, diagnosis of both infections based on microscopy has high specificity but low sensitivity [19,21,22]. Antibody-detecting serological tests offer higher sensitivity, at the expense of specificity, and have been shown to be useful in countries with low endemicity [19,22,23]. Finally, treatments for both infections are universally accepted with a high efficacy rate and low rate of adverse events. Praziquantel and ivermectin are the drugs of choice for treating schistosomiasis and strongyloidiasis, respectively [7,13].

In the last ten years, there has been a significant increase in migration patterns to the EU/EEA with some fluctuations in the volume and type of migration from year to year [24,25]. In 2017, migrants, here defined as being born abroad, made up 11% of this population, with 4% being born in another EU/EEA country and 7% originating from outside the EU/EEA [26]. There is an increased number of asylum applications with 56% of the 2,672,000 asylum decisions being positive between 2015 to 2017 [27]. Half of those denied asylum can be expected to leave, adding 580,000 to the EU/EEA's total number of irregular migrants [28].

There is a notable gap in data collection on the disease burden, public health management, and in the surveillance for imported diseases in migrants arriving from endemic areas to EU/EEA. Geographic differences in disease distribution between global regions, influenced by increasing migration and population mobility from high endemic to non-endemic areas, remains an ongoing challenge to surveillance programmes and hampers the implementation of health policies concerning migrant health screening strategies [29,30].

There have been several systematic reviews addressing how effective are approaches to migrant screening infectious diseases in Europe [31–33], however parasitic infections are not adequately covered. Therefore, given the recent increase in migrants to the EU/EEA from endemic countries, there is a need for public health guidelines on the optimal approach to screening for schistosomiasis and strongyloidiasis [34–36]. In this systematic review, we assessed the effectiveness (and cost-effectiveness) of screening and management of these two parasitic infections in migrant populations.

2. Methods

The review was one of six systematic reviews conducted under the auspices of a European Centre for Disease Prevention and Control (ECDC) project to develop guidance on screening for hepatitis C, hepatitis B, HIV, tuberculosis, vaccine-preventable diseases and parasitic infections in newly-arrived migrants to the EU/EEA [37]. The review group followed the Preferred Reporting Items for Systematic Reviews and Meta-Analyses (PRISMA) guidelines for the reporting of this systematic review [38]. The review protocol and methods assembled by a team of methodologists and clinicians with disease expertise was registered in Prospero (CRD42016045798) and published [39].

Our key research question was:

What are the most effective screening and treatment options for schistosomiasis and strongyloidiasis in migrant populations arriving from endemic regions in the EU/EEA?

To address this, we developed a logic model, prioritised outcomes important for the patient, and developed key questions along the evidence pathway (Appendix A). These key questions included:

(i) What are the best diagnostic tests to detect these infections non-endemic settings?
(ii) How effective are the drugs to treat them and what are the associated adverse events?
(iii) What are the most cost-effective screening and treatment options for schistosomiasis and strongyloidiasis in migrant populations from endemic regions in the EU/EEA?

2.1. Search Strategy and Selection Criteria

We searched for systematic reviews and meta-analyses in MEDLINE, Embase-ELSEVIER, the Cumulative Index to Nursing and Allied Health Literature (CINAHL), Epistemonikos, the Database of Abstracts of Reviews of Effects (DARE) and the Cochrane Database of Systematic Reviews (CDSR) for evidence on effectiveness. Our search used a combination of the key terms: 'Immigrant', '*Strongyloides*', 'Schistosomiasis', 'endemicity', 'prevalence', 'screening', 'migrant screening', 'mass screening', 'early detection', 'health impact assessment' and 'cost-effectiveness' (Appendix B). The primary inclusion populations were migrants and refugees. We considered as main outcomes: cure, mortality, morbidity, adverse effects, health equity, quality of life and test accuracy measures (sensitivity and specificity). Also, we searched the National Health System (NHS) Economic Evaluation Database, the Health Economic Evaluations Database, the Cost Effectiveness Analysis Registry and Google Scholar for evidence on cost-effectiveness. We also identified any reviews on prevalence of the two infections. We restricted the search to studies published between 1 January 1993 and 30 May 2016. We did not apply language restrictions, and where we identified more than one version of a systematic review, we included the most recent. For the economic evidence, systematic reviews and primary studies of resource use, costs or cost-effectiveness of screening for schistosomiasis or strongyloidiasis with or without treatment were identified using specific search terms including ("costs and cost analysis"; "cost effectiveness analysis"; "costs.tw"; "cost$.mp"; "cost effective$.tw"; "cost-benefit analys$.mp" "health care costs.mp") combined with clinical criteria. We reported all the costs in the local currency of the study setting or country, and in Euros using the Cochrane methods group purchasing power parity currency conversion calculator for the given year [40]. We also searched grey literature for published guidelines and reports on screening and prevention programme from the United States (U.S.) Centers for Disease Control and Prevention, ECDC, Joint United Nations Programme on HIV/AIDS (UNAIDS) and World Health Organization (WHO).

2.2. Additional Included Studies

Due to the limited evidence obtained from the initial search, we conducted an updated systematic search of six databases (MEDLINE, Embase-ELSEVIER, CINAHL, CDSR, DARE, Cochrane CENTRAL and Latin American Literature in Health Sciences—LILACS). We included relevant primary studies on diagnostic or screening tools for schistosomiasis (January 2010–February 2017) and strongyloidiasis (January 2012–February 2017). References of included primary studies were searched to identify other relevant studies.

2.3. Study Selection, Quality Assessment, and Synthesis

We included systematic reviews and evidence-based review guidelines which addressed each key question. When no systematic review was identified, we used primary studies. Two team members independently screened the titles and abstracts, followed by full-text assessments for eligibility of studies on prevalence, screening and treatment effectiveness, and related key questions (Eric Agbata, Nadia Montero) and of studies on cost-effectiveness (Nick Rowbotham, Rachael Morton). Disagreements were resolved by consensus or the involvement of a third author (AR). We assessed the methodological quality of reviews using AMSTAR [41] or Newcastle–Ottawa Scale [42] for reviews and observational studies respectively. We assessed the methodological quality of included primary studies on diagnostic effectiveness using the Quality Assessment of Diagnostic Accuracy Studies (QUADAS II) tool [43]. Synthesis of the studies and assessment of the certainty of the evidence for systematic reviews and individual studies was performed using GRADE (Grading of Recommendations Assessment, Development and Evaluation) methods, including Summary of Findings tables and Evidence to Decision tables [37]. For cost-effectiveness studies, we extracted the following data: economic study design (e.g., cost–utility analysis, Markov model), description of the case base population, the intervention and comparator, the absolute and relative difference in resource use and cost-effectiveness (e.g., incremental net benefit (INB) or incremental cost-effectiveness ratio (ICER).

3. Results

The first systematic search yielded, after removal of duplicates, 662 systematic reviews for which we screened titles and abstracts. Of the 26 systematic reviews selected for full-text screening, we included 11 systematic reviews which focused on the efficacy of diagnosis and treatment of schistosomiasis ($n = 8$) and strongyloidiasis ($n = 3$) (Figure 1) [19,44–53]. The updated systematic search for diagnostic testing accuracy studies for schistosomiasis yielded after de-duplication 1961 citations for the screening of titles and abstracts. Of the 30 articles selected for full-text screening, we included seven primary studies (Figure 2) [54–60]. One more primary research was identified later and included [61]. Another systematic search performed for diagnostic testing accuracy evidence for strongyloidiasis yielded 497 records after de-duplication; titles and abstracts were screened, and of the 24 papers selected for full-text screening, we included three primary studies (Figure 3) [62–64]. For the economic evidence, the search strategy yielded 160 studies after de-duplication. We retrieved 20 studies after title and abstract screening, of which six studies (four decision-analytic models for economic evaluation and two costing studies) were finally included—four for strongyloidiasis and two for schistosomiasis (Figure 4) [65–70]. Overall, we included 28 reviews and studies in this systematic review (Tables 1–3).

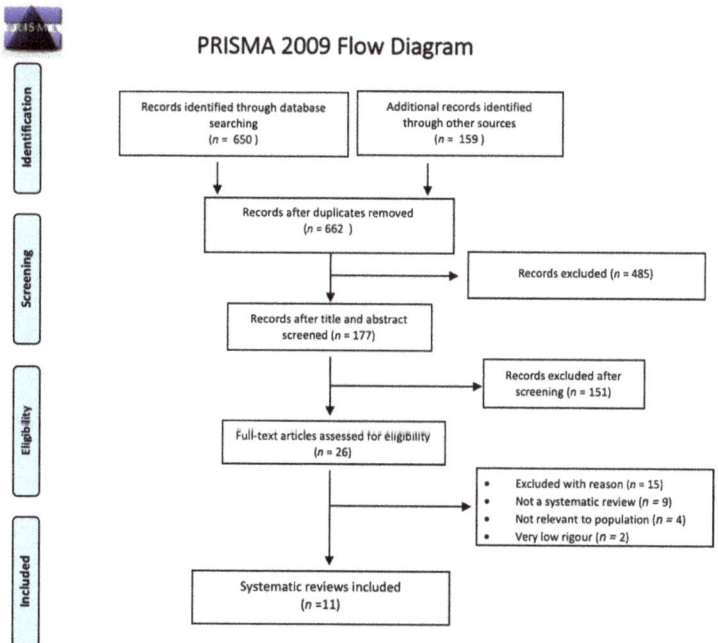

Figure 1. The Preferred Reporting Items for Systematic Reviews and Meta-Analyses (PRISMA) flow diagram for selection of systematic reviews on diagnostic accuracy and treatment efficacy for schistosomiasis and strongyloidiasis, (January 1993–May 2016).

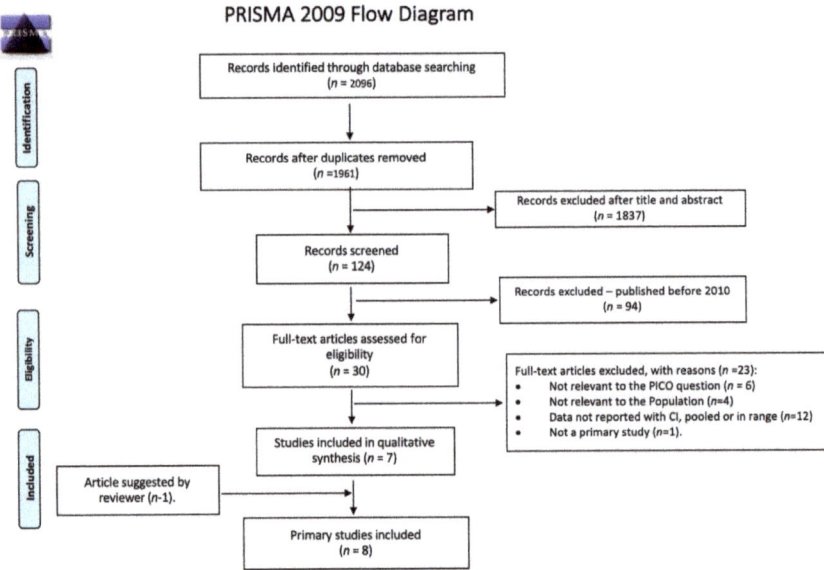

Figure 2. PRISMA flow diagram for selection of primary studies on diagnostic accuracy for schistosomiasis, January 2010–February 2017.

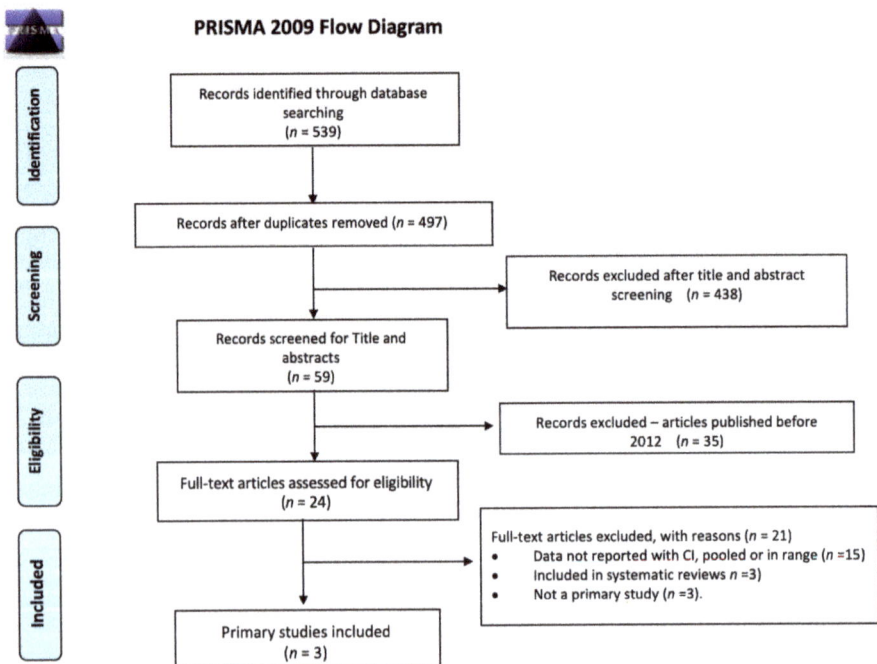

Figure 3. PRISMA flow diagram for selection of primary studies on diagnostic accuracy on strongyloidiasis, (January 2012–February 2017).

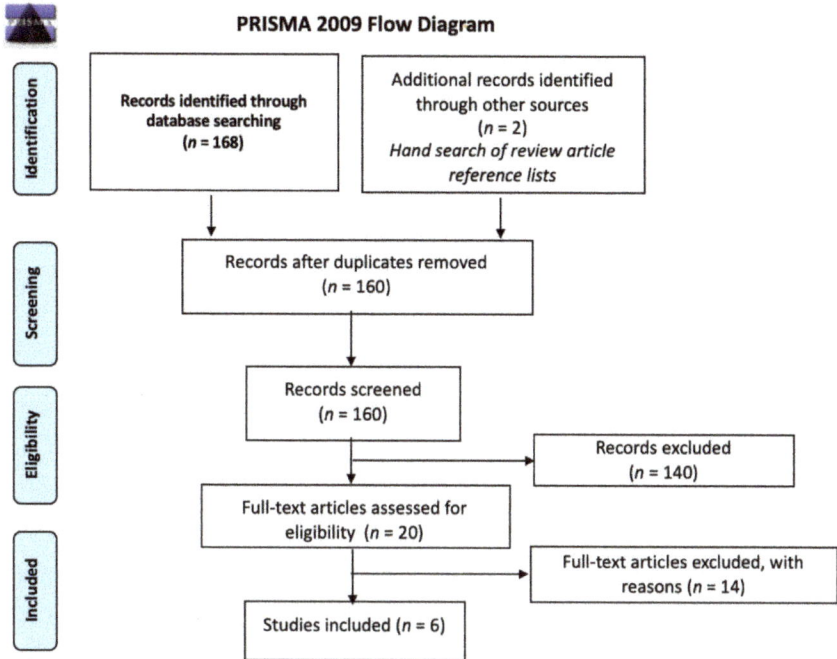

Figure 4. PRISMA flow diagram for selection of cost-effectiveness studies for schistosomiasis and strongyloidiasis, 1993–2016. DARE: Database of Abstracts of Reviews of Effects; NHS EED: National Health Service Economic Evaluation Database; Tufts CEA: Tufts Medical Centre Cost-Effectiveness Analysis Registry.

Table 1. Characteristics of included studies on diagnostic test effectiveness for schistosomiasis and strongyloidiasis, January 1993–February 2017.

Study	Quality	Design	Population	Intervention/Outcomes	Results
\multicolumn{6}{l}{Included systematic reviews of diagnostic tests to detect schistosomiasis}					
Danso Appiah et al., 2016 [53]	AMSTAR: 11/11 GRADE: low to moderate-quality evidence	Systematic review and meta-analysis	Preschool children and infants, school-aged children or adults from high-/low-prevalence locations	Intervention: POC CCA for Sc. mansoni Outcomes: detection of egg-positive urine—sensitivity/specificity (95% CI)	Sensitivity/specificity (95% CI) POC CCA (single standard) 90% (84–94)/56% (39–71); POC CCA (duplicate standard) 85% (80–88)/66% (53–76); POC CCA (triplicate standard) 91% (84–95)/56% (39–72)
Yang, et al., 2015 [50]	AMSTAR: 11/11 GRADE: low to moderate-quality evidence	Meta-analysis	Patients infected with schistosomiasis in endemic areas; mainly school children, Africa and China	Intervention: questionnaire screening for Schistosoma species. Outcomes: sensitivity/specificity (95% CI)	Sensitivity/specificity (95%CI) Sc. haematobium 85% (84–86)/94% (94–94); Sc. mansoni 46% (45–47)/81% (80–82); Sc. japonicum 82% (79–85)/59% (57–60)
Ochodo et al., 2015 [44]	AMSTAR: 11/11 GRADE: very low to low-quality evidence	Systematic review and meta-analysis of RCTs	Individuals with active infection with S. haematobium	Intervention: urine reagent strip tests; circulating antigen tests in urine/serum Outcomes: sensitivity/specificity (95% CI)	Sensitivity/specificity (95% CI) Sc. haematobium: microhaematuria 75% (71–79)/87% (84–90); proteinuria 61% (53–68)/82% (77–88); leukocyturia 58% (44–71)/61% (34–88); Sc. mansoni (CCA test) 89% (86–92)/55% (46–65)
King and Bertsch, 2013 [45]	AMSTAR: 11/11 GRADE: low-quality evidence	Systematic review and meta-analysis of surveys	Schools, communities with high/low prevalence, low intensity groups in Africa	Intervention: dipstick test Sc. haematobium. Outcomes: sensitivity and specificity (95% CI), diagnostic odds ratio (DOR)	Sensitivity/specificity (95% CI) Detection of egg-positive urine 81% (79–83)/89% (87–92). In high-prevalence settings 80% (78–83)/86% (82–90); lower in treated population 72% (61–78)/87% (81–94); in lower intensity population subgroups 65% (58–72)/82% (76–90)
Wang, et al., 2012 [46]	AMSTAR: 7/11 GRADE: very low- to low-quality evidence	Systematic review and meta-analysis of RCTs, retro-/pro-observational studies	Infected patients with schistosomiasis in control programmes in China	Intervention: IHA and ELISA. Outcomes: true positive rates, sensitivity/specificity (95% CI), DOR	Sensitivity/specificity (95% CI) IHA 75.6% (74–77)/73% (72–74) ELISA 84.9% (83–87)/50.4% (49.2–51.6) The DOR of IHA was 9.41 (95% CI: 5–18), and ELISA 4.78 (95% CI: 3.21–7.13)
\multicolumn{6}{l}{Included primary studies of diagnostic tests to detect schistosomiasis}					
Espirito-Santo et al., 2015 [57]	QUADAS-2: 11/14 GRADE: very low- to low-quality evidence	Cross-sectional epidemiological survey in areas of low prevalence of Sc. Mansoni	The estimated sample size required was 650 individuals; Barra Mansa City, Rio de Janeiro State, Brazil	Intervention: diagnostic assays: ELISA-IgG/ELISA-IgM/IFT-IgM/qPCR in faeces. Outcomes: sensitivity/specificity (95% CI.)	Sensitivity/specificity (95% CI) KK 13.8% (4–32)/99.8% (99.0–100); ELISA-IgG 66.7% (48–82)/91.5% (89–94); ELISA-IgM 81.8% (64–93)/82% (79–85); IFT-IgM 78.8% (61–91)/57.7% (84.8–90); qPCR in faeces 51.7% (32–71)/92.6% (90–95); qPCR in serum 12.1% (3–28)/99.1% (98–99)
Espirito-Santo et al., 2014a [60]	QUADAS-2: 12/14 GRADE: very low- to low-quality evidence	Cross-sectional study	City of Barra Mansa, Rio de Janeiro State, Brazil, with an estimated prevalence of 1%	Intervention: diagnostic assays: ELISA-IgG and ELISA-IgM. Outcomes: sensitivity/specificity (95% CI); PPV, NPV	Sensitivity/specificity (95%CI) ELISA-IgG 60.0% (15–95)/89.1% (86.2–91.5); ELISA-IgM 60.0 (15–95)/79.2% (75.6–82.5) PPV/NPV (95%CI): ELISA-IgG 4.6% (1–13)/99.6% (98–100); ELISA-IgM 2.5% (0.5–7); NPV 99.6% (98.4–100.0)

Table 1. *Cont.*

Study	Quality	Design	Population	Intervention/Outcomes	Results
Espirito-Santo et al., 2014b [56]	QUADAS-2:13/14 GRADE: very low- to low-quality evidence	Cross-sectional epidemiological survey	7000 inhabitants located in the outskirts of Barra Mansa, Rio de Janeiro, Brazil	Intervention: qPCR in serum or faeces. Outcomes: sensitivity/specificity (95% CI); PPV, NPV	Sensitivity/specificity (95% CI): qPCR in faeces 80.0% (28–99)/92.4% (90–94); qPCR in serum 20.0% (0.5–71.6)/98.8 (97–99) PPV/NPV (95% CI): qPCR in faeces 8.0% (2–19)/99.8% (99–100); qPCR in serum 12.5% (0.3–52.7)/99.3% (98.2–99.8)
Lodh et al., 2013 [55]	QUADAS-2:12/14 GRADE: very low- to low-quality evidence	Cross-sectional case study	Filtered urine specimens from infected and not-infected patients in Zambia	Intervention: qPCR ELISA IgG in serum or faeces; filtered Urine PCR. Outcomes: sensitivity/specificity (95% CI); PPV, NPV	Sensitivity/specificity (95%CI): KK test 57% (45–68)/100% (69–100); CCA rapid test 65% (56–77)/60% (26–88); PCR 100% (95–100)/100% (69–100) PPV/NPV: KK test 100%/23%; CCA rapid test 93%/19%; PCR 100%/100%.
Kinkel et al., 2012 [54]	QUADAS-2:12/14 GRADE: very low- to low-quality evidence	Retrospective comparative diagnostic study: performance of 8 serological tests for Schistosoma spp	Serum specimens from infected patients and those without the infection in low-prevalence locations or non-endemic settings (Germany)	Intervention: serological assays: IFAT, ELISA-CA, ELISA-AWA, ELISA-SEA, IHA, ELISA-NovaTec, ELISA-DRG and ELISA-Viramed. Outcomes: sensitivity and specificity (95% CI)	Sensitivity/specificity-(95% CI): IFAT 75.7% (58–98)/98.1% (92–99); ELISA-CA 40.5% (25–59)/95.2% (89–98); ELISA-AWA 54.1% (37–70)/100% (95.6–100); ELISA-SEA-75.7% (58–98)/97.1% (91–99); IHA 73.0% (55.6–85.6)/99.0% (94.0–100); ELISA-NovaTec 64.9% (47–79)/99 (94–100); ELISA-DRG 78.3% (61.3–89.6)/88.4 (80–94); ELISA-Viramed 67.6% (50–81)/76.9% (67–84).
De Frotas et al., 2011 [58]	QUADAS-2:12/14 GRADE: very low- to low-quality evidence	Cross-sectional survey	Stool and serum specimens from infected and not infected patients, low-endemic setting in Brazil	Intervention: serological assays, ELISA IgG Outcomes: sensitivity and specificity (95%CI)	Sensitivity/specificity (95% CI): ELISA-IgG 100% (68–100)/72.9% (67–78). PPV/NPV (95% CI): ELISA-IgG 26.0% (18–36) / 100% (97–100).
Silveira et al., 2016 [59]	QUADAS-2:12/14 GRADE: very low- to low-quality evidence	Evaluation of the CCA test to diagnose *Sc. mansoni* in Minas Gerais State, Brazil.	Infected individuals in regions with moderate to high prevalence	Intervention: CCA-immuno-chromatographic test. Outcomes: sensitivity/specificity (95% CI)	Sensitivity/specificity (95% CI): CCA-ICT 68.7% (54–81)/97.6% (87–99)
Beltrame et al., 2017 [61]	QUADAS-2:12/14 GRADE: very low- to low-quality evidence	Accuracy of parasitological and immunological tests for the screening of human schistosomiasis in immigrants and refugees from African countries	Frozen serum specimens from recent African asylum seekers that were routinely screened for schistosomiasis in Italy	Intervention: urine CCA; Bordier-ELISA, Western Blot IgG, ICT IgG-IgM, microscopy compared with composite reference standard. Outcomes: sensitivity/specificity (95% CI)	Sensitivity/specificity (95% CI): Urine CCA 29% (22–37)/95% (91–97); Bordier-ELISA 71% (63–78)/99.6% (98–100); Western blot IgG 92% (86–96)/94% (90–97); ICT IgG-IgM 96% (91–99)/83% (77–87); microscopy 45% (37–54)/100%
Included systematic reviews for diagnostic effectiveness for strongyloidiasis					
Campo Polanco et al., 2014 [51]	AMSTAR: 11/11 GRADE: moderate-quality evidence	Systematic review and meta-analysis	Individuals with active/chronic infection	Intervention: Baermann method, agar plate, direct faecal smear examination and formol-ether concentration technique. Outcome: sensitivity and specificity (95% CI)	Sensitivity: Baermann method (72%) with LR+228 and LR −0.32; APC 89%, LR +341 and LR −0.11; stool microscopy 21%, LR + 67 and LR −0.67; formol-ether concentration 48%, LR + 110 and LR −0.59. Specificity: 100% in all four tests. APC and Baermann method are best.

471

Table 1. Cont.

Study	Quality	Design	Population	Intervention/Outcomes	Results
Included systematic reviews of diagnostic tests to detect schistosomiasis					
Requena-Méndez et al., [19]	AMSTAR: 7/11 GRADE: low- to moderate-quality evidence	Systematic review	Individuals with active/chronic infection	Intervention: Baermann method, agar plate, direct faecal smear examination and formol-ether concentration technique, serological techniques. Outcome: sensitivity and specificity (95% CI)	No meta-analysis was undertaken. Sensitivity and specificity of different techniques were individually reported.
Included primary studies for diagnostic effectiveness for strongyloidiasis					
Bisoffi et al., 2014 [62]	QUADAS-2: 13/14 GRADE: low-quality evidence	Retrospective comparative diagnostic study to evaluate the performance of 5 tests for *St. stercoralis*.	Serum specimens from subjects with *St. stercoralis*; healthy people and patients with previous exposure	Intervention: IFAT, NIE-LIPS NIE-ELISA, IVD-ELISA and Bordier-ELISA Outcome: sensitivity and specificity (95% CI)	Sensitivity/specificity (95% CI): NIE-ELISA 75.4% (67-83)/94.8% (91-99); NIE-LIPS 85.1% (78-92)/100% (100-100); IFAT 93.9% (89-98)/92.2% (87-97); IVD-ELISA 91.2% (86-96)/99.1% (97.4-100.0); Bordier-ELISA 89.5% (84-95) 98.3% (96-100).
Rascoe et al., 2015 [63]	QUADAS-2: 10/14 GRADE: low-quality evidence	Retrospective comparative diagnostic study of 5 tests for the follow-up of patients infected with *St. stercoralis*	Serum samples positive for *St. stercoralis* and negative samples from United States residents with no history of foreign travel	Intervention: Ss-NIE-1 ELISA, Ss-NIE-1 Luminex. Outcome: sensitivity and specificity (95% CI)	Sensitivity/specificity (95% CI): Ss-NIE-1 ELISA 95% (92-97)/93% (90-96); Ss-NIE-1 Luminex 93% (88-96)/95% (93-97). The inter-assay coefficient of variation was determined to be 22% for the low-positive control serum and 10% for the medium-positive control serum.
Knopp et al., 2014 [64]	QUADAS-2: 11/14 GRADE: low-quality evidence	International standard randomised controlled trial	Children and adults residing in rural villages in the Bagamoyo District, Tanzania (endemic areas)	Intervention: Real-time PCR, FLOTAC technique, KK method. Outcome: sensitivity and specificity (95% CI)	Sensitivity/specificity (95% CI): PCR + pseudo-standard PCR 17.4 (8-31)/3.9 (89-97); Baermann + pseudo-standard 47 (23-72)/78.4 (72-84); PCR + multiple gold standard 30.9 (19.1-44.8)/100 (100-100); Baermann + multiple gold standard 83.6 (71.2-92.2)/100 (100-100)

AWA: adult worm antigen; AMSTAR: a tool for assessing the methodological quality of systematic reviews; APC: agar plate culture; CA: Cercarial antigen; CCA: circulatory cathodic antigen; CI: confidence interval; DOR: diagnostic odds ratio; GRADE: Grading of Recommendations, Assessment, Development and Evaluation; ELISA: enzyme-linked immunosorbent assay; FLOTAC: novel multivalent faecal egg count method; ICT: Immuno chromatographic test; IFAT: indirect fluorescent antibody technique; IHA: indirect haemagglutination; In Vitro Diagnostic kit; KK: Kato-Katz method; LIPS: luciferase immunoprecipitation system; LR+: positive likelihood ratio; LR −: negative likelihood ratio; NIE: a 31-kDa recombinant antigen; NovaTec Immundiagnostica, Dietzenbach, Germany; NPV: negative predictive value; POC: point-of-care; qPCR: quantitative PCR (real-time polymerase chain reaction); PPV: positive predictive value; RCT: randomised controlled trial; SEA: soluble egg antigen; Ss-NIE-1: a luciferase tagged recombinant protein of *St. stercoralis* for IgG and IgG4 specific antibodies; QUADAS-2: a tool for the quality assessment of diagnostic accuracy studies; Viramed®: Viramed Biotech, Planegg, Germany).

Table 2. Characteristics of included studies about efficacy of treatment for schistosomiasis and strongyloidiasis, 1993–2016.

Study	Quality	Design	Population	Intervention/Outcomes	Results
				Treatment efficacy of anti-Schistosoma drugs	
Kramer et al., 2014 [48]	AMSTAR: 11/11 Data in study: GRADE: high-quality evidence	Systematic review, fixed effects meta-analysis; Embase, MEDLINE (1966 to 2014), LILACS, Cochrane library, Cochrane infectious disease (1980–2014)	School-aged and young adults: 6–20 years (16 trials); 2–23 years (5 trials); Adults (2 trials). Participants setting: Rural areas in 15 sub-Saharan African countries; an urban setting in Saudi Arabia	Interventions: drugs used to treat urinary schistosomiasis: praziquantel, metrifonate, artesunate and/or in combination Outcome: parasitological cure or failure at 4 weeks; % egg reduction rate at 4 weeks	Praziquantel (single dose 40 mg/kg), egg reduction (60%) in urine achieved in 4–8 weeks (38 per 100 (95% CI: 26–54). Treatment failure: RR 0.42, (95% CI: 0.29–0.59), 864 participants, 7 trials Metrifonate (single dose 10 mg/kg) reduced egg excretion only marginally in comparison to placebo (RR 0.63, 95% CI: 0.54 to 0.73) 210 participants, 1 trial, at 8 months
Danso-Appiah et al., 2013 [47]	AMSTAR: 11/11 Data in study: GRADE: low- to moderate-quality evidence	Systematic review and meta-narrative of RCTs, RCTs of anti-Schistosoma drugs	Trials conducted in Africa (n = 36), South America (n = 15; all in Brazil) and the Middle East (n = 1). 52 trials enrolling 10,269 participants in endemic areas	Intervention: praziquantel 40 mg/kg, oxamniquine 40 mg/kg	Praziquantel (single dose 40 mg/kg) vs. placebo: reduced parasitological treatment failure at 1 month (69/100; RR = 3.13, 2 trials, 414 participants). Praziquantel (single dose 30 mg/kg): RR = 1.52, 3 trials, 521 participants. Higher doses: no significant difference. Oxamniquine (single dose 40 mg/kg) vs. Placebo: reduced parasitological treatment failure at 3 months in 2 trials (68/100; RR = 8.74).
Pérez del Villar et al., 2012 [49]	AMSTAR: 11/11 Data in study: not reported. GRADE: Moderate-quality evidence	Quantitative systematic review and meta-analysis	Healthy villagers who live in areas in Africa endemic for Sc. haematobium and Sc. mansoni and in China for Sc. japonicum	Intervention: prophylactic effect of artesunate or artemether vs. placebo against Sc. haematobium, Sc. mansoni and Sc. japonica infections. Outcomes: parasitological cure rate at 3–8 weeks; infection rate at 3–4 weeks after treatment.	Artesunate treatment (single dose: significantly lower cure rates than with praziquantel. Combined therapy of artesunate plus sulfadoxine-pyrimethamine: significantly less effective than praziquantel treatment Combination of artemisinin derivatives and praziquantel: higher cure rate than praziquantel monotherapy Artesunate or artemether: significantly better than a placebo.
				Treatment efficacy of drugs for strongyloidiasis	
Henriquez-Camacho et al., 2016 [52]	AMSTAR: 11/11 GRADE: Moderate-quality evidence	Systematic review of RCTs, controlled or uncontrolled interventional studies.	Individuals with chronic infections of St. stercoralis; Immuno-competent patients. All ages	Intervention: ivermectin (single/double dose) vs. albendazole or thiabendazole. Outcome: elimination of infection; parasitological cure (>2 negative stool samples, 5 weeks).	Ivermectin (single/double dose) vs. albendazole: parasitological cure was higher with ivermectin, 84/100 vs. 48/100 ivermectin (RR = 1.79). Ivermectin vs. thiabendazole: little or no difference in parasitological cure, 74/100 vs. 68/100), but adverse events were less common with ivermectin (RR = 0.31) than albendazole. No serious adverse events or death reported

AMSTAR: a tool for assessing the methodological quality of systematic reviews; GRADE: Grading of Recommendations, Assessment, Development and Evaluation; LILACS: Latin American Literature in Health Sciences; RCT: randomized clinical trial; RR: Relative Risk.

Table 3. Characteristics of included studies on cost-effectiveness of screening and treatment of schistosomiasis and strongyloidiasis, 1993–2016.

Study	Quality	Design	Population	Intervention/Outcomes	Results
Libman et al., 1993 [70]	NA	Retrospective-cross-sectional study with cost analysis	Cohort of individuals returning from the tropics and screened in a Canadian clinic 1981–1987. Costs in 1988 CAD	Stool examination + eosinophil count + serological studies for filariasis and schistosomiasis (gold standard) vs. stool examination + eosinophil count; vs. stool examination alone; vs. stool examination + serological studies; vs. eosinophil counts only. Outcome: difference in cost or resource use/cost effectiveness	Difference in resource use/costs: high-/low-prevalence locations. Costs per case of schistosomiasis and/or strongyloidiasis diagnosed for each strategy: (i) CAN$4674 [€4829]; (ii) CAN$6111 [€4829]; (iii) CAN$4788 [€3783]; (iv) CAN$3737 [€2953]; (v) CAN$3307 [€2613]. Cost-effectiveness (ICER or INB): no ICER calculated. Study did not include a decision analytic model
Muennig et al., 1999 [66]	NA	Decision analytic model	Large immigrant populations in which St. stercoralis is not endemic (one third of the sample population was from the state of New York). Costs in 1997 USD	No preventive intervention (watchful waiting) vs. universal screening vs. presumptive treatment with albendazole. Outcome: difference in cost or resource use/cost effectiveness (ICER or INB) per DALY averted	Difference in resource use/costs: gross costs: USD 11,086,181 [€7,228,785] for no intervention, USD 7,290,624 [€40,203,726] per year for treatment with albendazole, USD 40,547,651 [€40,203,726] for universal screening. Cost-effectiveness (ICER or INB): treatment with albendazole was cost saving compared with no intervention, universal screening had ICER of USD 159,236/DALY [€157,885/DALY averted]
Muennig et al., 2004 [67]	NA	Decision analytic model (Markov)	California and New York, two states with large immigrant populations in which St. stercoralis is not endemic. Costs in 2000 USD	Intervention: no intervention (watchful waiting) vs. 3 or 5 days of albendazole vs. eosinophil screening vs. ivermectin. Outcome: difference in cost or resource use/cost effectiveness (ICER or INB)	Difference in resource use/costs: costs per person: no intervention USD 1666 [€1611], albendazole 3 days USD 1674 [€1618], albendazole 5 days USD 1680 [€1624], screening USD 1684 [€1628], ivermectin USD 1688 [€1632]. Cost-effectiveness (ICER or INB): ICERs varied based on prevalence: albendazole USD 155–1584/QALY gained [€150–1531], albendazole 5 days USD 314–3175/QALY gained [€304–3069], ivermectin USD 848–8514/QALY gained [€820–8231]. Eosinophil was documented among all prevalence groups
King et al., 2011 [65]	AMSTAR	Systematic review of efficacy of schistosomiasis treatment with praziquantel (by dose), with a Markov model estimating cost-effectiveness of various dosing strategies	Non-migrants in endemic setting; population-based or sub-population-based (e.g., schools) drug treatment of Sc. haematobium or Sc. Mansoni. Costs in 2002 & 2008 USD	Intervention: No treatment vs. single dose of praziquantel per annual treatment vs. double dose. Outcome: difference in cost or resource use/cost effectiveness (ICER or INB)	Difference in resource use/costs: single dose lifetime cost: USD 23 [€19] per person; double dose: USD 46 [€35] per person. Cost-effectiveness (ICER or INB): single dose: ICER of USD 48 [€39] and USD 46 [€37] per QALY gained for Sc. mansoni and Sc. haematobium, respectively, compared with no treatment; double dose: ICERs of USD 291 [€236] and USD 433 [€351] per QALY gained respectively compared with single dose

Table 3. *Cont.*

Study	Quality	Design	Population	Intervention/Outcomes	Results
Worrell et al., 2015 [69]	NA	Cost analysis study	Cohort of children in Kenya assessed 2010–2011. Non-migrant settings. Costs in 2010 USD	Intervention: single KK (stool examination) vs. triplicate KK vs. POC CCA (urine dipstick) Outcome: difference in cost or resource use/cost effectiveness (ICER or INB)	Difference in resource use/costs: total costs per test: single KK USD 6.89 [€5], triplicate KK USD 17.54 [€14], POC CCA USD 7.26 [€6] Cost-effectiveness (ICER or INB): no ICER calculated, this was not a decision analysis study.
Maskery et al., 2016 [68]	NA	Cost analysis study; Markov model: discount rate of 3% over 60-year time horizon; costs in 2013 USD	Average annual cohort of 27,700 Asian refugees based on Department of Homeland Security data for 2002–2011, primarily from south-east Asia and the Middle East	Intervention: no screening or treatment vs. overseas albendazole and ivermectin treatment vs. domestic screening and treatment vs. overseas albendazole and domestic screening for strongyloidiasis. Outcome: difference in cost or resource use/cost effectiveness (ICER or INB)	Difference in resource use/costs, total costs per migrant (strongyloidiasis,): no treatment USD 5.99 [€5], overseas albendazole and ivermectin USD 15.12 [€12], domestic screening and treatment USD 138.36 [€108], overseas albendazole and domestic screening for Strongyloides infection USD 78.79 [€61]. Cost-effectiveness: ICERs per QALY gained: USD 2219 for "overseas albendazole and ivermectin", USD 32,706 [€25,422] for domestic screening and treatment, USD 18,167 [€14,121] for overseas albendazole followed by domestic screening for strongyloidiasis. All vs. no screening or treatment [€1723]

AMSTAR: A measurement tool to assess systematic reviews; CAD: Canadian dollars; CCA: circulatory cathodic antigen; GRADE: Grading of Recommendations, Assessment, Development and Evaluation; ICER: incremental cost-effectiveness ratio, INB: incremental net benefit; NA: Not Applicable KK: Kato–Katz; POC: point-of-care; USD: United States dollars.

3.1. Screening: Diagnostic Test Accuracy for Schistosomiasis

We assessed diagnostic and screening tools for *Schistosoma* spp. in five included systematic reviews [44–46,50,53] and eight individual studies [54–61]. The best performing tests were included in the GRADE summary of finding on diagnostic tools for screening schistosomiasis (Table 4 and Figure 5).

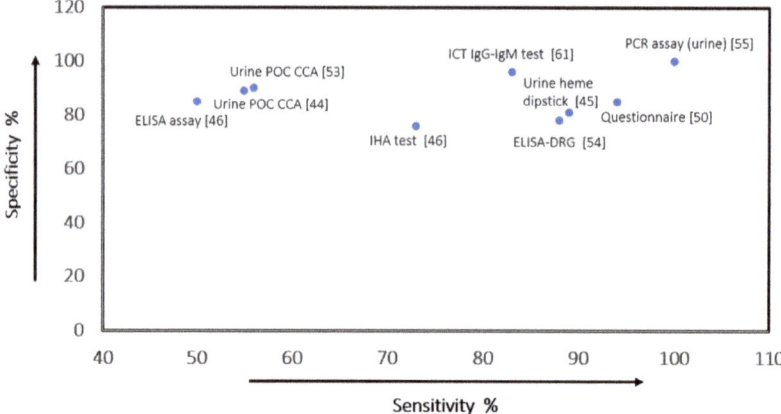

Figure 5. Scatter plot of sensitivity versus specificity values of the Index diagnostic tools for screening schistosomiasis.

3.1.1. Schistosoma Mansoni

A meta-analysis reported estimated sensitivity and specificity values of 89% (95% CI: 86–92) and 55% (95% CI: 46–55) respectively, for the urinary circulating cathodic antigen (CCA) assay that detects *Sc. mansoni* in endemic areas [44]. Another urinary CCA test for *Sc. mansoni* [53] reported sensitivity and specificity values of 90% (95% CI: 84–94) and 56% (95% CI: 39–71), respectively compared with the duplicate Kato–Katz (KK) test (moderate-quality evidence) (Table 4). From the included primary studies, PCR assay in urine was the best-performing diagnostic test for *Sc. mansoni* with a sensitivity of 100% (95% CI: 95–100) compared with the CCA test—65% (95% CI: 56–77) and KK test—57% (95% CI: 46–68) [55] (very low-quality evidence); the specificity of PCR assay in urine was 100% (95% CI: 69–100) (Table 4) [55]. Espírito-Santo et al. reported sensitivity and specificity of 80% (95% CI: 28–99) and 92.4% (95% CI: 90–94), respectively for quantitative PCR (qPCR) in faeces compared with the KK test (not included in the GRADE Summary of findings) [56].

In low-endemic settings, the best-performing diagnostic test was the IgM-ELISA assay with sensitivity and specificity values of, respectively, 82% (95% CI: 64–93) and 82% (95% CI: 79–85)-low-quality evidence (Table 1) [57]. In another study, the ELISA-DRG kit showed the best accuracy with sensitivity and specificity values of, respectively, 78% (95% CI: 61–90) and 95% (95% CI: 89–98) (Table 4) [54]. In a recent study on the accuracy of different screening tests for schistosomiasis in African migrants, the immuno chromatographic test (ICT) IgG-IgM showed the best accuracy, with sensitivity and specificity values of 96% (95% CI: 91–99) and 83% (95% CI: 77–87) (Table 4) [61]. In all the individual studies, the certainty of evidence was very low to low.

3.1.2. Schistosoma Haematobium

The urine heme dipsticks for the diagnosis of *Sc. haematobium* showed a mean sensitivity and specificity of 81% (95% CI: 73–83) and 89% (95% CI: 87–92), respectively, and were more accurate in high-prevalence than in low-prevalence settings -low-quality evidence (Table 4) [45]. Similarly, Ochodo et al. reported sensitivity and specificity values of 75% (95% CI: 71–79) and 87% (95% CI:

84–90)-low-quality evidence (Table 1) [44]. Furthermore, a meta-analysis on the diagnostic efficiency of questionnaire screening for schistosomiasis reported sensitivity and specificity values of 85% (95% CI: 84–86) and 94% (95% CI: 94–94) for *Sc. haematobium* infections (low-quality evidence) (Table 4) [50].

Kinkel et al. evaluated the accuracy of antibody-detection tests for diagnosis of imported *Sc. haematobium* [54]. The indirect haemagglutination (IHA) test with a sensitivity of 73% (95% CI: 56–86) and specificity of 99% (95% CI: 94–100) and the ELISA-DRG with a sensitivity of 78% (95% CI: 61–90) and specificity of 95% (95% CI: 89–98) demonstrated the best accuracy (certainty of evidence low) (Table 4) [54]. In another study, the ICT IgG-IgM test showed the best accuracy with sensitivity of 96% (95% CI: 91–99) and specificity of 83% (95% CI: 77–87) (Table 4) [61].

3.1.3. *Schistosoma Japonicum*

In a meta-analysis of the accuracy of antibody detection of *Sc. japonicum* infection in humans, pooled sensitivities and specificities were 76% (95% CI: 74–77) and 73% (95% CI: 72–74) for the IHA test and 85% (95% CI: 83–87) and 50% (95% CI: 49–52) for ELISA (Table 4) [46].

The evidence also suggests that accuracy of diagnostic tests for schistosomiasis depends on pre-test prevalence (Table 5). As prevalence increased (from 2.5% to 30%), the estimated number of false-positives per 1000 migrants tested decreased with all tests—from 47 to 34 (*Sc. haematobium/Sc. mansoni*) [54], 58 to 42 (*Sc. haematobium*) [44], 107 to 77 (*Sc. Haematobium*) [45] and 166 to 119—(*Sc. haematobium/Sc. mansoni*) [61] per 1000 for ELISA-DRG, questionnaire screening, urine heme dipsticks and ICT IgG-IgM, respectively. The estimated false-negative tests were between 0–6 and 0–73 per 1000 at 2.5% and 30% prevalence for all the tests. At 2.5% pre-test prevalence, the proportion of correctly diagnosed schistosomiasis infections in migrant populations was 100% for the urine PCR assay, 96% for the ICT IgG-IgM test, 90% for the urine POC CCA, 85% for the questionnaire screening and 84.9% for *Sc. japonicum* ELISA (Table 5).

3.2. *Screening: Diagnostic Test Accuracy for Strongyloidiasis*

We assessed diagnostic and screening tools for *St. stercoralis* in two included systematic reviews [19,51] and three individual studies (Tables 1 and 6) [62–64].

Table 4. GRADE summary of findings on diagnostic tools for screening schistosomiasis, 1993–2017.

Index Test at Median Test Prevalence in Study *	Sensitivity (95% CI)	Specificity (95% CI)	Post-Test Probability of a Positive Result (95% CI)	Post-Test Probability of a Negative Result (95% CI)	Number of Studies/ Participants	Certainty of Evidence (GRADE)	Reference Standard
PCR assay (filtered urine) at 89% prevalence—Sc. mansoni [55]	1.00 (0.95–1.00)	1.00 (0.69–1.00)	100% (96–100)	0% (37–0)	1/89	Very Low [a,b,c]	KK test—duplicate smears
Urine POC CCA test at 36% prevalence—Sc. mansoni [44]	0.89 (0.86–0.92)	0.55 (0.46–0.65)	53% (47–60)	10% (15–7)	15/6091	Very Low [a,b,c]	Stool microscopy
Urine POC CCA test at 30% prevalence—Sc. mansoni [53]	0.90 (0.84–0.94) [d]	0.56 (0.39–0.71) [d]	47% (37–58)	7% (15–3)	7/4584	Moderate [a,b]	KK test
Questionnaire screening 30% prevalence—Sc. haematobium [50]	0.85 (0.84–0.86) [d]	0.94 (0.94–0.94) [d]	86% (86–86)	6% (7–6)	12/41,412	Low [c,e]	Urine filtration/microscopy
ELISA-DRG (commercial kit) at 26% prevalence—All cases [54]	0.78 (0.61–0.90)	0.88 (0.80–0.94)	85% (65–95)	7% (13–4)	1/37	Very Low [c,e,f]	Stool/urine microscopy
Urine heme dipstick at 27% prevalence—Sc. haematobium [45]	0.81 (0.73–0.83) [d]	0.89 (0.87–0.92) [d]	73% (67–79)	7% (10–6)	98/126,119	Low [a,f,g]	Urine microscopy
ELISA at 24% prevalence—Sc. japonicum [46]	0.85 (0.83–0.87)	0.50 (0.49–0.52)	35% (34–36)	9% (10–7)	10/9014	Low [a,f,g]	KK and Miracidium hatching test
IHA at 12% prevalence—Sc. japonicum [46]	0.76 (0.72–0.74) [d]	0.73 (0.72–0.74) [d]	28% (26–28)	4% (5–5)	15/23,411	Low [a,b]	KK and Miracidium hatching test
ICT IgG-IgM test at 17% prevalence Sc. mansoni and Sc. haematobium [61]	0.96 (0.91–0.99)	0.83 (0.77–0.87)	13% (9–16)	0% (0–0)	1/373	Low [b,c]	Stool/urine microscopy/ composite standard.

Population: patients with schistosomiasis or stored sera; Settings: high-/low-endemic settings; Target condition: Schistosoma spp. Infections. GRADE: Grading of Recommendations, Assessment, Development and Evaluation. Tests—CCA: circulating cathodic antigen; CI: confidence interval; DRG: DRG Instruments, Marburg, Germany; ELISA: enzyme-linked immunosorbent assay; IHA: indirect haemagglutination; KK: Kato–Katz; POC: point-of-care. * Post-test probability of test was calculated at median test prevalence obtained from individual studies.

a   Heterogeneity across similar studies because of several factors; downgraded because of serious inconsistency.
b   Use of intermediate or surrogate outcomes rather than health outcomes, hence a source of serious indirectness.
c   Single study design, not a randomised control trial.
d   Sensitivity and specificity values obtained from multiple-field study.
e   Use of indirect comparisons; sample population not migrants, another source of indirectness.
f   Very low-quality of evidence (downgraded by 1) because of serious indirectness.
g   Studies were insufficient to provide summary estimates for CAA tests.

Table 5. Accuracy of diagnostic tools for schistosomiasis at different pre-test prevalence levels, January 2010–February 2017.

Index Test	True Positives Pre-Test Probability *			False Positives Pre-Test Probability *			True Negative Pre-Test Probability *			False Negative Pre-Test Probability *			% Infected Correctly Diagnosed
Test % Prevalence [a]	2.5%	10%	30%	2.5%	10%	30%	2.5%	10%	30%	2.5%	10%	30%	
PCR assay (filtered urine)—*Sc. mansoni* [55]	25	100	300	0	0	0	975	900	700	0	0	0	100%
ICT IgG-IgM test—*Sc. haematobium/Sc. mansoni* [61]	24	96	288	166	153	119	809	747	581	1	4	12	96%
Urine POC CCA test—*Sc. mansoni* [33]	23	90	270	429	396	308	546	504	392	2	10	30	90%
Questionnaire screening—*Sc. haematobium* [50]	21	85	255	58	54	42	917	846	658	4	15	45	85%
ELISA-DRG (commercial kit)—*Sc. haematobium/Sc. mansoni* [54]	20	78	235	47	43	34	928	857	666	5	22	65	78.3%
Urine heme dipstick—*Sc. haematobium* infections [45]	20	81	243	107	99	77	868	801	623	5	19	57	81.0%
ELISA—*Sc. japonicum* [46]	21	85	255	484	446	347	491	454	353	4	15	45	84.9%
IHA—*Sc. japonicum* [46]	19	76	227	263	243	189	712	657	511	6	24	73	75.6%

[a] Different pre-test prevalence or probability of having schistosomiasis in an at-risk population. * Data reported as effect per 1000 migrants tested. Tests: DRG: DRG Instruments, Marburg, Germany; ELISA: enzyme-linked immunosorbent assay; ICT: Immuno chromatographic test; IHA: Indirect haemagglutination; PCR: Polymerase chain reaction assay; POC: Point of care.

Table 6. GRADE summary of findings on diagnostic tools for screening strongyloidiasis, January 1993–February 2017.

Index Test—at 10% Prevalence *	Sensitivity (95% CI)	Specificity (95% CI)	Post-Test Probability of a Positive Result (95% CI)	Post-Test Probability of a Negative Result (95% CI)	Number of Studies/ Participants	Certainty of Evidence (GRADE)	Reference Standard
Baermann method [51]	0.72 (0.67–0.76) [a]	1.00 (1.00–1.00) [a]	100% (100–100)	3% (4–3)	9/2459	Moderate [b,c]	Combination of diagnostic tests
Agar plate—10% prevalence [51]	0.89 (0.86–0.92) [a]	1.00 (1.00–1.00) [a]	100% (100–100)	1% (2–1)	10/3563	Moderate [b,c]	Combination of diagnostic tests
NIE LIPS [62] [d]	0.85 (0.79–0.92)	0.95 (0.93–0.98)	65% (56–84)	2% (2–1)	1/399	Low [e,g]	Stool microscopy or culture
IVD ELISA—commercial test [62]	0.92 (0.87–0.97)	0.97 (0.96–0.99)	77% (71–92)	1% (1–0)	1/399	Low [e,h]	Stool microscopy
IFAT [62]	0.94 (0.90–0.98)	0.87 (0.83–0.91)	45% (37–55)	1% (1–0)	1/399	Low [e,h]	Stool microscopy and culture
Bordier-ELISA—commercial kit [62]	0.91 (0.86–0.96)	0.94 (0.91–0.96)	63% (52–77)	1% (2–0)	1/193	Low [e,h]	Kato-Katz, Flotac, and Baermann method
SS-NIE-1 ELISA [63]	0.95 (0.92–0.97)	0.93 (0.90–0.96)	60% (71–73%)	1% (1–0)	1/583	Low [f,g,i]	Stool microscopy and culture

Notes: Population: patients with strongyloidiasis or sera infected with *St. stercoralis*; Settings: low-/high-endemic areas; Target condition: strongyloidiasis (test prevalence 10%). Cost effectiveness: serological testing may be cost-effective relative to stool and eosinophil testing for both strongyloidiasis and schistosomiasis, because of superior test performance characteristics. Tests: ELISA: enzyme-linked immunosorbent assay; GRADE: Grading of Recommendations, Assessment, Development and Evaluation; IFAT: indirect fluorescent antibody technique; IVD: Invitro diagnostic test; LIPS: luciferase immunoprecipitation system; NIE: a 31-kDa recombinant antigen from *St. stercoralis*. * Post-test probability of test was calculated at 10% prevalence for all the tests.

[a] Sensitivity and specificity values obtained from a multiple-field study.
[b] Evidence was downgraded because of serious inconsistencies and heterogeneity.
[c] Heterogeneity between studies; use of intermediate or surrogate outcomes rather than health outcomes.
[d] Test result with a primary standard.
[e] Absence of a reliable gold standard for diagnosis of *S. stercoralis* infection. The review did not describe the specific gold standard used in the included studies for each test.
[f] Single study design.
[g] Samples were classified according to a composite reference standard, a procedure suggested for evaluation of diagnostic tests when there is no gold standard.
[h] Use of intermediate or surrogate outcomes rather than health outcomes.
[i] The inter-assay coefficient of variation was determined to be 22% for the low-positive control serum and 10% for the medium-positive control serum.

The best conventional diagnostic tools for *St. stercoralis* have been agar plate culture with a sensitivity and specificity of 89% (95% CI: 86–92) and 100% (95% CI: 100–100) respectively, and the Baermann method with a sensitivity and specificity of 72% (95% CI: 67–76) and 100% (95% CI: 100–100) respectively (moderate certainty of evidence) [51]. Knopps et al. reported a much lower sensitivity value of 31% (95% CI: 19.1–44.8) for PCR in stools compared with a combination of stool-based methods as the gold standard; specificity was 100% (95% CI: 100–100) [64].

Serological antibody detection methods have demonstrated greater sensitivity compared with classical parasitological techniques [19]. Bisoffi et al. reported the accuracy of five serological tests for detection of strongyloidiasis [62]. The sensitivity and specificity values were: 85% (95% CI: 79–92) and 100% (95% CI: 100–100) for the luciferase-immunoprecipitation system (LIPS) using 31-kD recombinants antigen from *St. stercoralis* (NIE); 75% (95% CI: 66–83) and 95% (95% CI: 91–99) for the NIE-ELISA (using the same antigen); 91% (95% CI: 86–96) and 99% (95% CI: 97–100) for the IVD-ELISA; 90% (95% CI: 84–95) and 98% (95% CI: 96–100) for the Bordier-ELISA; and 94% (95% CI: 90–98) and 92% (95% CI: 87–97) for the indirect fluorescent antibody technique (IFAT) (low certainty of evidence) [62] (Figure 6). Rascoe et al. reported comparable values for two new recombinant antigens in antibody detection assays: SS-NIE-1 ELISA with sensitivity of 95% (95% CI: 92–97) and specificity of 93% (95% CI: 90–96), and Ss-NIE-1 Luminex with sensitivity of 93% (95% CI: 86–96) and specificity of 95% (95% CI: 93–97) (Table 6) [63].

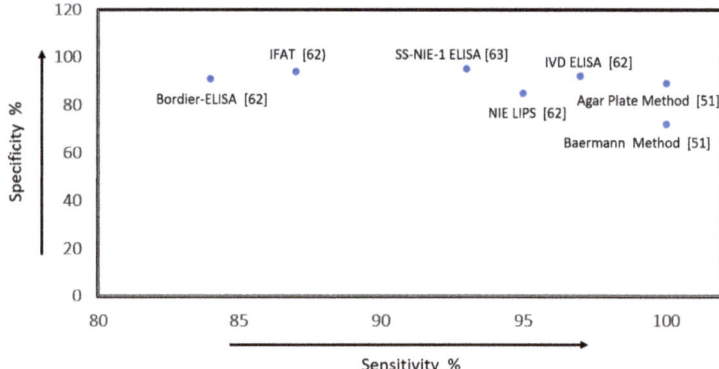

Figure 6. Scatter plot of sensitivity versus specificity values of the Index diagnostic tools for screening strongyloidiasis.

As with schistosomiasis, estimates of false-positive tests per 1000 tested decreased with increasing pre-test prevalence, from 29 to 21, 58 to 42 and 68 to 49 for IVD-ELISA, Bordier-ELISA and SS-NIE-1 ELISA assays, respectively [62,63]. The estimated number of false-positive tests for the Baermann and Agar plate methods was 0 at all pre-test prevalence levels. Lower numbers of false-negatives were estimated for all the serological tests, for example, 1 and 15, and 2 and 24, per 1000 tests for SS-NIE-1 and IVD-ELISA at 2.5% and 30% prevalence levels compared with 3 and 33, and 7 and 84, per 1000 for the Agar plate and Baermann methods. At 2.5% pre-test prevalence, the proportion of correctly diagnosed *Strongyloides* infections in migrant populations was 95% for the SS-NIE-1 ELISA, 93.8% for IFAT, 92% for IVD-ELISA and 90.7% for Bordier-ELISA, compared with 72% and 89% for the Baermann and Agar plate methods (Table 7).

3.3. Treatment Efficacy: Schistosomiasis and Strongyloidiasis

We evaluated four included systematic reviews on treatment of schistosomiasis and strongyloidiasis (Tables 8 and 9) [47–49,52]. In a Cochrane review, the efficacy of praziquantel (single 40 mg/kg dose) showed much lower parasitological failure in urine (<53%) at 1 to 2 months (RR = 0.42;

95% CI: 0.29–0.58) compared with placebo [48]. The proportion of people cured with praziquantel varied substantially between trials, from 22.5% to 83.3%, but was higher than 60% in five of the seven trials [48]. Similarly, in another Cochrane review, parasitological cure rate for *Sc. mansoni* infection at one month with praziquantel (single 40 mg/kg dose) varied substantially across studies, ranging from 52% to 92% in Brazil in 2006 and 2007, for example parasitological cure 66% more in intervention group compared with placebo (RR 3.13; 95% CI: 1.03–9.53) (Table 8) [47]. Pérez del Villar et al. compared the efficacy of praziquantel and artemisinin derivatives and reported that artesunate showed significantly lower cure rates than praziquantel 30% vs. 61% (RR 0.49 (0.28–0.75)) [49]. Artemeter monotherapy (6mg/kg single dose) reduced *Sc. Japonicum* infection rates in patients (RR = 0.25; 95% CI: 0.16–0.40). However, a combination of artemisinin derivatives plus praziquantel showed higher cure rates than praziquantel monotherapy (RR = 1.25; 95% CI: 1.09–1.37) in areas with intense transmission (moderate certainty of evidence) (Table 8) [49]. No significant adverse events were reported.

Table 7. Accuracy of diagnostic tools for strongyloidiasis at different pre-test prevalence levels, 2012–February 2017.

Index tests	True-Positives Pre-Test Probability [a]			False-Positives Pre-Test Probability [a]			True-Negatives Pre-Test Probability [a]			False-Negatives Pre-Test Probability [a]			% Infected Correctly Diagnosed
Test % Prevalence [b]	2.5%	10%	30%	2.5%	10%	30%	2.5%	10%	30%	2.5%	10%	30%	
Baermann method [51]	18	72	216	0	0	0	975	900	700	7	28	84	72%
Agar plate [51]	22	89	267	0	0	0	975	900	700	3	11	33	89%
NIE-LIPS [62]	21	85	255	49	45	35	926	855	665	4	15	45	85.1%
IVD-ELISA (commercial test) [62]	23	92	276	29	27	21	946	873	679	2	8	24	92%
IFAT [62]	23	94	282	127	117	91	848	783	609	2	6	18	93.8%
Bordier-ELISA (commercial kit) [62]	23	91	272	58	54	42	917	846	658	2	9	28	90.7%
SS-NIE-1 ELISA [63]	24	95	285	68	63	49	907	837	651	1	5	15	95%

ELISA: enzyme-linked immunosorbent assay; IFAT: indirect fluorescent antibody technique; IVD: Invitro diagnostic test; LIPS: luciferase immunoprecipitation system; NIE: 31-kDa recombinant antigen from *St. stercoralis*.

[a] Data reported as effect per 1000 migrants tested.
[b] pre-test prevalence or probability of having schistosomiasis in an at-risk population.

Table 8. GRADE summary of findings of different schistosomiasis treatments vs. placebo, 2010–2016.

Outcomes	Anticipated Absolute Effects [a] (95% CI)		Relative Chance of Cure (95% CI)	Number of Participants/Studies	Certainty of the Evidence (GRADE)
	Risk with Placebo per 1000	Cure with Intervention Drug			
Parasitological failure at 1 to 2 months (praziquantel 40 mg/kg single dose) [48]	908	381 (263–562)	RR 0.42 (0.29 to 0.58)	864/7 RCTs	High
Parasitological cure at 1 month [b]—*Sc. mansoni* infections (praziquantel 40 mg/kg single dose) [47]	337	1000 (347–1000)	RR 3.13 (1.03–9.53)	414/2 RCTs	Moderate [c]
Microhaematuria at 8 weeks (praziquantel 40 mg/kg single dose) [48]	281	149 (93–236)	RR 0.53 (0.33–0.84)	119/1 RCT	Low [d,e,f]
Infection rate of *Sc. japonicum* (artemether monotherapy 6 mg/kg) [49]	175	44 (28–70)	RR 0.25 (0.16–0.40)	8051/13 RCTs	Moderate [c]
Parasitological cure rate of *Schistosoma species*. (Artesunate—monotherapy (4 mg/kg daily for three consecutive days)) [49]	615 *	302 (172–459)	RR 0.49 (0.28–0.75)	800/7 RCTs	Moderate [c]
Adverse events, minor (praziquantel 40 mg/kg single dose) [49]	None	None	Not estimable	1591/9 RCTs	Low [d]

CI: confidence interval; GRADE: Grading of Recommendations, Assessment, Development and Evaluation; RR: risk ratio; RTC: randomized controlled trial. * praziquantel 40 mg/kg once.

[a] The risk in the intervention group per 1000 persons treated (95% CI) was based on the assumed risk in the comparison group and the relative effect of the intervention (and its 95% CI).
[b] Treatment of only *Sc. mansoni* infections reported.
[c] Downgraded by 1 for indirectness: only two trials from limited settings evaluated this comparison.
[d] The trial was under-powered; downgraded by 1.
[e] Only a single trial reported this outcome.
[f] Publication bias was unclear.

Table 9. GRADE summary of findings on ivermectin (200 mg/kg) vs. albendazole or thiabendazole for the treatment of strongyloidiasis, and certainty of evidence on treatment efficacy, benefits and harms, 2010–2016.

Outcomes	Anticipated Absolute Effects (95% CI)		Relative Chance of Cure (95% CI) [b]	Number of Participants/Studies	Certainty of the Evidence (GRADE)
	Cure with Comparator Drug per 1000 [a]	Cure with Intervention Drug—Ivermectin (200 mg/kg) [b]			
Cure overall assessed at 5 weeks—albendazole [52]	480	840 (720–980)	RR 1.79 (1.55–2.08)	478/4 RCTs	Moderate [d]
Adverse events assessed at 5 weeks—albendazole [52]	260	210 (150–290)	RR 0.80 (0.59–1.09)	518/4 RCTs	Low [c,g]
Cure overall assessed at 11 weeks—thiabendazole [52]	690	740 (660–820)	RR 1.07 (0.96–1.20)	467/3 RCTs	Moderate [e]
Adverse events assessed at 11 weeks—thiabendazole [52]	730	230 (150–360)	RR 0.31 (0.20–0.50)	507/3 RCTs	Moderate [f]

PICO—Patient or population: persons with Strongyloides stercoralis infection; Setting: south-east Asia, America and Europe; Intervention: ivermectin; Comparison: albendazole and thiabendazole. CI: confidence interval; GRADE: Grading of Recommendations, Assessment, Development and Evaluation; RR: risk ratio; RTC: randomized controlled trial.

[a] Albendazole or thiabendazole.
[b] The risk in the intervention group per 1000 persons treated (95% CI) was based on the assumed risk in the comparison group and the relative effect of the intervention (and its 95% CI).
[c] No method of allocation concealment in two trials and no method of allocation described.
[d] Two trials did not conceal allocation and no method of allocation was described.
[e] Two trials did not conceal allocation and no method of allocation was described in one trial.
[f] Two trials did not conceal allocation and no method of allocation was described.
[g] Wide range of estimates in three trials could include substantive fewer events.

Only one systematic review was included which addressed the efficacy of ivermectin vs. albendazole or thiabendazole for treating chronic strongyloidiasis infection (Table 9) [52]. Parasitological cure determined with both serological and conventional techniques was higher with ivermectin (single-/double-dose) treatment than with albendazole 84% vs. 48% (RR = 1.79; 95% CI: 1.55–2.08) (moderate-quality evidence) [52]. When ivermectin was compared with thiabendazole, there was no distinction in parasitological cure, i.e., 74% vs. 68% (RR = 1.07; 95% CI: 0.96–1.2), but adverse events were less frequent with ivermectin (RR = 0.31; 95% CI: 0.20–0.50) than with thiabendazole [52] (moderate certainty of evidence). No serious adverse events or deaths were reported with either ivermectin or thiabendazole.

3.4. Resource use, Costs and Cost-Effectiveness

3.4.1. Strongyloidiasis

Three economic studies of moderate quality support a strategy of presumptive treatment for strongyloidiasis in migrants from high-risk backgrounds [66–68]. One study showed potential cost savings of universal treatment with albendazole compared with i) no intervention (watchful waiting); and compared with ii) universal stool-based screening; in migrant populations in the U.S. [66]. Sensitivity analyses indicated a best-case scenario of large savings from presumptive treatment, and a worst-case scenario in which treatment was still cost effective at the $30,000/QALY threshold (1997 U.S. dollars).

The second study on presumptive treatment for strongyloidiasis in migrants living in the U.S. in California and New York compared: i) presumptive treatment with albendazole for 3 or 5 days; ii) presumptive treatment with one dose of ivermectin; iii) treatment in those with documented eosinophilia; and iv) no intervention [67]. It indicated that presumptive treatment with ivermectin was cost-effective at a threshold of less than USD 10,000 (EUR 9667) per QALY across a range of prevalence values in migrants living in the U.S. [67]. This study did not include antibody detection among the diagnostic tools. At a prevalence higher than 10%, treatment with ivermectin cost less than USD 2000 (EUR 1983) per QALY. These results were robust across a wide range of sensitivity analyses [67].

The third more recent study on presumptive treatment for hookworm and strongyloidiasis in U.S.-bound Asian populations indicated that treatment in the destination country with albendazole and ivermectin was likely to be cost-effective relative to no screening or screening and treatment strategies in the country of origin among refugees from high-prevalence countries [68]. For strongyloidiasis, overseas treatment cost less than USD 40,000 (EUR 31,092) per QALY gained at prevalence greater than 1% and fell to less than USD 18,000 (EUR 13,991) per QALY gained at prevalence greater than 3%.

3.4.2. Schistosomiasis

There were no cost-effectiveness studies of screening and presumptive treatment in migrants at risk of schistosomiasis. In non-migrant populations, a recent costing study compared the costs of single and double KK tests with a urine dipstick test [69] for *Sc. haematobium* diagnosis in areas of high endemicity. The results of this preliminary costing study indicated similar costs of around USD 6–7 (EUR 5–6) per test for single KK stool and urine tests; however, the quality of evidence for resource use was low. A cost-effectiveness study by King et al. compared single-dose (40 mg/kg body weight) and double-dose (40 mg/kg doses separated by 2–8 weeks) presumptive treatment with praziquantel for schistosomiasis in high-prevalence (>40%) settings in Africa [65]. Double-dose praziquantel was found deemed to be highly cost-effective (ICER of less than USD 500 (EUR 471)/QALY) compared with single-dose treatment.

4. Discussion

The rationale for screening for strongyloidiasis and schistosomiasis in the EU/EEA and not other parasitic infections is based on the estimated prevalence of these parasitic infections among migrants from endemic countries; potential prevention of fatal complications through early case detection and treatment, and secondary transmission in asymptomatic patients based on a highly sensitive test and very effective and safe treatment [11,35,36,71]. Therefore, the implementation of a screening programme would allow early detection of the infection in individuals at risk, before they develop a severe condition which may justify the screening itself.

Although quality data on the prevalence of schistosomiasis and strongyloidiasis among migrant populations in the EU/EEA is limited, available data from endemic regions shows that prevalence of schistosomiasis is between 20% and 40% and prevalence of strongyloidiasis is between 10% and 40% [3–5]. However, there is a rationale for public health surveillance for schistosomiasis and strongyloidiasis to inform proper surveillance of mobile population from the regions [30]

Overall, systematic reviews showed that antibody-detecting serological tests are the most effective screening tests for detection of schistosomiasis and strongyloidiasis in low-endemicity settings, because they have higher sensitivity than conventional parasitological methods [19,44,45,50,53]. Newer serological tests were shown to be more effective than conventional techniques such as agar plate culture and the Baermann method for strongyloidiasis and KK for *Sc. mansoni*. These conventional techniques, as well as PCR, failed to detect infections of very low intensity [64] although they were more specific than serological techniques [51,54]. They are also labor-intensive and require skilled personnel and are therefore not recommended as the first option for screening [19]. In contrast, serological testing is easier to perform in health facilities than collecting and testing faecal samples and can also be combined with other infectious disease screening tests.

One limitation of antibody-detecting serological tests, particularly with schistosomiasis, is that they cannot differentiate current from past infections; however, with strongyloidiasis, antibody titres decline after treatment over time in most patients [62,72]. In addition, in immuno-compromised patients, the sensitivity of serological tests may be reduced, and other additional screening methods may be needed if serology is negative. In this regard, the utility of PCR assay as an alternative screening method in immunosuppressed patients deserves further investigation.

Specifically, for *Schistosoma* spp. infections, available evidence shows that the IgM-ELISA [57], IHA [46] and ICT IgG-IgM [61] tests were the most effective screening tests in low-endemicity countries. In some low endemicity settings, two serological tests are performed, and a case is considered to be positive if either test is positive; in others, a combination of ELISA testing and KK faecal examinations is used to improve the accuracy of detection. However, Beltrame et al. advocate the use of the ICT IgG-IgM test as a single screening test (negative predictive value >97%) [61].

For strongyloidiasis, available evidence (of very low to low quality) shows that antibody-detecting blood tests using a variety of antigen preparations have a better detection rate than conventional parasitological methods, with IVD-ELISA, Bordier-ELISA and NIE LIPS being the most accurate tests [62]. Limitations of these serological tests include the large number of infective larvae required, cross–reactions with other nematode infections and lower sensitivity in immuno-compromised patients [19,62]. New tests based on the recombinant antigen Ss-NIE-1, although slightly less sensitive, but currently considerably more expensive than other serological techniques, show excellent specificity [62,63] and, although not widely available, they may be useful when designing rapid tests [63].

For treatment of schistosomiasis, single-dose praziquantel is the drug of choice. Evidence from systematic reviews shows that treatment with praziquantel significantly increased parasitological cure and, achieved marked reductions in microhaematuria compared with placebo; praziquantel also has a very good safety profile [47,48]. For treatment of strongyloidiasis, there is evidence (of low to moderate quality) that ivermectin is more effective than albendazole [52] and evidence (of moderate quality) that ivermectin is as effective as thiabendazole, but much better tolerated; no difference in the efficacy of ivermectin was observed between endemic and non-endemic populations [52]. However, there are no studies on the potential harms of large-scale administration of ivermectin (although widespread experience with filariasis control is reassuring).

Implementing presumptive treatment either with ivermectin or praziquantel requires additional complex screening strategies to identify individuals with loiasis or neurocysticercosis for whom these drugs might be inappropriate [70,71] and recently published recommendations specify that immigrants arriving from endemic areas should undergo a thorough clinical screening before being given either praziquantel or albendazole [73]. In addition, ivermectin is not readily available in most endemic and non-endemic countries and has limited approval by regulatory authorities in the EU/EEA.

We found no studies evaluating the cost-effectiveness of schistosomiasis screening and treatment interventions in migrant populations. For schistosomiasis, no studies were available on the cost of screening tests based on antibody detection in the non-endemic setting. In endemic settings, double-dose praziquantel was deemed to be highly cost-effective compared with a single dose and was considered robust to plausible changes in parameter estimates [65]. Further economic studies are required to provide better data on the cost-effectiveness of a test-and-treat strategy for schistosomiasis in non-endemic countries. For strongyloidiasis, three studies indicated that presumptive treatment with albendazole or ivermectin was cost-saving or cost-effective, in migrants to the U.S. or in endemic settings [66–68]. The limitations of these studies may decrease the relevance of the results for migrant populations in the EU/EEA. Most of the economic studies identified were limited to Asian populations and not based on screening with antibody testing in a non-endemic setting. However, where the prevalence of schistosomiasis and strongyloidiasis is greater than 1% and the price of presumptive treatment is similar to that used in the economic evaluations identified in this review, presumptive treatment with ivermectin or albendazole is likely to be cost-effective for migrants to the EU/EEA.

The strengths of our study include the use of the GRADE methodology to evaluate the quality and strength of the evidence and effect size in the included studies. The primary outcomes—parasitological cure or failure for efficacy of treatment and accuracy for screening—were objective measures. The individual studies in the included systematic reviews originated from different regions and countries with moderate to high endemicity for both parasites, increasing the generalizability of the results.

We did not identify any systematic reviews or RCTs on screening for schistosomiasis and strongyloidiasis in newly arrived migrants to EU/EEA. RCTs on preventive screening are rare, and so we used a logic model approach, as recommended at US Task Force on Preventive Health Care, and present data on population prevalence, diagnostic accuracy, treatment effectiveness and cost-effectiveness [70,74]. Other limitations include the lack of accurate data on the prevalence of schistosomiasis and strongyloidiasis among migrants from endemic countries entering the EU/EEA and the lack of data on the cost-effectiveness of screening and treating migrants for these parasitic infections. Further studies evaluating the effectiveness and cost-effectiveness of screening intervention in migrant populations are warranted.

The results of this systematic review indicate that although the certainty of desirable over undesirable effects of screening mobile and high-risk migrant populations from endemic areas is low to moderate, there is a rationale for screening, particularly in immunosuppressed patients since there is a high value placed on uncertain but potentially life-preserving benefits as suggested elsewhere [75]. Both schistosomiasis and strongyloidiasis can become chronic and cause severe long-term complications if untreated and the health benefits of intervention therefore outweigh its potential harms. Effective diagnostic tests are available and treatments for both infections are efficacious, well tolerated and safe with few exceptions [48,52,54,62].

Presumptive single-dose therapy of strongyloidiasis with ivermectin for all migrants is likely to be cost-effective; however, the feasibility of this measure has not been demonstrated in clinical studies in non-endemic settings. Importantly, implementing presumptive treatment either with ivermectin for strongyloidiasis or praziquantel for schistosomiasis requires additional screening strategies to identify individuals for whom these drugs might be harmful.

The evidence suggest screening should target people arriving from endemic areas, but national screening strategies will need to be tailored to the specific context of individual EU/EEA countries and, in particular, the countries of origin of migrants to those countries. Although, there are no studies on the extent to which multiple screening tests for infectious diseases in migrants can improve cost-effectiveness, integrating innovative public health screening strategies for schistosomiasis and strongyloidiasis with other infectious diseases will improve surveillance data as well as reduce costs.

However, the optimal approach to delivery of screening will need to consider a global perspective, as well as depend on the health system context in individual EU/EEA countries. In this regard, addressing lack of access to healthcare for migrants, heterogeneity of screening strategies applicable in member states, and improving health professionals' knowledge and training of migrant related infectious diseases should improve the responsiveness of the public health care system with regards to coverage and uptake of screening at the level of primary health care.

Finally, although we consider that sufficient evidence exists to justify screening for strongyloidiasis and schistosomiasis immigrants coming to the EU/EEA from endemic areas, further assessment of the benefits and risks of screening and treatment is needed. More specifically, additional economic analysis is required, in particular to evaluate the costs of a test and treat strategy and to compare the cost-effectiveness of screening and of presumptive treatment.

5. Conclusions

This systematic review provides a compendium of indirect evidence that support the screening for strongyloidiasis and schistosomiasis in migrants coming from endemic areas to the EU/EEA, and particularly in immunosuppressed or at-risk-of immunosuppression patients.

Screening for strongyloidiasis and schistosomiasis should be considered based on serological testing in the absence of immunosuppression. Ivermectin and praziquantel have demonstrated a high efficacy, an excellent safety profile, and a potentially easy schedule for the treatment of strongyloidiasis and schistosomiasis. Economic modelling suggests presumptive single-dose treatment of strongyloidiasis with ivermectin for all migrants is likely cost-effective, but the feasibility of this strategy has yet to be demonstrated in clinical studies in non-endemic settings.

Author Contributions: Conceptualization, E.N.A., A.R.-M., P.A.-C., C.G. and K.P.; Methodology, E.N.A., A.R.-M., E.B., P.A.-C., R.L.M. and K.P.; Software, E.N.A., D.T.M., I.A.-R. and K.P.; Validation, E.N.A., A.T., D.T.M., I.A.-R., N.M. and Z.B.; Formal Analysis, E.N.A., N.M., I.A.-R., R.L.M., A.T., N.R. and Z.B.; Investigation, E.N.A., N.M., T.N., E.B., Z.B., A.R.-M. and R.L.M.; Resources, E.N.A., I.A.-R., T.N., P.A.-C. and K.P.; Data Curation, E.N.A., D.T.M., and I.A.-R.; Writing—Original Draft Preparation, E.N.A., A.R.-M., P.A.-C., R.L.M., and K.P.; Writing—Review & Editing, E.N.A., E.B., A.R.-M., P.A.-C., R.L.M., T.N., and K.P.; Visualization, E.N.A., A.R.-M., P.A.-C., R.L.M. and Z.B.; Supervision, E.N.A., A.R.-M., P.A.-C., R.L.M., T.N. and K.P.; Project Administration, E.N.A., A.R.-M., P.A.-C., T.N. and K.P.; Funding Acquisition, K.P., T.N., and P.A.-C.

Funding: European Health Group and the European Centre for Disease Prevention and Control (ECDC); FWC No ECDC/2015/016; Specific Contract No 1 ECD.5748. The ECDC has suggested experts for review working groups, requested progress reports and provided stakeholder feedback on the proposed protocols. The Barcelona Institute for Global Health (ISGlobal) Research group was supported by Agència de Gestió d'Ajuts Universitaris i de Recerca (AGAUR) (2014SGR26). The views expressed in this publication are those of the author(s) and not necessarily those of the Barcelona Institute for Global Health (ISGlobal) Research group.

Acknowledgments: We appreciate the contributions of Alain Mayhew, Research Associate, C.T. Lamont Primary Health Care Research Centre, Bruyère Research Institute, who facilitated the disease group meeting as well as offered technical guidance to the IP team. Eric N. Agbata is a doctoral candidate for the PhD in Methodology of Biomedical Research and Public Health (Department of Paediatrics, Obstetrics, Gynaecology and Preventive Medicine), Universidad Autònoma de Barcelona, Barcelona, Spain. His significant contributions to this project will form part of his thesis.

Conflicts of Interest: The authors declare no conflict of interest.

Appendix A. Logic Model—Analytic Framework for Screening and Treatment for Schistosomiasis and Strongyloidiasis in Migrants

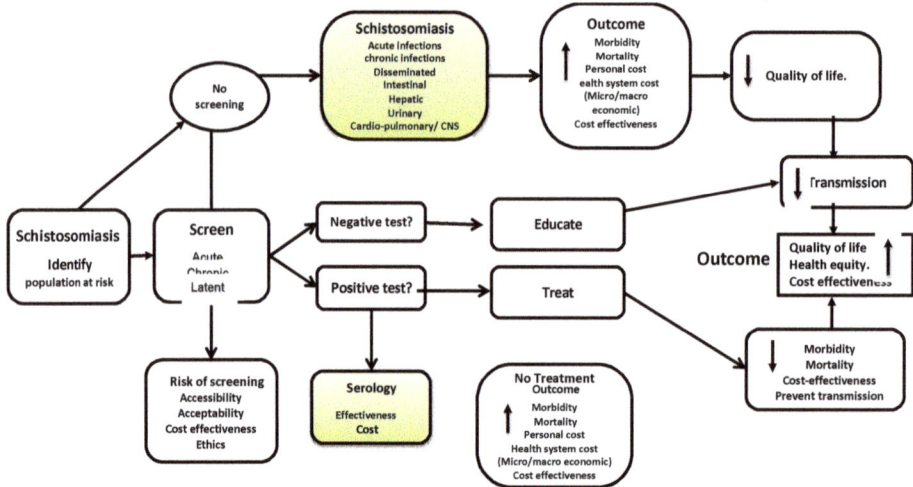

Figure A1. Analytic framework for screening and treatment of schistosomiasis in migrants.

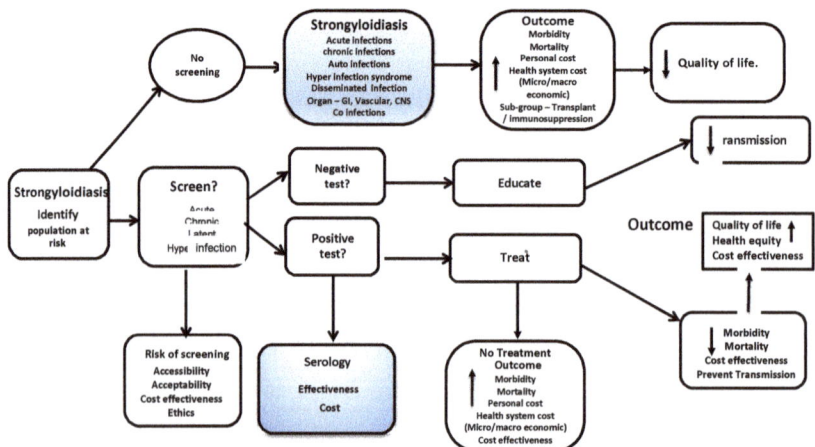

Figure A2. Analytic framework for screening and treatment of strongyloidiasis in migrants.

Appendix B. List of Sites and Literature Search Strategy

1. Literature search strategy for systematic review

The used search strategies for the identification of systematic reviews are listed here.

A. Database: Ovid MEDLINE(R) 1946 to Present with Daily Update
Search Date: 15 April 2016

---

1. exp Schistosoma/ (15595)
2. bilharzia$.tw. (2431)
3. exp Schistosomiasis/ (21432)

4. schistosom$.tw. (25367)
5. katayama fever$.tw. (30)
6. or/1–5 (30014)
7. Strongyloides/ (985)
8. Strongyloides stercoralis/ (1044)
9. Strongyloidiasis/ (3301)
10. strongyloid$.tw. (3988)
11. or/7–10 (4959)
12. 6 or 11 (34621)
13. exp Mass Screening/ (107821)
14. (screened or screening?) tw. (417896)
15. Early Diagnosis/ (19041)
16. (detected or detection? or diagnos$ or discover$ or indentif$) tw. (2972048)
17. exp Population Surveillance/ (56090)
18. (disease? adj2 surveillance) tw. (4053)
19. Contact Tracing/ (3521)
20. contact tracing tw. (1152)
21. or/13–20 (3301561)
22. meta analysis mp, pt. (91365)
23. review pt. (2035657)
24. search$ tw. (253765)
25. or/22–24 (2222329)
26. animals/ not (humans/ and animals/) (4194238)
27. 25 not 26 (2065589)
28. 12 and 21 and 27 (711)
29. 28 and (2010$ or 2011$ or 2012$ or 2013$ or 2014$ or 2015$ or 2016$) ed. (222)
30. remove duplicates from 29 (218)

****

B. Database: Embase <1980 to 2016 April 14>
Search Date: 15 April 2016

1. exp Schistosoma/ (19846)
2. bilharzia$.tw. (2115)
3. exp schistosomiasis/ (20241)
4. schistosom$.tw. (26744)
5. katayama fever$.tw. (10)
6. or/1–5 (33204)
7. Strongyloides/ (1220)
8. Strongyloides stercoralis/ (2315)
9. strongyloidiasis/ (3835)
10. strongyloid$.tw. (4704)
11. or/7–10 (6600)
12. 6 or 11 (39071)
13. exp mass screening/ (178654)
14. (screened or screening?).tw. (614882)
15. early diagnosis/ (82347)

16. parasite identification/ (13161)
17. ((case? or early or parasit$) adj5 (detected or detection? or diagnos$ or discover$ or egg or indentif$)).tw. (385884)
18. exp health survey/ (182738)
19. (disease? adj2 surveillance).tw. (5156)
20. contact examination/ (2830)
21. contact tracing.tw. (1448)
22. or/13–21 (1237076)
23. meta analys$.mp. (167508)
24. search$.tw. (362044)
25. review.pt. (2131214)
26. or/23–25 (2472677)
27. (exp animal/ or animal.hw. or nonhuman/) not (exp human/ or human cell/ or (human or humans) ti.) (5499319)
28. 26 not 27 (2251777)
29. 12 and 22 and 28 (455)
30. 29 and (2010$ or 2011$ or 2012$ or 2013$ or 2014$ or 2015$ or 2016$) dd. (195)
31. remove duplicates from 30 (190)

****

C. Database: EBSCO CINAHL <1970 to April 2016>
Search Date: 15 April 2016

Query   Limiters/Expanders   Last Run Via Results
S28   S24 AND S27   129
S27   S25 OR S26   2,596,403
S26   EM 2010 or EM 2011 or EM 2012 or EM 2013 or EM 2014 or EM 2015 or EM 2016   2,415,478
S25   PY 2010 or PY 2011 or PY 2012 or PY 2013 or PY 2014 or PY 2015 or PY 2016   2,346,296
S24   S9 AND S17 AND S23   253
S23   S18 OR S19 OR S20 OR S21 OR S22   221,252
S22   (TI meta analy * or AB meta analy *)   29,697
S21   (MH "Meta-Analysis")   24,939
S20   PT review   141,448
S19   PT systematic review   53,358
S18   (MH "Systematic Review")   37,435
S17   S10 OR S11 OR S12 OR S13 OR S14 OR S15 OR S16   1,246,183
S16   TX contact tracing   2230
S15   TX (disease * or population) N2 surveillance   23,893
S14   (MH "Population Surveillance+")   5949
S13   TX (detected or detection * or diagnos * or discover * or indentif *)   1,184,038
S12   (MH "Early Diagnosis")   4472
S11   TI ((screened or screening *) OR AB (screened or screening *))   78,236
S10   (MH "Health Screening+")   62,744
S9   S5 OR S8   5460
S8   S6 OR S7   4460
S7   TX strongyloid * 529
S6   (MH "Helminthiasis+")   4132
S5   S1 OR S2 OR S3 OR S4   1931
S4   TX katayama fever   25
S3   TX bilharzia *   175

S2   TX schistosome *   1871
S1   (MH "Schistosomiasis+")   756
****

D. Databases: Database of Abstracts of Reviews of Effects (DARE) and Cochrane Database of Systematic Reviews (CDSR)

Search Date: 15 April 2016

ID Search
#1   MeSH descriptor: [Schistosoma] explode all trees
#2   bilharzia *
#3   MeSH descriptor: [Schistosomiasis] explode all trees
#4   schistosom *
#5   katayama fever
#6   #1 or #2 or #3 or #4 or #5
#7   MeSH descriptor: [Strongyloides] this term only
#8   MeSH descriptor: [Strongyloides stercoralis] this term only
#9   MeSH descriptor: [Strongyloidiasis] this term only
#10 strongyloid *
#11 #7 or #8 or #9 or #10
#12 #6 or #11
#13 #12 in Other Reviews
#14 #12 in Cochrane Reviews (Reviews and Protocols)
****

2. Literature search strategy for systematic search for cost-effectiveness studies

The used search strategies for the identification of systematic reviews on cost-effectiveness are listed here.

A. Database: Ovid MEDLINE(R) Epub Ahead of Print <May Week 3 2016>, Ovid MEDLINE(R) 1946 to Present with Daily Update

Search Date: 31 May 2016

---

1.   exp Schistosoma/ (15714)
2.   bilharzia$.tw. (2438)
3.   exp Schistosomiasis/ (21583)
4.   schistosom$.tw. (25722)
5.   katayama fever$.tw. (30)
6.   or/1–5 (30381)
7.   Strongyloides/ (990)
8.   Strongyloides stercoralis/ (1056)
9.   Strongyloidiasis/ (3319)
10. strongyloid$.tw. (4079)
11. or/7–10 (5051)
12. 6 or 11 (35067)
13. exp Mass Screening/ (108535)
14. (screened or screening? or tested or testing or tests).tw. (1734474)
15. Early Diagnosis/ (19350)
16. (detected or detection? or diagnos$ or discover$ or indentif$).tw. (3053822)
17. exp Population Surveillance/ (56687)
18. (disease? adj2 surveillance).tw. (4195)

19. Contact Tracing/ (3563)
20. contact tracing.tw. (1176)
21. or/13–20 (4387118)
22. meta analysis.mp,pt. (96759)
23. review.pt. (2060867)
24. search$.tw. (266775)
25. guideline.pt. (15780)
26. guideline/ (15780)
27. guidelines as topic/ (34071)
28. practice guideline.pt. (21216)
29. practice guideline/ (21216)
30. practice guidelines as topic/ (91792)
31. (CPG or CPGs or guidance or guideline? or recommend$ or standard?).ti. (147179)
32. exp clinical pathway/ (5273)
33. exp clinical protocol/ (139345)
34. ((care or clinical) adj2 pathway?).tw. (5129)
35. or/22–34 (2572065)
36. 12 and 21 and 35 (960)
37. animals/ not (humans/ and animals/) (4215704)
38. 36 not 37 (838)
39. 38 and (2010$ or 2011$ or 2012$ or 2013$ or 2014$ or 2015$ or 2016$).ed. (271)
40. remove duplicates from 39 [reviews and guidelines] (261)
41. exp "costs and cost analysis"/ (197942)
42. cost$.mp. (467877)
43. cost effective$.tw. (83090)
44. cost benefit analys$.mp. (67319)
45. health care costs.mp. (37157)
46. or/41–45 (477217)
47. 12 and 21 and 46 (260)
48. animals/ not (humans/ and animals/) (4215704)
49. 47 not 48 (222)
50. 49 and (2010$ or 2011$ or 2012$ or 2013$ or 2014$ or 2015$ or 2016$).ed. (82)
51. remove duplicates from 50 (78)

****

B. Database: Embase <1974 to 2016 Week 22>
Search Date: 31 May 2016

1. exp Schistosoma/ (21727)
2. bilharzia$.tw. (2492)
3. exp schistosomiasis/ (21930)
4. schistosom$.tw. (29047)
5. katayama fever$.tw. (42)
6. or/1–5 (36157)
7. Strongyloides/ (1229)
8. Strongyloides stercoralis/ (2447)
9. strongyloidiasis/ (3986)
10. strongyloid$.tw. (4977)

11. or/7–10 (6962)
12. 6 or 11 (42352)
13. exp mass screening/ (182895)
14. (screened or screening? or tested or testing or tests).tw. (2429856)
15. early diagnosis/ (83110)
16. parasite identification/ (13222)
17. ((case? or early or parasit$) adj5 (detected or detection? or diagnos$ or discover$ or egg or indentif$)).tw. (405389)
18. exp health survey/ (184236)
19. (disease? adj2 surveillance).tw. (5253)
20. contact examination/ (2867)
21. contact tracing.tw. (1512)
22. or/13-21 (2999272)
23. meta analys$.mp. (170914)
24. search$.tw. (371898)
25. review.pt. (2163187)
26. guideline.pt. (0)
27. guideline/ (144)
28. guidelines as topic/ (229895)
29. practice guideline.pt. (0)
30. practice guideline/ (275502)
31. practice guidelines as topic/ (171091)
32. (CPG or CPGs or guidance or guideline? or recommend$ or standard?).ti. (203285)
33. exp clinical pathway/ (6983)
34. exp clinical protocol/ (75932)
35. ((care or clinical) adj2 pathway?).tw. (9455)
36. or/23–35 (2900847)
37. 12 and 22 and 36 (824)
38. (exp animal/ or animal.hw. or nonhuman/) not (exp human/ or human cell/ or (human or humans).ti.) (5865460)
39. 37 not 38 (678)
40. 39 and (2010$ or 2011$ or 2012$ or 2013$ or 2014$ or 2015$ or 2016$).dd. (304)
41. remove duplicates from 40 [reviews and guidelines] (295)
42. cost effectiveness analysis/ (114264)
43. cost.tw. (387431)
44. costs.tw. (208732)
45. or/42–44 (544771)
46. 12 and 22 and 45 (274)
47. (exp animal/ or animal.hw. or nonhuman/) not (exp human/ or human cell/ or (human or humans).ti.) (5865460)
48. 46 not 47 (223)
49. 48 and (2010$ or 2011$ or 2012$ or 2013$ or 2014$ or 2015$ or 2016$).dd. (115)
50. remove duplicates from 49 [costing] (111)

****

C. Databases: Database of Abstracts of Reviews of Effects (DARE) and Cochrane Database of Systematic Reviews (CDSR) and NHS EED
Search Date: 31 May 2016

ID	Search
#1	MeSH descriptor: [Schistosoma] explode all trees
#2	bilharzia*
#3	MeSH descriptor: [Schistosomiasis] explode all trees
#4	schistosom*
#5	katayama fever
#6	#1 or #2 or #3 or #4 or #5
#7	MeSH descriptor: [Strongyloides] this term only
#8	MeSH descriptor: [Strongyloides stercoralis] this term only
#9	MeSH descriptor: [Strongyloidiasis] this term only
#10	strongyloid*
#11	#7 or #8 or #9 or #10
#12	#6 or #11
#13	#12 in Other Reviews
#14	#12 in Cochrane Reviews (Reviews and Protocols)
#15	#12 in Economic Evaluations

****

D. Database: EBSCO CINAHL <1970 to May 2016>
Search Date: 31 May 2016

#	Query	Limiters/Expanders Last Run Via	Results
S38	S32 AND S37		38
S37	S9 AND S17 AND S36		76
S36	S34 OR S35		139,767
S35	TI (cost OR costs) OR AB (cost OR costs)		89,616
S34	(MH "Costs and Cost Analysis+")		82,915
S33	S29 AND S32		164
S32	S30 OR S31		2,653,954
S31	EM 2010 or EM 2011 or EM 2012 or EM 2013 or EM 2014 or EM 2015 or EM 2016		2,445,432
S30	PY 2010 or PY 2011 or PY 2012 or PY 2013 or PY 2014 or PY 2015 or PY 2016		2,403,611
S29	S9 AND S17 AND S28		307
S28	S18 OR S19 OR S20 OR S21 OR S22 OR S23 OR S24 OR S25 OR S26 OR S27		348,353
S27	TX (care or clinical) N2 pathway *		15,555
S26	TI (CPG or CPGs or guidance or guideline * or recommend * or standard *)		79,261
S25	(MH "Critical Path")		4120
S24	PT Practice Guidelines		9487
S23	(MH "Practice Guidelines")		53,690
S22	(TI meta analy * or AB meta analy *)		30,542
S21	(MH "Meta Analysis")		25,200
S20	PT review		144,019
S19	PT systematic review		53,350
S18	(MH "Systematic Review")		37,846
S17	S10 OR S11 OR S12 OR S13 OR S14 OR S15 OR S16		1,801,344
S16	TX contact tracing		2236
S15	TX (disease * or population) N2 surveillance		24,089
S14	(MH "Population Surveillance+")		6026
S13	TX (detected or detection * or diagnos * or discover * or identif *)		1,195,388
S12	(MH "Early Diagnosis")		4553
S11	TX (screened or screening * or tested or testing or tests)		1,102,848

S10   (MH "Health Screening+")   63,147
S9   S5 OR S8   5501
S8   S6 OR S7   4500
S7   TX strongyloid *   537
S6   (MH "Helminthiasis+")   4167
S5   S1 OR S2 OR S3 OR S4   1942
S4   TX katayama fever   24
S3   TX bilharzia *   175
S2   TX schistosome *   1881
S1   (MH "Schistosomiasis+")   764
****

E. Databases: PubMed
Search Date: 31 May 2016

(((((((schistosome * or bilharzia * or katayama or strongyloid *))) AND ((screened or screening * or tested or testing or tests)))) AND (((CPG or CPGs or guidance or guideline * or metaanalysis or meta-analysis or recommend * or review or standard or standards)))) AND ((publisher [3]))))) (8)

(((((((schistosome * or bilharzia * or katayama or strongyloid *))) AND ((screened or screening * or tested or testing or tests)))) AND (((cost or costs)))) AND ((publisher [3]))))) (2)
****

3. **Update Literature strategy for primary studies on diagnostic or screening tools for schistosomiasis.**

A. Database: Ovid MEDLINE(R)—1946 to February 2017.

1.   Schistosomiasis/ (13485)
2.   Schistosomiasis.mp. (24533)
3.   snail fever.mp. (10)
4.   schistosome *.mp. (5528)
5.   exp "Sensitivity and Specificity"/ (495027)
6.   sensitivity.tw. (638974)
7.   specificity.tw. (379605)
8.   ((pre-test or pretest) adj probability).tw. (1695)
9.   post-test probability.tw. (441)
10. predictive value$.tw. (85102)
11. likelihood ratio$.tw. (11639)
12. or/5–11 (1217873)
13. or/1–4 (26340)
14. 12 and 13 (1493)
15. limit 14 to humans (1112)
16. from 15 keep 1001–1112 (112)

A. Database: EMBASE—up to February 2017
#16   #14 AND 'human'/de AND [embase]/lim NOT [medline]/lim   308
#15   #14 AND 'human'/de   1489
#14   #5 AND #13   2534
#13   #6 OR #7 OR #8 OR #9 OR #10 OR #11 OR #12   1688887
#12   'sensitivity and sensibility'   982
#11   'sensitivity'   1132406
#10   'specificity'   719846
#9   'pretest posttest design'   2331

#8 'predictive value'   161458
#7 'likelihood ratio'   11832
#6 'diagnostic accuracy'   220669
#5 #1 OR #2 OR #3 OR #4   35984
#4 'snail fever'   9
#3 'schistosome'   4643
#2 'schistosoma'   25091
#1 'schistosomiasis'/exp   22890

B. Database: COCHRANE LIBRARY- up to February 2017
ID   Search   Hits
#1   MeSH descriptor: [Schistosomiasis] explode all trees   295
#2   Schistosomiasis   497
#3   snail fever   3
#4   schistosome *   50
#5   #1 or #2 or #3 or #4   506
#6   MeSH descriptor: [Diagnosis] explode all trees   298999
#7   diagno *   129750
#8   #6 or #7   367644
#9   #5 and #8   220

C. Database: CINAHL—up to February 2017
S12   S4 AND S11
S11   S5 OR S6 OR S7 OR S8 OR S9 OR S10
S10   likelihood ratio$
S9   predictive value$
S8   post-test probability
S7   sensitivity and specificity
S6   specificity
S5   sensitivity
S4   S1 OR S2 OR S3
S3   schistosoma
S2   schistosome *
S1   Schistosomiasis

D. Database: LILACS – up to February 2017
(tw:((tw:(esquistosomiasis)) OR (tw:(bilharziasis)) OR (tw:(schistosoma)))) AND (tw:((tw:(diagnostico)) OR (tw:(deteccion)))) AND (instance:"regional") AND (db:("LILACS" OR "colecionaSUS" OR "IBECS" OR "SES-SP" OR "MedCarib" OR "CUMED" AND clinical_aspect:("diagnosis") AND limit:("humans"))
****

4. Update Literature strategy for primary studies on diagnostic or screening tools for strongyloidiasis

A. Database: Ovid MEDLINE(R)—1946 to February 2017

1. Strongyloidiasis/ (3403)
2. Strongyloidiasis.mp. (3747)
3. Strongyloides stercoralis/ (1098)
4. Strongyloides stercoralis.mp. (2142)
5. or/1–4 (4376)
6. exp "Sensitivity and Specificity"/ (494358)
7. sensitivity.tw. (637846)

8. specificity.tw. (379066)
9. ((pre-test or pretest) adj probability).tw. (1689)
10. post-test probability.tw. (438)
11. predictive value$.tw. (84929)
12. likelihood ratio$.tw. (11613)
13. or/6–12 (1216076)
14. 5 and 13 (247)
15. limit 14 to humans (207)

B. Database: EMBASE—up to February 2017

No.   Query   Results
#14   #12 AND [embase]/lim NOT [medline]/lim AND 'human'/de   136
#13   #12 AND [embase]/lim NOT [medline]/lim   156
#12   #3 AND #11   472
#11   #4 OR #5 OR #6 OR #7 OR #8 OR #9 OR #10   1686971
#10   'diagnostic accuracy'   220414
#9   'likelihood ratio'   11815
#8   'predictive value'   161090
#7   'pretest posttest design'   2315
#6   'specificity'   719056
#5   'sensitivity'   1131076
#4   'sensitivity and sensibility'   981
#3   #1 OR #2   5662
#2   'strongyloides stercoralis'   3193
#1   'strongyloidiasis'/exp   4162

C. Database: COCHRANE LIBRARY—up to February 2017

ID   Search   Hits
#1   MeSH descriptor: [Strongyloidiasis] explode all trees   28
#2   Strongyloidiasis   53
#3   MeSH descriptor: [Strongyloides stercoralis] explode all trees   12
#4   Strongyloides stercoralis   47
#5   #1 or #2 or #3 or #4   72
#6   MeSH descriptor: [Diagnosis] explode all trees   298999
#7   diagno *   129739
#8   #6 or #7   367633
#9   #5 and #8   38

D. Database: CINAHL—up to February 2017

Términos de la búsqueda   Opciones de búsqueda
S11   (S4 OR S5 OR S6 OR S7 OR S8 OR S9) AND (S3 AND S10)
S10   S4 OR S5 OR S6 OR S7 OR S8 OR S9
S9   likelihood ratio$
S8   predictive value$
S7   post-test probability
S6   sensitivity and specificity
S5   specificity
S4   sensitivity
S3   S1 OR S2
S2   strongyloides stercoralis
S1   strongyloidiasis

E. Database: LILACS—up to February 2017

(tw:((tw:(estrongiloidiasis)) OR (tw:(Strongyloides stercoralis)))) AND (tw:((tw:(diagnostico)) OR (tw:(deteccion))))

****

References

1. Puthiyakunnon, S.; Boddu, S.; Li, Y.; Zhou, X.; Wang, C.; Li, J.; Chen, X. Strongyloidiasis—An insight into its global prevalence and management. *PLoS Negl. Trop. Dis.* **2014**, *8*, e3018. [CrossRef] [PubMed]
2. Riccardi, N.; Nosenzo, F.; Peraldo, F.; Sarocchi, F.; Taramasso, L.; Traverso, P.; Viscoli, C.; Di Biagio, A.; Derchi, L.E.; De Maria, A. Increasing prevalence of genitourinary schistosomiasis in Europe in the Migrant Era: Neglected no more? *PLoS Negl. Trop. Dis.* **2017**, *11*, e0005237. [CrossRef] [PubMed]
3. Murray, C.J.; Vos, T.; Lozano, R.; Naghavi, M.; Flaxman, A.D.; Michaud, C.; Ezzati, M.; Shibuya, K.; Salomon, J.A.; Abdalla, S.; et al. Disability-adjusted life years (DALYs) for 291 diseases and injuries in 21 regions, 1990–2010: A systematic analysis for the Global Burden of Disease Study 2010. *Lancet* **2012**, *380*, 2197–2223. [CrossRef]
4. King, C.H. Parasites and poverty: The case of schistosomiasis. *Acta Trop.* **2010**, *113*, 95–104. [CrossRef] [PubMed]
5. Zoni, A.C.; Catalá, L.; Ault, S.K. Schistosomiasis Prevalence and Intensity of Infection in Latin America and the Caribbean Countries, 1942–2014: A Systematic Review in the Context of a Regional Elimination Goal. *PLoS Negl. Trop. Dis.* **2016**, *10*, e0004493. [CrossRef] [PubMed]
6. Schar, F.; Trostdorf, U.; Giardina, F.; Khieu, V.; Muth, S.; Marti, H.; Vounatsou, P.; Odermatt, P. Strongyloides stercoralis: Global Distribution and Risk Factors. *PLoS Negl. Trop. Dis.* **2013**, *7*, e2288. [CrossRef] [PubMed]
7. Bisoffi, Z.; Buonfrate, D.; Montresor, A.; Requena-Mendez, A.; Munoz, J.; Krolewiecki, A.J.; Gotuzzo, E.; Mena, M.A.; Chiodini, P.L.; Anselmi, M.; et al. Strongyloides stercoralis: A plea for action. *PLoS Negl. Trop. Dis.* **2013**, *7*, e2214. [CrossRef]
8. Adenowo, A.F.; Oyinloye, B.E.; Ogunyinka, B.I.; Kappo, A.P. Impact of human schistosomiasis in sub-Saharan Africa. *Braz. J. Infect. Dis.* **2015**, *19*, 196–205. [CrossRef]
9. Hotez, P.J.; Alvarado, M.; Basanez, M.G.; Bolliger, I.; Bourne, R.; Boussinesq, M.; Brooker, S.J.; Brown, A.S.; Buckle, G.; Budke, C.M.; et al. The global burden of disease study 2010: Interpretation and implications for the neglected tropical diseases. *PLoS Negl. Trop. Dis.* **2014**, *8*, e2865. [CrossRef] [PubMed]
10. Beltrame, A.; Buonfrate, D.; Gobbi, F.; Angheben, A.; Marchese, V.; Monteiro, G.B.; Bisoffi, Z. The hidden epidemic of schistosomiasis in recent African immigrants and asylum seekers to Italy. *Eur. J. Epidemiol.* **2017**. [CrossRef]
11. Khan, K.; Sears, J.; Chan, A.; Rashid, M.; Greenaway, C.; Stauffer, W.; Narasiah, L.; Pottie, K. Canadian Collaboration for Immigrant and Refugee Health (CCIRH). Strongyloides and Schistosoma: Evidence review for newly arriving immigrants and refugee. In *The Canadian Collaboration for Immigrant and Refugee Health. Appendix 8: Intestinal Parasites*; Canadian Medical Association Journal: Ottawa, ON, Canada, 2011.
12. Wilson, J.M.G.; Jungner, G.; Organization, W.H. *Principles and Practice of Screening for Disease*; World Health Organization: Geneva, Switzerland, 1968.
13. Colley, D.G.; Bustinduy, A.L.; Secor, W.E.; King, C.H. Human schistosomiasis. *Lancet* **1969**, *383*, 2253–2264. [CrossRef]
14. Deniaud, F.; Rouesse, C.; Collignon, A.; Domingo, A.; Rigal, L. Failure to offer parasitology screening to vulnerable migrants in France: Epidemiology and consequences. *Sante (Montrouge, France)* **2010**, *20*, 201–208. (In French)
15. Ross, A.G.; McManus, D.P.; Farrar, J.; Hunstman, R.J.; Gray, D.J.; Li, Y.S. Neuroschistosomiasis. *J. Neurol.* **2012**, *259*, 22–32. [CrossRef] [PubMed]
16. Buonfrate, D.; Requena-Mendez, A.; Angheben, A.; Munoz, J.; Gobbi, F.; Van Den Ende, J.; Bisoffi, Z. Severe strongyloidiasis: A systematic review of case reports. *BMC Infect. Dis.* **2013**, *13*, 78. [CrossRef] [PubMed]
17. Kim, J.H.; Kim, D.S.; Yoon, Y.K.; Sohn, J.W.; Kim, M.J. Donor-Derived Strongyloidiasis Infection in Solid Organ Transplant Recipients: A Review and Pooled Analysis. *Transp. Proc.* **2016**, *48*, 2442–2449. [CrossRef] [PubMed]

18. Berry, A.; Paris, L.; Boissier, J.; Caumes, E. Schistosomiasis Screening of Travelers to Corsica, France. *Emerg. Infect. Dis.* **2016**, *22*, 159. [CrossRef] [PubMed]
19. Requena-Mendez, A.; Chiodini, P.; Bisoffi, Z.; Buonfrate, D.; Gotuzzo, E.; Munoz, J. The laboratory diagnosis and follow up of strongyloidiasis: A systematic review. *PLoS Negl. Trop. Dis.* **2013**, *7*, e2002. [CrossRef]
20. Greaves, D.; Coggle, S.; Pollard, C.; Aliyu, S.H.; Moore, E.M. Strongyloides stercoralis infection. *BMJ* **2013**, *347*, f4610. [CrossRef]
21. Deniaud, F.; Legros, P.; Collignon, A.; Prevot, M.; Domingo, A.; Ayache, B. Targeted screening proposed in 6 migrant worker housing units in Paris in 2005: Feasibility and impact study. *Sante Publique* **2008**, *20*, 547–559. (In French) [CrossRef]
22. Chernet, A.; Kling, K.; Sydow, V.; Kuenzli, E.; Hatz, C.; Utzinger, J.; van Lieshout, L.; Marti, H.; Labhardt, N.D.; Neumayr, A. Accuracy of diagnostic tests for Schistosoma mansoni infection in asymptomatic Eritrean refugees: Serology and POC-CCA against stool microscopy. *Clin. Infect. Dis.* **2017**. [CrossRef]
23. Weerakoon, K.G.; Gobert, G.N.; Cai, P.; McManus, D.P. Advances in the Diagnosis of Human Schistosomiasis. *Clin. Microbiol. Rev.* **2015**, *28*, 939–967. [CrossRef] [PubMed]
24. Agbata, E.N.; Padilla, P.F.; Agbata, I.N.; Armas, L.H.; Sola, I.; Pottie, K.; Alonso-Coello, P. Migrant Healthcare Guidelines: A Systematic Quality Assessment. *J. Immigr. Minor. Health* **2018**. [CrossRef] [PubMed]
25. Eurostat. Eurostat migr_resfirst, m.r. Residence permits statistics. Available online: https://ec.europa.eu/eurostat/documents/2995521/9333446/3-25102018-AP-EN.pdf/3fa5fa53-e076-4a5f-8bb5-a8075f639167 (accessed on 19 December 2018).
26. European Centre for Disease Prevention and Control. *Monitoring implementation of the Dublin Declaration on Partnership to Fight HIV/AIDS in Europe and Central Asia: 2017 Progress Report Stockholm*; European Centre for Disease Prevention and Control: Stockholm, Sweden, 2017.
27. Eurostat. Eurostat migr_asydcfsta, t. Asylum quarterly report. Available online: https://ec.europa.eu/eurostat/statistics-explained/pdfscache/13562.pdf (accessed on 19 December 2018).
28. European Parliament. EU Migrant Crisis: Facts and Figures. 2017. Available online: http://www.europarl.europa.eu/news/en/headlines/society/20170629STO78630/eu-migrant-crisis-facts-and-figures (accessed on 19 December 2018).
29. Gushulak, B.D.; MacPherson, D.W. Population mobility and health: An overview of the relationships between movement and population health. *J. Travel Med.* **2004**, *11*, 171–178. [CrossRef] [PubMed]
30. Beknazarova, M.; Whiley, H.; Ross, K. Strongyloidiasis: A disease of socioeconomic disadvantage. *Int. J. Environ. Res. Public Health* **2016**, *13*, 517. [CrossRef] [PubMed]
31. Seedat, F.; Hargreaves, S.; Nellums, L.B.; Ouyang, J.; Brown, M.; Friedland, J.S. How effective are approaches to migrant screening for infectious diseases in Europe? A systematic review. *Lancet Infect. Dis.* **2018**, *18*, e259–e271. [CrossRef]
32. Kortas, A.; Polenz, J.; von Hayek, J.; Rüdiger, S.; Rottbauer, W.; Storr, U.; Wibmer, T. Screening for infectious diseases among asylum seekers newly arrived in Germany in 2015: A systematic single-centre analysis. *Public Health* **2017**, *153*, 1–8. [CrossRef] [PubMed]
33. Aldridge, R.W.; Yates, T.A.; Zenner, D.; White, P.J.; Abubakar, I.; Hayward, A.C. Pre-entry screening programmes for tuberculosis in migrants to low-incidence countries: A systematic review and meta-analysis. *Lancet Infect. Dis.* **2014**, *14*, 1240–1249. [CrossRef]
34. Carballo, M.; Hargreaves, S.; Gudumac, I.; Maclean, E.C. Evolving migrant crisis in Europe: Implications for health systems. *Lancet Glob. Health* **2017**, *5*, e252–e253. [CrossRef]
35. Karki, T.; Napoli, C.; Riccardo, F.; Fabiani, M.; Dente, M.G.; Carballo, M.; Noori, T.; Declich, S. Screening for infectious diseases among newly arrived migrants in EU/EEA countries-varying practices but consensus on the utility of screening. *Int. J. Environ. Res. Public Health* **2014**, *11*, 11004–11014. [CrossRef]
36. Semenza, J.C.; Carrillo-Santisteve, P.; Zeller, H.; Sandgren, A.; van der Werf, M.J.; Severi, E.; Pastore Celentano, L.; Wiltshire, E.; Suk, J.E.; Dinca, I.; et al. Public Health needs of migrants, refugees and asylum seekers in Europe, 2015: Infectious disease aspects. *Eur. J. Public Health* **2016**, *26*, 372–373. [CrossRef]
37. Schunemann, H.J.; Wiercioch, W.; Brozek, J.; Etxeandia-Ikobaltzeta, I.; Mustafa, R.A.; Manja, V.; Brignardello-Petersen, R.; Neumann, I.; Falavigna, M.; Alhazzani, W.; et al. GRADE Evidence to Decision (EtD) frameworks for adoption, adaptation, and de novo development of trustworthy recommendations: GRADE-ADOLOPMENT. *J. Clin. Epidemiol.* **2017**, *81*, 101–110. [CrossRef] [PubMed]

38. Moher, D.; Liberati, A.; Tetzlaff, J.; Altman, D.G.; Group, P. Preferred reporting items for systematic reviews and meta-analyses: The PRISMA statement. *PLoS Med.* **2009**, *6*, e1000097. [CrossRef] [PubMed]
39. Pottie, K.; Mayhew, A.D.; Morton, R.L.; Greenaway, C.; Akl, E.A.; Rahman, P.; Zenner, D.; Pareek, M.; Tugwell, P.; Welch, V.; et al. Prevention and assessment of infectious diseases among children and adult migrants arriving to the European Union/European Economic Association: A protocol for a suite of systematic reviews for public health and health systems. *BMJ Open* **2017**, *7*, e014608. [CrossRef] [PubMed]
40. Shemilt, I.; Thomas, J.; Morciano, M. A web-based tool for adjusting costs to a specific target currency and price year. *Evid. Policy A J. Res. Debate Pract.* **2010**, *6*, 51–59. [CrossRef]
41. Shea, B.J.; Grimshaw, J.M.; Wells, G.A.; Boers, M.; Andersson, N.; Hamel, C.; Porter, A.C.; Tugwell, P.; Moher, D.; Bouter, L.M. Development of AMSTAR: A measurement tool to assess the methodological quality of systematic reviews. *BMC Med. Res. Methodol.* **2007**, *7*, 10. [CrossRef] [PubMed]
42. The Newcastle-Ottawa Scale (NOS) for Assessing the Quality of Nonrandomised Studies in Meta-Analyses. Available online: http://www.ohri.ca/programs/clinical_epidemiology/oxford.asp (accessed on 19 December 2018).
43. Whiting, P.F.; Rutjes, A.W.; Westwood, M.E.; Mallett, S.; Deeks, J.J.; Reitsma, J.B.; Leeflang, M.M.; Sterne, J.A.; Bossuyt, P.M. QUADAS-2: A revised tool for the quality assessment of diagnostic accuracy studies. *Ann. Intern. Med.* **2011**, *155*, 529–536. [CrossRef] [PubMed]
44. Ochodo, E.A.; Gopalakrishna, G.; Spek, B.; Reitsma, J.B.; van Lieshout, L.; Polman, K.; Lamberton, P.; Bossuyt, P.M.M.; Leeflang, M.M.G. Circulating antigen tests and urine reagent strips for diagnosis of active schistosomiasis in endemic areas. *Cochrane Database Syst. Rev.* **2015**. [CrossRef]
45. King, C.H.; Bertsch, D. Meta-analysis of Urine Heme Dipstick Diagnosis of *Schistosoma haematobium* Infection, Including Low-Prevalence and Previously-Treated Populations. *PLoS Negl. Trop. Dis.* **2013**, *7*, e2431. [CrossRef]
46. Wang, W.; Li, Y.; Li, H.; Xing, Y.; Qu, G.; Dai, J.; Liang, Y. Immunodiagnostic efficacy of detection of Schistosoma japonicum human infections in China: A meta analysis. *Asian Pac. J. Trop. Med.* **2012**, *5*, 15–23. [CrossRef]
47. Danso-Appiah, A.; Olliaro, P.L.; Donegan, S.; Sinclair, D.; Utzinger, J. Drugs for treating Schistosoma mansoni infection. *Cochrane Database Syst. Rev.* **2013**. [CrossRef]
48. Kramer, C.V.; Zhang, F.; Sinclair, D.; Olliaro, P.L. Drugs for treating urinary schistosomiasis. *Cochrane Database Syst. Rev.* **2014**. [CrossRef] [PubMed]
49. Pérez del Villar, L.; Burguillo, F.J.; López-Abán, J.; Muro, A. Systematic Review and Meta-Analysis of Artemisinin Based Therapies for the Treatment and Prevention of Schistosomiasis. *PLoS ONE* **2012**, *7*, e45867. [CrossRef] [PubMed]
50. Yang, F.; Tan, X.D.; Liu, B.; Yang, C.; Ni, Z.L.; Gao, X.D.; Wang, Y. Meta-analysis of the diagnostic efficiency of the questionnaires screening for schistosomiasis. *Parasitol. Res.* **2015**, *114*, 3509–3519. [CrossRef] [PubMed]
51. Campo Polanco, L.; Gutierrez, L.A.; Cardona Arias, J. Diagnosis of Strongyloides Stercoralis infection: Meta-analysis on evaluation of conventional parasitological methods (1980–2013). *Rev. Esp. Salud Publica* **2014**, *88*, 581–600. (In French) [CrossRef] [PubMed]
52. Henriquez-Camacho, C.; Gotuzzo, E.; Echevarria, J.; White, A.C., Jr.; Terashima, A.; Samalvides, F.; Pérez-Molina, J.A.; Plana, M.N. Ivermectin versus albendazole or thiabendazole for Strongyloides stercoralis infection. *Cochrane Database Syst. Rev.* **2016**. [CrossRef] [PubMed]
53. Danso-Appiah, A.; Minton, J.; Boamah, D.; Otchere, J.; Asmah, R.H.; Rodgers, M.; Bosompem, K.M.; Eusebi, P.; De Vlas, S.J. Accuracy of point-of-care testing for circulatory cathodic antigen in the detection of schistosome infection: Systematic review and meta-analysis. *Bull. World Health Organ.* **2016**, *94*, 522–533. [CrossRef] [PubMed]
54. Kinkel, H.F.; Dittrich, S.; Baumer, B.; Weitzel, T. Evaluation of eight serological tests for diagnosis of imported schistosomiasis. *Clin. Vaccine Immunol.* **2012**, *19*, 948–953. [CrossRef]
55. Lodh, N.; Mwansa, J.C.; Mutengo, M.M.; Shiff, C.J. Diagnosis of Schistosoma mansoni without the stool: Comparison of three diagnostic tests to detect Schistosoma [corrected] mansoni infection from filtered urine in Zambia. *Am. J. Trop. Med. Hyg.* **2013**, *89*, 46–50. [CrossRef]
56. Espirito-Santo, M.C.; Alvarado-Mora, M.V.; Dias-Neto, E.; Botelho-Lima, L.S.; Moreira, J.P.; Amorim, M.; Pinto, P.L.; Heath, A.R.; Castilho, V.L.; Goncalves, E.M.; et al. Evaluation of real-time PCR assay to detect Schistosoma mansoni infections in a low endemic setting. *BMC Infect. Dis.* **2014**, *14*, 558. [CrossRef]

57. Espirito-Santo, M.C.; Alvarado-Mora, M.V.; Pinto, P.L.; Sanchez, M.C.; Dias-Neto, E.; Castilho, V.L.; Goncalves, E.M.; Chieffi, P.P.; Luna, E.J.; Pinho, J.R.; et al. Comparative Study of the Accuracy of Different Techniques for the Laboratory Diagnosis of Schistosomiasis Mansoni in Areas of Low Endemicity in Barra Mansa City, Rio de Janeiro State, Brazil. *Biomed. Res. Int.* **2015**, *2015*, 135689. [CrossRef]
58. da Frota, S.M.; Carneiro, T.R.; Queiroz, J.A.; Alencar, L.M.; Heukelbach, J.; Bezerra, F.S. Combination of Kato-Katz faecal examinations and ELISA to improve accuracy of diagnosis of intestinal schistosomiasis in a low-endemic setting in Brazil. *Acta Trop.* **2011**, *120* (Suppl. 1), S138–S141. [CrossRef] [PubMed]
59. Silveira, A.M.; Costa, E.G.; Ray, D.; Suzuki, B.M.; Hsieh, M.H.; Fraga, L.A.; Caffrey, C.R. Evaluation of the CCA Immuno-Chromatographic Test to Diagnose Schistosoma mansoni in Minas Gerais State, Brazil. *PLoS Negl. Trop. Dis.* **2016**, *10*, e0004357. [CrossRef] [PubMed]
60. Espirito-Santo, M.C.; Sanchez, M.C.; Sanchez, A.R.; Alvarado-Mora, M.V.; Castilho, V.L.; Goncalves, E.M.; Luna, E.J.; Gryschek, R.C. Evaluation of the sensitivity of IgG and IgM ELISA in detecting Schistosoma mansoni infections in a low endemicity setting. *Eur. J. Clin. Microbiol. Infect. Dis.* **2014**, *33*, 2275–2284. [CrossRef] [PubMed]
61. Beltrame, A.; Guerriero, M.; Angheben, A.; Gobbi, F.; Requena-Mendez, A.; Zammarchi, L.; Formenti, F.; Perandin, F.; Buonfrate, D.; Bisoffi, Z. Accuracy of parasitological and immunological tests for the screening of human schistosomiasis in immigrants and refugees from African countries: An approach with Latent Class Analysis. *PLoS Negl. Trop. Dis.* **2017**, *11*, e0005593. [CrossRef] [PubMed]
62. Bisoffi, Z.; Buonfrate, D.; Sequi, M.; Mejia, R.; Cimino, R.O.; Krolewiecki, A.J.; Albonico, M.; Gobbo, M.; Bonafini, S.; Angheben, A.; et al. Diagnostic accuracy of five serologic tests for Strongyloides stercoralis infection. *PLoS Negl. Trop. Dis.* **2014**, *8*, e2640. [CrossRef] [PubMed]
63. Rascoe, L.N.; Price, C.; Shin, S.H.; McAuliffe, I.; Priest, J.W.; Handali, S. Development of Ss-NIE-1 recombinant antigen based assays for immunodiagnosis of strongyloidiasis. *PLoS Negl. Trop. Dis.* **2015**, *9*, e0003694. [CrossRef] [PubMed]
64. Knopp, S.; Salim, N.; Schindler, T.; Karagiannis Voules, D.A.; Rothen, J.; Lweno, O.; Mohammed, A.S.; Singo, R.; Benninghoff, M.; Nsojo, A.A.; et al. Diagnostic accuracy of Kato-Katz, FLOTAC, Baermann, and PCR methods for the detection of light-intensity hookworm and Strongyloides stercoralis infections in Tanzania. *Am. J. Trop. Med. Hyg.* **2014**, *90*, 535–545. [CrossRef] [PubMed]
65. King, C.H.; Olbrych, S.K.; Soon, M.; Singer, M.E.; Carter, J.; Colley, D.G. Utility of Repeated Praziquantel Dosing in the Treatment of Schistosomiasis in High-Risk Communities in Africa: A Systematic Review. *PLoS Negl. Trop. Dis.* **2011**, *5*, e1321. [CrossRef] [PubMed]
66. Muennig, P.; Pallin, D.; Sell, R.L.; Chan, M.-S. The Cost Effectiveness of Strategies for the Treatment of Intestinal Parasites in Immigrants. *N. Engl. J. Med.* **1999**, *340*, 773–779. [CrossRef]
67. Muennig, P.; Pallin, D.; Challah, C.; Khan, K. The cost-effectiveness of ivermectin vs. albendazole in the presumptive treatment of strongyloidiasis in immigrants to the United States. *Epidemiol. Infect.* **2004**, *132*, 1055–1063. [CrossRef]
68. Maskery, B.; Coleman, M.S.; Weinberg, M.; Zhou, W.; Rotz, L.; Klosovsky, A.; Cantey, P.T.; Fox, L.M.; Cetron, M.S.; Stauffer, W.M. Economic Analysis of the Impact of Overseas and Domestic Treatment and Screening Options for Intestinal Helminth Infection among US-Bound Refugees from Asia. *PLoS Negl. Trop. Dis.* **2016**, *10*, e0004910. [CrossRef] [PubMed]
69. Worrell, C.M.; Bartoces, M.; Karanja, D.M.; Ochola, E.A.; Matete, D.O.; Mwinzi, P.N.; Montgomery, S.P.; Secor, W.E. Cost analysis of tests for the detection of Schistosoma mansoni infection in children in western Kenya. *Am. J. Trop. Med. Hyg.* **2015**, *92*, 1233–1239. [CrossRef] [PubMed]
70. Libman, M.D.; MacLean, J.D.; Gyorkos, T.W. Screening for schistosomiasis, filariasis, and strongyloidiasis among expatriates returning from the tropics. *Clin. Infect. Dis.* **1993**, *17*, 353–359. [CrossRef] [PubMed]
71. CDC. *Guidelines for Overseas Presumptive Treatment of Strongyloidiasis, Schistosomiasis, and Soil-Transmitted Helminth Infections*; CDC: Atlanta, GA, USA, 2013.
72. Buonfrate, D.; Sequi, M.; Mejia, R.; Cimino, R.O.; Krolewiecki, A.J.; Albonico, M.; Degani, M.; Tais, S.; Angheben, A.; Requena-Mendez, A.; et al. Accuracy of five serologic tests for the follow up of Strongyloides stercoralis infection. *PLoS Negl. Trop. Dis.* **2015**, *9*, e0003491. [CrossRef] [PubMed]

73. Zammarchi, L.; Bonati, M.; Strohmeyer, M.; Albonico, M.; Requena-Méndez, A.; Bisoffi, Z.; Nicoletti, A.; García, H.H.; Bartoloni, A. Screening, diagnosis and management of human cysticercosis and T. solium taeniasis: Technical recommendations by the COHEMI project study group. *Trop. Med. Int. Health* **2017**, *2*, 881–894. [CrossRef] [PubMed]
74. Jonas, D.E.; Ferrari, R.M.; Wines, R.C.; Vuong, K.T.; Cotter, A.; Harris, R.P. Evaluating evidence on intermediate outcomes: Considerations for groups making healthcare recommendations. *Am. J. Prev. Med.* **2018**, *54*, S38–S52. [CrossRef] [PubMed]
75. Atkins, D.; Best, D.; Briss, P.A.; Eccles, M.; Falck-Ytter, Y.; Flottorp, S.; Guyatt, G.H.; Harbour, R.T.; Haugh, M.C.; Henry, D. Grading quality of evidence and strength of recommendations. *BMJ* **2004**, *328*, 1490.

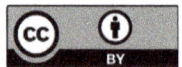

© 2018 by the authors. Licensee MDPI, Basel, Switzerland. This article is an open access article distributed under the terms and conditions of the Creative Commons Attribution (CC BY) license (http://creativecommons.org/licenses/by/4.0/).

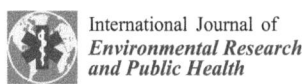

Article

For What Illnesses Do Asylum Seekers and Undocumented Migrant Workers in Israel Seek Healthcare? An Analysis of Medical Visits at a Large Urgent Care Clinic for the Uninsured in Tel Aviv

Elizabeth B. Moran [1], Mark A. Katz [1,2,3], Orel-Ben Ari [2], Nadav Davidovitch [3] and Oren Zwang [2,*]

[1] University of Michigan, School of Public Health, Ann Arbor, MI 48104, USA; ebmoran@umich.edu (E.B.M.); katzmar@post.bgu.ac.il (M.A.K.)
[2] Terem Urgen Care, Jerusalem 91000, Israel; orelbenari@gmail.com
[3] Ben Gurion University of the Negev, School of Public Health, Beer-Sheva 84102, Israel; nadavd@bgu.ac.il
* Correspondence: refugeedoctor@gmail.com; Tel.: +972-52-705-1747

Received: 6 December 2018; Accepted: 13 January 2019; Published: 16 January 2019

Abstract: In 2017, there were nearly 80,000 asylum seekers and undocumented migrant workers in Israel, most of whom did not have health insurance. We evaluated trends in medical visits of asylum seekers and undocumented migrant workers who presented to Terem Refugee Clinic (TRC), a large clinic in Tel Aviv available only to uninsured residents of Israel. Data were collected from electronic medical records at TRC from 2013–2017. Diagnoses were grouped into categories using ICD-10-equivalent diagnosis codes. We used a chi-squared test for trends to test the significance of trends 2013 to 2017. There were 99,569 medical visits from 2013 to 2017 at TRC. Visits were lowest in 2013 (11,112), and relatively stable from 2014–2017 (range: 19,712–23,172). Most visits were among adults aged 18–35 (41.2%) and children <2 years old (23.7%). Only 3% of visits were from patients aged >50. The percentage of infectious disease diagnoses decreased over the study period, from 9.4% of all diagnoses in adults in 2014 to 5.2% in 2017, and from 32.0% of all diagnoses in children in 2013 to 19.4% in 2017. The annual percentage of respiratory diagnoses in children and adults 18–35 years of age, musculoskeletal in all adults, and digestive in adults except women ≥35 years old increased. Over time, asylum seekers and undocumented migrant workers visited TRC with fewer infectious diseases diagnoses overall but more respiratory diseases, including acute respiratory infections and more musculoskeletal diseases.

Keywords: refugee; health; migration; chronic disease; infectious disease

1. Introduction

The number of international migrants worldwide has risen significantly in recent years and now totals approximately 258 million people, which includes 25.4 million refugees and 3.1 million asylum seekers [1]. Both refugees and asylum seekers flee their country because of persecution, war or violence. Refugees have been granted legal status and receive protection and assistance from their host country, whereas asylum seekers are awaiting legal recognition as refugees [2]. Migrant workers are persons who are employed in a country of which they are not a citizen. Undocumented migrant workers do not have legal permission to reside and work in their host country and do not benefit from legal protections [3]. Asylum seekers tend to include families and individuals of a range of ages and undocumented migrant workers tend to be young men [2,3]. The health of these refugees, asylum seekers, and undocumented migrant workers is crucial for reasons including human rights, public health, the economic stability of their communities, and the stability of the healthcare systems in the countries in which they reside [4]. Refugees and other immigrants tend to arrive to new countries mostly healthy, but their health often deteriorates over time—a pattern referred to as the "healthy immigrant effect" that has been described in several countries, including in North America and in Europe [5–8]. In addition, over time, the health problems of refugees and asylum seekers tend to shift from mostly acute infectious illnesses to chronic diseases, such as cardiovascular disease and diabetes [5].

In the last decade, Israel has experienced a marked increase in the number of asylum seekers and undocumented migrant workers. From 2006 to 2012, over 60,000 asylum seekers, primarily from Eritrea and South Sudan, arrived in Israel by way of the Sinai Peninsula, and as of the end of 2017, 35,659 were still living in the country, most of whom were residing in South Tel Aviv [9–12]. In addition, according to the Israeli Population and Immigration Authority, by the end of June 2018, an estimated 19,250 migrant workers were living in Israel after their initial visas and work-related health insurance had expired [10]. Asylum seekers are not covered under Israel's national health insurance fund, but they have the option to buy private health insurance. Many asylum seekers do not enroll in these plans due to the high cost. Legal migrant workers are required to have health insurance, whereas undocumented migrant workers often do not have health insurance.

While refugee health has been studied in high-income countries in Europe and North America, very little is known about the health and healthcare use practices of uninsured residents, asylum seekers, and undocumented migrant workers in Israel. In this study, we describe the demographic characteristics and clinical visits of asylum seekers and undocumented migrant workers at Terem Refugee Clinic (TRC), a clinic in Tel Aviv available only to uninsured residents of Israel, from 2013 through 2017.

2. Materials and Methods

This serial cross-sectional study was conducted using visit data from TRC, a clinic located in the Tel Aviv Central Bus Station, which was opened in 2013 in order to serve exclusively asylum seekers and other undocumented, uninsured residents in Israel. Terem is a private organization that operates a network of urgent care centers in Israel, nearly all of which serve the general Israeli population, who are insured under Israel's system of universal coverage. TRC is an exception, funded by the Government of Israel through a contract from the Ministry of Health to serve the uninsured. In order to receive care at TRC, patients must show identification specific to asylum seekers or migrant workers. For asylum seekers, this identification is a conditional release document from the Ministry of the Interior. For migrant workers, this identification is a passport with an expired working visa. Treatment is not provided to Israeli citizens or tourists.

Terem provides the staffing and infrastructure for the urgent care clinic, including an electronic medical record system, evidence-based protocols for treatment of frequent diagnoses, point-of-care laboratory and radiology services, diagnostic equipment, and treatment supplies. The TRC, like many urgent care clinics, provides services including and beyond what may be available at most general practitioners' offices, but short of what is typical for a hospital-based emergency department. Diagnostic services include vital signs, doctor's examination, point-of-care laboratory, electrocardiography, radiology, and limited ultrasound. Treatment services include oral and parenteral medicines, respiratory inhalations, suturing, incision-drainage and similar bedside procedures, and casting. Unavailable at TRC are CT scans, magnetic resonance imaging, and thrombolytics, and patients who need services such as these are sent to one of two local hospitals. For every urgent care visit, patients pay a flat rate of 20 NIS (approximately USD 5.50), which includes triage with vital signs taken by a paramedic, a doctor's examination, blood tests, radiology imaging, and bedside procedures as clinically indicated. While patient country of origin is not recorded as part of routine clinic visits, based on the staff's experience at TRC, the vast majority of patients at TRC are Eritrean, with Sudanese a distant second.

We evaluated the electronic medical records for all patient visits at TRC from 1 January 2013 through 31 December 2017. For each medical visit, we extracted data on the patient's age, sex, discharge status, and diagnosis.

At the end of every patient visit at TRC, doctors choose at least one diagnosis from a list of 623 possible diagnoses (see Supplementary Table S1). In order to better understand the main reasons for patient visits, we matched each diagnosis with its equivalent ICD-10 code and then assigned each of the 623 diagnoses to one of 22 diagnostic categories. These 22 categories were largely based on ICD-10 body-system categories that were used in a previous study of healthcare in refugees in Switzerland [7]. Some ICD-10 organ-system categories, such as respiratory diseases and digestive system diseases, include acute infections, such as acute respiratory infections and gastroenteritis (Supplementary Table S1). For discharge diagnoses that did not fit clearly into one of the 22 disease categories, two TRC medical doctors (O.Z., M.K.) agreed on the appropriate disease category by consensus. In order to not count individual patient visits multiple times if the visits were associated with multiple diagnoses, we only included the first diagnosis in our main analysis. However, we also performed a separate analysis that included all diagnoses to evaluate for significant differences in trends reported in this paper.

Doctors at TRC refer patients presenting with symptoms suspicious for tuberculosis (TB) or patients with exposure to known TB cases to a government-funded, regional TB center in Israel, where more extensive TB testing and treatment is offered. In addition, because TRC is an urgent care clinic without all the services of a hospital emergency room, doctors refer patients who need more intensive medical treatment to an area hospital, sometimes by ambulance. As part of our analysis, we also examined whether patient visits ended with a referral to the regional TB clinic or a discharge to the hospital.

We analyzed data for changes in the age and gender distribution of patients treated at the clinic over time, changes in the percentage of patients discharged to hospital and referred to tuberculosis clinic over time, and changes in top diagnosis groups over time. The unit of time used in the analysis was the calendar year. We used a chi-squared test for trends (Cochran–Armitage test for trend) to determine statistical significance. A p-value less than 0.05 in the chi-squared test for trends indicated that the trend in the variable from 2013 to 2017 was statistically significant. R version 3.4.3 was used for this analysis.

The Ethical Review Committee of Ben-Gurion University of the Negev approved this study.

3. Results

3.1. Overall Patient Visits and Age Distribution

Over the five years, there were 99,569 visits to TRC. Visits were lowest in 2013 (11,112) and relatively stable from 2014–2017 (range: 19,712–23,172). Overall, most clinic visits were among adults aged 18–35 (41.2%) and among children under 2 years of age (23.7%). Relatively few clinic visits occurred in patients older than 50 years of age (3.0%) (Table 1). Over the five years, the age distribution of patient visits varied slightly. The percentage of patients under 2 years old and patients 18–35 years old decreased from 2013 to 2017, while the percentage of patients 2–5 years old, 5–18 years old, 35–50 years old, and 50 years old and older increased.

Table 1. Patient characteristics and medical visit outcomes at Terem Refugee Clinic, 2013–2017.

Population Attributes	Total N (%)	2013 N (%)	2014 N (%)	2015 N (%)	2016 N (%)	2017 N (%)	p^T
Total	99,569	11,112	19,712	23,172	22,673	22,900	
Age [1]							
Under 2 years	23,593 (23.7)	2928 (26.3)	5803 (29.4)	6197 (26.7)	4721 (20.8)	3944 (17.2)	<0.001
2–5 years	13,224 (13.3)	828 (7.4)	1992 (10.1)	3217 (13.9)	3423 (15.1)	3764 (16.4)	<0.001
5–18 years	4450 (4.5)	344 (3.1)	697 (3.5)	1000 (4.3)	1065 (4.7)	1344 (5.9)	<0.001

Table 1. Cont.

Population Attributes	Total N (%)	2013 N (%)	2014 N (%)	2015 N (%)	2016 N (%)	2017 N (%)	p^T
18–35 years	41,038 (41.2)	5366 (48.3)	8414 (42.7)	9396 (40.5)	9225 (40.7)	8637 (37.7)	<0.001
35–50 years	14,299 (14.4)	1388 (12.5)	2368 (12.0)	2847 (12.3)	3504 (15.4)	4192 (18.3)	<0.001
50 and over	2955 (3.0)	256 (2.3)	434 (2.2)	513 (2.2)	733 (3.2)	1017 (4.4)	<0.001
Male:Female [2]							
Children	1.1	1.1	1.1	1.1	1.1	1.1	n.s.
Adults	1.3	1.7	1.6	1.4	1.2	1.1	<0.001
Referred to hospital	2359 (2.3)	260 (2.3)	411 (2.1)	441 (1.9)	500 (2.2)	747 (3.3)	<0.001
Referred to TB clinic	498 (0.5)	58 (0.5)	47 (0.2)	89 (0.4)	101 (0.4)	203 (0.9)	<0.001

[T] p-value calculated using chi-squared test for trend in proportions. Trend was defined as changes in percentages in each category over the time, 2013–2017. Denominator used is the total number of patient visits that year denoted at the top of the column. Not calculated for age. [1] Age groups are inclusive at the low end and exclusive at the high end. [2] Denominator used for trends for ratio male:female was the total number of patient visits that year for children and the total number of patient visits that year for adult. TB: Tuberculosis. "n.s." means non-significant, indicating a p-value > 0.05.

3.2. Gender

Among all clinic visits, 44,580 (44.8%) were among females and 53,989 (55.2%) were among males. The overall male:female ratio for all visits was 1.1 for children under 18 years old and 1.3 for adults. Although the male:female ratio for children did not change significantly over time, the male:female ratio for adults decreased from 1.7 in 2013 to 1.1 in 2017 (p for trend <0.00001).

3.3. Hospital and TB Clinic Referrals

Overall, 2359 (2.4%) of all patient visits ended in a hospital referral (Table 1). The percentage of patients referred to the hospital varied from a low of 1.9% in 2015 to a high of 3.3% in 2017 (p for trend <0.00001). Over the five years, the most common diagnoses for patient visits that ended in hospital referral were upper respiratory infection (11.7%), cough (4.5%), unspecified abdominal pain (3.6%), and bronchitis (3.0%). The median age of patients referred to the hospital was 25.5 years (interquartile range 2.2–32.5) and most patients (55.6%) were male.

Over the five years, 498 (0.5%) of all patient visits ended with a referral to the regional TB clinic (Table 1). The percentage of patients referred to the TB clinic for further diagnostics ranged from a low of 0.2% in 2014, to a high of 0.9% in 2017 (p for trend <0.00001). The median age of patients referred to the TB clinic was 26.2 (IQR 2.4–33.0) and 282 (56.6%) were male.

3.4. Diagnositic Categories

For the five-year period, the most common diagnoses for children were respiratory diseases (35.1% of diagnoses), infectious diseases (21.4%), skin diseases (12.7%), digestive system diseases (10.0%), and eye and ear diseases (7.3%) (Table 2). These diagnostic groups did not differ by gender for children. Compared to younger children, children older than 5 years old had a higher percentage of injuries and accidents, which was the third most common diagnosis in children over 5 years old (21.5%). The percentage of diagnoses in children categorized as respiratory diseases increased from 25.9% in 2013 to 35.3% in 2017 and overtook infectious diseases as the top diagnosis group in 2014 (p for trend <0.00001). Conversely, the percentage of infectious disease diagnoses in children decreased over time, from 32.0% in 2013 (the most common diagnosis) to 19.4% in 2017 (the second most-common diagnosis) (p for trend <0.00001) (Figure 1).

In contrast to children, over the five-year period, adults 18 years of age and older were most commonly diagnosed with respiratory diseases (26.3%), digestive system diseases (12.7%), musculoskeletal diseases (9.6%), injuries and accidents (8.5%), and skin diseases (7.5%). There were differences in the most common diagnostic groups between men and women, but respiratory diseases were the top diagnostic group across all age groups of men and women (Table 2). Women aged 18 to 35 were commonly diagnosed with genitourinary diseases (10.5%) and pregnancy-related conditions

(8.3%). Women aged 35 and older were also commonly diagnosed with genitourinary conditions (7.3%). Men were most commonly diagnosed with conditions relating to injury and accidents (12.0% in males 18–35 and 10.1% in males 35 and older); for women, these diagnoses were much less common.

As in children, in adults, the percentage of diagnoses categorized as infectious diseases decreased from 2013 to 2017 for both males and females in all age groups (p for trend <0.005 for all) (Figure 1). By contrast, the percentage of diagnoses categorized as digestive system diseases and musculoskeletal diseases increased from 2013 to 2017 for both males and females in all age groups (p for trend <0.01 for all), with the exception of digestive system diseases in women aged 35 and older, where it remained the third most common diagnosis over time.

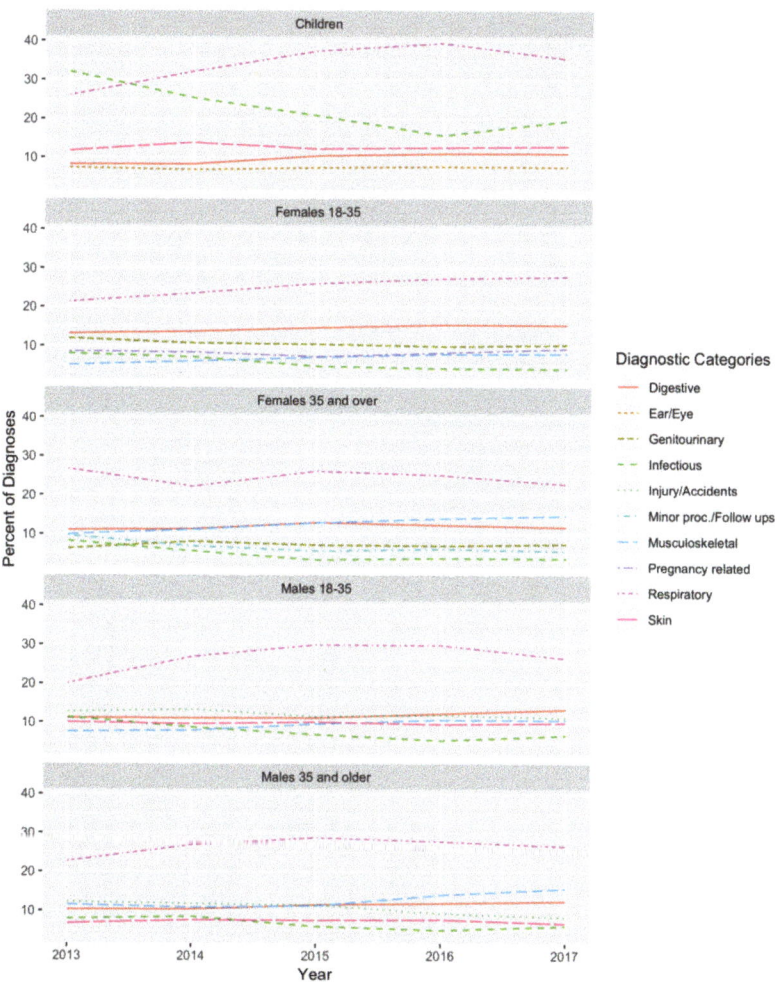

Figure 1. Percent of total diagnoses in each diagnostic category by age and gender over time.

Of the 99,569 patient visits, 13.6% had more than one diagnosis recorded. For reasons described in the above methods section, our main analysis included only the first of these diagnoses when counting the frequency of diagnostic groups. When we analyzed the data including all diagnoses per patient instead of including only the first one, the top five diagnosis groups in children and in adults remained the same, with two exceptions: In women 18–35 years old, pregnancy-related conditions, which were the fourth-most common diagnosis category in the main analysis, became the third most common diagnostic category, and genitourinary diseases, which were the third-most common diagnosis category, became the fourth most common diagnosis (data not shown).

Table 2. Top five diagnostic categories of Terem Refugee Clinic patient visits, 2013–2017.

Rank	Children * <18 Years Old N (%)	Adults 18–34		Adults 35 and Older	
		Females N (%)	Males N (%)	Females N (%)	Males N (%)
Total	41,267	19,782	21,256	5242	12,012
1.	Respiratory 14,490 (35.1)	Respiratory 5085 (25.7)	Respiratory 5750 (27.1)	Respiratory 1268 (24.2)	Respiratory 3219 (26.8)
2.	Infectious 8827 (21.4)	Digestive 2888 (14.6)	Injury/Accidents 2555 (12.0)	Musculoskeletal 699 (13.3)	Musculoskeletal 1566 (13.0)
3.	Skin 5241 (12.7)	Genitourinary 2068 (10.5)	Digestive 2484 (11.7)	Digestive 692 (12.0)	Digestive 1377 (11.5)
4.	Digestive 4123 (10.0)	Pregnancy 1636 (8.3)	Skin 2070 (9.7)	Genitourinary 382 (7.3)	Injury/Accidents 1217 (10.1)
5.	Eye and Ear 3027 (7.3)	Musculoskeleta 11,387 (7.0)	Musculoskeletal 1961 (9.2)	Minor Procedures and Follow-Ups 325 (6.2)	Skin 866 (7.2)

* Data for children under 18 years old are combined for males and females.

4. Discussion

In our study, the first to describe the trends in demographics and medical visits of asylum seekers and uninsured migrant workers in Israel, at the largest urgent care clinic in the country serving this population, we found that over a five-year period, most people who came to TRC were children less than 2 years old and young adults. Over time, patients presented to the clinic with fewer infectious diseases overall, and more musculoskeletal diagnoses. In addition, there were more respiratory and, to a lesser extent, digestive system diagnoses. By 2017, the disease visit profile at TRC was quite similar to disease visit profiles described in other clinics in Israel that serve the general Israeli population [13].

The trends from diagnostic categories data showed evidence of a decreasing burden of infectious diseases among asylum seekers and undocumented migrants. We found that over time, the percentage of overall infectious disease diagnoses decreased in both children and adults. However, there was a relative increase in respiratory and digestive diseases, which include some acute infections, but this increase was considerably less than the decrease in infectious diseases. During the same time period, there was an increase in the relative percentage of diagnoses more reflective of chronic, noncommunicable illnesses, such as musculoskeletal disease in adults. Medical treatment of refugees and immigrants frequently focuses on treating infectious diseases, and screening and care for chronic disease conditions is often limited [12]. This focus leads to an increased burden of undiagnosed and untreated chronic diseases, as these conditions worsen and require more intensive treatment [14]. In addition to the chronic diseases that refugees and immigrants already have on arrival to their new country, shifts in lifestyle, such as changes in diet and lack of exercise, can lead to the development of new chronic diseases in this population [15]. Currently, there is minimal governmental support in Israel for longitudinal ambulatory care of undocumented residents with chronic diseases. However, our findings suggest that chronic diseases are a large, growing problem in this population. If more resources were dedicated to this problem, this community would likely be healthier and have fewer long-term complications, and costs to the overall healthcare system would be alleviated in future years.

The clinic had a relatively low overall percentage of hospital referrals (2.3%) over the five-year period. This percentage of hospitals referrals at the TRC clinic was much lower than the percentage of hospital referrals cited in a previous study that described data from 2008 to 2011 from public clinics serving uninsured asylum seekers and uninsured migrant workers in Israel (40%) [16]. However, that study included data from clinics which have limited onsite diagnostic and treatment capacity compared to TRC. The fact that the clinic is equipped to perform on-site lab testing, X-rays, casting, intravenous treatments, and other interventions likely reduces hospital referrals and in turn reduces potential hospital costs among a population with very limited ability to pay large hospital bills. Therefore, the relatively low number of hospital referrals in our study is likely a reflection of the greater treatment capacity at TRC and is unlikely to indicate improved health in the population over time. The increase in hospital referrals found in 2017 compared to all prior years may reflect a change in the internal TRC guidelines for hospital referrals, which were implemented in 2016.

Throughout the five-year period, a high percentage of clinic visits among males 18 years and older was related to injuries and accidents. This finding was also described in the refugee population in Switzerland [7]. Asylum seekers and undocumented migrants have limited legal status, and therefore limited employment options. Migrant workers and asylum seekers often take jobs with working conditions that are hazardous and unsafe, leading to injuries and accidents [7,16]. In Israel, many asylum seekers and undocumented migrant workers are employed in restaurants, construction sites, and cleaning—settings which can be prone to injuries.

Tuberculosis continues to cause high levels of morbidity and mortality globally. The vast majority of patients at TRC are from two countries, Eritrea and Sudan, where TB is endemic [17,18]. In Israel, all asylum seekers who arrived through the Sinai Peninsula were screened for TB upon arrival with a Mantoux test, and referred to free, government-funded TB treatment centers [19]. Factors like language barriers, lack of familiarity with the medical system, and suboptimal case reporting and tracking infrastructure are known barriers to TB care and treatment in other settings [20] and may be relevant barriers to TB care in the asylum seeker and migrant worker populations in Israel. In our study, a small percentage of patient visits were referred from TRC to the regional TB treatment center every year. TRC does not receive regular communication about whether referred patients are actually seen at the TB center, and, if so, whether TB was confirmed and treated. Thus, potential TB infections in the population presenting to TRC are likely the result of patients not receiving proper treatment upon entry due to barriers to care, reactivation of latent TB, or TB infection acquired in Israel.

Every year from 2014 to 2017, there were progressively fewer children under 2 years of age presenting to TRC, as a percentage of all clinic visits per year. This change could be a result of more parents purchasing health insurance for their very young children. A change in Israeli health care policy in 2016 lowered premiums for children's health insurance regardless of their parents' legal status in Israel [21]. This decrease in cost could have led more asylum seekers and uninsured migrant workers to enroll their children in a health insurance plan through one of the existing national health funds operating within the Israeli National Health Insurance Law.

Over the five-year period, fewer young adults aged 18 to 35 attended the clinic. This demographic change could reflect the ongoing process of "voluntary" migration from Israel encouraged by the Israeli government. According to informal interviews with NGOs working with asylum seekers in Israel, the healthiest individuals in the population preferentially take on migration.

Finally, over the five-year period, relatively higher percentage of women used the clinic compared to men, which may reflect the fact that more men are receiving health insurance through work. In addition, more women may be using the clinic for reproductive health needs, including pregnancy care and contraception consultations. Finally, this trend may reflect an increase in the number of men leaving Israel through resettlement campaigns.

5. Conclusions

This study was able to use a robust electronic medical record (EMR) system to evaluate trends in the healthcare use of asylum seekers and undocumented migrant workers in Israel. Because the EMR has been in place since the clinic opened in 2013, we were able to evaluate trends from the clinic's first year for a five-year period.

This study had limitations, which were mostly related to the availability of data and the coding of the data. We grouped discharge diagnoses by ICD-10 disease categories, some of which include some overlap between infectious and chronic diseases; for example, some infectious diseases, such as acute upper respiratory infection, are included in an ICD-10 organ system disease category, respiratory diseases. This approach to coding makes it more difficult to draw conclusions about trends in infectious relative to chronic diseases. While there was no change in coding instructions for physicians at the clinic that would explain varying disease trends, the broad nature of the ICD-10 categories limits our ability to draw broad conclusions about disease trends.

TRC does not collect information on country of origin and time spent in Israel and, therefore, we were not able to evaluate the relationship of these two variables to trends in clinic visits. We were not able to link patient visits to individuals and, therefore, we could not determine how many times the same individual went to the clinic. In addition, our study population may not accurately represent the greater population of asylum seekers and undocumented migrants in Israel, due to its location in Tel Aviv and the convenience sample of patients treated at TRC. In addition, our study population may not accurately represent the entire population of asylum seekers and undocumented migrants in Israel. Some asylum seekers and undocumented workers in Tel Aviv and in Israel likely receive their medical care in clinics other than TRC. This study serves as one snapshot of the medically attended healthcare trends of this population. We did not have access to data from urgent care clinics attended by Israeli citizens and legal residents in Tel Aviv or elsewhere in Israel. Therefore, we could not compare trends in demographics or discharge diagnoses between the population that attended the Terem Clinic and the general Israeli population—citizens and legal residents—attending other clinics in in Tel Aviv or Israel. Undertaking this kind of comparison would be an important future direction for research.

Additionally, because we lacked follow-up data on TB referrals, we could not evaluate trends in the incidence of TB among patients at TRC. The ICD-10 disease categories we used do not clearly distinguish between infectious and non-infectious diseases. For example, some acute respiratory and gastrointestinal infections are included in the ICD-10 disease categories of respiratory system diseases and digestive system diseases, respectively, and are therefore not included in our definition of infectious diseases. Trends in demographics used a chi-squared test for linear trend analysis that may have reported significance due to large sample size instead of due to robust evidence of a linear trend. Some of the trends reported may be better fit by a nonlinear trend.

Asylum seekers and undocumented migrant workers presented to TRC with decreasing infectious disease diagnoses and increasing chronic diseases diagnoses from 2013 to 2017. Future research on asylum seeker and undocumented migrant health should include data from other clinics and hospitals serving this population in Israel.

Supplementary Materials: The following are available online at http://www.mdpi.com/1660-4601/16/2/252/s1, Table S1: Terem diagnoses categorized based on ICD-10 system.

Author Contributions: Conceptualization, M.A.K. and N.D.; Formal Analysis, O.B.-A. and N.D.; Data Curation, E.B.M., M.A.K. and O.B.-A.; Project Administration, O.Z.; Funding Acquisition, O.Z.

Funding: Funding for Elizabeth Moran was provided by Office of Global Public Health at University of Michigan School of Public Health (Gelman Global Scholars Award), Mary Sue and Kenneth Coleman Global Experience Scholarship, and Raoul Wallenberg International Summer Travel Award.

Acknowledgments: The authors would like to thank the Ben Gurion University/University of Michigan Israel Initiative for its support in this collaboration.

Conflicts of Interest: The authors declare no conflict of interest.

References

1. The UN Refugee Agency. *Global Trends: Forced Displacement in 2016*; The UN Refugee Agency: Geneva, Switzerland, 2016.
2. Nicholson, F.; Kumin, J. *A Guide to International Refugee Protection and Building State Asylum Systems*; Inter-Parliamentary Union: Geneva, Switzerland; United Nations High Commissioner for Refugees: Geneva, Switzerland, 2017.

3. Simon, J.; Kiss, N.; Laszewsja, A.; Mayer, S. *Public Health Aspects of Migrant Health: A Review of the Evidence on Health Status for Labour Migrants in the European Region*; WHO Regional Office for Europe: Copenhagen, Denmark, 2015.
4. Gushulak, B.D.; MacPherson, D.W. Globalization of Infectious Diseases: The Impact of Migration. *Clin. Infect. Dis.* **2004**, *38*, 1742–1748. [CrossRef] [PubMed]
5. Gushulak, B.D.; Pottie, K.; Roberts, J.H.; Torres, S.; DesMeules, M. Migration and health in Canada: Health in the global village. *Can. Med. Assoc. J.* **2011**, *183*, E952–E958. [CrossRef] [PubMed]
6. Hyman, I. *Immigration and Health: Reviewing Evidence of the Healthy Immigrant Effect in Canada*; Joint Centre of Excellence for Research on Immigration and Settlement: Toronto, ON, Canada, 2007.
7. Bischoff, A.; Schneider, M.; Denhaerynck, K.; Battegay, E. Battegay Health and ill health of asylum seekers in Switzerland: An epidemiology study. *Eur. J. Public Health* **2009**, *19*, 59–64. [CrossRef] [PubMed]
8. Nyiri, P.; Eling, J. A specialist clinic for destitute asylum seekers and refugees in London. *Br. J. Gen. Pract.* **2012**, *62*, 599–600. [CrossRef] [PubMed]
9. Pew Reseach Center. Number of Refugees and Asylum Seekers in Israel from 2005 to 2015. *Statista-The Statistics Portal*. Available online: https://www-statista-com.proxy.lib.umich.edu/statistics/742491/israel-number-of-refugees/ (accessed on 29 May 2018).
10. Population and Migration Authority of Israel. נתוני זרים בישראל *(Report on Foreign Workers in Israel)*; Population and Migration Authority of Israel: Jerusalem, Israel, 2018.
11. The African Refugee Development Center. African Refugees in Israel. 2017. Available online: https://www.ardc-israel.org/refugees-in-israel (accessed on 4 June 2018).
12. The UN Refugee Agency. *Global Focus 2017 Year End Report: Israel*; The UN Refugee Agency: Geneva, Switzerland, 2017.
13. CBS (Central Bureau of Statistics and State of Israel). *Health Survey 2009. General Findings*; Publication No. 1500; CBS (Central Bureau of Statistics and State of Israel): Jerusalem, Israel, 2013.
14. Amara, A.H.; Aljunid, S.M. Noncommunicable diseases among urban refugees and asylum-seekers in developing countries: A neglected health care need. *Glob. Health* **2014**, *10*, 1–14. [CrossRef] [PubMed]
15. Singh, G.K.; Siahpush, M. Ethnic-Immigrant Differentials in Health Behaviors, Morbidity, and Cause-Specific Mortality in the United States: An Analysis of Two National Data Bases. *Hum. Biol.* **2016**, *74*, 83–109. [CrossRef]
16. Mor, Z.; Raveh, Y.; Lurie, I.; Leventhal, A.; Gamzu, R.; Davidovitch, N.; Benari, O.; Grotto, I. Medical condition and care of undocumented migrants in ambulatory clinics in Tel Aviv, Israel: Assessing unmet needs. *BMC Health Serv. Res.* **2017**, *17*, 1–6. [CrossRef] [PubMed]
17. World Health Organization. *Tuberculosis Country Reports. TB Burden Estimates and Country-Reported TB Data: Eritrea*; World Health Organization: Geneva, Switzerland, 2016.
18. World Health Organization. *Tuberculosis country Reports. TB Burder Estimates and Country-Reported TB Data: Sudan*; World Health Organization: Geneva, Switzerland, 2016.
19. Eisenberg, J.R.; Lidji, M.; Gelfer, E.; Zehavi, N.; Grotto, I.; Mor, Z. Same but Different: Tuberculosis Treatment and Care Among Migrants from Different Countries of Origin in Israel. *Lung* **2014**, *192*, 863–867. [CrossRef] [PubMed]
20. World Health Organization. *Tuberculosis Control in Migrant Populations: Guiding Principles and Proposed Actions*; World Health Organization: Geneva, Switzerland, 2016.
21. *Provision of Health Services to Minors Who Are in Israel and Are Not Insured by the National Health Insurance Law*; Health Minister Director: Jerusaelm, Israel, 2016.

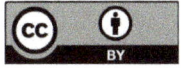

© 2019 by the authors. Licensee MDPI, Basel, Switzerland. This article is an open access article distributed under the terms and conditions of the Creative Commons Attribution (CC BY) license (http://creativecommons.org/licenses/by/4.0/).

MDPI
St. Alban-Anlage 66
4052 Basel
Switzerland
Tel. +41 61 683 77 34
Fax +41 61 302 89 18
www.mdpi.com

International Journal of Environmental Research and Public Health Editorial Office
E-mail: ijerph@mdpi.com
www.mdpi.com/journal/ijerph

www.ingramcontent.com/pod-product-compliance
Lightning Source LLC
LaVergne TN
LVHW071933080526
838202LV00064B/6603